Developmental Hematopoiesis

METHODS IN MOLECULAR MEDICINE™

John M. Walker, *Series Editor*

105. **Developmental Hematopoiesis:** *Methods and Protocols,* edited by *Margaret H. Baron, 2005*
104. **Stroke Genomics:** *Methods and Reviews,* edited by *Simon J. Read and David Virley, 2005*
103. **Pancreatic Cancer:** *Methods and Protocols,* edited by *Gloria H. Su, 2005*
102. **Autoimmunity:** *Methods and Protocols,* edited by *Andras Perl, 2004*
101. **Cartilage and Osteoarthritis:** *Volume 2, Structure and In Vivo Analysis,* edited by *Frederic De Ceuninck, Massimo Sabatini, and Philippe Pastoureau, 2004*
100. **Cartilage and Osteoarthritis:** *Volume 1, Cellular and Molecular Tools,* edited by *Massimo Sabatini, Philippe Pastoureau, and Frederic De Ceuninck, 2004*
99. **Pain Research:** *Methods and Protocols,* edited by *David Z. Luo, 2004*
98. **Tumor Necrosis Factor:** *Methods and Protocols,* edited by *Angelo Corti and Pietro Ghezzi, 2004*
97. **Molecular Diagnosis of Cancer:** *Methods and Protocols, Second Edition,* edited by *Joseph E. Roulston and John M. S. Bartlett, 2004*
96. **Hepatitis B and D Protocols:** *Volume 2, Immunology, Model Systems, and Clinical Studies,* edited by *Robert K. Hamatake and Johnson Y. N. Lau, 2004*
95. **Hepatitis B and D Protocols:** *Volume 1, Detection, Genotypes, and Characterization,* edited by *Robert K. Hamatake and Johnson Y. N. Lau, 2004*
94. **Molecular Diagnosis of Infectious Diseases,** *Second Edition,* edited by *Jochen Decker and Udo Reischl, 2004*
93. **Anticoagulants, Antiplatelets, and Thrombolytics,** edited by *Shaker A. Mousa, 2004*
92. **Molecular Diagnosis of Genetic Diseases,** *Second Edition,* edited by *Rob Elles and Roger Mountford, 2004*
91. **Pediatric Hematology:** *Methods and Protocols,* edited by *Nicholas J. Goulden and Colin G. Steward, 2003*
90. **Suicide Gene Therapy:** *Methods and Reviews,* edited by *Caroline J. Springer, 2004*
89. **The Blood–Brain Barrier:** *Biology and Research Protocols,* edited by *Sukriti Nag, 2003*
88. **Cancer Cell Culture:** *Methods and Protocols,* edited by *Simon P. Langdon, 2003*
87. **Vaccine Protocols,** *Second Edition,* edited by *Andrew Robinson, Michael J. Hudson, and Martin P. Cranage, 2003*
86. **Renal Disease:** *Techniques and Protocols,* edited by *Michael S. Goligorsky, 2003*
85. **Novel Anticancer Drug Protocols,** edited by *John K. Buolamwini and Alex A. Adjei, 2003*
84. **Opioid Research:** *Methods and Protocols,* edited by *Zhizhong Z. Pan, 2003*
83. **Diabetes Mellitus:** *Methods and Protocols,* edited by *Sabire Özcan, 2003*
82. **Hemoglobin Disorders:** *Molecular Methods and Protocols,* edited by *Ronald L. Nagel, 2003*
81. **Prostate Cancer Methods and Protocols,** edited by *Pamela J. Russell, Paul Jackson, and Elizabeth A. Kingsley, 2003*
80. **Bone Research Protocols,** edited by *Miep H. Helfrich and Stuart H. Ralston, 2003*
79. **Drugs of Abuse:** *Neurological Reviews and Protocols,* edited by *John Q. Wang, 2003*
78. **Wound Healing:** *Methods and Protocols,* edited by *Luisa A. DiPietro and Aime L. Burns, 2003*
77. **Psychiatric Genetics:** *Methods and Reviews,* edited by *Marion Leboyer and Frank Bellivier, 2003*
76. **Viral Vectors for Gene Therapy:** *Methods and Protocols,* edited by *Curtis A. Machida, 2003*
75. **Lung Cancer:** *Volume 2, Diagnostic and Therapeutic Methods and Reviews,* edited by *Barbara Driscoll, 2003*
74. **Lung Cancer:** *Volume 1, Molecular Pathology Methods and Reviews,* edited by *Barbara Driscoll, 2003*

METHODS IN MOLECULAR MEDICINE™

Developmental Hematopoiesis

Methods and Protocols

Edited by

Margaret H. Baron, MD, PhD

Department of Medicine (Hematology-Oncology), Mount Sinai School of Medicine, New York, NY

HUMANA PRESS ✵ TOTOWA, NEW JERSEY

999 Riverview Drive, Suite 208
Totowa, New Jersey 07512

www.humanapress.com

This publication is printed on acid-free paper. ∞
ANSI Z39.48-1984 (American Standards Institute) Permanence of Paper for Printed Library Materials.

Production Editor: C. Tirpak
Cover design by Patricia F. Cleary

Cover Illustration: From Fig. 5, Chapter 25, "Dynamic In Vivo Imaging of Mammalian Hemataovascular Development Using Whole Embryo Culture," by Elizabeth A. V. Jones, Margaret H. Baron, Scott E. Fraser, and Mary E. Dickinson.

For additional copies, pricing for bulk purchases, and/or information about other Humana titles, contact Humana at the above address or at any of the following numbers: Tel.: 973-256-1699; Fax: 973-256-8341; E-mail: humana@humanapr.com; or visit our Website: www.humanapress.com

Printed in the United States of America. 10 9 8 7 6 5 4 3 2 1

ISSN 1543-1894
E-ISBN 1-58829-296-7

Library of Congress Cataloging-in-Publication Data

Developmental hematopoiesis : methods and protocols / edited by Margaret H. Baron.
p. ; cm. -- (Methods in molecular medicine ; 105)
Includes bibliographical references and index.
ISBN 1-58829-296-7 (alk. paper)
1. Hematopoietic system--Growth--Laboratory manuals. 2. Developmental biology--Laboratory manuals. [DNLM: 1. Hematopoiesis--genetics. 2. Embryo Research. 3. Hematopoietic Stem Cells--cytology. 4. Models, Animal. 5. Molecular Biology--methods. WH 140 D612 2005] I. Baron, Margaret H. II. Series.
QP92.D48 2005
616.1'5--dc22

2004008992

Preface

During the past few decades, technical and conceptual breakthroughs have led to a virtual revolution in developmental biology. In part through cross-species comparisons and multidisciplinary approaches (combining, for example, classical embryology, genetics, molecular biology, and systems biology), major questions have often been redefined and examined from new angles and with innovative tools. Analyses using such model systems as *Drosophila*, *Xenopus*, zebrafish, chick, human, and mouse have underscored the remarkable extent to which molecular and genetic pathways are conserved across species and throughout embryonic, fetal, and adult development. What we learn from the embryo, then, is not only of fundamental interest, but may well have future practical applications in the clinic.

A number of excellent volumes, including several in this series (e.g., *Hematopoietic Stem Cell Protocols*, Klug and Jordan, eds., 2002), have surveyed methods used in the study of hematopoiesis—the processes by which the multiple lineages of the blood form from stem and progenitor cells during ontogeny and throughout the entire life of the animal. These collections of protocols have focused largely on the postnatal cells of mouse and human. Our understanding of hematopoietic development, however, has benefitted enormously from investigations in a variety of organisms at different stages of ontogeny. It is my hope that *Developmental Hematopoiesis* will serve as a starting point for students, postdocs, and more experienced investigators who have not previously studied hematopoietic development, as well as for those who wish to extend the scope of their work to another model organism. Several chapters depart from the standard format of this series, presenting an overview of useful approaches rather than a set of protocols. All of the chapters, however, contain a Notes section intended to provide practical advice not readily obtained from the standard literature.

Part I deals with genetic approaches to hematopoietic development. Each of these deals with the mouse, but the general approaches and concepts are broadly applicable to other systems. For more in-depth coverage of these areas, the reader may wish to consult *Mouse Genetics and Transgenics: A Practical Approach*, Jackson and Abbott eds., 2000. Part II covers two transplantation systems that can be used to follow the determination of cell fate following introduction of embryonic or fetal hematopoietic stem/progenitor cells into mice. Although these cells fail to effect long-term multilineage hematopoietic reconstitution of adult hosts, they do engraft in and reconstitute the hematopoietic systems of conditioned newborn recipients, indicating that they have the potential to function in adults and suggesting that they may need to mature (for example, to express certain homing receptors) during development.

Intrauterine transplantation has not yet been exploited for this purpose, but is likely to provide a second option for assessing developmental outcomes. Both transplantation approaches rely heavily on flow cytometric (FACS) methods for purification of stem cell populations and analysis of cell fate outcomes, and a chapter on flow cytometric analysis of hematopoietic development has thus been included here. Transplantation approaches using adult mouse recipients are described in detail in *Hematopoietic Stem Cell Protocols*, Klug and Jordan eds., 2002.

Part III covers those model systems most widely used for investigating the formation of hematopoietic cells and tissues. The protocols include molecular and cellular assays; explant, organ, and cell culture; and whole animal approaches, including in vivo imaging. The developmental biology of hematopoiesis can be approached from numerous perspectives: ontogeny; cell fate specification [which lineage(s) will form from a given stem/progenitor cell]; signal transduction; gene regulation; cell migrations and interactions with other cells; changes that occur in stem cells (presumably allocated during embryogenesis) as the animal ages. From fruit flies to humans, blood cells form in several distinct phases during development. The earliest ("primitive") hematopoietic cell types are distinct from the later, "definitive" cells and, in general, arise in different (possibly multiple) regions within the developing animal. Maturation of stem and progenitor cells may occur in a location physically far removed from their site of origin. Each model system has unique advantages and limitations and is generally best suited to study certain types of biological problems. For more general information about the development of particular organisms, the reader is referred to well-known practical manuals published elsewhere, such as those from Cold Spring Harbor Press: *Manipulating the Mouse Embryo*, Third Edition, Nagy et al., 2003; *Early Development of Xenopus laevis: A Laboratory Manual*, Sive, Grainger, and Harland, eds., 2000; and *Drosophila: A Laboratory Handbook, Second Edition*, Ashburner, Hawley, and Golic, eds., 2004. *Zebrafish: A Practical Approach*, Nusslein-Volhard and Dahm, eds., 2002. Two other volumes from Humana Press cover the production of transgenic mice or frogs, and may be of interest to readers of *Developmental Hematopoiesis*; they are *Transgenic Mouse Methods and Protocols*, Hofker and van Deursen, 2002 and *Transgenic Xenopus: Microinjection Methods and Developmental Neurobiology*, Seidman and Soreq 1996.

Bioinformatics and functional genomics approaches for studying stem cells and their supporting stromal cells are outlined in Part IV. The Stem Cell Database (SCDb) has been discussed in a number of recent reviews, and a new, expanded version will be released shortly. The chapter included here touches briefly on SCDb, but focuses on the Stromal Cell Database (StroCDB). However, these approaches are generally applicable to any developing system. Global genomics technologies are particularly exciting: they hold the promise of eventually permitting the assembly of molecular components of the cell into pathways and networks that should afford an understanding of the regulation of cell fate specification at the "systems" level.

I thank the authors for their contributions to this book and the many colleagues whose stimulating discussions have helped to shape my own interest in developmental hematopoiesis. Special thanks go to Dr. John Walker, the series editor, to Nicole Furia, Editorial Assistant at Humana Press, and to Thomas Lanigan, the publisher.

Margaret H. Baron, MD, PhD

Contents

Preface v
Contributors xi

Part I: Genetic Approaches

1 Gene-Targeting and Transgenic Strategies for the Analysis of Hematopoietic Development in the Mouse
Hanna K. A. Mikkola and Stuart H. Orkin 3

2 Inducible Transgene Expression in Mouse ES Cells
David T. Ting, Michael Kyba, and George Q. Daley 23

3 Quantitative Trait Analysis in the Investigation of Function and Aging in Hematopoietic Stem Cells
Hans-Willem Snoeck 47

Part II: Analysis of Cell Fate Outcomes in Transplantation Models

4 Flow Cytometric Analysis of Hematopoietic Development
Edward F. Srour and Mervin C. Yoder 65

5 Reconstitution of Hematopoiesis Following Intrauterine Transplantation of Stem Cells
Elisabeth H. Javazon, Aziz M. Merchant, Enrico Danzer, and Alan W. Flake 81

6 Reconstitution of Hematopoiesis Following Transplantation Into Neonatal Mice
Scott A. Johnson and Mervin C. Yoder 95

Part III: Animal Models

Drosophila

7 Hemocyte Development During *Drosophila* Embryogenesis
Robert A. Schulz and Nancy Fossett 109

Xenopus

8 Tracking and Programming Early Hematopoietic Cells in *Xenopus* Embryos
Maggie Walmsley, Aldo Ciau-Uitz, and Roger Patient 123

9 Fate Mapping Hematopoietic Lineages in the *Xenopus* Embryo
Mary Constance Lane and Michael D. Sheets 137

10 Analyses of Immune Responses to Ontogeny-Specific Antigens Using an Inbred Strain of *Xenopus laevis* (J Strain)
Yumi Izutsu and Mitsugu Maéno ***149***

11 Use of Flow Cytometry and Combined DNA/Surface Staining for Analysis of Hematopoietic Development in the *Xenopus* Embryo
James B. Turpen ***159***

Zebrafish

12 Analysis of Hematopoietic Development in the Zebrafish
Noëlle N. Paffett-Lugassy and Leonard I. Zon ***171***

13 Imaging Early Macrophage Differentiation, Migration, and Behaviors in Live Zebrafish Embryos
Philippe Herbomel and Jean-Pierre Levraud ***199***

Chick

14 In Vivo Methods to Analyze Cell Origins, Migrations, Homing, and Interactions in the Blood, Vascular, and Immune Systems of the Avian and Mammalian Embryo
Françoise Dieterlen-Lièvre, Sophie Creuzet, and Josselyne Salaün ***215***

Mouse

15 Mouse Embryonic Explant Culture System for Analysis of Hematopoietic and Vascular Development
Margaret H. Baron and Deanna Mohn ***231***

16 Hematopoietic Stem Cell Enrichment From the AGM Region of the Mouse Embryo
Catherine Robin and Elaine Dzierzak ***257***

17 Hematopoietic Stem Cell Development During Mouse Embryogenesis
Julien Y. Bertrand, Sebastien Giroux, Ana Cumano, and Isabelle Godin ***273***

18 Analysis of Hematopoietic Progenitors in the Mouse Embryo
James Palis and Anne Koniski ***289***

19 In Vivo and In Vitro Assays of Thymic Organogenesis
Julie Gordon, Valerie A. Wilson, Billie A. Moore-Scott, Nancy R. Manley, and C. Clare Blackburn ***303***

20 Retroviral Transduction in Fetal Thymic Organ Culture
Bronwyn M. Owens, Robert G. Hawley, and Lisa M. Spain ***311***

21 Expansion and Differentiation of Immature Mouse and Human Hematopoietic Progenitors
Helmut Dolznig, Andrea Kolbus, Cornelia Leberbauer, Uwe Schmidt, Eva-Maria Deiner, Ernst W. Müllner, and Hartmut Beug ***323***

22 A New Clonal Assay System for Lymphoid and Myeloid Lineages
Hiroshi Kawamoto and Yoshimoto Katsura ***345***

23 Hematopoietic and Endothelial Development of Mouse Embryonic Stem Cells in Culture
Kyunghee Choi, Yun Shin Chung, and Weh Jie Zhang ***359***

24 Analysis of the Vascular Potential of Hematopoietic Stem Cells
Steven M. Guthrie, Sergio Caballero, Robert N. Mames, Maria B. Grant, and Edward W. Scott ***369***

25 Dynamic In Vivo Imaging of Mammalian Hematovascular Development Using Whole Embryo Culture
Elizabeth A.V. Jones, Margaret H. Baron, Scott E. Fraser, and Mary E. Dickinson ***381***

26 Fluorescent Protein–Cell Labeling and Its Application in Time-Lapse Analysis of Hematopoietic Differentiation
Matthias Stadtfeld, Florencio Varas, and Thomas Graf ***395***

Human

27 Analysis of Hematopoietic Development During Human Embryonic Ontogenesis
Manuela Tavian and Bruno Péault ***413***

28 Hematopoietic Development of Human Embryonic Stem Cells in Culture
Xinghui Tian and Dan S. Kaufman ***425***

PART IV: BIOINFORMATICS AND FUNCTIONAL GENOMICS

29 A Functional Genomics Approach to Hematopoietic Stem Cell Regulation
Jason A. Hackney and Kateri A. Moore ***439***

Index 453

Contributors

MARGARET H. BARON • *Departments of Medicine (Hematology-Oncology), Molecular Cell and Developmental Biology, Ruttenberg Cancer Center, and Icahn Center for Gene Therapy and Molecular Medicine, Mount Sinai School of Medicine, New York, NY*

JULIEN Y. BERTRAND • *Unité du Développement des Lymphocytes, Institut Pasteur, Paris, France*

HARTMUT BEUG • *Institute of Molecular Pathology, Vienna, Austria*

C. CLARE BLACKBURN • *Institute for Stem Cell Research, University of Edinburgh, Edinburgh, UK*

SERGIO CABALLERO • *Program in Stem Cell Biology, Shands Cancer Center, University of Florida, Gainesville, FL*

KYUNGHEE CHOI • *Department of Pathology and Immunology, Washington University School of Medicine, St. Louis, MO*

YUN SHIN CHUNG • *Department of Pathology and Immunology, Washington University School of Medicine, St. Louis, MO*

ALDO CIAU-UITZ • *Institute of Genetics, University of Nottingham, Nottingham, UK*

SOPHIE CREUZET • *Laboratoire d'Embryologie cellulaire et moléculaire du CNRS et Collège de France, Nogent-sur-Marne cedex, France*

ANA CUMANO • *Unité du Développement des Lymphocytes, Institut Pasteur, Paris, France*

GEORGE Q. DALEY • *Division of Hematology/Oncology, Children's Hospital, Boston, MA*

ENRICO DANZER • *Children's Institute for Surgical Science, Children's Hospital of Philadelphia, Philadelphia, PA*

EVA-MARIA DEINER • *Institute of Molecular Pathology, Vienna, Austria*

MARY E. DICKINSON • *Biological Imaging Center, Department of Biology, California Institute of Technology, Pasadena, CA*

FRANÇOISE DIETERLEN-LIÈVRE • *Laboratoire d'Embryologie cellulaire et moléculaire du CNRS et Collège de France, Nogent-sur-Marne cedex, France*

HELMUT DOLZNIG • *Institute of Clinical Pathology, Medical University of Vienna, Vienna, Austria*

ELAINE DZIERZAK • *Department of Cell Biology and Genetics, Erasmus University Medical Center, Rotterdam, The Netherlands*

ALAN W. FLAKE • *Children's Institute for Surgical Science, Children's Hospital of Philadelphia, Philadelphia, PA*

NANCY FOSSETT • *Holland Laboratory, American Red Cross, Rockville, MD*

SCOTT E. FRASER • *Biological Imaging Center, Department of Biology, California Institute of Technology, Pasadena, CA*

Sebastien Giroux • *Hématopoïèse et cellules souches, INSERM U362, Institut Gustave Roussy-PR1, Villejuif, France*
Isabelle Godin • *Hématopoïèse et cellules souches, INSERM U362, Institut Gustave Roussy-PR1, Villejuif, France*
Julie Gordon • *Department of Genetics, University of Georgia, Athens, GA*
Thomas Graf • *Department of Developmental and Molecular Biology, Albert Einstein College of Medicine, Bronx, NY*
Maria B. Grant • *Program in Stem Cell Biology, Shands Cancer Center, University of Florida, Gainesville, FL*
Steven M. Guthrie • *Program in Stem Cell Biology, Shands Cancer Center, University of Florida, Gainesville, FL*
Jason A. Hackney • *Department of Molecular Biology, Princeton University, Princeton, NJ*
Robert G. Hawley • *Department of Anatomy and Cell Biology, The George Washington University, Washington, DC*
Philippe Herbomel • *Unité Macrophages et Développement de l'Immunité, Institut Pasteur, Paris, France*
Yumi Izutsu • *Graduate School of Science, Niigata University, Niigata, Japan*
Elisabeth H. Javazon • *Children's Institute for Surgical Science, Children's Hospital of Philadelphia, Philadelphia, PA*
Scott A. Johnson • *Herman B. Wells Center for Pediatric Research, Indiana University School of Medicine, Indianapolis, IN*
Elizabeth A.V. Jones • *Department of Chemical Engineering and Biological Imaging Center, Department of Biology, California Institute of Technology, Pasadena, CA*
Yoshimoto Katsura • *Department of Cell Regeneration and Transplantation, Nihon University School of Medicine and Department of Molecular Immunopathology, School of Medicine, Tokyo Medical and Dental University, Tokyo, Japan*
Dan S. Kaufman • *Stem Cell Institute and Department of Medicine, University of Minnesota, Minneapolis, MN*
Hiroshi Kawamoto • *Laboratory for Lymphocyte Development, RIKEN Research Center for Allergy and Immunology, Yokohama, Japan*
Andrea Kolbus • *Department of Gynecological Endocrinology, Medical University of Vienna, Vienna, Austria*
Anne Koniski • *Department of Pediatrics and Center for Human Genetics and Molecular Pediatric Disease, University of Rochester Medical Center, Rochester, NY*
Michael Kyba • *Center for Developmental Biology, UT Southwestern Medical Center, Dallas, TX*
Mary Constance Lane • *Department of Biomolecular Chemistry, University of Wisconsin School of Medicine, Madison, WI*
Cornelia Leberbauer • *Max F. Perutz Laboratories–The University Departments at the Vienna Biocenter, Institute of Medical Biochemistry, Medical University of Vienna, Vienna, Austria*

Jean-Pierre Levraud • *Unité Macrophages et Développement de l'Immunité, Institut Pasteur, Paris, France*

Mitsugu Maéno • *Faculty of Science, Niigata University, Niigata, Japan*

Robert N. Mames • *Program in Stem Cell Biology, Shands Cancer Center, University of Florida, Gainesville, FL*

Nancy R. Manley • *Department of Genetics, University of Georgia, Athens, GA*

Aziz M. Merchant • *Children's Institute for Surgical Science, Children's Hospital of Philadelphia, Philadelphia, PA*

Hanna K. A. Mikkola • *Department of Pediatric Oncology, Dana-Farber Cancer Institute, Children's Hospital, and Harvard Medical School, Boston, MA*

Deanna Mohn • *Department of Medicine (Hematology-Oncology), Mount Sinai School of Medicine, New York, NY*

Kateri A. Moore • *Department of Molecular Biology, Princeton University, Princeton, NJ*

Billie A. Moore-Scott • *Department of Genetics, University of Georgia, Athens, GA*

Ernst W. Müllner • *Max F. Perutz Laboratories–The University Departments at the Vienna Biocenter, Institute of Medical Biochemistry, Medical University of Vienna, Vienna, Austria*

Stuart H. Orkin • *Howard Hughes Medical Institute, Department of Pediatric Oncology, Dana-Farber Cancer Institute, Children's Hospital, and Harvard Medical School, Boston, MA*

Bronwyn M. Owens • *Beth Israel Deaconess Medical Center, Harvard Medical School, Boston, MA*

Noëlle N. Paffett-Lugassy • *Department of Pediatric Oncology, Children's Hospital, Boston, MA*

James Palis • *Department of Pediatrics and Center for Human Genetics and Molecular Pediatric Disease, University of Rochester Medical Center, Rochester, NY*

Roger Patient • *Institute of Genetics, University of Nottingham, Nottingham, UK*

Bruno Péault • *Department of Pediatrics, Rangos Research Center, Children's Hospital, Pittsburgh, PA*

Catherine Robin • *Department of Cell Biology and Genetics, Erasmus University Medical Center, Rotterdam, The Netherlands*

Josselyne Salaün • *Laboratoire d'Embryologie cellulaire et moléculaire du CNRS et Collège de France, Nogent-sur-Marne cedex, France*

Uwe Schmidt • *Institute of Immunology, Medical University of Vienna, Vienna, Austria*

Robert A. Schulz • *Department of Biochemistry and Molecular Biology, The University of Texas M. D. Anderson Cancer Center, Houston, TX*

Edward W. Scott • *Program in Stem Cell Biology, Shands Cancer Center, University of Florida, Gainesville, FL*

Michael D. Sheets • *Department of Biomolecular Chemistry, University of Wisconsin School of Medicine, Madison, WI*

Hans-Willem Snoeck • *Carl Icahn Center for Gene Therapy and Molecular Medicine, Mount Sinai School of Medicine, New York, NY*

Lisa M. Spain • *National Institute of Diabetics, Digestive Diseases, and Kidney (NIDDK), National Institutes of Health, Bethesda, MD*

Edward F. Srour • *Herman B. Wells Center for Pediatric Research, Indiana University School of Medicine, Indianapolis, IN*

Matthias Stadtfeld • *Department of Developmental and Molecular Biology, Albert Einstein College of Medicine, Bronx, NY*

Manuela Tavian • *Inserm U506, Hôpital Paul Brousse, Villejuif, France*

Xinghui Tian • *Stem Cell Institute and Department of Medicine, University of Minnesota, Minneapolis, MN*

David T. Ting • *Harvard-M.I.T. Program in Health Sciences and Technology, Harvard Medical School, Boston, MA*

Florencio Varas • *Center for Genomic Regulation (C.R.G.), Barcelona, Spain*

Maggie Walmsley • *Institute of Genetics, University of Nottingham, Nottingham, UK*

Valerie A. Wilson • *Institute for Stem Cell Research, University of Edinburgh, Edinburgh, UK*

Mervin C. Yoder • *Herman B. Wells Center for Pediatric Research, Indiana University School of Medicine, Indianapolis, IN*

Weh Jie Zhang • *Department of Pathology and Immunology, Washington University School of Medicine, St. Louis, MO*

Leonard I. Zon • *Howard Hughes Medical Institute, Department of Pediatric Oncology, Dana-Farber Cancer Institute, Children's Hospital, and Harvard Medical School, Boston, MA*

Color Plates

Color Plates 1–10 appear as an insert following p. 80

PLATE 1 Fig. 5. A schematic demonstrating of the various routes of IUHCT. (*See* full caption on p. 88, Chapter 5.)

PLATE 2 Fig. 3. Immunolocalization of lozenge and U-shaped in *Drosophila* blood cells using confocal microscopy. (*See* full caption on p. 119, Chapter 7.)

PLATE 3 Fig. 2. Examples of murine hematopoietic colonies. (*See* full caption on p. 297, Chapter 18.)

PLATE 4 Fig. 4. Areas of neovascularization in the retina. (*See* full caption on p. 377, Chapter 24.)

PLATE 5 Fig. 5. Immunohistochemistry of kidney tissue sections. (*See* full caption on p. 377, Chapter 24.)

PLATE 6 Fig. 5. Expression of GFP in Primitive Erythroblasts. (*See* full caption on p. 389, Chapter 25.)

PLATE 7 Fig. 2. Differentiation of myeloid progenitors visualized by fluorescence time-lapse microscopy. (*See* full caption on p. 398, Chapter 26.)

PLATE 8 Fig. 6. Fluorescent intensities of three GFP variants and of RFP determined with the different filters. (*See* full caption on p. 403, Chapter 26.)

PLATE 9 Fig. 7. CFP and GFP can be separated using the Yellow GFP filter. (*See* full caption on p. 406, Chapter 26.)

PLATE 10 Fig. 8. The JP1/JP2 filter combination facilitates separation of GFP and YFP. (*See* full caption on p. 407, Chapter 26.)

I

Genetic Approaches

1

Gene Targeting and Transgenic Strategies for the Analysis of Hematopoietic Development in the Mouse

Hanna K. A. Mikkola and Stuart H. Orkin

Summary

The generation of gene-targeted and transgenic mouse models facilitates the in vivo study of mammalian gene function. Advances in technologies to engineer the mouse genome have extended the choice of gene manipulation from straightforward gene inactivation or overexpression to detailed modification of gene expression pattern, structure, and function in desired cell types and at specific times. Combining conventional/conditional, knockout/knockin, inducible, and even reversible gene manipulation strategies provides the investigator with the freedom to design an optimal model to study the function of a gene in a specific organ system during development or in postnatal life. To maximize success, however, the requirements and limitations of each approach need to be considered. This chapter provides an overview of gene targeting strategies that are available for manipulation of the mouse genome. We emphasize approaches that aid the investigation of the development and function of the hematopoietic system in the mouse.

Key Words: Gene targeting; transgenic mouse; knockout; knockin; chimera; conditional gene targeting; Cre recombinase; ES cell; homologous recombination.

1. Introduction

The development of gene-targeting strategies applied to mouse embryonic stem (ES) cells has greatly facilitated the study of in vivo function of mammalian genes. The generation of a mouse model affords the opportunity to assess gene function in a physiological context during development and in adult life. However, each in vivo model is informative only to the stage at which expression of the relevant gene product is required for survival of the mouse. To bypass embryonic lethality and facilitate the analysis of gene function in specific organ systems, it has been crucial to improve gene targeting strategies to allow tissue-specific and inducible gene manipulation.

Gene-targeted mouse models have been instrumental in identifying critical regulators of blood cell development. Through knockout studies, molecular regulators directing commitment to the hematopoietic program and differentiation to various blood cell lin-

From: *Methods in Molecular Medicine, Vol. 105: Developmental Hematopoiesis: Methods and Protocols.*
Edited by: M. H. Baron © Humana Press Inc., Totowa, NJ

eages have been defined. However, many of the knockout models fail to produce an essential component of the hematopoietic system and thus are embryonic lethal, precluding further analysis of the phenotype at later stages of development or during postnatal life. Although many of the key regulators that were identified through knockout studies are also likely to play an important role in adult hematopoiesis, straightforward extrapolation of gene function from the embryo to adult may not be feasible because of differences between the embryonic and adult hematopoietic programs. Adult hematopoiesis is centered in the bone marrow (BM) where pluripotential hematopoietic stem cells (HSCs) that have the ability to self-renew and differentiate, give rise to lineage-restricted progenitors and ultimately to terminally differentiated hematopoietic cells in the circulation, thymus and spleen. Hematopoiesis during embryogenesis is instead characterized by transient waves of hematopoietic activity in several anatomical locations. The purpose of early hematopoiesis is to produce red blood cells that are required for proper oxygen delivery to the embryo and to generate hematopoietic stem cells that will establish postnatal hematopoiesis in the bone marrow. The hematopoietic stem cell, as defined by the ability to reconstitute BM hematopoiesis of an irradiated adult recipient, is a relatively late product of embryonic hematopoiesis. The first hematopoietic progenitors are found already at E 7–8 in the yolk sac, whereas the first rare HSCs are found at the aorta–gonad–mesonephros region several days later, at approx E 10.5–11 ***(1–3)***. Furthermore, it is not until E 12.5 that expansion of HSCs takes place in the fetal liver and not until birth that HSCs colonize the bone marrow. The first requirement of early hematopoiesis is to produce primitive (also called embryonic) nucleated erythrocytes in the yolk sac; in their absence, embry-onic lethality occurs between E 9.5–11 ***(4–6)***. Seeding of the fetal liver by hematopoietic progenitors establishes the definitive (or adult) hematopoietic program, leading to the production of adult-type red cells, megakaryocytes, and white blood cells. Disruption of the definitive hematopoietic program leads to lethality at E 11–13 ***(7,8)***. Likewise, development of an intact vascular system is essential for blood cell function and survival of the embryo past E 10.5 ***(9–11)***. Thus, any severe defects affecting primitive or definitive hematopoietic progenitors or the vascular system need to be circumvented to assess the role of a given gene in the development and function of HSCs. Conversely, a defect in HSCs in postnatal hematopoiesis impairs the entire hematopoietic system and precludes analysis of gene function in specific lineages, unless the gene can be inactivated after a critical stage in development has taken place. Thus, generations of several different gene targeted mouse models are often necessary to elucidate the role of the gene both during embryonic and adult hematopoiesis.

2. Materials

1. Gene-targeting construct.
2. Mouse ES cells.
3. ES cell culture reagents.
4. Electroporation equipment.
5. Mouse colonies (blastocyst donor females, stud males, vasectomized males, pseudopregnant females).
6. Blastocysts.
7. Microinjection equipment.

(For details, *see* **refs. *12–15***).

3. Methods

3.1. Selection of the Gene-Targeting or Transgenic Strategy

Gene-targeting and transgenic strategies may be used to inactivate, overexpress, or modify genes in the mouse (**Fig. 1**; **refs.** ***12–15***). The manipulation of the gene can be directed to all tissues of the body or to selected cell types, or to a specific time in the life of the animal.

3.1.1. Knockout Mouse

A knockout mouse represents a loss of function mouse model and is generated by disrupting the gene of interest by introducing deoxyribonucleic acid (DNA) sequences through homologous recombination in mouse ES cells. Upon injection into blastocysts and implantation into foster mothers, the targeted ES cells can contribute to all cell types in the embryo and adult, including germ cells. Germline transmission of the targeted allele and interbreeding of heterozygous animals leads to production of homozygous knockout animals that lack the targeted gene product in all tissues of the body. The phenotype of the animals displays the impact of the gene on mouse development and physiology.

3.1.2. Transgenic Mouse

A transgenic mouse represents a gain of function mouse model and is usually designed to overexpress a gene of interest. By choosing an ubiquitous, tissue-specific or regulatable promoter, the expression of the transgene may be directed in space and time.

Several strategies may be chosen to express transgenes in an inducible fashion. These include the tet-on, tet-off, and ecdysone systems, in which the inducer and the responsive gene are introduced separately ***(16–20)***. An alternative approach is to use promoter elements that respond directly to an inducer, such as the interferon inducible Mx promoter ***(21)*** or fusion protein systems, in which the transgene is coupled with a modified ligand-binding domain of the estrogen or glucocorticoid receptors ***(22–25)***. These fusion proteins are inactive until the appropriate ligand is added.

3.1.3. Knockin Mouse

Expression of introduced sequences may also be achieved by generating a knockin mouse (**Fig. 1A**). In this instance, foreign sequences are introduced into a given locus by homologous recombination. This strategy can be used to express transgenes from known regulatory elements or to modify rather than merely inactivate the targeted gene. Knockin alleles are generally expressed precisely as the endogenous gene where the sequences are introduced. Knockin of a marker gene under the regulatory elements of the gene of interest offers a valuable tool for monitoring gene expression. Markers such as *Escherichia coli* β-galactosidase (lacZ), green fluorescent protein (GFP), or inert cell surface molecules (e.g., inactive human CD4) are particularly useful in this regard ***(26–31)***. Expression of markers may be detected by immunohistochemistry or flow cytometry. The availability of such knockin strains obviates the need for gene-specific antibodies and permits detection of gene expression at the single cell level.

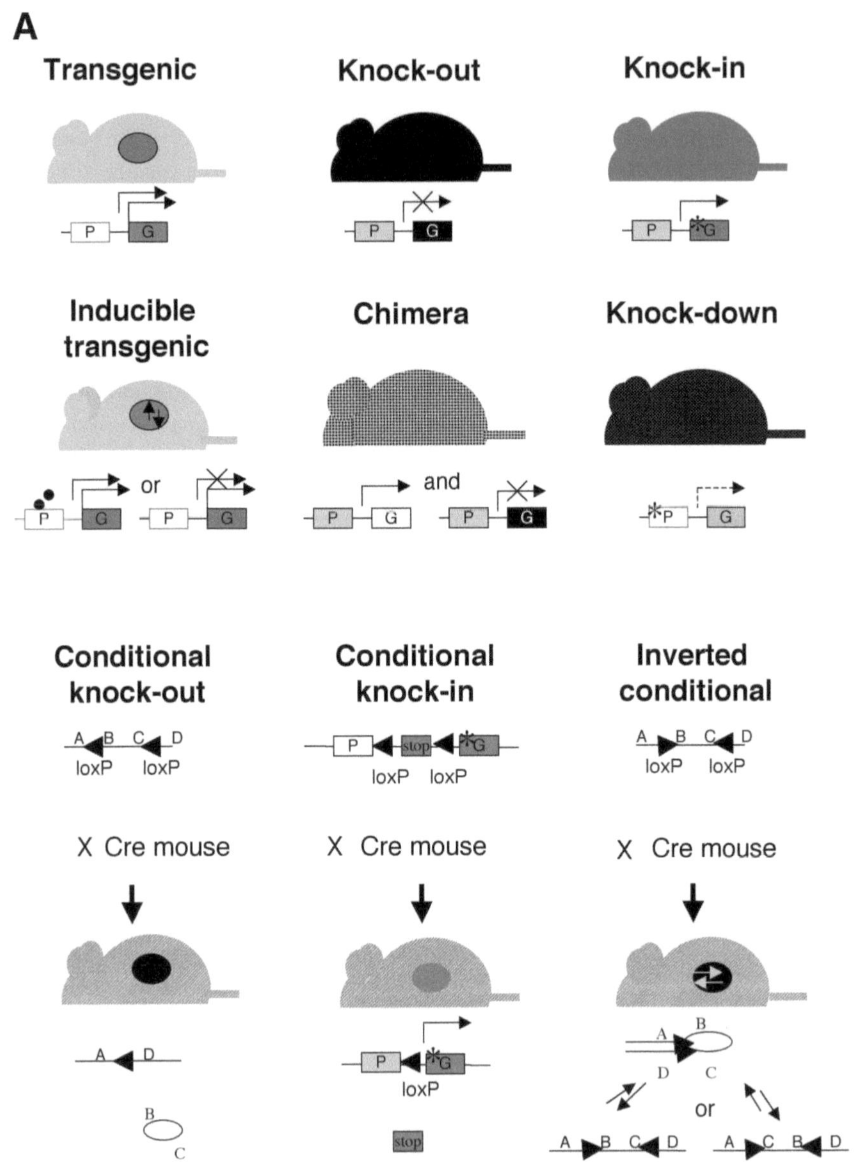

Fig. 1. Gene-targeting and transgenic animal models. **(A)** Transgenic mice may be engineered to express novel gene sequences from ubiquitous, tissue-specific, or inducible promoters. Gene-targeted mice may be designed to inactivate or modify the function (knockout or knockin, respectively) or expression level (knockdown) of the gene in all cells of the body, or conditionally in selected tissues and times. A tissue-specific role for a gene product may be revealed in the context of an intact animal by generating chimeric mice or reversibly targeted mice (inverted conditional). P, promoter; G, transgene or targeted gene; *, gene modification; arrows, gene expression. *(Continued on next page.)*

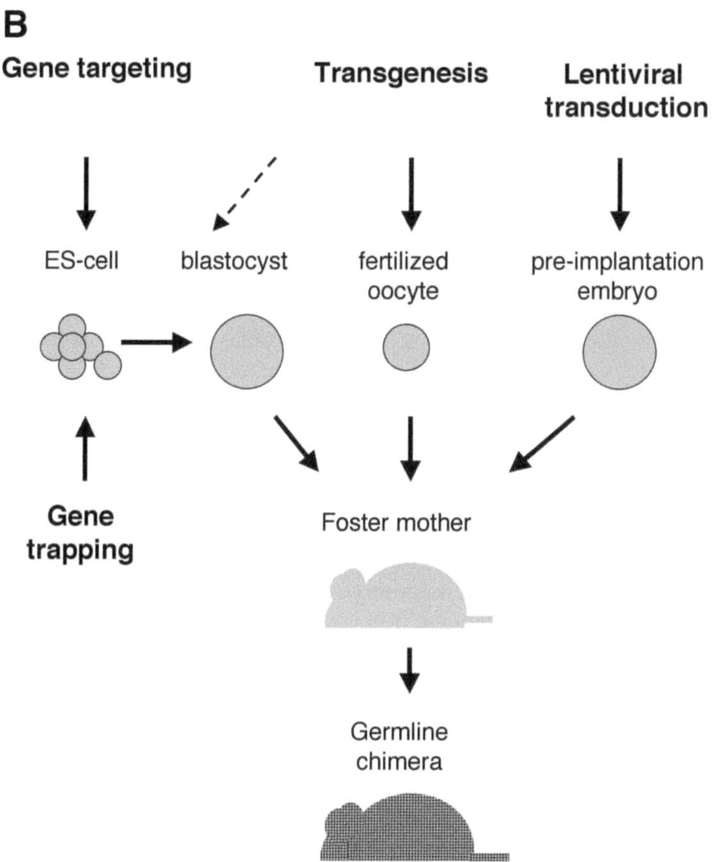

Fig. 1. *(Continued)* **(B)** The mouse ES cell genome can be modified by directed gene targeting via homologous recombination or by random targeting using retroviral gene trapping. The modified ES cells are injected into blastocysts that are implanted into pseudopregnant females and contribute to normal embryonic development. Transgenic mice may be generated by conventional transgenesis using DNA microinjection into fertilized oocytes (or electroporation of the transgenic construct to ES cells) or through lentiviral transgenesis by transducing pre-implantation embryos that develop to term in foster mothers. Germline transmission of the modified cells creates a mouse strain with mutated genome.

Depending on the design of the knockin construct, introduction of sequences into the locus may generate a null or hypomorphic allele of the endogenous gene. Likewise, the knockin strategy may be used to modify the endogenous gene by creating single base substitutions or deletions and offers a valuable tool to study the correlation of structure and function of the gene product in vivo ***(32,33)***.

3.1.4. Knockdown Mouse

Gene-targeting strategies can also be applied to modify the *cis*-regulatory elements of a gene in an effort to identify sequences critical for gene activation or maintenance. By this approach, alleles may be inactivated, phenocopying knockout mutations, or impaired in their expression, leading to the generation of knockdown mutants ***(34)***.

3.1.5. Chimeric Mouse

Inactivation, modification, or overexpression of a critical gene often results in embryonic lethality. In this case, the mouse model may be of limited utility for assessing the requirement for gene function in specific organ systems. Fortunately, additional strategies offer the means to circumvent or delay embryonic lethality. Chimera analysis provides a powerful method to investigate the ability of the gene targeted ES cells to contribute to specific tissues within the context of an intact animal. To use this approach one must select double knockout ES cells through successive gene targeting or selection in high G418 (for neoresistant heterozygous cells), if the gene of interest is located on an autosome ***(15,35)***. The ES cells are injected into blastocysts and the contribution of the introduced cells is followed in the resulting chimeras. This strategy circumvents embryonic lethality as normal cells from the host blastocyst will generally rescue the developing chimeric embryo ***(36–39)***. The knockout cells will contribute only to those tissues/cell types for which they are competent to develop. By choosing an ES cell line that expresses a different marker than the cells derived from the blastocyst, the contribution of the knockout cells can be monitored. The markers that are useful in studying contribution of targeted cells to the hematopoietic system include hemoglobin variants, GPI-1 isoenzymes, CD45 alleles, lacZ, and GFP ***(37–39)***. Chimera analysis is especially useful in demonstrating a cell autonomous function of the gene (*also see* **Notes 1** and **2**).

3.1.6. Conditional Knockout

The development of conditional gene-targeting strategies based on sequence-specific recombinases permits exquisite manipulation of the mouse genome (**Fig. 1A**). Conditional targeting relies on the introduction of recombinase recognition sequences into a gene locus in an “innocuous” region (**Fig. 2**). Expression of a sequence-specific recombinase leads to excision of DNA sequences between two recognition sites, if these sites are oriented similarly in the locus. If oriented in an opposed fashion, expression of the recombinase leads to inversion rather than excision. Two recombinase systems, Cre-loxP and Flp-frt, are currently in use ***(40–43)***. The majority of studies to date have used the Cre-loxP system. To generate a conditional knockout allele, loxP sites are introduced so as to flank an essential region of the target gene. Cre recombinase is introduced into the conditional strain from a separate mouse that expresses Cre from known regulatory elements. With a suitable Cre-expressing strain, deletion of the gene of interest may be controlled spatially and/or temporally ***(21,44–65)*** (**Table 1**).

3.1.7. Conditional Knockin

The Cre-loxP strategy may also be applied for conditional expression of genes in a transgenic or knockin model (**Fig. 1A**). A “stopper” fragment flanked by loxP

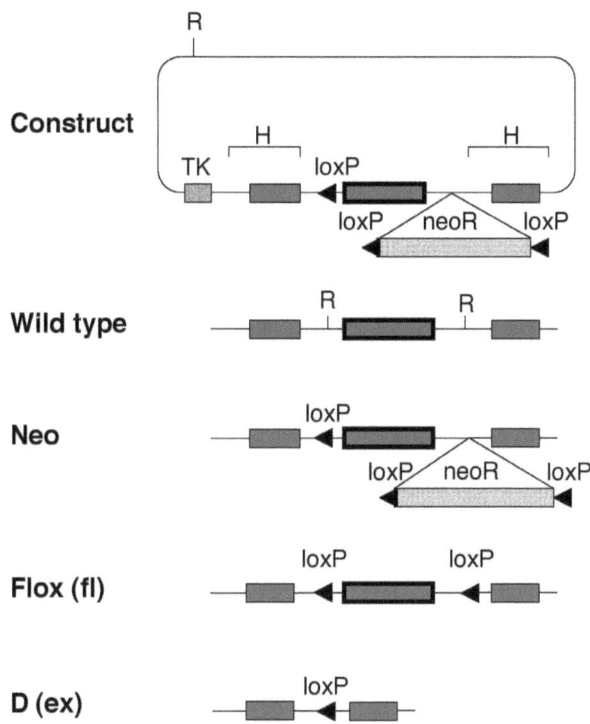

Fig. 2. Engineering a conditionally targeted locus. A conditional gene-targeting construct contains a positive selection marker (for selection of homologous recombinants) flanked by two loxP sites and two homologous arms (for directing homologous recombination into wild type locus) A third loxP site is placed flanking a critical region of the gene providing the option to inactivate or modify the gene. The negative selection marker, thymidine kinase gene (for counterselection of random integrants), and unique restriction site (for linearization of the construct) are placed outside the homologous regions. Homologous recombination generates a targeted allele that contains the neo-resistance gene, which may be removed by transient Cre expression to yield the floxed allele where the critical region of the gene is flanked by two lox P sites. Recombination between two remaining loxP sites results in deletion of the gene fragment and inactivation or modification of the gene. R, restriction enzyme site; TK, thymidine kinase gene; neoR, neomycin resistance gene; H, homologous arm; arrowheads, loxP sites; grey boxes, exons.

sequences is introduced into the construct to block gene expression ***(66)***. After Cre-mediated deletion of the stopper fragment expression of the downstream gene sequences is permitted. By breeding with an inducible or tissue-specific Cre strain, transgene expression may be controlled temporally or spatially. This strategy has been especially useful in studying "toxic" transgenes, such as oncoproteins/fusion proteins, where it is critical to bypass the deleterious effects of the gene product during development ***(67)***.

Table 1
Some Cre-Expressing Transgenic Mouse Lines

Cre Mouse	Strategy	Deletion	Notes	References
GATA1	Transgene	General or red cells, megakaryocytes, mast cells and eosinophils	Early embryonic excision more common	***44,45***
Tie 2	Transgene	Endothelial and hematopoietic cells	Some excision in heart	***53,54***
Tie 1	Transgene	Endothelial cells	Some excision in hematopoietic cells	***46***
GPIIb	Transgene	Embryonic hematopoietic cells	Efficient excision in YS, AGM, FL, but partial in BM	***47***
GPIIb	Knockin	Megakaryocytes	Low efficiency	***47***
vav	Transgene	Hematopoietic cells	Some excision in testis and ovary	***52,65***
Lysozyme	Knockin	Macrophages, granulocytes		***63***
CD2	Transgene	Lymphoid cells	Efficient in T-cells, partial in B-cells	***56,65***
LCK	Transgene	T-cells	Excision at the DN stage	***57–60***
MMTV	Transgene	Secretory tissues and some hematopoietic cells	Developmental and puberty induced	***61,62***
CD19	Knockin	B-cells	Bly pre-B-cells	***51,55***
CD19	Knockin	Inducible (tamoxifen) in B-cells	>80% of B-cells in high doses	***50***
Mx	Transgene	Inducible (interferon or pIpC)	Efficient in hematopoitic cells, partial in other tissue	***21,48,49***

3.1.8. Inverted Conditional

Recombination of a conditional knockout or knockin allele targeted with two loxP sites that are oriented in the same direction is an irreversible event. However, the loxP strategy may also be used to modify the gene in a reversible fashion (**Fig 1A**). By introducing loxP sites in opposed orientations, an inversion event takes place and the two loxP sites are retained. As such, inversion may occur in a successive fashion. Since the inversion is reversible, at equilibrium half of the alleles should be in the inverted (or inactive) configuration and half in the normal (active) configuration, unless there is a selective advantage for one of the two orientations. The inverted conditional may circumvent lethality by altering the equilibrium of the configurations and may simultaneously reveal a selective advantage or disadvantage for the modified gene function in specific cell types *(49,68)*.

3.2. Generation of a Transgenic Mouse

3.2.1. Transgenic Construct

The oldest and usually least time-consuming strategy to modify the mouse genome is to generate a transgenic mouse. The transgenic construct contains a promoter element, cDNA for the gene of interest (usually coupled with an intron to enhance expression levels) and a polyadenylation (poly A) signal *(12)*. Insulator sequences may be incorporated into the transgene construct to minimize position effects on transgene expression. It is advisable to remove plasmid sequences from the construct by restriction digestion, as plasmid sequences flanking the transgenes may negatively influence transgene expression, and linearization of the construct increases the efficiency of transgenesis.

3.2.2. DNA Microinjection

The transgenic construct is injected into the pronucleus of a fertilized oocyte, which is then reimplanted into a foster mother (**Fig 1B**, *also see* **Notes 3** and **4**). The resulting mice are founders (F_0). After microinjection, transgene DNA is integrated into the genome in multiple copies in tandem, although in some instances single copy transgenics may be obtained. As the integration site and copy number of the transgene often affect the expression of the transgene, screening of several individual mouse lines is frequently required to obtain a desired expression pattern. Confirmation of the phenotype in independent transgenic mouse lines is important to exclude nonspecific phenotypes owing to improper transgene regulation or activation/inactivation of endogenous genes at the integration site.

3.3. Generation of a Gene-Targeted Mouse

3.3.1. Knockout Construct

A gene-targeting construct for homologous recombination in ES cells contains a selectable marker gene flanked by two arms of homologous genomic sequence (generally more than 2 kb in both arms; **Fig. 2**; **refs.** ***13,15***). The homologous arms direct recombination with the endogenous gene and introduce the selectable marker (or other gene sequences) into the genome of the ES cell, thereby modifying the endogenous gene.

Integration and expression of the positive selection marker (e.g., neomycin resistance gene, NeoR, driven by a promoter, e.g., phosphoglycerate kinase [PGK]) facilitates the recovery of ES cells that have incorporated the DNA construct. A negative selection marker (e.g., thymidine kinase gene, TK) is frequently placed outside the homologous region to enrich for homologous, as opposed to random, integrants. Cells that incorporate the TK gene (i.e., random integrants) are sensitive to ganciclovir, whereas those that do not (i.e., homologous recombinants) are resistant. In practice, enrichment for homologous recombinants with the TK-counterselective system is modest ***(69,70)***. The targeting vector can be constructed by adding the neoresistance gene and TK sequences into a subcloned homologous sequence or by adding regions of the homologous sequence to a plasmid that already contains the neo and TK genes.

The precise design of the targeting construct is important. The specific structural features of the given gene are relevant to designing a targeting vector, especially if a null allele is sought. On occasion, removal of the initiator ATG or placement of the neomycin-resistance cassette near the 5'- end of the gene may not ablate expression of functional protein from the locus if downstream ATGs are present or alternatively spliced products may be generated. The basic principles of designing a gene-targeting construct based on homologous recombination are the same for knockout and knockin models. The nuances of the design of targeting constructs are beyond the scope of this brief review (*see* **Note 5**; **refs. *13,15***).

3.3.4. Conditional Knockout Construct

The design of a conditional gene-targeting vector requires even more attention than that of a conventional knockout construct ***(14)***. The neomycin resistance gene and recombination sites (e.g., loxP sites) must be placed flanking a critical region of the gene (**Fig. 2**). These elements are generally placed in introns or untranslated regions of the locus so as not to perturb proper expression of the locus. In the gene-targeting vector, three loxP sites are introduced: two flanking the neomycin resistance gene, allowing for selection of the targeted ES-cells, and a third one positioned beyond a critical region of the gene. All three loxP sites must be oriented in the same direction for excision to occur. The neomycin cassette is flanked by loxP sites because it is often desirable to remove the neomycin resistance gene and its promoter by transient Cre expression to ensure minimal interference from external sequences in the function of the gene. The goal is to select for ES cell clones in which the recombination event had occurred only between the loxP sites flanking the neo gene, and where the critical gene sequence remains intact and flanked by two remaining loxP sites.

3.3.5. Cre Mice

Cre mice can be generated by transgenesis or through a knockin strategy. Although the generation of a transgenic mouse may be faster and technically easier, the specificity of transgene expression may be compromised by poorly defined promoter elements or by unexpected expression of a transgene. Knockin of Cre sequences into a locus by homologous recombination ensures more faithful and regulated expression and is generally preferable ***(51)***. However, if the expression level from the locus is low, the extent of deletion may not precisely follow the expression of the endogenous gene ***(47)***. Several tissue specific or inducible Cre mice are available to study the function of conditionally targeted genes at various stages of blood and immune system (**Table 1**; **refs. *21,44–65***).

3.3.6. Knockin Construct

A knockin construct is designed to express novel sequences from the regulatory elements of the locus or to introduce subtle mutations into the endogenous gene, which continues to be expressed by its own promoter. In the first case, to facilitate proper expression of the transgene, the placement of the targeted sequence in the construct is crucial. In the second case, the goal is to modify the endogenous gene by altering specific regions of the genomic clone in the construct by mutagenesis. In both cases it is advisable to flank the selection marker by loxP sites that allow the deletion of unnecessary foreign sequences that could be deleterious for the expression or function of the gene product.

3.3.7. Conditional Knockin Construct

A conditional knockin construct is generated by introducing a loxP flanked 1.3-kb stopper fragment between the promoter and the modified gene/transgene ***(66)***, thus rendering the gene "dormant." The stopper fragment causes premature translation termination, and additionally introduces a false translation initiation site and a 5' splice donor site, thereby ensuring that the gene product is not synthesized. Upon Cre expression, the stopper fragment is deleted and the gene is transcribed and translated.

3.3.8. Manipulation of Mouse ES Cells

Mouse embryonic stem cells used for gene targeting are typically male ES cells derived from a 129 background (e.g., CJ7, J1, and R1), although female ES cells and other strains have also been used ***(71)***. The ES cells are cultured on mouse embryonic fibroblasts, in the presence of leukemia inhibitory factor to maintain pluripotentiality. The gene-targeting construct is electroporated into the ES cells and homologous recombinants are selected in G418 (for neoresistance) and ganciclovir (for absence of TK). Correctly targeted clones are identified by Southern blot or polymerase chain reaction (PCR). In practice, it is advisable to perform karyotypic analysis of clones prior to blastocyst injection. Clones with abnormal karyotypes contribute poorly to the germline of chimeras and should be discarded.

3.3.9. Blastocyst Injection and Generation of Chimeric Mice

Blastocysts are obtained from hormone primed (5 U of pregnant mare's serum i.p. 1 wk prior to ES cell injection followed by 5 U of human chorionic gonadotropin i.p. 48 h later) young (3–4 wk) C57Bl6 females at 3.5 d after coitus. Up to 10 to 12 targeted ES cells are generally injected into single blastocysts, which are then implanted in pseudopregnant (i.e., mated with vasectomized males) C57Bl6 females. Relative contribution of the targeted ES cells in the offspring may be monitored by coat color (e.g., 129 ES cells, agouti; C57Bl6 blastocyst, black). Germline transmission is verified by breeding highly chimeric animals and observing agouti pups. The germline chimeras are expected to be males if male ES cells were used for targeting. Southern blotting or PCR is used to confirm transmission of the targeted allele.

3.4. Optimization the Use of Conditional Knockout Technology

3.4.1. Analysis of Cre Activity and Gene Deletion in Conditionally Targeted Mice

Although conditional gene targeting offers tremendous potential for spatially and/or temporally specific gene manipulation, the interpretation of the phenotypes may be complicated by unexpected expression of Cre recombinase in the Cre mice. Cre expression may be nonspecific because of position effects or limitations in the selected promoter elements. Not uncommonly, the promoter may also be active at an early stage during mouse development, resulting in extensive deletion in multiple tissues. On the other hand, Cre expression may be variegated (or mosaic), resulting in only partial excision in the desired cell type. This may lead to incomplete penetrance of the phenotype. To assess the phenotype, the extent of Cre-mediated excision must be evaluated. This may be accomplished at the DNA level (Southern blot or semiquantitative PCR) by monitoring the excision of the targeted gene, or by use of a reporter allele in the breeding. Although Southern blot is semiquantitative, it requires more DNA than PCR-based assays. A three primer PCR method that amplifies both intact gene-targeted (floxed, fl), deleted (ex) and wild-type alleles in one reaction provides an estimate of excision frequency, but is not strictly quantitative owing to amplification efficiency differences between primer pairs *(48)*. "Reporter" or indicator alleles offer an alternative approach to monitoring Cre-mediated excision, particularly at the single cell level. Indicator mouse strains have been generated by introducing a loxP flanked stopper fragment and a marker gene in a widely expressed locus, e.g., the ROSA26 locus *(72–74)*. Expression of the marker gene such as lacZ, GFP, and enhanced yellow fluorescent protein is activated upon Cre-mediated removal of the stopper fragment and can be monitored by immunohistochemistry or flow cytometry *(44,65,74–76)*. The marker locus is introduced into a conditional knockout background by breeding the conditional, Cre-expressing, and reporter strains. Because the accessibility of targeted loci for Cre-mediated deletion may vary, deletion of the marker gene may not directly reflect deletion in the gene of interest. Furthermore, it is possible that presence of multiple loxP sites in the genome may lead to rare, but unexpected, genetic rearrangements. Alternatively, the reporter gene can be introduced in the locus of the targeted gene *(77)*.

3.4.2. Induction of Gene Deletion in the Adult Hematopoietic System

Advances in conditional gene targeting have facilitated temporal control of gene inactivation, allowing for the first time comparison of gene requirements in embryonic and postnatal hematopoiesis in vivo. The interferon inducible MxCre mouse is particularly effective in inducing conditional gene deletion in the hematopoietic and immune systems in the adult mouse. Hence, it is widely used to study the role of conditionally targeted genes in the adult. The Mx promoter is silent unless activated by interferon, or the interferon inducer poly(I):poly(C) [pIpC]. Some leakiness of Cre expression may be detected, presumably owing to endogenous interferon expression. The inducer is administered intraperitoneally in neonates or adult mice allowing control of timing of the deletion by the investigator. Although protocols to induce the Mx promoter vary between studies, three injections of 250 μg of pIpC to seven injections of 450 μg every other day have been used successfully in adult mice. This results in efficient gene deletion in the hematopoietic and immune system and partial deletion in other tissues, whereas brain tissue remains unexcised ***(21,48,49)***. Because of the requirement for an intact hematopoietic system for the survival of the adult mouse, it is difficult in practice to maintain 100% gene deletion in the BM with genes that are essential for adult hematopoiesis. Not uncommonly, an initially strong hematopoietic phenotype may disappear after a few weeks as repopulation of the hematopoietic system by rare unexcised hematopoietic stem cells can occur. Incomplete excision complicates the evaluation of the phenotype. The strong selection pressure for rare unexcised hematopoietic stem cells may be circumvented by generation of mice with chimeric BM by transplantation ***(48)*** Here, gene-targeted BM and support/competitor BM that can be distinguished by cell surface markers and/or DNA analyses are transplanted into irradiated recipients. The support BM ensures the production of all blood cell lineages and survival of the mouse and thus obviates the pressure to expand rare unexcised progenitors or HSCs from gene-targeted BM. CD45 alleles can be used to distinguish between the gene targeted hematopoietic cells, support cells and host cells. Gene-targeted mice from the 129/C57bl6 background express the CD45.2 allele on the surface of all nucleated hematopoietic cells. Congenic C57Bl6.sjl mice that express the CD45.1 allele may be used as a competitor (and/or recipients), and an F1 heterozygote (CD45.1/CD45.2) from C57bl6.sjl and C57bl6 intercross or C57bl6.sjl and 129 intercross as recipients. Although 129 and C57bl6 express the same CD45 allele and allow transplantation without major immunological mismatch, if other mouse strains are used, the expression of correct CD45 alleles and MHC molecules has to be verified ***(78)***.

Analysis of CD45 alleles on the surface of hematopoietic cells facilitates detection and purification of each BM population in different hematopoietic organs and cell types by flow cytometry. Thus the kinetics of development or disappearance of cells lacking the gene of interest can be addressed reliably. By using BM containing the inducible MxCre transgene, multiple recipients with the same BM composition may be generated. After the induction of gene deletion in a subgroup of the mice, the role of the particular gene can be addressed in a controlled fashion.

Another advantage of using BM transplantation prior to induction of gene excision is the ability to isolate the hematopoietic compartment from other tissues and restrict the deletion or modification of the gene in the hematopoietic system. This may be useful in studying the function of a widely expressed gene specifically within the hematopoietic system. Likewise, it is possible to bypass a strong hematopoietic phenotype by rescuing conditional knockout animals by transplantation of wild type BM cells prior to induction, thereby allowing phenotypic analysis of the gene function in other organ systems.

4. Notes

1. An alternative means for circumventing or delaying embryonic lethality in knockout embryos relies on lineage restricted transgene rescue ***(79,80)***. The knockout strain is bred with a transgenic mouse that expresses the gene of interest (or another gene that rescues the pathway) in a particular manner. Use of a tissue-specific promoter may lead to rescue of the knockout phenotype in a subset of cells/tissues.

2. A complementary in vitro approach to study the developmental potential of the targeted ES cells is to use ES cell in vitro differentiation *(81,82)*.
3. Transgenic construct may alternatively be introduced into mouse ES cells by electroporation and stable transformants then injected into blastocysts, from which mouse chimeras are generated (**Fig. 1B**).
4. Another way to introduce transgenes into ES cells or preimplantation embryos and produce transgenic mice is to use transduction by lentiviral vectors (**Fig. 1B**). The power of lentiviral transgenesis relies on efficient transduction and ability to sustain stable, tissue specific transgene expression from internal promoters through development *(83,84)*.
5. A possible alternative to obtaining a targeted ES cell line is the "gene trap" technology (**Fig. 1B**, **refs.** *72,85*). Gene trap is based on random integration of a retroviral vector with a positive selection marker into the ES cell genome. The selection marker is expressed only if it integrates into a locus that is active in ES cells and thus facilitates the recovery of a targeted ES cell line. Several gene trap libraries containing a large set of targeted genes are available (e.g., tikus.gsf.de and baygenomic.ucsf.edu). Each gene trap clone needs to be analyzed individually to determine the effect of the integration of foreign sequences on gene expression. Sometimes, a null allele is generated in the gene trap. Often, a hypomorphic mutation is created. Both may be useful for functional studies.
6. Cre recombinase can be also introduced into hematopoietic cells by viral transduction whereafter the phenotype of the modified hematopoietic cells may be studied by in vitro assays, or in vivo after BM transplantation *(86)*.

References

1. Palis, J., Robertson, S., Kennedy, M., Wall, C., and Keller, G. (1999) Development of erythroid and myeloid progenitors in the yolk sac and embryo proper of the mouse. *Development* **126,** 5073–5084.
2. Medvinsky, A. and Dzierzak, E. (1996) Definitive hematopoiesis is autonomously initiated by the AGM region. *Cell* **86,** 897–906.
3. Muller, A. M., Medvinsky, A., Strouboulis, J., Grosveld, F., and Dzierzak, E. (1994) Development of hematopoietic stem cell activity in the mouse embryo. *Immunity* **1,** 291–301.
4. Shivdasani, R. A., Mayer, E. L., and Orkin, S. H. (1995) Absence of blood formation in mice lacking the T-cell leukaemia oncoprotein tal-1/SCL. *Nature* **373,** 432–434.
5. Robb, L., Elwood, N. J., Elefanty, A. G., Kontgen, F., Li, R., Barnett, L. D., and Begley, C. G. (1996) The scl gene product is required for the generation of all hematopoietic lineages in the adult mouse. *EMBO J.* **15,** 4123–4129.
6. Fujiwara, Y., Browne, C. P., Cunniff, K., Goff, S. C., and Orkin, S. H. (1996) Arrested development of embryonic red cell precursors in mouse embryos lacking transcription factor GATA-1. *Proc. Natl. Acad. Sci. USA* **93,** 12,355–12,358.
7. Wang, Q., Stacy, T., Binder, M., Marin-Padilla, M., Sharpe, A. H., and Speck, N. A. (1996) Disruption of the Cbfa2 gene causes necrosis and hemorrhaging in the central nervous system and blocks definitive hematopoiesis. *Proc. Natl. Acad. Sci. USA* **93,** 3444–3449.
8. Okuda, T., van Deursen, J., Hiebert, S. W., Grosveld, G., and Downing, J. R. (1996) AML1, the target of multiple chromosomal translocations in human leukemia, is essential for normal fetal liver hematopoiesis. *Cell* **84,** 321–330.
9. Dickson, M. C., Martin, J. S., Cousins, F. M., Kulkarni, A. B., Karlsson, S., and Akhurst, R. J. (1995) Defective haematopoiesis and vasculogenesis in transforming growth factor-beta 1 knockout mice. *Development* **121,** 1845–1854.

10. Oshima, M., Oshima, H., and Taketo, M. M. (1996) TGF-beta receptor type II deficiency results in defects of yolk sac hematopoiesis and vasculogenesis. *Dev. Biol.* **179,** 297–302.
11. Wang, L. C., Kuo, F., Fujiwara, Y., Gilliland, D. G., Golub, T. R., and Orkin, S. H. (1997) Yolk sac angiogenic defect and intra-embryonic apoptosis in mice lacking the Ets-related factor TEL. *EMBO J.* **16,** 4374–4383.
12. Hammess, A. and Schedl, A. (2000) Generation of transgenic mice from plasmids, BACs and YACs, in *Mouse Genetics and Transgenics* (Jackson, I. J. and Abbott, C. M., eds.), Oxford University Press Inc., New York.
13. Plagge, A., Kelsey, G., and Allen, N. (2000) Direct mutagenesis in embryonic stem cells, in *Mouse Genetics and Transgenics* (Jackson, I. J., and Abbott, C. M., eds.), Oxford University Press Inc., New York.
14. Torres, R. M. and Sauer, B. (1997) *Laboratory Protocols for Conditional Gene Targeting.* Oxford University Press, New York.
15. Conner, D. A. (2000) Manipulating the mouse genome, in *Current Protocols in Molecular Biology* (Ausubel, F. M., Brent, R., Kingston, R. E., Moore, D. D., Seidman, J. G., Smith, J. A., and Struhl, K., eds.), John Wiley & Sons, New York.
16. Gossen, M. and Bujard, H. (1992) Tight control of gene expression in mammalian cells by tetracycline-responsive promoters. *Proc. Natl. Acad. Sci. USA* **89,** 5547–5551.
17. Furth, P. A., St Onge, L., Boger, H., Gruss, P., Gossen, M., Kistner, A., et al. (1994) Temporal control of gene expression in transgenic mice by a tetracycline-responsive promoter. *Proc. Natl. Acad. Sci. USA* **91,** 9302–9306.
18. Schonig, K., Schwenk, F., Rajewsky, K., and Bujard, H. (2002) Stringent doxycycline dependent control of CRE recombinase in vivo. *Nucleic Acids Res.* **30,** e134.
19. Kistner, A., Gossen, M., Zimmermann, F., Jerecic, J., Ullmer, C., Lubbert, H., et al. (1996) Doxycycline-mediated quantitative and tissue-specific control of gene expression in transgenic mice. *Proc. Natl. Acad. Sci. USA* **93,** 10,933–10,938.
20. St-Onge, L., Furth, P. A., and Gruss, P. (1996) Temporal control of the Cre recombinase in transgenic mice by a tetracycline responsive promoter. *Nucleic Acids Res.* **24,** 3875–3877.
21. Kuhn, R., Schwenk, F., Aguet, M., and Rajewsky, K. (1995) Inducible gene targeting in mice. *Science* **269,** 1427–1429.
22. Feil, R., Brocard, J., Mascrez, B., LeMeur, M., Metzger, D., and Chambon, P. (1996) Ligand-activated site-specific recombination in mice. *Proc. Natl. Acad. Sci. USA* **93,** 10,887–10,890.
23. Brocard, J., Warot, X., Wendling, O., Messaddeq, N., Vonesch, J. L., Chambon, P., et al. (1997) Spatio-temporally controlled site-specific somatic mutagenesis in the mouse. *Proc. Natl. Acad. Sci. USA* **94,** 14,559–14,563.
24. Brocard, J., Feil, R., Chambon, P., and Metzger, D. (1998) A chimeric Cre recombinase inducible by synthetic, but not by natural ligands of the glucocorticoid receptor. *Nucleic Acids Res.* **26,** 4086–4090.
25. Zheng, B., Zhang, Z., Black, C. M., de Crombrugghe, B., and Denton, C. P. (2002) Ligand-dependent genetic recombination in fibroblasts : a potentially powerful technique for investigating gene function in fibrosis. *Am. J. Pathol.* **160,** 1609–1617.
26. Mansour, S. L., Thomas, K. R., Deng, C. X., and Capecchi, M. R. (1990) Introduction of a lacZ reporter gene into the mouse int-2 locus by homologous recombination. *Proc. Natl. Acad. Sci. USA* **87,** 7688–7692.
27. Elefanty, A. G., Begley, C. G., Metcalf, D., Barnett, L., Kontgen, F., and Robb, L. (1998) Characterization of hematopoietic progenitor cells that express the transcription factor SCL, using a lacZ "knockin" strategy. *Proc. Natl. Acad. Sci. USA* **95,** 11,897–11,902.

28. Elefanty, A. G., Begley, C. G., Hartley, L., Papaevangeliou, B., and Robb, L. (1999) SCL expression in the mouse embryo detected with a targeted lacZ reporter gene demonstrates its localization to hematopoietic, vascular, and neural tissues. *Blood* **94,** 3754–3763.
29. North, T. E., de Bruijn, M. F., Stacy, T., Talebian, L., Lind, E., Robin, C., et al. (2002) Runx1 expression marks long-term repopulating hematopoietic stem cells in the midgestation mouse embryo. *Immunity* **16,** 661–672.
30. de Bruijn, M. F., Ma, X., Robin, C., Ottersbach, K., Sanchez, M. J., and Dzierzak, E. (2002) Hematopoietic stem cells localize to the endothelial cell layer in the midgestation mouse aorta. *Immunity* **16,** 673–683.
31. Chung, Y. S., Zhang, W. J., Arentson, E., Kingsley, P. D., Palis, J., and Choi, K. (2002) Lineage analysis of the hemangioblast as defined by FLK1 and SCL expression. *Development* **129,** 5511–5520.
32. Crispino, J. D., Lodish, M. B., Thurberg, B. L., Litovsky, S. H., Collins, T., Molkentin, J. D., et al. (2001) Proper coronary vascular development and heart morphogenesis depend on interaction of GATA-4 with FOG cofactors. *Genes Dev.* **15,** 839–844.
33. Chang, A. N., Cantor, A. B., Fujiwara, Y., Lodish, M. B., Droho, S., Crispino, J. D., et al. (2002) GATA-factor dependence of the multitype zinc-finger protein FOG-1 for its essential role in megakaryopoiesis. *Proc. Natl. Acad. Sci. USA* **99,** 9237–9242.
34. McDevitt, M. A., Shivdasani, R. A., Fujiwara, Y., Yang, H., and Orkin, S. H. (1997) A "knockdown" mutation created by cis-element gene targeting reveals the dependence of erythroid cell maturation on the level of transcription factor GATA-1. *Proc. Natl. Acad. Sci. USA* **94,** 6781–6785.
35. Mortensen, R. M., Conner, D. A., Chao, S., Geisterfer-Lowrance, A. A., and Seidman, J. G. (1992) Production of homozygous mutant ES cells with a single targeting construct. *Mol. Cell Biol.* **12,** 2391–2395.
36. Pevny, L., Simon, M. C., Robertson, E., Klein, W. H., Tsai, S. F., D'Agati, V., et al. (1991) Erythroid differentiation in chimaeric mice blocked by a targeted mutation in the gene for transcription factor GATA-1. *Nature* **349,** 257–260.
37. Pevny, L., Lin, C. S., D'Agati, V., Simon, M. C., Orkin, S. H., and Costantini, F. (1995) Development of hematopoietic cells lacking transcription factor GATA-1. *Development* **121,** 163–172.
38. Porcher, C., Swat, W., Rockwell, K., Fujiwara, Y., Alt, F. W., and Orkin, S. H. (1996) The T cell leukemia oncoprotein SCL/tal-1 is essential for development of all hematopoietic lineages. *Cell* **86,** 47–57.
39. Saleque, S., Cameron, S., and Orkin, S. H. (2002) The zinc-finger proto-oncogene Gfi-1b is essential for development of the erythroid and megakaryocytic lineages. *Genes Dev.* **16,** 301–306.
40. Gu, H., Marth, J. D., Orban, P. C., Mossmann, H., and Rajewsky, K. (1994) Deletion of a DNA polymerase beta gene segment in T cells using cell type-specific gene targeting. *Science* **265,** 103–106.
41. Fiering, S., Kim, C. G., Epner, E. M., and Groudine, M. (1993) An "in-out" strategy using gene targeting and FLP recombinase for the functional dissection of complex DNA regulatory elements: analysis of the beta-globin locus control region. *Proc. Natl. Acad. Sci. USA* **90,** 8469–8473.
42. Dymecki, S. M., and Tomasiewicz, H. (1998) Using Flp-recombinase to characterize expansion of Wnt1-expressing neural progenitors in the mouse. *Dev. Biol.* **201,** 57–65.
43. Vooijs, M., van der Valk, M., te Riele, H., and Berns, A. (1998) Flp-mediated tissue-specific inactivation of the retinoblastoma tumor suppressor gene in the mouse. *Oncogene* **17,** 1–12.

44. Mao, X., Fujiwara, Y., and Orkin, S. H. (1999) Improved reporter strain for monitoring Cre recombinase-mediated DNA excisions in mice. *Proc. Natl. Acad. Sci. USA* **96,** 5037–5042.
45. Jasinski, M., Keller, P., Fujiwara, Y., Orkin, S. H., and Bessler, M. (2001) GATA1-Cre mediates Piga gene inactivation in the erythroid/megakaryocytic lineage and leads to circulating red cells with a partial deficiency in glycosyl phosphatidylinositol-linked proteins (paroxysmal nocturnal hemoglobinuria type II cells) *Blood* **98,** 2248–2255.
46. Gustafsson, E., Brakebusch, C., Hietanen, K., and Fassler, R. (2001) Tie-1-directed expression of Cre recombinase in endothelial cells of embryoid bodies and transgenic mice. *J. Cell Sci.* **114,** 671–676.
47. Emambokus, N. R. and Frampton, J. (2003) The glycoprotein IIb molecule is expressed on early murine hematopoietic progenitors and regulates their numbers in sites of hematopoiesis. *Immunity* **19,** 33–45.
48. Mikkola, H. K., Klintman, J., Yang, H., Hock, H., Schlaeger, T. M., Fujiwara, Y., et al. (2003) Haematopoietic stem cells retain long-term repopulating activity and multipotency in the absence of stem-cell leukaemia SCL/tal-1 gene. *Nature* **421,** 547–551.
49. Roberts, C. W., Leroux, M. M., Fleming, M. D., and Orkin, S. H. (2002) Highly penetrant, rapid tumorigenesis through conditional inversion of the tumor suppressor gene Snf5. *Cancer Cell* **2,** 415–425.
50. Han, H., Tanigaki, K., Yamamoto, N., Kuroda, K., Yoshimoto, M., Nakahata, T., et al. (2002) Inducible gene knockout of transcription factor recombination signal binding protein-J reveals its essential role in T versus B lineage decision. *Int. Immunol.* **14,** 637–645.
51. Rickert, R. C., Roes, J., and Rajewsky, K. (1997) B lymphocyte-specific, Cre-mediated mutagenesis in mice. *Nucleic Acids Res.* **25,** 1317–1318.
52. Georgiades, P., Ogilvy, S., Duval, H., Licence, D. R., Charnock-Jones, D. S., Smith, S. K., et al. (2002) vavCre transgenic mice: a tool for mutagenesis in hematopoietic and endothelial lineages. *Genesis* **34,** 251–256.
53. Forde, A., Constien, R., Grone, H. J., Hammerling, G., and Arnold, B. (2002) Temporal Cre-mediated recombination exclusively in endothelial cells using Tie2 regulatory elements. *Genesis* **33,** 191–197.
54. Kisanuki, Y. Y., Hammer, R. E., Miyazaki, J., Williams, S. C., Richardson, J. A., and Yanagisawa, M. (2001) Tie2-Cre transgenic mice: a new model for endothelial cell-lineage analysis in vivo. *Dev. Biol.* **230,** 230–242.
55. Horcher, M., Souabni, A., and Busslinger, M. (2001) Pax5/BSAP maintains the identity of B cells in late B lymphopoiesis. *Immunity* **14,** 779–790.
56. Wilson, T. J., Cowdery, H. E., Xu, D., Kola, I., and Hertzog, P. J. (2002) A human CD2 minigene directs CRE-mediated recombination in T cells in vivo. *Genesis* **33,** 181–184.
57. Cheung, A. M., Hande, M. P., Jalali, F., Tsao, M. S., Skinnider, B., Hirao, A., et al. (2002) Loss of Brca2 and p53 synergistically promotes genomic instability and deregulation of T-cell apoptosis. *Cancer Res.* **62,** 6194–6204.
58. Takeda, K., Kaisho, T., Yoshida, N., Takeda, J., Kishimoto, T., and Akira, S. (1998) Stat3 activation is responsible for IL-6-dependent T cell proliferation through preventing apoptosis: generation and characterization of T cell-specific Stat3-deficient mice. *J. Immunol.* **161,** 4652–4660.
59. Takahama, Y., Ohishi, K., Tokoro, Y., Sugawara, T., Yoshimura, Y., Okabe, M., et al. (1998) Functional competence of T cells in the absence of glycosylphosphatidylinositol-anchored proteins caused by T cell-specific disruption of the Pig-a gene. *Eur. J. Immunol.* **28,** 2159–2166.

60. Hennet, T., Hagen, F. K., Tabak, L. A., and Marth, J. D. (1995) T-cell-specific deletion of a polypeptide N-acetylgalactosaminyl-transferase gene by site-directed recombination. *Proc. Natl. Acad. Sci. USA* **92,** 12,070–12,074.
61. Wagner, K. U., Wall, R. J., St-Onge, L., Gruss, P., Wynshaw-Boris, A., Garrett, L., et al. (1997) Cre-mediated gene deletion in the mammary gland. *Nucleic Acids Res.* **25,** 4323–4330.
62. Wagner, K. U., Claudio, E., Rucker, E. B., 3rd, Riedlinger, G., Broussard, C., Schwartzberg, P. L., et al. (2000) Conditional deletion of the Bcl-x gene from erythroid cells results in hemolytic anemia and profound splenomegaly. *Development* **127,** 4949–4958.
63. Clausen, B. E., Burkhardt, C., Reith, W., Renkawitz, R., and Forster, I. (1999) Conditional gene targeting in macrophages and granulocytes using LysMcre mice. *Transgenic Res.* **8,** 265–277.
64. Schwenk, F., Kuhn, R., Angrand, P. O., Rajewsky, K., and Stewart, A. F. (1998) Temporally and spatially regulated somatic mutagenesis in mice. *Nucleic Acids Res.* **26,** 1427–1432.
65. de Boer, J., Williams, A., Skavdis, G., Harker, N., Coles, M., Tolaini, M., et al. (2003) Transgenic mice with hematopoietic and lymphoid specific expression of Cre. *Eur. J. Immunol.* **33,** 314–325.
66. Lakso, M., Saucr, B., Mosinger, B., Jr., Lee, E. J., Manning, R. W., Yu, S. H., et al. (1992) Targeted oncogene activation by site-specific recombination in transgenic mice. *Proc. Natl. Acad. Sci. USA* **89,** 6232–6236.
67. Higuchi, M., O'Brien, D., Kumaravelu, P., Lenny, N., Yeoh, E. J., and Downing, J. R. (2002) Expression of a conditional AML1-ETO oncogene bypasses embryonic lethality and establishes a murine model of human t(8;21) acute myeloid leukemia. *Cancer Cell* **1,** 63–74.
68. Lam, K. P., Kuhn, R., and Rajewsky, K. (1997) In vivo ablation of surface immunoglobulin on mature B cells by inducible gene targeting results in rapid cell death. *Cell* **90,** 1073–1083.
69. Capecchi, M. R. (1980) High efficiency transformation by direct microinjection of DNA into cultured mammalian cells. *Cell* **22,** 479–488.
70. Mansour, S. L., Thomas, K. R., and Capecchi, M. R. (1988) Disruption of the proto-oncogene int-2 in mouse embryo-derived stem cells: a general strategy for targeting mutations to non-selectable genes. *Nature* **336,** 348–452.
71. Auerbach, W., Dunmore, J. H., Fairchild-Huntress, V., Fang, Q., Auerbach, A. B., Huszar, D., et al. (2000) Establishment and chimera analysis of 129/SvEv- and C57BL/6-derived mouse embryonic stem cell lines. *Biotechniques* **29,** 1024–1028, 1030, 1032.
72. Friedrich, G., and Soriano, P. (1991) Promoter traps in embryonic stem cells: a genetic screen to identify and mutate developmental genes in mice. *Genes Dev.* **5,** 1513–1523.
73. Zambrowicz, B. P., Imamoto, A., Fiering, S., Herzenberg, L. A., Kerr, W. G., and Soriano, P. (1997) Disruption of overlapping transcripts in the ROSA beta geo 26 gene trap strain leads to widespread expression of beta-galactosidase in mouse embryos and hematopoietic cells. *Proc. Natl. Acad. Sci. USA* **94,** 3789–3794.
74. Soriano, P. (1999) Generalized lacZ expression with the ROSA26 Cre reporter strain. *Nat. Genet.* **21,** 70–71.
75. Mao, X., Fujiwara, Y., Chapdelaine, A., Yang, H., and Orkin, S. H. (2001) Activation of EGFP expression by Cre-mediated excision in a new ROSA26 reporter mouse strain. *Blood* **97,** 324–326.
76. Constien, R., Forde, A., Liliensiek, B., Grone, H. J., Nawroth, P., Hammerling, G., et al. (2001) Characterization of a novel EGFP reporter mouse to monitor Cre recombination as demonstrated by a Tie2 Cre mouse line. *Genesis* **30,** 36–44.

77. Theis, M., de Wit, C., Schlaeger, T. M., Eckardt, D., Kruger, O., Doring, B., et al. (2001) Endothelium-specific replacement of the connexin43 coding region by a lacZ reporter gene. *Genesis* **29,** 1–13.
78. Hashimoto, F., Sugiura, K., Inoue, K., and Ikehara, S. (1997) Major histocompatibility complex restriction between hematopoietic stem cells and stromal cells in vivo. *Blood* **89,** 49–54.
79. Visvader, J. E., Fujiwara, Y., and Orkin, S. H. (1998) Unsuspected role for the T-cell leukemia protein SCL/tal-1 in vascular development. *Genes Dev.* **12,** 473–479.
80. Sanchez, M. J., Bockamp, E. O., Miller, J., Gambardella, L., and Green, A. R. (2001) Selective rescue of early haematopoietic progenitors in Scl(-/-) mice by expressing Scl under the control of a stem cell enhancer. *Development* **128,** 4815–4827.
81. Wiles, M. V. and Keller, G. (1991) Multiple hematopoietic lineages develop from embryonic stem (ES) cells in culture. *Development* **111,** 259–267.
82. Weiss, M. J., Keller, G., and Orkin, S. H. (1994) Novel insights into erythroid development revealed through in vitro differentiation of GATA-1 embryonic stem cells. *Genes Dev.* **8,** 1184–1197.
83. Lois, C., Hong, E. J., Pease, S., Brown, E. J., and Baltimore, D. (2002) Germline transmission and tissue-specific expression of transgenes delivered by lentiviral vectors. *Science* **295,** 868–872.
84. Pfeifer, A., Ikawa, M., Dayn, Y., and Verma, I. M. (2002) Transgenesis by lentiviral vectors: lack of gene silencing in mammalian embryonic stem cells and preimplantation embryos. *Proc. Natl. Acad. Sci. USA* **99,** 2140–2145.
85. Friedrich, G. and Soriano, P. (1993) Insertional mutagenesis by retroviruses and promoter traps in embryonic stem cells. *Methods Enzymol.* **225,** 681–701.
86. Potocnik, A. J., Brakebusch, C., and Fassler, R. (2000) Fetal and adult hematopoietic stem cells require beta1 integrin function for colonizing fetal liver, spleen, and bone marrow. *Immunity* **12,** 653–663.

2

Inducible Transgene Expression in Mouse Stem Cells

David T. Ting, Michael Kyba, and George Q. Daley

Summary

Embryonic stem (ES) cells serve as a potentially unlimited source of cells and tissues to treat a number of genetic and malignant diseases. The differentiation of these cells into specific cell types is an area of very active investigation. One method of manipulating ES cell differentiation is through the alteration of gene expression. There are a multitude of different methods for expressing a target gene in ES cells, but most are limited in their ability to provide spatial, temporal, and quantitative control of gene expression. These properties are important because many developmentally interesting genes are regulated in at least one of these ways. This chapter will address these limitations through the use of an ES cell line with a doxycycline-inducible transgene system. A characterization of this inducible transgene system will be discussed, as well as the use of this system to develop ES-derived long-term engrafting hematopoietic stem cells. This demonstration is one of many possible uses for this powerful and versatile system.

Key Words: Embryonic stem (ES) cell; genetic modification; inducible transgene; tet operon; rtTA; hematopoiesis.

1. Introduction

1.1. ES Cells as Research Tool and Potential Therapy

Since their identification and isolation in 1981 by Evans and Kaufman *(1)* and Martin *(2)*, there have been major advances in genetically modifying ES cells, allowing for the ability to manipulate cellular processes involved in embryonic development. These innovations not only provide for a very powerful research tool to study development but also the capability to develop cellular therapies for a myriad of diseases. The key to unlocking the potential of ES cells is the ability to control the development of these cells into the desired cell or tissue type. The most popular strategies to control ES cell fate are to manipulate culture conditions or to alter gene expression. The former is accomplished with variations in exogenous factors, including cytokines,

From: *Methods in Molecular Medicine, Vol. 105: Developmental Hematopoiesis: Methods and Protocols.*
Edited by: M. H. Baron © Humana Press Inc., Totowa, NJ

media, serum, or growth in different spatial organizations, such as through embryoid body (EB) formation. The latter can be done through a combination of different gene transfer modalities, including viral vectors, homologous recombination, and/or recombinase-based approaches. This chapter will discuss the development of a doxycycline-dependent inducible gene expression system using a combination of targeted homologous recombination and Cre-lox recombinase techniques. We will also discuss the use of this inducible expression system in the context of generating and propagating long-term engrafting hematopoietic stem cells (HSCs) from ES cells.

1.2. Comparison of Different Gene Expression Systems

There have been a number of different approaches developed for expressing a desired gene of interest in ES cells. One of the most common and easiest approaches for transferring a gene is through viral vector systems. The first genetic modifications of ES cells were done with retroviruses ***(3,4)***. Recombinant retroviruses integrate into the ES cell genome, making a provirus that is able to express the gene of interest in cells derived from these cells; however, upon further development and differentiation, proviruses are often found to be silenced through two major mechanisms: 1) methylation of the provirus genome, and 2) transacting repressive factors that bind to the long terminal repeats of the viral promoter ***(5)***. There are a number of groups who have attempted, with varying degrees of success, to develop modified retroviruses ***(6–8)*** and lentiviruses ***(9–13)*** to circumvent the issue of gene silencing.

Another limitation of using retroviruses is the inability to effectively control the quantitative, spatial, and/or temporal expression of the gene of interest. There have been several viral systems that have been developed to control gene expression with the addition of a chemical inducer. One inducible system developed by Jin and Blau uses the F36V mutant of FK506-binding protein's (FKBP's) dimerization domain fused to the cytoplasmic domain of c-Mpl, which in the presence of AP20187 causes dimerization of the fusion protein and activation of c-Mpl ***(14,15)***. Other groups have incorporated the more frequently used tetracycline inducible system in their retroviral constructs, as will be discussed in more detail ***(10,13,16)***.

An alternative to viral gene transfer in ES cells emerged when the constitutively active *hprt* locus was targeted through homologous recombination in 1987 by Doetschman et al. ***(17)*** and Thomas and Capecchi ***(18)***. Further refinements were later made to target nonselectable genes by Mansour et al. ***(19)*** and Schwartzberg et al. ***(20)***. These discoveries revolutionized ES cell genetic manipulation and allowed the generation of numerous transgenic and knockout ES cell lines and mice. Despite its tremendous utility, homologous recombination is a relatively inefficient method and is burdensome when trying to retarget a given locus with different gene insertions. Strategies to improve the latter include the "hit and run" ***(21–23)***, "tag and exchange" ***(24,25)***, and "plug and socket" ***(26)*** protocols, but they are all constrained by the inefficiency of homologous recombination. The discovery of the Cre-lox recombinase system solved this problem of inefficient gene insertion and allowed for effective retargeting of a specified locus ***(27–30)***. The combination of homologous recombination and the Cre-lox system provides a reliable and flexible gene transfer method.

Although this method is more labor intensive and less efficient than viral transduction modalities, there are a couple of key advantages to this system. The first advantage is that homologous recombination can be targeted to a precise locus allowing for control of the gene of interest by an endogenous gene regulatory system. Targeting a tissue specific gene regulatory system allows spatial and temporal control of gene expression. The second advantage is the ability to target the inducible locus to a location that has a lower propensity for silencing.

The latest advance in ES gene expression systems has been the ability to control expression with an exogenously added factor. This has been coupled to the Cre-lox recombination system to generate conditional knockouts and knockins. In the case of the conditional knockout system, a target gene is engineered with flanking loxP sites, and upon Cre-recombinase expression, the gene of interest is excised. A conditional knockin involves the elimination of an artificial stop codon placed in the gene of interest using the same strategy resulting in target gene expression. Both of these systems have been recently modified to allow for control of Cre-mediated recombination by a steroid exogenous factor such as tamoxifen ***(31–42)***. The system works by expressing a fusion protein of Cre and a mutated ligand-binding domain of the estrogen receptor [ER(T)] This fusion protein is retained in the cytoplasm because of the ER(T), but migrates into the nucleus when the exogenous factor tamoxifen is added and binds ER(T). Once in the nucleus, Cre can then mediate excision of the loxP-targeted site. This system allows for both spatial and temporal control of gene expression, but it lacks quantitative control and reversibility. However, this system has less background activity than other inducible systems and can exert a complete knockout of gene expression.

A more common inducible system employed in ES cells uses the *Escherichia coli* tetracycline resistance operon. This system uses the binding affinity of the tetracycline repressor protein (TetR) to its operon (TetO) to deliver a transcription activator to drive the expression of a target gene. The first system developed involved the fusion of the C-terminal portion of the herpes simplex virus transcription activator VP16 to TetR to make the tetracycline transactivator (tTA), which in the presence of doxycycline releases the fusion protein from its target and turns off gene expression ***(43)***. The same group later created a VP16 fusion with a mutated TetR that bound TetO in the presence of doxycycline, which stimulated expression of a target gene ***(44)***. This VP16-mutated TetR fusion was named the reverse tetracycline transactivator (rtTA; *see* **Note 1**). These systems have proven useful in controlling gene expression in eukaryotic cells in vitro ***(43–48)*** as well as in transgenic mice in vivo ***(49–52)***. Although there is some background activity in this system, the level of expression can be accurately titrated in a reversible fashion. These properties of the doxycycline inducible system were most suitable for our applications in hematopoiesis. We will demonstrate how we developed and used the doxycycline inducible gene expression system in the context of generating ES-derived hemotopoietic stem cells (HSCs).

1.3. Implications of Inducible Transgene Expression in the Development of HSCs

There have been various studies on the effect of diminished or eliminated expression of a specific gene on the development of HSCs using gene knockout and/or conditional knockout systems ***(39,53–60)***. However, the use of an inducible system to understand the effects of a specified gene's expression on developmental hematopoiesis has not been extensively used. Era and Witte used the tet-off system to study the effect of Bcr-Abl on hematopoietic differentiation of ES cells ***(48)***. The tTA- and Tet-responsive Bcr-Abl were not targeted to a particular gene, but stable integrants were obtained using successive rounds of clone selection. In this system, Bcr-Abl drove proliferation of multipotent cells and myeloid progenitors while suppressing erythroid progenitor development. This effect was reversed when Bcr-Abl expression was stopped with the addition of doxycycline. A distinct tet-inducible transgene system in ES cells was designed by Niwa et al. to investigate the POU transcription factor Oct-3/4 ***(47)***. In this study, an ES cell line named ZHTc6 was created from CGR8 ES cells using random integration of both the tTA and the inducible transgene constructs. Doxycycline repressed Oct-3/4 expression within 24 h. After 48 h in the absence of doxycycline, Oct-3/4 expression reached approx 50% higher levels than wild-type ES cells. Experiments performed with this ES cell line showed that a defined range of Oct-3/4 expression regulated the pluripotent or trophoblastic fate of ES cells. In another set of experiments, the same ES cell line was modified with a super-targeting vector to replace Oct-3/4 with STAT3F, a dominant interfering mutant of the transcription factor signal transducer and activator of transcription (STAT)3 ***(46)***. STAT3 was shown to be necessary for ES cell self-renewal, which was inhibited by STAT3F expression. An inducible system was necessary for this study because constitutive expression of STAT3F precluded the isolation of a viable ES cell.

Our system differs from the previous two examples in three ways. First, we have targeted the transactivator and the inducible tet operator into loci that have previously been shown to be favorable transgene expression sites. This bypasses the problem of silencing and allows us to maintain a homogenous population of cells with consistent properties. Furthermore, because the targeted sites are known, they can be easily retargeted if the system requires modifications. Second, we use the rtTA instead of the tTA, which allows us to drive gene expression by adding doxycycline, (so called "dox-on") The "dox-on" system offers the advantages of controlling the timing and amount of target gene expression and avoids the potential adverse effects of a constitutively active transgene and/or the toxic effect of continuous doxycycline administration to suppress gene expression. Third, we use a lox-in strategy that affords us the ability to easily and efficiently insert any gene of interest into the inducible locus rather than requiring the inefficient retargeting of a site by homologous recombination.

We have found that the inducible system provided some fortuitous advantages in our attempts to develop long-term engrafting HSCs using HoxB4 as our transgene ***(61)***. HoxB4 was selected because it had previously been shown that several homeobox (Hox) genes were expressed in definitive HSCs and not in the nonrepopulating hematopoietic progenitors found in the yolk sac of developing embryos ***(62,63)***. In our system, the timing of HoxB4 expression during a critical window was important for developing definitive HSCs in vitro. Interestingly, experiments showed that continued expression of HoxB4 was not necessary after bone marrow engraftment of these cells in vivo. This avoids the need for continuous doxycycline administration to animals, which prevents the possible in vivo adverse effects of doxycycline, constitutive expression of HoxB4, and/or constant high levels of activated transactivator. In addition to enabling us to model blood transplantation from ES cells, manipulation of HoxB4 suggests it can trigger a cell fate switch from primitive to definitive hematopoietic potential.

In addition to HoxB4, we are also investigating whether the regulated expression of other genes, including Stat5 and SCL/tal-1, in this system will enhance the development of definitive HSCs from ES cells. Stat5 is a signal transducer that has been shown to be important in hematopoiesis by various groups ***(64–71)*** and was particularly interesting to us because of its implication as a downstream effector in the transforming ability of Bcr-Abl ***(72–77)***. These properties made it an attractive target for inducible expression to provide nononcogenic proliferation of ES-derived HSCs. SCL/tal-1 expression was chosen because it has been shown to be important in early hematopoiesis by a number of groups in a variety of species ***(39,54,55,78–88)***. Furthermore, using a tamoxifen-inducible Cre-lox knockin system, SCL/tal-1 has been shown to be critical before d 4 of ES differentiation into hematopoietic cells on OP9 ***(39)***. Another group has recently shown that SCL/tal-1 is essential for the generation of HSCs and differentiation of erythroid and megakaryocytic precursors, but dispensable for certain HSC functions including self-renewal and bone marrow engraftment ***(58)***. The demonstrated importance of the temporal aspects of SCL/tal-1 expression made it an appropriate gene for investigation using our inducible system. These examples delineate the versatility and power of this inducible system to provide important insights into the genetic regulation of hematopoietic development and to advance experimental models of cell transplantation therapies.

2. Materials

2.1. Generation of ES Cell Lines With Inducible Transgene Expression From Ainv15 Targeting Cells

1. Standard deoxyribonucleic acid (DNA) restriction enzyme and ligation kits.
2. Targeting plasmid with loxP site in between the Pgk1 promoter-ATG and the gene of interest (*see* **Note 2**).
3. Cre expression plasmid: pSalk-Cre (generously provided by Stephen O'Gorman; *see* **Note 2**).
4. Electroporation apparatus: Bio-Rad gene pulser with capacitance extender.
5. Neo-resistant murine embryonic fibroblasts (store at –80°C).
6. ES cell media: DME, 15% fetal calf serum approved for ES cell maintenance (Stem Cell Technologies, Vancouver, B.C., Canada), LIF 1000 U/mL, 0.1 m*M* nonessential amino acids (Gibco), 0.1 m*M* β-mercaptoethanol, 2 m*M* glutamine, penicillin/streptomycin (Gibco; store at 4°C).
7. Selection agent: G418 (Neo^r).
8. 0.25% Trypsin/ethylenediamine tetraacetic acid (EDTA; store at –20°C).
9. Polymerase chain reaction (PCR) machine and standard PCR kit (Taq based).
10. PCR primers: LoxinF: 5'-ctagatctcgaaggatctggag-3' LoxinR: 5'-atactttctcggcaggagca-3'.

2.2. Characterization of Inducible ES Cell Line

1. Doxycycline powder (Sigma) dissolved in water (store at –20°C).
2. Method for detecting gene expression levels (e.g., fluorescence-activated cell sorting [FACS], immunoblot, or reverse transcription [RT]-PCR).

2.3. Induction of Target Gene HoxB4 and Culture of EB-Derived Cells on OP9 to Develop Definitive Hematopoietic Stem Cells

1. 0.25% Trypsin–EDTA.
2. EB differentiation medium: Iscove's modified Dulbecco's medium, 15% fetal calf serum approved for ES cell differentiation (Stem Cell Technologies, Vancouver, B.C., Canada), 50 μg/mL ascorbic acid (Sigma), 200 μg/mL iron-saturated transferring (Sigma), 4.5 m*M* monothioglycerol (Sigma), 2 m*M* glutamine, penicillin/streptomycin (Gibco; store at 4°C).
3. Eight-well multichannel pipetor.
4. Non-tissue culture-treated dishes, 15 cm.
5. Rotating shaker.
6. Doxycycline powder (Sigma) dissolved in water (store at –20°C).
7. 10X Collagenase/DNAse I mixture: 10 mg/mL collagenase IV (Sigma) + 800 U/mL DNAse I mixture (use as 10X; store at –20°C).
8. Cell dissociation buffer (Gibco 13151-014).
9. OP9 Stroma cell line (store at –80°C; **ref.** ***89***).
10. OP9 Culture VFTS media: Iscove's modified Dulbecco's medium /10% IFS, 100 ng/mL stem cell factor, 40 ng/mL vascular endothelial growth factor, 40 ng/mL thrombopoietin, and 100 ng/mL Flt-3 ligand (Cytokines from Peprotech; store at 4°C).
11. 0.04% Trypsin–EDTA.

2.4. Therapeutic Transplantation of ES-derived Cells In Vivo

1. MSCV-IRES-GFP retrovirus or other retrovirus expressing a marker that can be followed in vivo.
2. Syngeneic mice 129 Ola/Hsd (Harlan Laboratories).

3. Methods

3.1. Generation of ES Cell Lines With Inducible Transgene Expression From Ainv15-Targeting Cells

Our system was built by gene targeting through a combination of homologous recombination and the Cre-lox recombinase system. The original ES cell line was created from a male, HPRT-deficient ES cell line E14-Tg5 and was generously provided by Wutz et al. ***(90,91)***. The original system (**Fig. 1**) had rtTA-nls ***(44)*** integrated at the ubiquitously expressed ROSA 26 locus ***(92)*** and used doxycycline-induced gene expression and green fluorescent protein (GFP) co-expression from a bidirectional promoter consisting of seven TetO sites flanked by minimal promoters derived from cyto-megalovirus (CMV) ***(93)***. Although this original system was successful in the study of Xist's role in chromosomal silencing, inducible expression levels of genes that we inserted into the system were significantly reduced in ES-derived differentiated cells. We determined that inverting the orientation of the inducible locus in relation to the HPRT locus and eliminating the co-inducible GFP reporter successfully corrected the problem of transgene silencing with differentiation. The reengineered cell line was named Ainv15 (**Fig. 1**; **ref.** ***94***) The maintenance of inducible gene expression is evident in the positive expression of HoxB4 in different stages of differentiation as seen by immunoblot analysis (**Fig. 2**).

The targeting vector for Cre-lox recombination (**Fig. 1**) is on a pBS backbone and contains two primary features: 1) A Pgk1 promoter and translation initiation codon (ATG) to restore neo^r function upon recombination into the inducible gene locus,

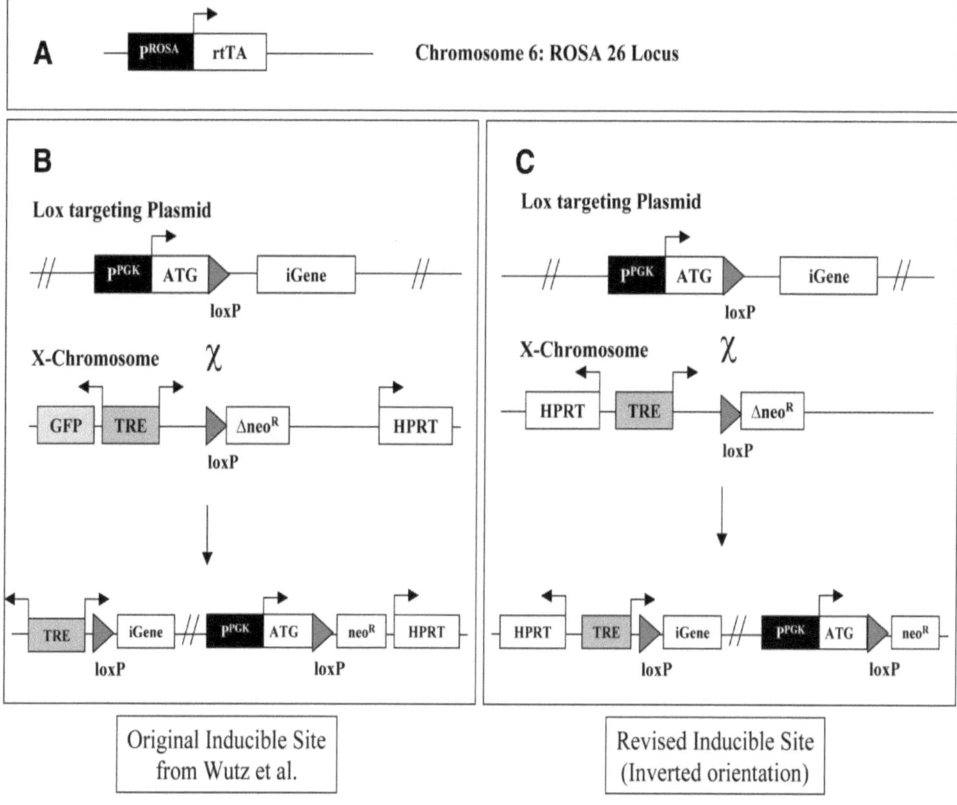

Fig. 1. Comparative schematic of inducible transgene systems. **(A)** Chromosome 6 carries the reverse tetracycline transactivator (rtTA) integrated into the constitutive and ubiquitously expressed ROSA26 locus. **(B,C)** The X chromosome carries the inducible gene locus 5' to the HPRT gene. The general strategy for inserting a gene into the inducible locus involves a lox-in (shown by the symbol chi) of the targeting plasmid. This restores neomycin resistance by providing a start codon (ATG) and the PGK promoter/enhancer to the formerly nonfunctional Δ neoR gene, which provides a method for positive selection. The gene of interest is integrated downstream of the tetracycline responsive element, which provides for doxycycline inducible expression of the gene. **(B)** The original configuration designed by Wutz et al. also has the tetracycline responsive element driving expression of a GFP reporter gene. After integration, the inducible gene locus is separated by several kilobases of plasmid sequence and the neoR gene from the constitutively active HPRT locus. This locus configuration was associated with silencing of gene expression in differentiated products of ES cells. **(C)** To correct this problem, the orientation was inverted relative to HPRT and the GFP reporter was eliminated. This places the inducible gene closer to the HPRT locus and precludes the silencing of the inducible gene. PROSA, ROSA26 enhancer/promoter; PPGK, phospho-glycero-kinase enhancer/promoter; ATG, start codon for the neo gene; loxP, Cre-recombinase recognition sequence; Δneo, deletion mutant of the neomycin (G418) resistance gene; //, plasmid sequence.

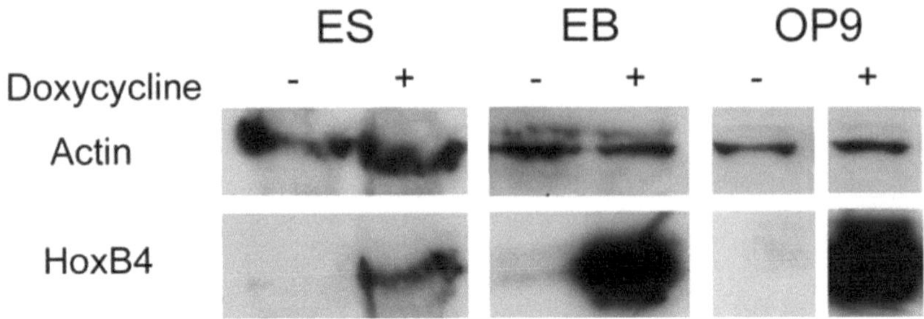

Fig. 2. HoxB4 induction in undifferentiated and differentiated ES cells. Immunoblot of HoxB4 (27 kDa) followed by second probing for actin (42 kDa) from cell lysates of inducible HoxB4 ES cells before and after differentiation in EBs and culture on OP9 stroma cells. HoxB4 expression is insignificant without doxycycline induction in ES cells, EBs, and in OP9 cultures. In the presence of doxycycline at 1 mg/mL, there is marked HoxB4 expression in the ES, EB, and OP9 cultures. This demonstrates that the inducible locus is not silenced upon differentiation of the ES cells.

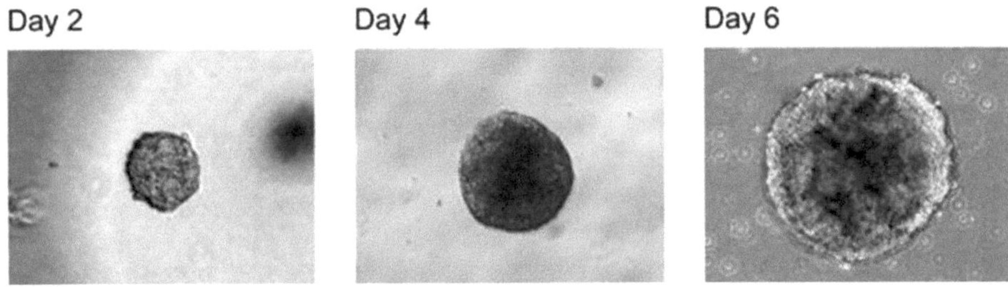

Fig. 3. Growth of EBs at 40X magnification. ES cells are dispersed in hanging drops on d 0 and are allowed to grow until d 2. The EBs are then collected, pooled in a 10-cm dish, and cultured with continuous rotation. At d 4, doxycycline is added to the media to drive expression of HoxB4. At d 6, EBs are harvested and dissociated for plating on OP9. Representative EBs are shown at d 2, 4, and 6 after initial plating.

(which provides a selection method for positive loxin of the gene of interest), and 2) The transgene (in our case HoxB4) with polyadenylation sequence so the loxP site is engineered between the Pgk1 promoter-ATG and the gene of interest. Using the lox targeting plasmid, the gene of interest can now be inserted into the inducible locus of Ainv15. This is accomplished through co-electroporation of the targeting plasmid and a suitable Cre-expression plasmid, selection of positive recombinants using **G418,** and confirmation of integrants with PCR (*see* **Note 2**). The procedure is as follows:

1. Add 8×10^6 Ainv15 cells in 800 μL of phosphate-buffered saline (PBS) with 20 μg each of the targeting plasmid carrying the inducible gene of interest and CRE-expression plasmid.

2. Add the mixture to an electroporation cell and electroporate at room temperature on the Bio-Rad gene pulser with capacitance extender using the settings: 200 Ω, 0.25 V.
3. Add the electroporated cells to a 10-cm dish carrying neo-resistant MEFs at 80 to 90% confluence in ES cell media (MEFs are plated the day before).
4. The next day, add **G418** (350 μg/mL) and maintain selection until resistant colonies appear around d 10 to 14. The cells will be very dense the first few days, and medium should be changed twice per day. After most cells have died off, feeding can be done once a day.
5. After 10 to 14 d, flood the dish with 10 to 15 mL of PBS and pick individual colonies using a P20 pipetman. Transfer to 100 μL of 0.25% trypsin–EDTA in an Eppendorf tube and disrupt the colony by gently pipetting up and down. Incubate at 37°C for 2 min and again disrupt any aggregates by pipetting. Add 900 μL of ES cell medium and collect the cells of the colony by centrifugation. Aspirate media and trypsin and resuspend cells in appropriate amount of ES cell medium. Replate the suspension onto fresh MEFs in 12-well dishes.
6. Confirm integration through PCR by using primers that amplify across the loxP site to give a band of approx 420 bp on ethidium bromide agarose gel electrophoresis. The primers are, for LoxinF, 5'-ctagatctcgaaggatctggag-3', and for LoxinR, 5'-atactttctcggcaggagca-3'. The PCR cycle conditions are as follows: 45 s at 95°C, 1 min at 60°C, and 1 min at 72°C; repeat cycle 29X. Promega PCR buffer with 1.25 m*M* $MgCl_2$ should be used with Taq polymerase.
7. Colonies that are positive can be cultured further from the 12-well dishes by using 0.25% trypsin–EDTA and plating on fresh semiconfluent MEFs on an appropriately sized tissue culture dish or flask.

3.2. Characterization of Inducible ES Cell Line

Induction of target gene expression can be started at different times and stages of differentiation; however, the amount and timing of expression can only be controlled if the inducible system has been fully characterized. This characterization was performed using GFP as the inducible gene. One question was whether doxycycline diffusion in different culturing methods was a limiting factor in expression kinetics. EB formation (one method for differentiating ES cells that will be discussed in the next section) creates a multilayer structure that may influence the diffusion kinetics of doxycycline. Images of EBs at different developmental stages are found in **Fig. 3**. Based on confocal images of inducible GFP EBs, doxycycline reaches all cells of the EB by 14 h of incubation in 1 μg/mL of doxycycline (**Fig. 4**). FACS analyses demonstrate faster expression kinetics in monolayer ES cell culture than in EB culture with maximal GFP expression reached in 8 and 14 h, respectively (**Fig. 5A**). This difference in gene expression in monolayer and multilayer culturing conditions should be considered when using this system. Moreover, there may be variations in gene expression in different parts of the embryoid body. The initial lag in GFP positivity is probably the result of three factors: 1) The time required for doxycycline to penetrate the cell membrane and increase intracellular concentration above a critical threshold for rtTA binding; 2) The time required to initiate the transcription and translation of GFP; 3) The time required to synthesize enough GFP to be detectable by FACS. Analysis of GFP expression levels over time shows a sigmoid relationship (**Fig. 5B**), but in this situation the lag in expression is confined to doxycycline membrane diffusion kinetics and the time required to synthesize GFP. The nonlinear increase after the initial lag is either the result of an exponential increase in intracellular doxy-

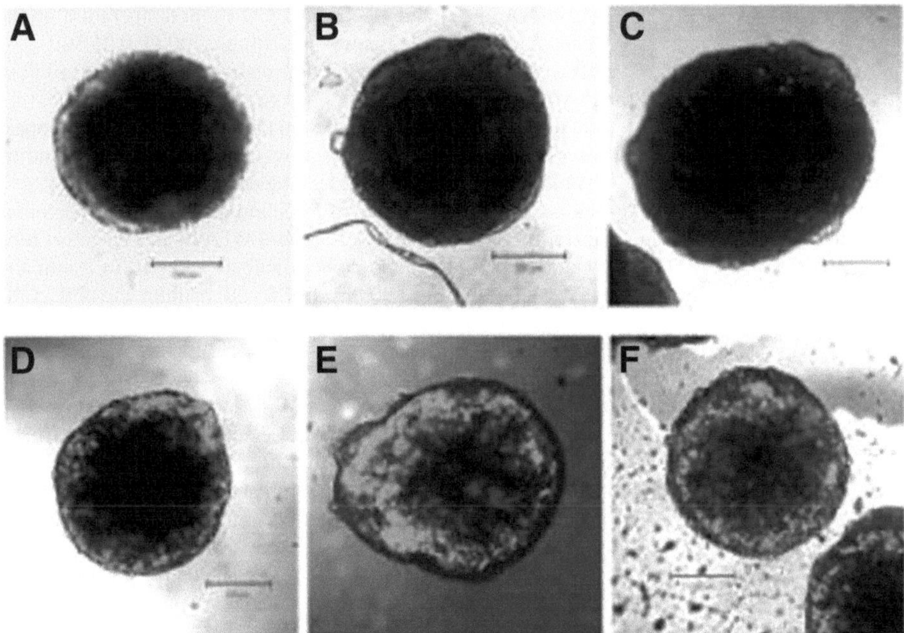

Fig. 4. Midsection confocal image of d 6 EBs from inducible GFP ES cells in the presence of 1 μg/mL of doxycycline for 0 h (**A**), 4 h (**B**), 6 h (**C**), 14 h (**D**), 24 h (**E**), and 48 h (**F**). The above EBs were also dissociated and analyzed by FACs. At 4 h, there was 10% GFP positivity and at 14 h, there was 80% positivity. These data indicate that doxycycline can penetrate into all of the cells of the EB within 14 h. Note that the non-GFP-positive area in the middle of the EB is a developmental cyst. The bar represents 200 μm.

cycline concentration or a cooperative mechanism for rtTA-driven GFP expression. A cooperative mechanism is supported by analysis of the doxycycline concentration dependence of GFP expression (**Fig. 6**). The sigmoidal curve is indicative of a cooperative process and is consistent with the design of the system. There are seven TetO sites located between the minimal promoters that allow for multiple rtTA binding to the bidirectional promoter unit. Because there is only one inducible transgene per cell, the proportional increase of activated rtTA with doxycycline concentration causes a non-linear increase in transgene expression. Lastly, **Fig. 7** shows the decay of GFP expression over time when doxycycline is removed after 24 h in 1 μg/mL. There is an initial rise in GFP expression over 10 h, probably the result of one or more of the following: 1) Transactivator remaining bound to the promoter unit; 2) Residual transcript that continues to be translated; 3) A lag for intracellular concentration of doxycycline to decrease to non-activating levels; and 4) The relatively long half-life of GFP. The induction kinetics between different transgenes is expected to be comparable; however, there will be more variation in the off kinetics between different transgenes because of inherent differences in protein half-lives. This characterization

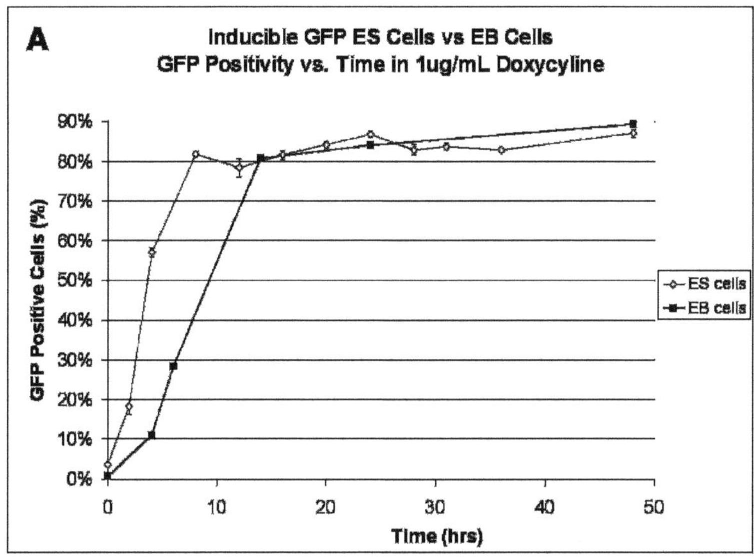

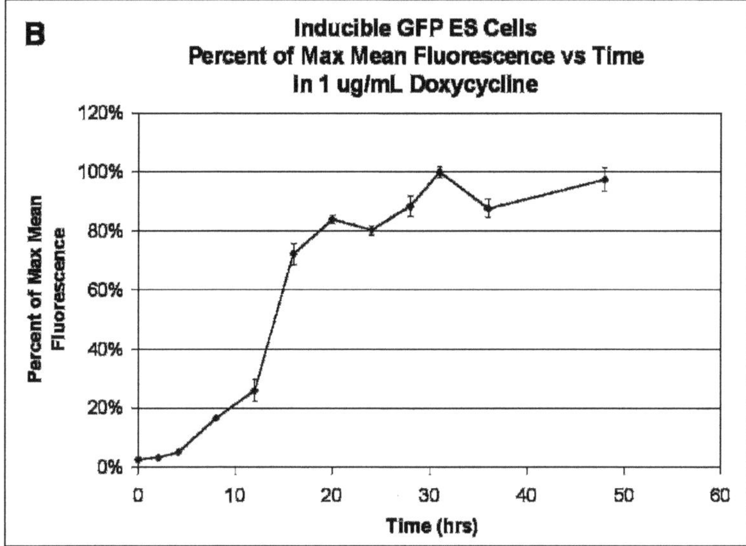

Fig. 5. Induction kinetics of inducible GFP in Ainv15 ES cell line at 1 μg/mL of doxycycline. (**A**) Percent of GFP-positive cells over time. Maximum number of cells with positive GFP expression in both EBs and ES cells is reached by 14 h of incubation; however, GFP positivity increases more rapidly in ES cell culture than in the EBs. 100% GFP positivity is not reached because 10% of the cells are MEFs. The initial lag is caused by 1) the time required for doxycycline to penetrate the cell membrane and increase intracellular concentration above a critical concentration for rtTA binding, 2) the time required to initiate the transcription and translation of GFP, and 3) the time required to synthesize enough GFP to be detectable by FACS.

(Continued on next page)

Fig. 5. *(Continued)* (**B**) Mean GFP fluorescence over time. There is an initial lag in mean fluorescence because of the diffusion of doxycycline into the cell and the time required to initiate GFP synthesis. The following rapid increase of GFP synthesis per cell suggests that either the intracellular doxycycline concentration is rapidly increasing in a non-linear fashion or that the doxycycline–rtTA complex increases the rate of GFP expression through a cooperative mechanism. A steady-state level of GFP in ES culture is reached after approx 24 h.

of the inducible system demonstrates that the timing and level of expression can be accurately controlled, which is essential in the majority of processes during development. This provides a more accurate method of investigating the role of specific genes in development as well as a reproducible and controllable method of engineering a particular tissue or cell type with induced gene expression.

3.3. Induction of Target Gene HoxB4 and Culture of EB-Derived Cells on OP9 Stroma to Develop Definitive HSCs

The characterization of the inducible system demonstrates the ability to have consistent control of gene expression in ES and ES-derived cells. The use of this system will vary depending on the genes and developmental processes investigated. We will discuss an example of using this system in the context of developing ES-derived HSCs. This was achieved through inducible expression of HoxB4 and a combination of culturing methods. The culturing method we used involved EB formation ***(95–97)*** followed by co-culture on the OP9 stromal cell line ***(89)***. Induction of HoxB4 is performed at the time when the hemangioblast commits to the primitive HSC, which is from d 4 to 6 of EB development. The EBs were then dissociated and plated on OP9 stromal cells in the presence of a unique set of cytokines and various doxycycline concentrations. Experiments to determine whether doxycycline concentration variation correlated with HoxB4 expression levels and, consequently, phenotypic changes in OP9 cultured cells are summarized in **Fig. 8**. As shown, HoxB4 levels can be carefully controlled with variations in doxycycline concentration (**Fig. 9A**). The number of ES-derived cells growing on OP9 increased with increasing HoxB4 levels (**Fig. 9**). This demonstrates the ability of HoxB4 to drive proliferation of these ES-derived cells. Moreover, previous experiments have shown that induced HoxB4 expression in these ES-derived cells results in the development of the definitive HSC ***(61)***. These conclusions were drawn from in vitro data showing a shift from embryonic (β-H1) to adult (β-major) globin and the increase in the known homing genes CXCR-4 and TEL, which is consistent with definitive hematopoiesis. Furthermore, colony-forming cell (CFC) assays showed an increase in the numbers of the multipotential progenitor colony-forming unit-granulocyte erythroid megakaryocyte macrophage (CFU-GEMM), which produces myeloid and erythroid lineage cells. This was further supported by data delineating a HoxB4-dependent increase in the surface marker phenotypes Sca-1 ***(98–107)*** and CD41/c-kit ***(108,109)***, which have been implicated as possible surface phenotypes for the definitive HSC (**Fig. 9C**). These results are suggestive of the successful development and propagation of ES-derived definitive HSCs.

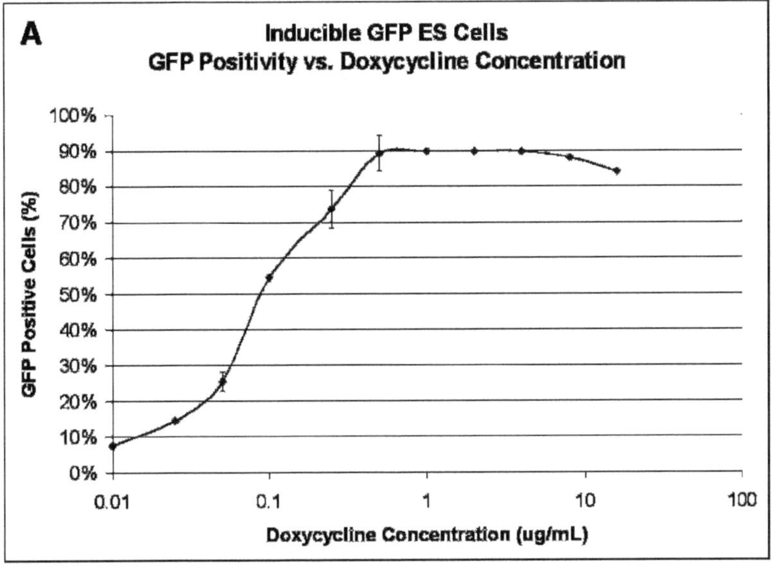

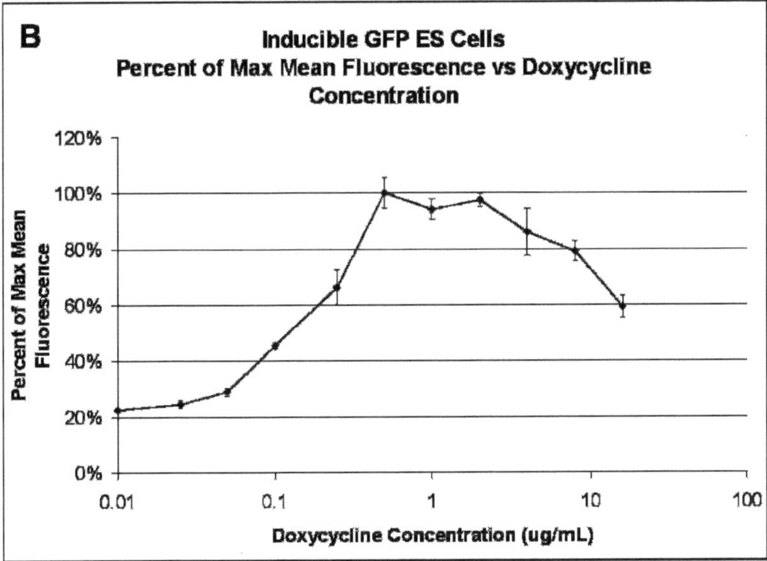

Fig. 6. Induced GFP expression dependence on doxycycline concentration. **(A)** Percentage positivity vs concentration shows that the kinetics of doxycycline penetration into ES cells is concentration dependent. After 24 h, all of the ES cells are induced at a concentration of 0.5 mg/mL. 100% GFP positivity is not reached because 10% of the cells are MEFs. **(B)** The sigmoidal curve is consistent with a cooperative mechanism for GFP expression. With increasing doxycycline concentration, more rtTAs bind the promoter unit and work synergistically to increase the rate of GFP expression in a nonlinear fashion. Above 2 mg/mL of doxycycline, there is toxicity from either doxycycline or rtTA as indicated by the dropping fluorescence levels.

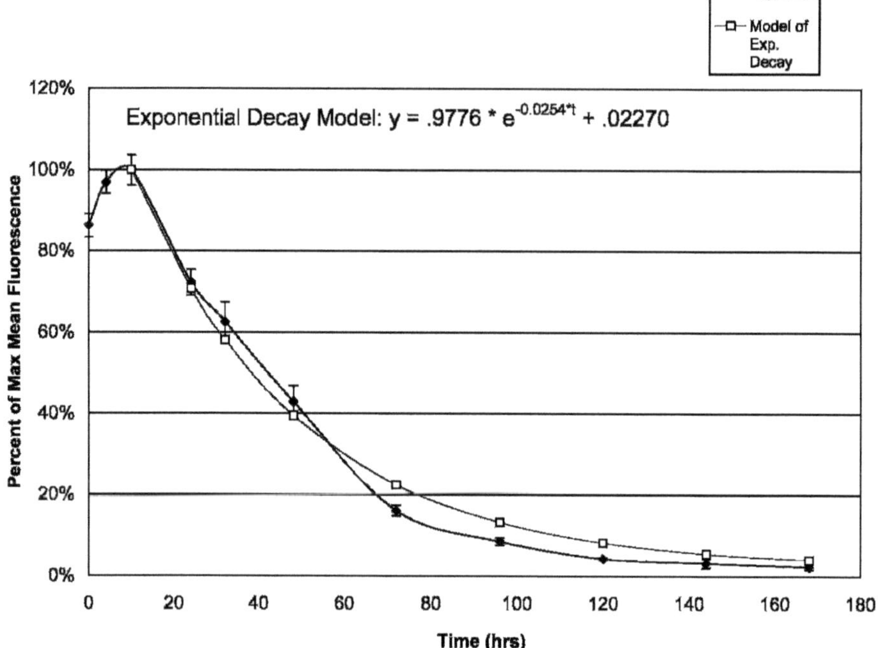

Fig. 7. Off kinetics of GFP expression after incubation with 1 μg/mL of doxycycline over 24 h. The decay kinetics will be unique to each transgene because proteins will have differing half-lives. GFP is a relatively long-lived protein and persists for over 5 d. In the graph, it is notable that there is an initial rise in GFP expression in the first 10 h as the result of a combination of untranslated RNA, delay of rtTA unbinding from the promoter unit, and the time for intracellular doxycycline concentrations to drop. A model of exponential decay of GFP after the initial 10-h rise in fluorescence is graphed. The decay model fits relatively well with a time constant of 0.0254 1/h and a half-life for GFP of around 27 h.

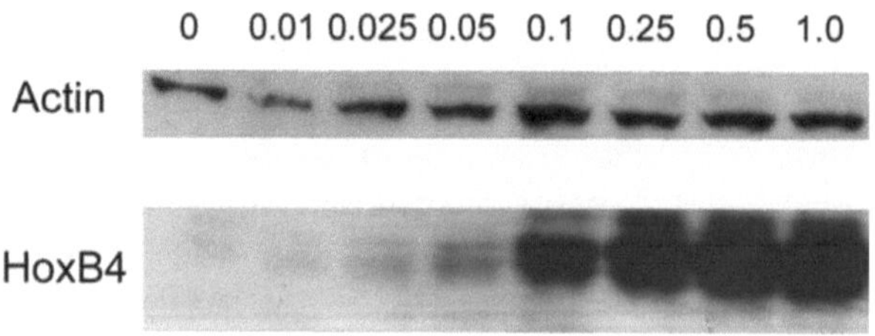

Fig. 8. Titration of HoxB4 levels with increasing concentrations of doxycycline in OP9 culture. Cell lysates of inducible HoxB4 d 6 EB-derived cells growing on OP9 at different doxycycline concentrations were subjected to immunoblot for HoxB4 (27 kDa) with second probing for actin (42 kDa) There is no detectable basal level of HoxB4 expression in the system without doxycycline, and the expression levels of HoxB4 can be titrated with doxycycline up to an apparent maximum of 0.5 μg/mL of doxycycline.

1. Starting from a confluent ES culture in a 25-cm^2 T-flask, trypsinize culture with 0.25% trypsin/EDTA for 10 to 15 min at 37°C.
2. Add 5 mL of EB differentiation media to the culture and disrupt any cell clumps with a pipettor. Incubate cells for 45 min at 37°C to allow MEFs to re-attach, while the majority of the ES cells will be retained in suspension.
3. Count cells and make suspension of 10,000 cells/mL in EB differentiation medium.
4. Make as many hanging drops as possible with the multichannel pipettor of 10 μL (100 cells/drop) on 15-cm nontissue culture-treated dishes (*see* **Note 3**).
5. Incubate for 2 d at 37°C (d 0–2) inverted so that drop is hanging.
6. On d 2, flood Petri dishes with 10 to 15 mL of PBS, collect in a 15-mL tube, and allow the EBs to sediment by gravity for 3 min.
7. Aspirate PBS, resuspend EBs in 10 mL of EB differentiation medium, and put into 10-cm bacterial Petri dish bottom with 10-cm tissue culture dish top.
8. Place on rotator at 50 rpm in a dedicated 37°C/5% CO_2 incubator.
9. Feed the cultures every 2 d with a half media exchange.
10. On d 4, add 1 μL of doxycycline (1 mg/mL) directly to the EB media in the rotating dish to make a final concentration of 1 μg/mL (*see* **Note 4**).
11. On d 6, collect the EBs in a 15-mL tube and dissociate EBs by washing with PBS, incubating with 900 μL of PBS and with 100 μL of 10X collagenase/DNase I mixture at 37°C for 15 to 20 min, and then pipetting the EBs against the wall of the tube.
12. Add 4 mL of cell dissociation buffer (Gibco 13151-014), mix cells, and then pellet the cells in a centrifuge.
13. Resuspend in PBS and repeat procedure from **step 2** until EB is sufficiently dissociated (usually requires two treatments total).
14. Resuspend in OP9 culture VFTS media and plate cells on 80% confluent OP9 stroma cells in appropriate sized flask (*see* **Note 5**).
15. Add appropriate amount of doxycycline (1 mg/mL) to make final concentration 1 μg/mL.
16. Discrete semiadherent colonies should begin to form within 3 to 4 d.
17. Split cells onto fresh OP9 when confluent through trypsinization with 0.04% trypsin/EDTA for 5 to 10 min.

3.4. Therapeutic Transplantation of ES-Derived Cells In Vivo

The in vitro data indicating that induced HoxB4 expression develops the definitive HSC was confirmed in vivo with bone marrow transplantation studies ***(61)***. Long-term engraftment studies were performed in 2- to 3-mo-old isogenic 129 Ola/Hsd mice. To follow the ES-derived iHox cells in vivo, the cells were infected with a GFP-expressing retrovirus, sorted, and recultured on OP9 cells before transplantation. Transplants were performed in lethally irradiated mice (1000 cGy of γ- irradiation) with approx 2×10^6 cells of OP9 cultured cells injected via lateral tail vein. GFP expression was seen in primary mice up to 15 wk after transplant and in secondary mice more than 5 mo after transplant. Interestingly, induction after transplant was not necessary for long-term engraftment, which suggests that HoxB4 is required at a specific time in development to guide a cell towards the definitive HSC fate. This finding demonstrates the value and power of the inducible system as a developmental research tool and a reliable method for modeling cell therapies.

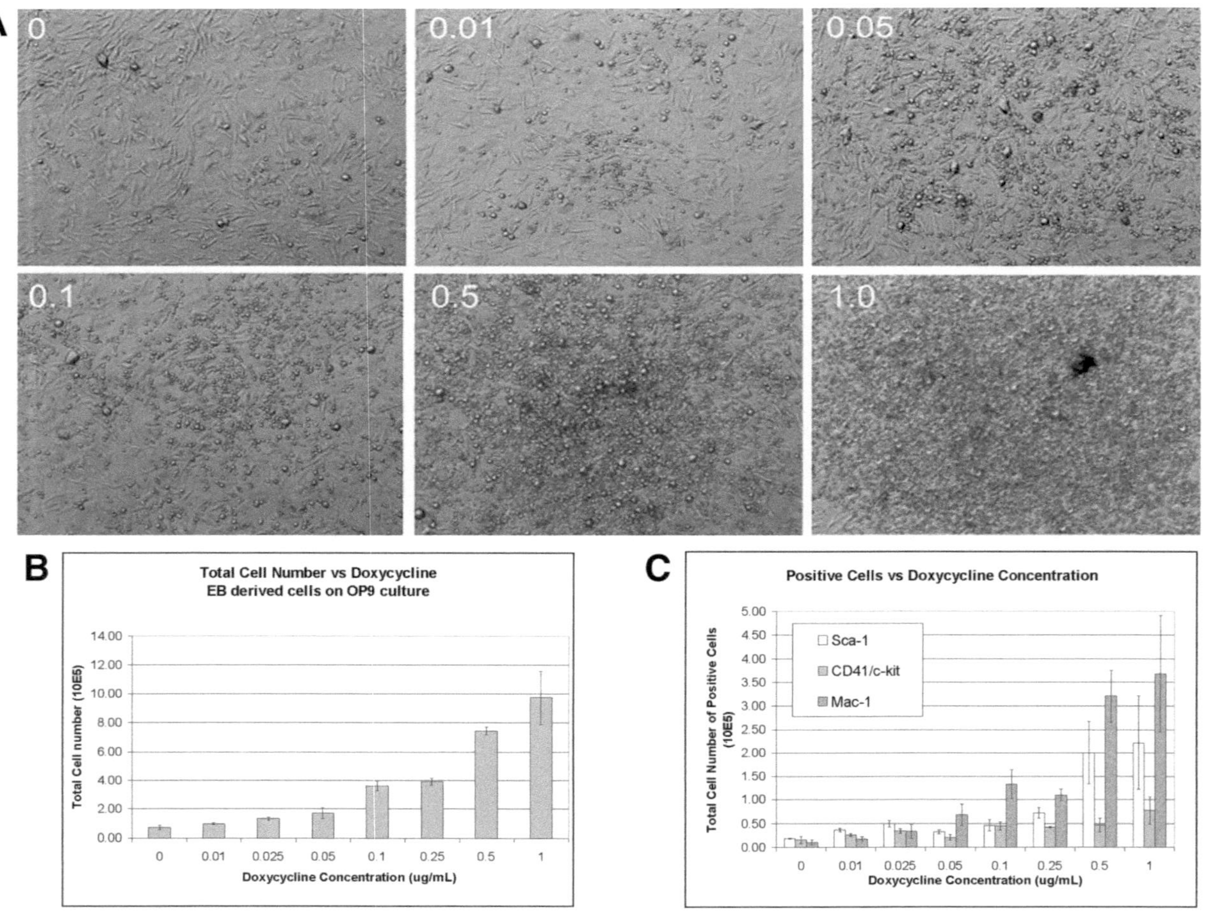

A
0
0.01
0.05
0.1
0.5
1.0
B
Total Cell Number vs Doxycycline
EB derived cells on OP9 culture
Total Cell number (10E5)
14.00
12.00
10.00
8.00
6.00
4.00
2.00
0.00
0
0.01
0.025
0.05
0.1
0.25
0.5
1
Doxycycline Concentration (ug/mL)
C
Positive Cells vs Doxycycline Concentration
Sca-1
CD41/c-kit
Mac-1
Total Cell Number of Positive Cells (10E5)
5.00
4.50
4.00
3.50
3.00
2.50
2.00
1.50
1.00
0.50
0.00
0
0.01
0.025
0.05
0.1
0.25
0.5
1
Doxycycline Concentration (ug/mL)

Fig. 9. *(Opposite)* Effect of varying induced levels of HoxB4 gene expression on ES-derived cells co-cultured on OP9. **(A)** Images at 40X of OP9 cultures at different doxycycline concentrations. As shown, the density of ES-derived cells (small round cells) increases dramatically with increases in doxycycline concentration. **(B)** Total cell number vs doxycycline concentration. With increasing doxycycline, cell number increases rapidly up to 1 mg/mL. **(C)** Total cell number of positive cells stained for either Sca-1, CD41 + c-kit, or Mac-1. Sca-1 and CD41 + c-kit are two surface phenotypes that have recently been suggested to indicate the definitive HSC. As doxycycline concentration increases, the detectable level of both sets of markers also increases. Increasing HoxB4 expression appears to affect Sca-1 positive population more than the CD41/c-kit double positive population. Mac-1 was included as a marker of myeloid lineage cells because it had been previously shown that expression of this marker increases with induction of HoxB4.

4. Notes

1. In this protocol, the rtTA-nls is used as the transactivator and a bidirectional minimal promoter derived from CMV is used to express the target gene. The nls stands for nuclear localization signal, which was created to target the rtTA to the nucleus and improve transactivation. This variation was shown to provide enrichment of rtTA in the nucleus. One problem of the first rtTA and tTA was the toxicity of constitutive expression of these transactivators. This has been improved by diminishing the VP16 portion to 12 amino acids, which was shown to be better tolerated at higher intracellular concentrations *(45)*. Others have generated an autoregulatory system with the transactivators to reduce toxicity *(110)*. In addition, work has been performed to modify the rtTA to be more sensitive to doxycycline and to have lower background activity. Urlinger et al. have demonstrated new rtTA mutants that operate at doxycycline concentrations 10 times less than the original rtTA and have undetectable background expression *(111)*. Other groups have fused TetR to another transcriptional activator E2F4 as an alternative to tTA and rtTA *(112)*. There have been many other modifications and refinements to the system, including variations in promoter systems *(113)* and alterations in transactivator DNA binding specificities *(114)*.
2. The lox-targeting plasmid we generated was derived from pPGK-loxP-Xist *(90,91)*, which was generously provided by Anton Wutz and Rudolf Jaenisch. This was modified using pNEO-EGFP, which is no longer available from Clontech. The Cre-expression plasmid pSalk-Cre was generously provided by Stephen O'Gormon. There are a number of other plasmids that are commercially available to generate a lox-targeting plasmid and a Cre-expression plasmid. It is only important to maintain the location of the loxP site in relation to the transgene and the PGK1 promoter-ATG.
3. EBs can be made with more than 100 cells/drop or with larger drop sizes if EBs fail to properly form or grow to a desirable size.
4. Doxycycline induction concentration and times will vary depending on quantitative, temporal, and spatial characteristics desired in expressing a gene of interest.
5. Optional FACS sorting of blast populations with surface markers such as CD41, c-kit, CD34, or Sca-1 can be done before plating on OP9 culture to enrich the cultures for hematopoietic blast cells.

Acknowledgments

This work was supported by fellowships from the Howard Hughes Medical Institute (D.T.), the Alberta Heritage Foundation for Medical Research (M.K.), and the Canadian Institutes of Health Research (M.K.) Research in the principal investigator's laboratory was supported by grants from the National Institutes of Health and the National Science Foundation. G.Q.D. is the Birnbaum Scholar of the Leukemia & Lymphoma Society of America.

References

1. Evans, M. J. and Kaufman, M. (1981) Establishment in culture of pluripotential cells from mouse embryos. *Nature* **292,** 154–156.
2. Martin, G. R. (1981) Isolation of a pluripotent cell line from early mouse embryos cultured in medium conditioned by teratocarcinoma stem cells. *Proc. Natl. Acad. Sci. USA* **78,** 7634–7638.
3. Robertson, E., Bradley, A., Kuehn, M., and Evans, M. (1986) Germ-line transmission of genes introduced into cultured pluripotential cells by retroviral vector. *Nature* **323,** 445–448.
4. Kuehn, M. R., Bradley, A., Robertson, E. J., and Evans, M. J. (1987) A potential animal model for Lesch-Nyhan syndrome through introduction of HPRT mutations into mice. *Nature* **326,** 295–298.
5. Cherry, S. R., Biniszkiewicz, D., van Parijs, L., Baltimore, D., and Jaenisch, R. (2000) Retroviral expression in embryonic stem cells and hematopoietic stem cells. *Mol. Cell Biol.* **20,** 7419–7426.
6. Robbins, P. B., Yu, X. J., Skelton, D. M., Pepper, K. A., Wasserman, R. M., Zhu, L., et al. (1997) Increased probability of expression from modified retroviral vectors in embryonal stem cells and embryonal carcinoma cells. *J. Virol.* **71,** 9466–9474.
7. Hildinger, M., Eckert, H. G., Schilz, A. J., John, J., Ostertag, W., and Baum, C. (1998) FMEV vectors: both retroviral long terminal repeat and leader are important for high expression in transduced hematopoietic cells. *Gene Ther.* **5,** 1575–1579.
8. Ketteler, R., Glaser, S., Sandra, O., Martens, U. M., and Klingmuller, U. (2002) Enhanced transgene expression in primitive hematopoietic progenitor cells and embryonic stem cells efficiently transduced by optimized retroviral hybrid vectors. *Gene Ther.* **9,** 477–487.
9. Hamaguchi, I., Woods, N. B., Panagopoulos, I., Andersson, E., Mikkola, H., Fahlman, C., et al. (2000) Lentivirus vector gene expression during ES cell-derived hematopoietic development in vitro. *J. Virol.* **74,** 10,778–10,784.
10. Kafri, T., van Praag, H., Gage, F. H., and Verma, I. M. (2000) Lentiviral vectors: regulated gene expression. *Mol. Ther.* **1,** 516–521.
11. Ramezani, A., Hawley, T. S., and Hawley, R. G. (2000) Lentiviral vectors for enhanced gene expression in human hematopoietic cells. *Mol. Ther.* **2,** 458–469.
12. Pfeifer, A., Ikawa, M., Dayn, Y., and Verma, I. M. (2002) Transgenesis by lentiviral vectors: lack of gene silencing in mammalian embryonic stem cells and preimplantation embryos. *Proc. Natl. Acad. Sci. USA* **99,** 2140–2145.
13. Vigna, E., Cavalieri, S., Ailles, L., Geuna, M., Loew, R., Bujard, H., and Naldini, L. (2002) Robust and efficient regulation of transgene expression in vivo by improved tetracycline-dependent lentiviral vectors. *Mol. Ther.* **5,** 252–261.
14. Jin, L., Siritanaratkul, N., Emery, D. W., Richard, R. E., Kaushansky, K., Papayannopoulou, T., et al. (1998) Targeted expansion of genetically modified bone marrow cells. *Proc. Natl. Acad. Sci. USA* **95,** 8093–8097.
15. Jin, L., Zeng, H., Chien, S., Otto, K. G., Richard, R. E., Emery, D. W., and Blau, C. A. (2000) In vivo selection using a cell-growth switch. *Nat. Genet.* **26,** 64–66.

16. Hofmann, A., Nolan, G. P., and Blau, H. M. (1996) Rapid retroviral delivery of tetracycline-inducible genes in a single autoregulatory cassette. *Proc. Natl. Acad. Sci. USA* **93,** 5185–5190.
17. Doetschman, T., Gregg, R. G., Maeda, N., Hooper, M. L., Melton, D. W., Thompson, S., et al. (1987) Targetted correction of a mutant HPRT gene in mouse embryonic stem cells. *Nature* **330,** 576–578.
18. Thomas, K. R. and Capecchi, M. R. (1987) Site-directed mutagenesis by gene targeting in mouse embryo-derived stem cells. *Cell* **51,** 503–512.
19. Mansour, S. L., Thomas, K. R., and Capecchi, M. R. (1988) Disruption of the proto-oncogene int-2 in mouse embryo-derived stem cells: a general strategy for targeting mutations to non-selectable genes. *Nature* **336,** 348–352.
20. Schwartzberg, P. L., Goff, S. P., and Robertson, E. J. (1989) Germ-line transmission of a c-abl mutation produced by targeted gene disruption in ES cells. *Science* **246,** 799–803.
21. Hasty, P., Ramirez-Solis, R., Krumlauf, R., and Bradley, A. (1991) Introduction of a subtle mutation into the Hox-2.6 locus in embryonic stem cells. *Nature* **350,** 243–246.
22. Valancius, V. and Smithies, O. (1991) Testing an "in-out" targeting procedure for making subtle genomic modifications in mouse embryonic stem cells. *Mol. Cell Biol.* **11,** 1402–1408.
23. Rudolph, U., Brabet, P., Hasty, P., Bradley, A., and Birnbaumer, L. (1993) Disruption of the G(i2) alpha locus in embryonic stem cells and mice: a modified hit and run strategy with detection by a PCR dependent on gap repair. *Transgenic Res.* **2,** 345–355.
24. Askew, G. R., Doetschman, T., and Lingrel, J. B. (1993) Site-directed point mutations in embryonic stem cells: a gene-targeting tag-and-exchange strategy. *Mol. Cell Biol.* **13,** 4115–4124.
25. Stacey, A., Schnieke, A., McWhir, J., Cooper, J., Colman, A., and Melton, D. W. (1994) Use of double-replacement gene targeting to replace the murine alpha-lactalbumin gene with its human counterpart in embryonic stem cells and mice. *Mol. Cell Biol.* **14,** 1009–1116.
26. Detloff, P. J., Lewis, J., John, S. W., Shehee, W. R., Langenbach, R., Maeda, N., and Smithies, O. (1994) Deletion and replacement of the mouse adult beta-globin genes by a "plug and socket" repeated targeting strategy. *Mol. Cell Biol.* **14,** 6936–6943.
27. Sauer, B. (1998) Inducible gene targeting in mice using the Cre/lox system. *Methods* **14,** 381–392.
28. Hadjantonakis, A. K., Pirity, M., and Nagy, A. (1999) Cre recombinase mediated alterations of the mouse genome using embryonic stem cells. *Methods Mol. Biol.* **97,** 101–122.
29. Le, Y. and Sauer, B. (2000) Conditional gene knockout using cre recombinase. *Methods Mol. Biol.* **136,** 477–485.
30. Nagy, A. (2000) Cre recombinase: the universal reagent for genome tailoring. *Genesis* **26,** 99–109.
31. Zhang, Y., Riesterer, C., Ayrall, A. M., Sablitzky, F., Littlewood, T. D., and Reth, M. (1996) Inducible site-directed recombination in mouse embryonic stem cells. *Nucleic Acids Res.* **24,** 543–548.
32. Danielian, P. S., Muccino, D., Rowitch, D. H., Michael, S. K., and McMahon, A. P. (1998) Modification of gene activity in mouse embryos in utero by a tamoxifen-inducible form of Cre recombinase. *Curr. Biol.* **8,** 1323–1326.
33. Verrou, C., Zhang, Y., Zurn, C., Schamel, W. W., and Reth, M. (1999) Comparison of the tamoxifen regulated chimeric Cre recombinases MerCreMer and CreMer. *J. Biol. Chem.* **380,** 1435–1438.

34. Indra, A. K., Warot, X., Brocard, J., Bornert, J. M., Xiao, J. H., Chambon, P., and Metzger, D. (1999) Temporally-controlled site-specific mutagenesis in the basal layer of the epidermis: comparison of the recombinase activity of the tamoxifen-inducible Cre-ER(T) and Cre-ER(T2) recombinases. *Nucleic Acids Res.* **27,** 4324–4327.
35. Chiba, H., Chambon, P., and Metzger, D. (2000) F9 embryonal carcinoma cells engineered for tamoxifen-dependent Cre-mediated site-directed mutagenesis and doxycycline-inducible gene expression. *Exp. Cell Res.* **260,** 334–339.
36. Fuhrmann-Benzakein, E., Garcia-Gabay, I., Pepper, M. S., Vassalli, J. D., and Herrera, P. L. (2000) Inducible and irreversible control of gene expression using a single transgene. *Nucleic Acids Res.* **28,** E99.
37. Imai, T., Jiang, M., Kastner, P., Chambon, P., and Metzger, D. (2001) Selective ablation of retinoid X receptor alpha in hepatocytes impairs their lifespan and regenerative capacity. *Proc. Natl. Acad. Sci. USA* **98,** 4581–4586.
38. Imai, T., Jiang, M., Chambon, P., and Metzger, D. (2001) Impaired adipogenesis and lipolysis in the mouse upon selective ablation of the retinoid X receptor alpha mediated by a tamoxifen-inducible chimeric Cre recombinase (Cre-ERT2) in adipocytes. *Proc. Natl. Acad. Sci. USA* **98,** 224–228.
39. Endoh, M., Ogawa, M., Orkin, S., and Nishikawa, S.-I. (2002) SCL/tal-1-dependent process determines a competence to select the definitive hematopoietic lineage prior to endothelial differentiation. *EMBO J.* **21,** 6700–6708.
40. Guo, C., Yang, W., and Lobe, C. G. (2002) A Cre recombinase transgene with mosaic, widespread tamoxifen-inducible action. *Genesis* **32,** 8–18.
41. Hayashi, S., and McMahon, A. P. (2002) Efficient recombination in diverse tissues by a tamoxifen-inducible form of Cre: a tool for temporally regulated gene activation/inactivation in the mouse. *Dev. Biol.* **244,** 305–318.
42. Petrich, B. G., Molkentin, J. D., and Wang, Y. (2003) Temporal activation of c-Jun N-terminal kinase in adult transgenic heart via cre-loxP-mediated DNA recombination. *FASEB J.* **19,** 19.
43. Gossen, M. and Bujard, H. (1992) Tight control of gene expression in mammalian cells by tetracycline-responsive promoters. *Proc. Natl. Acad. Sci. USA* **89,** 5547–5551.
44. Gossen, M., Freundlieb, S., Bender, G., Muller, G., Hillen, W., and Bujard, H. (1995) Transcriptional activation by tetracyclines in mammalian cells. *Science* **268,** 1766–1769.
45. Baron, U., Gossen, M., and Bujard, H. (1997) Tetracycline-controlled transcription in eukaryotes: novel transactivators with graded transactivation potential. *Nucleic Acids Res.* **25,** 2723–2729.
46. Niwa, H., Burdon, T., Chambers, I., and Smith, A. (1998) Self-renewal of pluripotent embryonic stem cells is mediated via activation of STAT3. *Genes Dev.* **12,** 2048–2060.
47. Niwa, H., Miyazaki, J., and Smith, A. G. (2000) Quantitative expression of Oct-3/4 defines differentiation, dedifferentiation or self-renewal of ES cells. *Nat. Genet.* **24,** 372–376.
48. Era, T. and Witte, O. N. (2000) Regulated expression of P210 Bcr-Abl during embryonic stem cell differentiation stimulates multipotential progenitor expansion and myeloid cell fate. *Proc. Natl. Acad. Sci. USA* **97,** 1737–1742.
49. Furth, P. A., St Onge, L., Boger, H., Gruss, P., Gossen, M., Kistner, A., Bujard, H., and Hennighausen, L. (1994) Temporal control of gene expression in transgenic mice by a tetracycline-responsive promoter. *Proc. Natl. Acad. Sci. USA* **91,** 9302–9306.
50. Bjornsson, J. M., Andersson, E., Lundstrom, P., Larsson, N., Xu, X., Repetowska, E., Humphries, R. K., et al. (2001) Proliferation of primitive myeloid progenitors can be reversibly induced by HOXA10. *Blood* **98,** 3301–3308.

51. Schonig, K., Schwenk, F., Rajewsky, K., and Bujard, H. (2002) Stringent doxycycline dependent control of CRE recombinase in vivo. *Nucleic Acids Res.* **30,** e134.
52. Moody, S. E., Sarkisian, C. J., Hahn, K. T., Gunther, E. J., Pickup, S., Dugan, K. D., et al. (2002) Conditional activation of Neu in the mammary epithelium of transgenic mice results in reversible pulmonary metastasis. *Cancer Cell* **2,** 451–461.
53. Shalaby, F., Rossant, J., Yamaguchi, T. P., Gertsenstein, M., Wu, X. F., Breitman, M. L., et al. (1995) Failure of blood-island formation and vasculogenesis in Flk-1 deficient mice. *Nature* **376,** 62–66.
54. Shivdasani, R. A., Mayer, E. L., and Orkin, S. H. (1995) Absence of blood formation in mice lacking the T-cell leukaemia oncoprotein tal-1/SCL. *Nature* **373,** 432–434.
55. Porcher, C., Swat, W., Rockwell, K., Fujiwara, Y., Alt, F. W., and Orkin, S. H. (1996) The T cell leukemia oncoprotein SCL/tal-1 is essential for development of all hematopoietic lineages. *Cell* **86,** 47–57.
56. Shalaby, F., Ho, J., Stanford, W. L., Fischer, K.-D., Schuh, A. C., Schwartz, L., et al. (1997) A requirement for Flk1 in primitive and definitive hematopoiesis and vasculogenesis. *Cell* **89,** 981–990.
57. North, T., Gu, T. L., Stacy, T., Wang, Q., Howard, L., Binder, M., et al. (1999) Cbfa2 is required for the formation of intra-aortic hematopoietic clusters. *Development* **126,** 2563–2575.
58. Mikkola, H. K. A., Klintman, J., Yang, H., Hock, H., Schlaeger, T. M., Fujiwara, Y., et al. (2003) Haematopoietic stem cells retain long-term repopulating activity and multipotency in the absence of stem-cell leukaemia SCL/tal-1 gene. *Nature* **421,** 547–551.
59. Cho, S. K., Bourdeau, A., Letarte, M., and Zuniga-Pflucker, J. C. (2001) Expression and function of CD105 during the onset of hematopoiesis from Flk1(+) precursors. *Blood* **98,** 3635–3642.
60. Lacaud, G., Gore, L., Kennedy, M., Kouskoff, V., Kingsley, P., Hogan, C., et al. (2002) *Runx1* is essential for hematopoietic commitment at the hemangioblast stage of development in vitro. *Blood* **100,** 458–468.
61. Kyba, M., Perlingeiro, R. C., and Daley, G. Q. (2002) HoxB4 confers definitive lymphoid-myeloid engraftment potential on embryonic stem cell and yolk sac hematopoietic progenitors. *Cell* **109,** 29–37.
62. Sauvageau, G., Landsdorp, P. M., Eaves, C. J., Hogge, D. E., Dragowska, W. H., Reid, D. S., et al. (1994) Differential expression of homeobox genes in functionally distinct $CD34^+$ subpopulations of human bone marrow cells. *Proc. Natl. Acac. Sci. USA* **91,** 12,223–12,227.
63. McGrath, K. E. and Palis, J. (1997) Expression of homeobox genes, including an insulin promoting factor, in the murine yolk sac at the time of hematopoietic initiation. *Mol. Reprod. Dev.* **48,** 145–153.
64. Onishi, M., Nosaka, T., Misawa, K., Mui, A. L.-F., Gorman, D., McMahon, M., et al. (1998) Identification and characterization of a constitutively active STAT5 mutant that promotes cell proliferation. *Mol. Cell Biol.* **18,** 3871–3879.
65. Moriggl, R., Topham, D. J., Teglund, S., Sexl, V., McKay, C., Wang, D., et al. (1999) Stat5 activation is uniquely associated with cytokine signaling in peripheral T cells. *Immunity* **10,** 249–259.
66. Socolovsky, M., Fallon, A. E. J., Wang, S., Brugnara, C., and Lodish, H. F. (1999) Fetal anemia and apoptosis of red cell progenitors in $Stat5a^{-/-}5b^{-/-}$ mice: a direct role for Stat5 in $Bcl\text{-}X_L$ induction. *Cell* **98,** 181–191.

67. Schwaller, J., Parganas, E., Wang, D., Cain, D., Aster, J. C., Williams, I. R., et al. (2000) Stat5 is essential for the myelo- and lymphoproliferative disease induced by TEL/JAK2. *Mol. Cell* **6,** 693–704.
68. Bradley, H. L., Hawley, T. S., and Bunting, K. D. (2002) Cell intrinsic defects in cytokine responsiveness of STAT5-deficient hematopoietic stem cells. *Blood* **100,** 3983–3989.
69. Bunting, K. D., Bradley, H. L., Hawley, T. S., Moriggi, R., Sorrentino, B. P., and Ihle, J. N. (2002) Reduced lymphomyeloid repopulating activity from adult bone marrow and fetal liver of mice lacking expression of STAT5. *Blood* **99,** 479–487.
70. Snow, J. W., Abraham, N., Ma, M. C., Abbey, N. W., Herndier, B., and Goldsmith, M. A. (2002) STAT5 promotes multilineage hematolymphoid development in vivo through effects on early hematopoietic progenitor cells. *Blood* **99,** 95–101.
71. Buitenhuis, M., Baltus, B., Lammers, J.-W. J., Coffer, P. J., and Koenderman, L. (2003) Signal transducer and activator of transcription 5a (STAT5a) is required for eosinophil differentiation of human cord blood-derived CD34+ cells. *Blood* **101,** 134–142.
72. Carlesso, N., Frank, D. A., and Griffin, J. D. (1996) Tyrosyl phosphorylation and DNA binding activity of signal transducers and activators of transcription (STAT) proteins in hematopoietic cell lines transformed by Bcr/Abl. *J. Exp. Med.* **183,** 811–820.
73. Frank, D. A. and Varticovski, L. (1996) BCR/abl leads to the constitutive activation of Stat proteins, and shares an epitope with tyrosine phosphorylated Stats. *Leukemia* **10,** 1724–1730.
74. Ilaria, R. L. J. and Etten, R. A. V. (1996) P210 and P190(BCR/ABL) induce the tyrosine phosphorylation and DNA binding activity of multiple specific STAT family members. *J. Biol. Chem.* **271,** 31,704–31,710.
75. Shuai, K., Halpern, J., Hoeve, J. T., Rao, X., and Sawyers, C. L. (1996) Constitutive activation of STAT5 by the BCR-ABL oncogene in chronic myelogenous leukemia. *Oncogene* **13,** 247–254.
76. Nieborowska-Skorska, M., Wasik, M. A., Slupianek, A., Salomoni, P., Kitamura, T., Calabretta, B., and Skorski, T. (1999) Signal transducer and activator of transcription (STAT)5 activation by BCR/ABL is dependent on intact Src homology SH)3 and SH2 domains of BCR/ABL and is required for leukemogenesis. *J. Exp. Med.* **189,** 1229–1242.
77. Hoover, R. R., Gerlach, M. J., Koh, E. Y., and Daley, G. Q. (2001) Cooperative and redundant effects of STAT5 and Ras signaling in BCR/ABL transformed hematopoietic cells. *Oncogene* **20,** 5826–5835.
78. Robb, L., Elwood, N. J., Elefanty, A. G., Kontgen, F., Li, R., Barnett, L. D., and Begley, C. G. (1996) The scl gene product is required for the generation of all hematopoietic lineages in the adult mouse. *EMBO J.* **15,** 4123–4129.
79. Drake, C. J., Brandt, S. J., Trusk, T. C., and Little, C. D. (1997) TAL1/SCL is expressed in endothelial progenitor cells/angioblasts and defines a dorsal-to-ventral gradient of vasculogenesis. *Dev. Biol.* **192,** 1–30.
80. Elefanty, A. G., Begley, C. G., Metcalf, D., Barnett, L., Kontgen, F., and Robb, L. (1998) Characterization of hematopoietic progenitor cells that express the transcription factor SCL, using a lacZ "knock-in". *Proc. Natl. Acad. Sci. USA* **95,** 11,897–11,902.
81. Gering, M., Rodaway, A. R., Gottgens, B., Patient, R. K., and Green, A. R. (1998) The SCL gene specifies haemangioblast development from early mesoderm. *EMBO J.* **17,** 4029–4045.
82. Mead, P. E., Kelley, C. M., Hahn, P. S., Piedad, O., and Zon, L. I. (1998) SCL specifies hematopoietic mesoderm in *Xenopus* embryos. *Development* **125,** 2611–2620.

83. Elefanty, A. G., Begley, C. G., Hartley, L., Papaevangeliou, B., and Robb, L. (1999) SCL expression in the mouse embryo detected with a targeted lacZ reporter gene demonstrates its localization to hematopoietic, vascular, and neural tissues. *Blood* **94,** 3754–3763.
84. Robertson, S. M., Kennedy, M., Shannon, J. M., and Keller, G. (2000) A transitional stage in the commitment of mesoderm to hematopoiesis requiring the transcription factor SCL/tal-1. *Development* **127,** 2447–2459.
85. Mead, P. E., Deconinck, A. E., Huber, T. L., Orkin, S. H., and Zon, L. I. (2001) Primitive erythropoiesis in the Xenopus embryo: the synergistic role of LMO-2, SCL and GATA-binding proteins. *Development* **128,** 2301–2308.
86. Chung, Y. S., Zhang, W. J., Arentson, E., Kingsley, P. D., Palis, J., and Choi, K. (2002) Lineage analysis of the hemangioblast as defined by FLK1 and SCL expression. *Development* **129,** 5511–5520.
87. Ema, M., Faloon, P., Zhang, W. J., Hirashima, M., Reid, T., Stanford, W. L., et al. (2003) Combinatorial effects of Flk1 and Tal1 on vascular and hematopoietic development in the mouse. *Development* **17,** 380–393.
88. Hall, M. A., Curtis, D. J., Metcalf, D., Elefanty, A. G., Sourris, K., L, L. R., Gothert, J. R., et al. (2003) The critical regulator of embryonic hematopoiesis, SCL, is vital in the adult for megakaryopoiesis, erythropoiesis, and lineage choice in CFU-S12. *Proc. Natl. Acad. Sci. USA* **100,** 992–997.
89. Nakano, T., Kodama, H., and Honjo, T. (1994) Generation of lymphohematopoietic cells from embryonic stem cells in culture. *Science* **265,** 1098–1101.
90. Wutz, A. and Jaenisch, R. (2000) A shift from reversible to irreversible X inactivation is triggered during ES cell differentiation. *Mol. Cell* **5,** 695–705.
91. Wutz, A., Rasmussen, T. P., and Jaenisch, R. (2002) Chromosomal silencing and localization are mediated by different domains of Xist RNA. *Nat. Genet.* **30,** 167–174.
92. Zambrowicz, B. P., Imamoto, A., Fiering, S., Herzenberg, L. A., Kerr, W. G., and Soriano, P. (1997) Disruption of overlapping transcripts in the ROSA beta geo 26 gene trap strain leads to widespread expression of beta-galactosidase in mouse embryos and hematopoietic cells. *Proc. Natl. Acad. Sci. USA* **94,** 3789–3794.
93. Baron, U., Freundlieb, S., Gossen, M., and Bujard, H. (1995) Co-regulation of two gene activities by tetracycline via a bidirectional promoter. *Nucleic Acids Res.* **23,** 3605–3606.
94. Kyba, M., Perlingeiro, R. C. R., and Daley, G. Q. (2003) Development of hematopoietic repopulating cells from embryonic stem cells, in *Methods in Enzymology* (Wassarman, P. M. and Keller, G. M., eds.), pp. 114–129.
95. Martin, G. R. and Evans, M. J. (1975) Differentiation of clonal lines of teratocarcinoma cells: formation of embryoid bodies in vitro. *Proc. Natl. Acad. Sci. USA* **72,** 1441–1445.
96. Doetschman, T. C., Eistetter, H., Katz, M., Schmidt, W., and Kemler, R. (1985) The in vitro development of blastocyst-derived embryonic stem cell lines: formation of visceral yolk sac, blood islands and myocardium. J *Embryol. Exp. Morphol.* **87,** 27–45.
97. Schmidt, R. M., Bruyns, E., and Snodgrass, H. R. (1991) Hematopoietic development of embryonic stem cells in vitro: cytokine and receptor gene expression. *Genes Dev.* **5,** 718–740.
98. Spangrude, G. J., Heimfeld, S., and Weissman, I. L. (1988) Purification and Characterization of Mouse Hematopoietic Stem Cells. *Science* **241,** 58–62.
99. Uchida, N. and Weissman, I. L. (1992) Searching for hematopoietic stem cells: evidence that Thy-1.1lo Lin- Sca-1+ cells are the only stem cells in C57BL/Ka-Thy-1.1 bone marrow. *J. Exp. Med.* **175,** 175–184.

100. Jurecic, R., Van, N. T., and Belmont, J. W. (1993) Enrichment and functional characterization of Sca-1+WGA+, Lin-WGA+, Lin-Sca-1+, and Lin-Sca-1+WGA+ bone marrow cells from mice with an Ly-6a haplotype. *Blood* **82,** 2673–2683.
101. Uchida, N., Aguila, H. L., Fleming, W. H., Jerabek, L., and Weissman, I. L. (1994) Rapid and sustained hematopoietic recovery in lethally irradiated mice transplanted with purified Thy-1.1lo Lin-Sca-1+ hematopoietic stem cells. *Blood* **83,** 3758–3779.
102. Morrison, S. J., Hemmati, H. D., Wandycz, A. M., and Weissman, I. L. (1995) The purification and characterization of fetal liver hematopoietic stem cells. *Proc. Natl. Acac. Sci. USA* **92,** 10,302–10,306.
103. Osawa, M., Nakamura, K., Nishi, N., Takahasi, N., Tokuomoto, Y., Inoue, H., and Nakauchi, H. (1996) In vivo self-renewal of c-Kit+ Sca-1+ Lin(low/-) hemopoietic stem cells. *J. Immunol.* **156,** 3207–3214.
104. Morrison, S. J., Wandycz, A. M., Hemmati, H. D., Wright, D. E., and Weissman, I. L. (1997) Identification of a lineage of multipotent hematopoietic progenitors. *Development* **124,** 1929–1939.
105. Ma, X., Robin, C., Ottersbach, K., and Dzierzak, E. (2002) The Ly-6A (Sca-1) GFP transgene is expressed in all adult mouse hematopoietic stem cells. *Stem Cells* **20,** 514–521.
106. Hanson, P., Mathews, V., Marrus, S. H., and Graubert, T. A. (2003) Enhanced green fluorescent protein targeted to the Sca-1 (Ly-6A) locus in transgenic mice results in efficient marking of hematopoietic stem cells in vivo. *Exp. Hematol.* **31,** 159–167.
107. Ito, C. Y., Li, C. Y., Bernstein, A., Dick, J. E., and Stanford, W. L. (2003) Hematopoietic stem cell and progenitor defects in Sca-1/Ly-6A-null mice. *Blood* **101,** 517–523.
108. Mitjavila-Garcia, M. T., Cailleret, M., Godin, I., Nogueira, M. M., Cohen-Solal, K., Schiavon, V., et al. (2002) Expression of CD41 on hematopoietic progenitors derived from embryonic hematopoietic cells. *Development* **129,** 2003–2013.
109. Mikkola, H. K., Fujiwara, Y., Schlaeger, T. M., Traver, D., and Orkin, S. H. (2003) Expression of CD41 marks the initiation of definitive hematopoiesis in the mouse embryo. *Blood* **101,** 508–516.
110. Shockett, P., Difilippantonio, M., Hellman, N., and Schatz, D. G. (1995) A modified tetracycline-regulated system provides autoregulatory, inducible gene expression in cultured cells and transgenic mice. *Proc. Natl. Acad. Sci. USA* **92,** 6522–6526.
111. Urlinger, S., Baron, U., Thellmann, M., Hasan, M. T., Bujard, H., and Hillen, W. (2000) Exploring the sequence space for tetracycline-dependent transcriptional activators: novel mutations yield expanded range and sensitivity. *Proc. Natl. Acad. Sci. USA* **97,** 7963–7968.
112. Akagi, K., Kanai, M., Saya, H., Kozu, T., and Berns, A. (2001) A novel tetracycline-dependent transactivator with E2F4 transcriptional activation domain. *Nucleic Acids Res.* **29,** E23.
113. Chung, S., Andersson, T., Sonntag, K. C., Bjorklund, L., Isacson, O., and Kim, K. S. (2002) Analysis of different promoter systems for efficient transgene expression in mouse embryonic stem cell lines. *Stem Cells* **20,** 139–145.
114. Baron, U., Schnappinger, D., Helbl, V., Gossen, M., Hillen, W., and Bujard, H. (1999) Generation of conditional mutants in higher eukaryotes by switching between the expression of two genes. *Proc. Natl. Acad. Sci. USA* **96,** 1013–1018.

3

Quantitative Trait Analysis in the Investigation of Function and Aging of Hematopoietic Stem Cells

Hans-Willem Snoeck

Summary

Extensive genetically determined quantitative variation exists in the number and function of hematopoietic stem cells in inbred mouse strains. Furthermore, aging of hematopoietic stem cells is genetically determined. Gene identification of quantitative trait loci involved in the regulation and aging of hematopoietic stem cells would provide novel insights into regulatory mechanisms that are relevant in vivo and may be clinically important. Here we describe strategies for mapping and gene identification of quantitative trait loci applied to traits contributing to the regulation of hematopoietic stem cells.

Key Words: Hematopoietic stem cell; quantitative trait locus; aging; inbred mice; genetic trait.

1. Introduction

The mechanisms responsible for the regulation of self-renewal and differentiation of hematopoietic stem cells (HSCs) in vivo are unclear ***(1,2)***. The observation that the total HSC number differs in different strains of inbred mice provides strong evidence that these mechanisms are, in part, genetically determined ***(3–8)***. A powerful approach to begin to dissect regulation of the HSC compartment is the investigation of genetically determined variation by quantitative trait analysis. Quantitative traits are traits that vary continuously across genetically different individuals and are inherited in a non-Mendelian fashion because of the contribution of multiple loci to the phenotype. These loci are called quantitative trait loci, or QTL ***(9–11)***. Here we will briefly review quantitative genetic variation in the biology of HSC in inbred mice and discuss the rationale for pursuing this approach, followed by an overview of mapping strategies that are relevant to the investigation of the quantitative variation in the HSC compartment and an outline of potential strategies for gene identification for QTL.

From: *Methods in Molecular Medicine, Vol. 105: Developmental Hematopoiesis: Methods and Protocols.*
Edited by: M. H. Baron © Humana Press Inc., Totowa, NJ

2. Genetic Variation in the Hematopoietic Stem Cell Compartment in Inbred Mouse Strains

In embryo-aggregated chimeric DBA/2-C57BL/6 mice, DBA/2-derived stem cells contribute significantly and stably to hematopoiesis in young adults, but upon aging, C57BL/6-derived hematopoiesis becomes predominant, if not exclusive. A key finding from these studies was that because the microenvironment in these chimeric mice was identical for both DBA/2- and C57BL/6-derived stem cells, stem cell-intrinsic mechanisms underlie these differences *(3,4)*. Consistent with the observations in allophenic mice, the number of putative HSC as determined by competitive repopulation tends to increase with aging in C57BL/6 mice, whereas in other mouse strains, such a BALB/c and DBA/2, repopulating HSC numbers decrease upon aging *(12)*. Upon serial transplantation, however, the repopulation capacity of C57BL/6-derived HSC also declines *(12,13)*. The difference in age-related changes in HSC between C57BL/6 and other mouse strains is, therefore, quantitative rather than qualitative. Linkage analysis for repopulation capacity in vivo is difficult because of histoincompatibility between genetically different sources of competing HSC and any potential recipient mouse strain. Efforts have been undertaken to identify genetic variation in the HSC compartment of young and old inbred mice, using in vitro assays, and to perform linkage analysis to map relevant QTL. Putative stem cell pool size, as determined by the d 35 cobblestone area-forming cell assay (CAFCd35), varies widely among inbred mouse strains, and is higher in young DBA/2 than in young C57BL/6 mice *(5)*. Loci involved in the regulation of HSC frequency were mapped to mouse chromosome 18 using the CAFCd35 assay *(5)*, and to chromosome 1 using another surrogate HSC assay, the long-term culture initiating cell assay *(8)*. With age, CAFCd35 expand in C57BL/6 mice but decrease in DBA/2 *(14,15)*. This is consistent with the fact that, upon aging, HSC function in vivo is better preserved in C57BL/6 than in other mouse strains. A locus on chromosome 2 was found to contribute to the expansion of CAFCd35 in C57BL/6 mice *(15)*. A QTL contributing to lifespan was also found in this region of chromosome 2 (70 cM) *(16)*. It is interesting to note that C57BL/6 is one of the longest-living mouse strains, suggesting a role for the HSC compartment in the regulation of longevity. Further supporting the idea of a link between the kinetics of the hematopoietic stem and progenitor cell compartment and longevity is the observation that cycling of bone marrow progenitor cells correlates inversely with life span in BXD recombinant inbred mouse strains, and that both traits map to the same regions on chromosomes 7 and 11 *(16)*. Using the number of HSC as determined by phenotype as a surrogate marker for the repopulation capacity, QTL were identified on chromosomes 2, 4, and 7 in one study *(6)* and on chromosome 17 in another study *(7)*. Other traits that show mouse strain-dependent variation include the efficiency of mobilization of progenitor cells to the peripheral blood (chromosomes 2 and 11; **ref.** *17)* and the responsiveness of primitive progenitor cells to the early-acting cytokines (chromosome 2 and X; **ref.** ***6***. It is interesting to note that three groups of investigators mapped at least five traits roughly to same region in the middle of the terminal half of chromosome 2: responsiveness of HSC to early-acting cytokines *(6)*, the number of lin-Sca++kit+ cells *(6)*, the efficiency of mobilization of HSC *(17)*, the expansion of CAFC35 with age *(14)*, and lifespan *(16)*. These results may suggest that at least some of these traits are not independent from one another, and again raise the possibility of a link between longevity and HSC.

3. Rationale for Investigating Quantitative Genetic Variation in the HSC Compartment

Identification of the genes contributing to traits such as HSC pool size, efficiency of mobilization of HSC, aging of HSC, and longevity would shed light on the regulation of HSC and on the potential contribution of HSC to longevity. These are obviously medically relevant traits. The identification of QTL in the mouse system may have clinical relevance, as susceptibility to many diseases and the efficacy of therapeutic modalities are polygenic or complex traits in humans. Some QTL, such as those contributing to susceptibility of type I diabetes *(18)* and to systemic lupus erythematosus *(19)*, map to similar locations in mice and humans. Analyzing QTL in a genetically tractable organism such as the mouse, followed by a more focused search for linkage with orthologous loci in humans, is thus a valid strategy. Furthermore, gene identification of a QTL can reveal the involvement of genes in the regulation of HSC that could not be or were not yet identified as regulatory genes for HSC using knockout approaches.

4. Strategies for Linkage Analysis of QTL Affecting the Biology of HSCs

There are four classical approaches to performing linkage analysis of quantitative traits in inbred mice. These involve the use of backcross, intercross, advanced intercross, and recombinant inbred mice *(20–23)*. A fifth approach, involving chromosome substitution strains, was recently proposed *(24)*.

4.1. Backcross, Intercross, and Advanced Intercross Designs

In a strategy involving backcrossing, two inbred mouse strains with a quantitatively different phenotype for a given trait are intercrossed, followed by backcrossing of the F1 offspring onto one of the parental strains (**Fig. 1**). In the strategy involving intercrossing, F1 mice are intercrossed to obtain a set of F2 mice (**Fig. 2**). To produce advanced intercross mice, F2 mice are crossed semirandomly, to avoid inbreeding, so that more recombinations are accumulated for linkage analysis. The N2 (backcross), F2 (intercross), or advanced intercross mice are then phenotyped and genotyped for polymorphic markers. If a trait is polygenic, then a continuum of values will be observed across the respective populations. Genotyping all the individual progeny for markers that show allelic variation between the parental strains (either single nucleotide polymorphisms or simple sequence repeats) will allow the detection of associations between trait values and marker genotype, and in this way demonstrate to which set of markers a QTL is linked. To reduce the genotyping effort, selective genotyping of the individuals at the extremes of the phenotypic spectrum can be performed *(20,23)*. Although these three approaches are in general considered to be the best to detect and map QTL, they have several disadvantages for quantitative traits involving HSC. For instance, they rely on randomly segregating populations, so each recombinant is unique

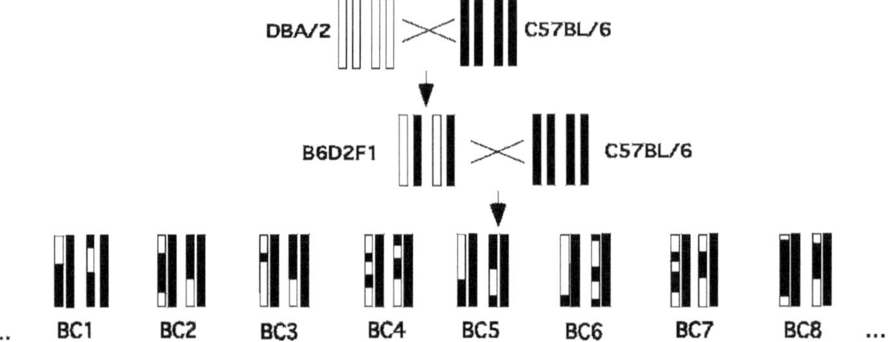

Fig. 1. Schematic representation of the generation of a set of backcross (BC) mice using C57BL6 mice as the background strain.

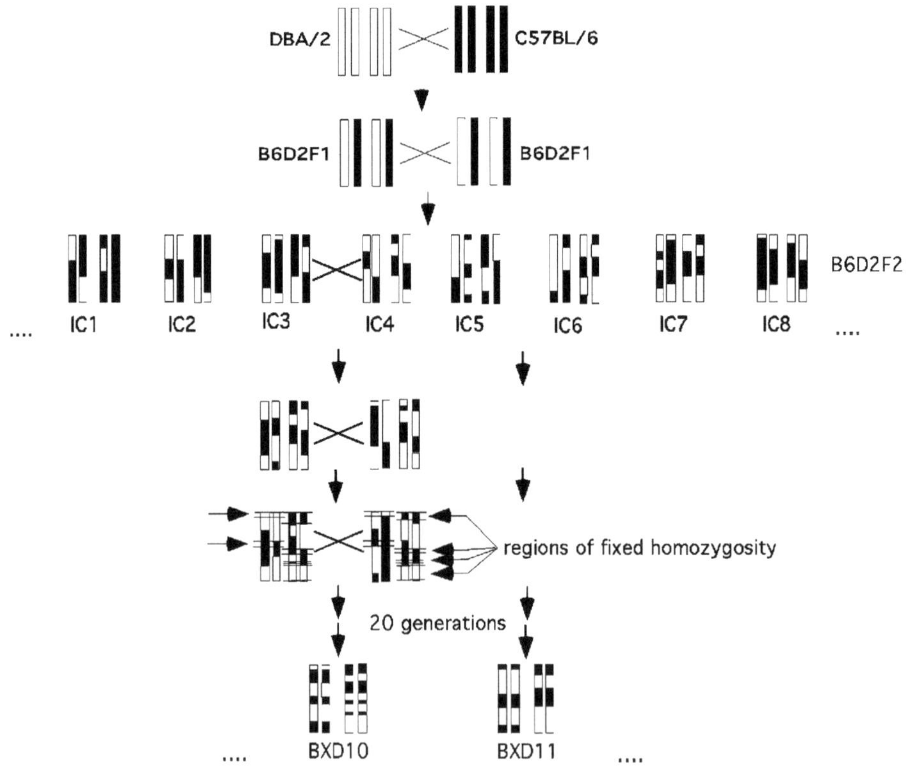

Fig. 2. Schematic representation of the generation of a set of B6D2F2 intercross (IC) mice. These intercross mice are then inbred for 20 generations to obtain a set of BXD recombinant inbred mice.

and can only be phenotyped once. This is a problem if a technically complex trait is measured or when HSC pooled from several identical mice are required to obtain a reliable measurement of the trait under study. For example, measuring the responsiveness of putative HSC to cytokines involves harvesting bone marrow, if possible from several genetically identical mice, labeling with antibodies, cell sorting and culture. The multiple manipulations involved introduce a significant error. The impact of phenotyping errors on linkage analysis is significant, unless extremely large numbers of progeny are tested ***(9–11,20,23)***.

4.2. Recombinant Inbred Strains

4.2.1. Description

In the setting of the analysis of QTL involved in the regulation of HSC, recombinant inbred (RI) strains offer particular advantages ***(22,23)***. RI strains are commercially available and were generated by repeated inbreeding of F2 mice derived from two parental inbred strains. After 20 generations of inbreeding, a set of RI strains is obtained (**Fig. 2**). The genome of the individual RI strains of the set is composed of a patchwork of homozygous chromosome segments derived from either progenitor strain, with each of the RI lines having a unique combination of "patches" from the progenitor. Each RI strain will have the genotype of one or of the other progenitor at a given locus. RI strains are named by the short form of the name of one progenitor, followed by "X" and the short of form of the name of the other progenitor, and by the strain number. RI strains derived from C57BL/6 and DBA/2 mice are thus called BXD strains.

4.2.2. Available Sets of RI Strains

Several sets of RI strains have been developed over the last decades. At least 15 RI strains have to be analyzed to have some chance of identifying a QTL with large effect ***(10)***. In many sets, however, insufficient numbers of individual strains have been generated for QTL analysis. A list of available RI strains can be found at http://jaxmice.jax.org/info/recombinant.html. The most frequently used RI strains are the BXD (35 strains), AXB (25 strains), and BXA (24 strains) sets, (AXB and BXA have A/J and C57BL/6J mice as progenitors). A large number of markers, mostly simple sequence repeats, that are polymorphic between C57BL/6 and DBA/2 and between A and C57BL/6 mice have been identified, so that these markers are spaced by 1 to 2 cM. These are the only large RI sets that are readily available. Other sets, such as AKXD (with AKR and DBA/2 mice as progenitors), are cryopreserved. When choosing between different sets of RI strains for linkage analysis of traits related to the HSC compartment, the mouse strain-dependent variation in the phenotype of HSC has to be taken into account as well. HSC are enriched in the lin-Sca1++kit+ population of the bone marrow. There is allelic variation in the Sca1 (Ly6A/E) gene, of which two alleles are known, Ly6A/E^a and Ly6A/E^b. All the repopulating stem cells are within the lin-Sca1+ population in Ly6A/E^b mice (such as C57BL/6, DBA/2, BXD RI strains, and AKR), whereas only a minority of the stem cells are Sca1+ in Ly6A/E^a mouse strains (such as A, CBA, C3H and BALB/c) ***(25)***. Therefore, it is difficult to compare data obtained from RI strains that show allelic variation at the Ly6A/E locus when isolation or detection of HSC using the expression of Sca1 is involved in generating the data. BXD RI strains are therefore currently the most interesting set for linkage analysis of QTL contributing to the regulation of the HSC compartment.

4.2.3. Linkage Analysis Using Recombinant Inbred Strains

4.2.3.1. Phenotyping of RI Strains

Linkage analysis is performed by determining the relevant trait in each of the strains of a set of RI strains, which results in a strain-distribution pattern (SDP) of trait values *(23,26)*. A typical feature of the SDP for a multigenic or complex trait across a set of RI strains is that the phenotypic spread among RI strains may be wider than between the two progenitor strains. This occurs when each of the progenitor strains has a mixture of positively and negatively acting alleles. Some of the RI strains can then display more extreme phenotypes than the progenitor strains, if they have accumulated most of the positive or most of the negative alleles for that trait from the progenitor strains. Phenotypic spread among BXD strains thus actually represents the phenotypic spread in the F2 generation, and not of the progenitor strains *(10,23)*. Therefore, if quantitative variation is observed for a trait among inbred mouse strains, it is justifiable to attempt linkage analysis using BXD RI strains, even when the progenitors, C57BL/6 and DBA/2, happen to have a similar phenotype for this trait.

4.2.3.2. Statistical Analysis

The association of the SDP of the trait under study with the SDP of polymorphic markers is statistically analyzed. There are several software packages available to analyze the data *(27)*. Map ManagerQTb29ppc software developed by Manley *(27)* is user-friendly, can analyze data generated in RI strains, and allows permutation testing (*see* **Subheading 4.2.3.3.**). This software statistically analyzes the linkage of a given trait with previously typed polymorphic loci in the RI strains. This allows assignment of a trait to a corresponding map position and the calculation of statistical significance. The SDP of the marker genotypes across the set of RI strains is available in genetic maps, which can be downloaded from mapping databases such as www.nervenet.org/papers/bxn.html *(28)* or from http://www.informatics.jax.org/searches/riset_form.shtml and imported into Map Manager. QTL analysis can now be performed online using a website (http://webqtl.org/cgi-bin/WebQTL.py), where the data are analyzed using the algorithms implemented in the MapManager software. This website also allows comparing and correlating a given SDP with other sets of phenotypic and expression data generated in RI strains. A subroutine of the Map Manager QT software and of WebQTL, using computationally efficient regression equations, is used for determining the location of QTLs. The probability of linkage between a trait under study and previously mapped genotypes is estimated at 1-cM intervals along the entire genome, except for the Y chromosome. This is called interval mapping.

4.2.3.3. Genome-Wide Significance Levels

Although a detailed description of the statistical analysis implemented in the MapManager software and in WebQTL is beyond the scope of this review (for more details, *see* **refs. *26, 29,*** and ***30***), a discussion of the significance levels necessary to accept linkage is useful, however. The statistical interpretation of linkage data is complicated by multiple testing when the SDP of the trait under investigation is compared with the SDP of multiple polymorphic markers. A concordance between the SDP of the trait under study and the SDP of a given marker may appear significant at the p = 0.05 level. This is called a point-wise significance level. However, because this test is repeated across the genome on hundreds to thousands of markers, the probability of finding an association at this significance level somewhere in the genome is very high and can be calculated to occur on average once per chromosome when a dense genetic map is assumed ***(29)***. A point-wise significance cutoff of 0.05 would therefore clearly yield a large number of false QTL. A point-wise p-value of 0.05 thus corresponds to a much higher genome-wide p-value and more stringent significance cutoff values are required. Linkage data also are expressed by a logarithm of odds score or LOD score. A LOD score is the log of the ratio between the probability of obtaining the observed data under the hypothesis of linkage with a marker and the probability of obtaining these data under the null hypothesis of no linkage. The LOD score follows a chi-square distribution for a large numbers of individuals tested, and can be converted to a chi-square value by multiplying by 4.61. This is the likelihood ratio statistic (LRS), which is provided by the Map Manager software and on the WebQTL site. The associated p-value actually represents the probability of obtaining a given LOD score or LRS value by coincidence. A good and probably the best way to determine which LRS or point-wise p-values indicate significant linkage is permutation analysis ***(30)***. Here, the genome-wide probability of obtaining the observed linkage by random chance corresponding to a given genome-wide error threshold is calculated using a nonparametric permutation method. The peak LOD score or LRS value of the correctly ordered data obtained in the study is compared with the peak LOD scores or LRS values computed for 5000 random permutations of the same data while maintaining the same genetic map during all the permutations of the experimental data. Thus, if in only one in a thousand random permutations a given LOD score is exceeded, then the genome-wide probability of a false-positive would be approx 0.001 when this LOD score is used as a significance threshold. This is considered highly significant linkage. A genome-wide p-value of 0.05 is considered significant linkage, whereas $p = 0.5$ error threshold is considered,"suggestive" of a QTL ***(30)***. In a typical experiment, suggestive linkage will require a LOD score of more than 2.2, whereas an LOD score of more than 3.6 will generally indicate significant linkage. This will correspond to point-wise p-values of approx 0.001 and 0.0001, respectively. Permutation analysis is implemented in the Map Manager software and is automatically performed in WebQTL.

4.2.4. Advantages and Limitations of RI Strains for QTL Analysis

Because RI strains are homozygous in all their loci, they can be propagated and expanded indefinitely. Therefore, multiple independent phenotype measurements can be performed so that a mean and a standard error, based on independent measurements in multiple identical individuals, can be associated with each genotype. This can enormously reduce the measurement error and is especially useful for aging studies because stochastic and environmental variation in lifespan can be significant.

Furthermore, using RI strains, multiple individuals can be pooled to obtain sufficient numbers of rare cells, such as putative HSC. Mapping can be performed for both recessive and dominant loci because all the RI strains are homozygous in all their loci. There is no need for genotyping because dense genetic maps of polymorphic markers are available, making the use of RI strains both cost and time efficient. A final advantage is that a locus in RI strains will be transmitted, on average, through four generations before it is fixed to homozygosity ***(20,23)***. The resolving power in terms of map location of RI strains is thus fourfold higher than in a backcross design if the same number of animals is used. Because mapping resolution depends on the number of recombinations in the population under study, this immediately shows a disadvantage of RI strains as well. The investigator can breed as many backcross or F2 mice as needed to obtain a desired mapping resolution and statistical power, whereas in RI strains, the number of strains available is limited. Many QTL may therefore be missed, and only a few QTL with large effect will be detected. These QTL will be mapped with a relatively low resolution, in an interval of 20 to 40 cM. Furthermore, closely linked QTL with effects in the same direction will be interpreted as one large QTL. If this is the case, then this will become obvious when fine-mapping is attempted (*see* **Subheading 5.2.**). Conversely, if a chromosome segment contains several QTL with opposite effect on the phenotype, these will go undetected. Finally, it is important to realize that, in general, the contribution of a QTL to a phenotype tends to be overestimated. Because probably only a small fraction of the many QTL contributing to a trait are detected, it is only those QTL whose contribution happens to be pushed over the significance cut-off by random background variation in the phenotype in a given experiment that are identified. Many weak QTL are therefore not confirmed in subsequent rounds of linkage analysis. However, confirmation of a QTL in an independent linkage experiment would strongly increase the confidence in the existence and location of the QTL, even if the QTL is only mapped with a suggestive level of significance in each independent experiment ***(10)***.

4.3. Chromosome Substitution Strains (CSS)

CSS carry one entire chromosome from one mouse strain on the genetic background of another mouse strain ***(24)***. They are produced by repeated backcrossing onto the background strain while selecting at each generation offspring that have not undergone recombination in one chromosome. After ten generations, the backcrossed mice are considered heterosomic for one chromosome, and homozygous in all other loci. One round of inbreeding then yields homozygous CSS. Phenotypic analysis of a set of CSS covering all chromosomes will immediately indicate the chromosomal location of a QTL. The advantages are similar to those of RI strains, with the added benefit that the statistical problem of multiple testing is less important here, simplifying statistical analysis and making false positives less likely. One disadvantage of RI strains is exacerbated in CSS, however. If multiple QTL are located on the same chromosome, then these will be interpreted as one large QTL if they act in the same direction, or may be missed if their contributions cancel each other. CSS are a good starting point to construct congenic mice (*see* **Subheading 5.1.1.**). Only reciprocal CSS derived from C57BL/6 and A mice are currently available, however ***(24)***.

5. Gene Identification of QTL

Gene identification of QTL contributing to the regulation of HSC has not been achieved yet. A theoretical outline of how to proceed with gene identification of these QTL is given here.

5.1. Confirming a QTL: Congenic Mice

The first step in gene identification of a QTL is to confirm the presence and the location of the QTL by constructing congenic mice ***(9–11,20,23)***. Congenic mice have a homozygous chromosome segment of one inbred strain (the donor) on the genetic background of another inbred strain (the acceptor).

5.1.1. Generation of Congenic Mice

Construction of congenic mice normally requires one generation of outcrossing, 10 generations of backcrossing onto the acceptor strain, followed by one round of inbreeding. Selection is performed in each backcross generation by genotyping for two markers flanking the region of interest. More than 98% of the genome is of acceptor background after ten generations if selection is performed for a 20-cM segment (B6D2-chromosome no. in **Fig. 3**). Ideally, reciprocal congenics should be constructed. The production of congenic mice can be sped up by selecting offspring with the lowest degree of heterozygosity for recipient strain markers (as part of a normal distribution around an expected degree of heterozygosity at each backcross generation), while retaining the markers in the region of interest of donor origin in a heterozygous state. Using this protocol, called a marker-assisted selection protocol, congenics can be made in five generations ***(31,32)***. In this protocol, backcross offspring is genotyped for a limited number of markers scattered throughout the genome. Markers for which homozygosity has been fixed do not have to be tested anymore in the subsequent backcross generations, so that the number of markers to be tested decreases by at least 50% per generation. Because animals with the highest level of acceptor strain homozygosity will be selected, the number of markers to be tested will in fact be reduced by more than 50% per generation. Because a selected male can breed with several females, males are exclusively selected at each generation for backcrossing. Models using optimized numbers of offspring and markers based on computer simulations suggest that genotyping 16 offspring per generation is sufficient ***(31)***. This process can be sped up further by using an appropriate RI strain as the donor (**Fig. 3**). On average, 50% of the loci are homozygously derived from each of the progenitors in any RI strain. Therefore, one more round of breeding can be omitted and the number of markers to be tested is reduced by another 50%. It may even be possible to a choose a BXD strain that has the appropriate chromosome segment of DBA/2 origin, and more than 50% of the remainder of the genome of C57BL/6 origin, which may reduce the number of markers to be tested even further. After four generations of marker-assisted selection, homozygous mice are obtained by one round of inbreeding (**Fig. 3**). Genotyping, and even breeding, can be outsourced to Charles River Laboratories (Wilmington, MA; http://www.criver.com/) or to the Jackson Laboratory (Bar Harbor, ME; http://www.jax.org/). Primers to detect simple sequence repeats and appropriate genotyping protocols can be purchased from Research Genetics (Huntington, AL; http://www.resgen.com/).

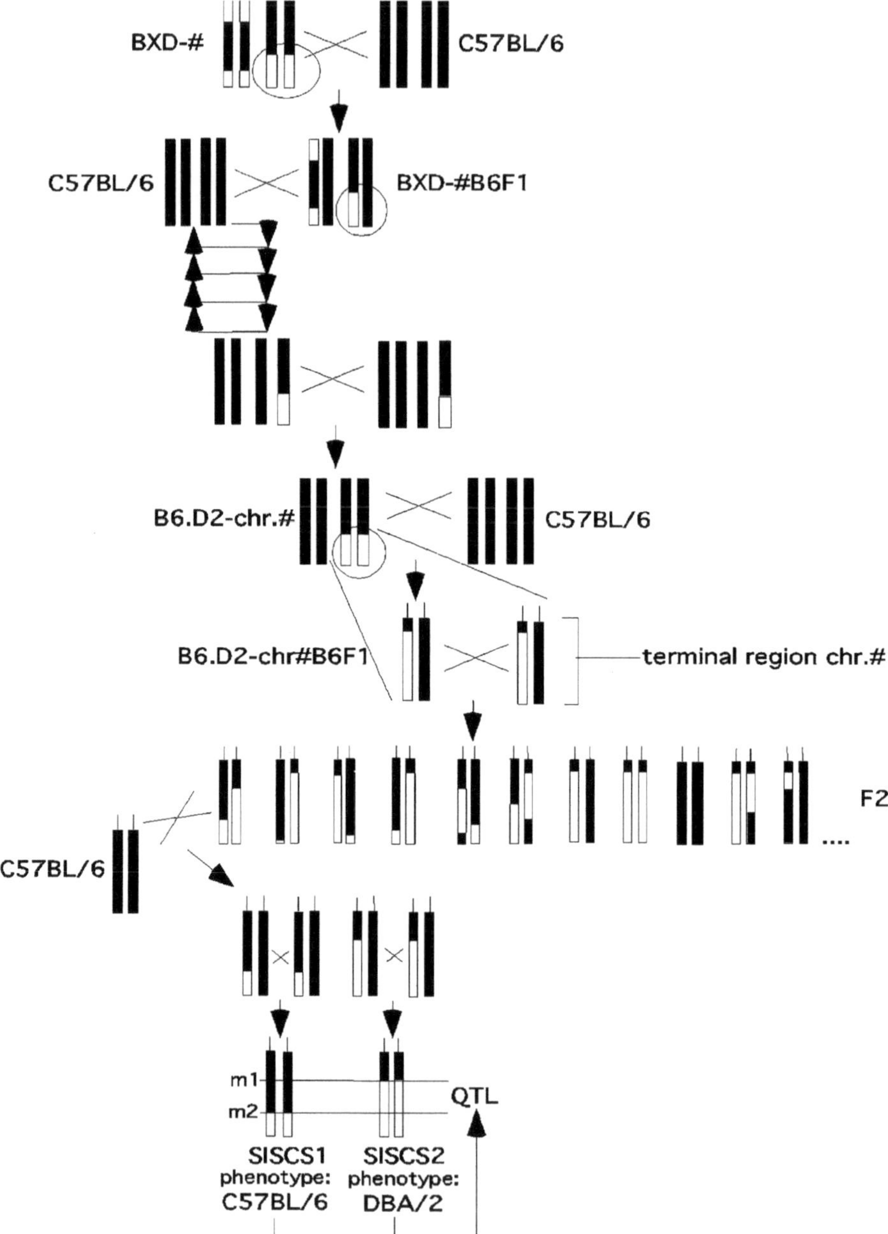

Fig. 3. Schematic representation of the generation of B6.D2 congenic mice, where a segment of a DBA/2 chromosome is introgressed into the C57BL/6 background, starting from an appropriate BXD recombinant inbred strain. The introgressed chromosome segment (terminal region of chr. no. in the figure) can be further subdivided by producing SISCS, which allows fine mapping of the QTL of interest.

5.1.2. Analysis of Congenic Mice

Congenic mice are homozygous and can be propagated indefinitely. This will allow not only confirmation of the location of a QTL but also testing for biologically and technically more complex traits such as competitive repopulation capacity. Linkage analysis in the context of HSC is typically performed using in vitro assays that are believed to be surrogate assays for stem cell function in vivo ***(5–8)***. Examples are the CAFCd35 assay ***(5)***, the long-term culture-initiating cell assay (8), and the enumeration of HSC as defined by phenotype ***(6,7)***. The gold standard for measuring stem cell number and function in vivo is competitive repopulation ***(33)***. There is currently no in vitro assay that unequivocally reflects competitive repopulation capacity. Linkage analysis for competitive repopulation capacity is impossible because of the genetic, and, therefore, the immunological heterogeneity of the progeny to be tested. The construction of mice congenic for a chromosome segment that is believed to contribute to quantitative variation in a surrogate HSC assay will thus allow evaluation of whether the same locus also affects repopulation capacity in vivo. The congenic mice will be histocompatible with the background strain because only 1 to 2% of their genome is donor-strain derived. When the background strain is C57BL/6, allelic variation at the CD45 locus can be used to differentiate the competing cell populations. Note that when the introgressed region (i.e., the region of the donor strain that is bred onto the genetic background of the acceptor strain) contains the major histocomptability complex region or known regions containing minor histocompatibility regions, congenic and background mice will not be histocompatible. It is therefore prudent to perform mixed lymphocyte reactions before initiating repopulation studies.

The location of many QTL related to the hematopoietic system has now been confirmed in congenic mice ***(6,14)***. However, if a phenotype cannot be reproduced in the congenics, then, assuming that the QTL was correctly mapped, epistasis with QTL outside the introgressed region is the most plausible explanation ***(9–11,26)***. Epistasis is the genetic interaction in which the combined effect of two or more loci exceeds the sum of the effect of the individual loci. It is unknown how frequent significant epistatic interactions are in quantitative trait variation, and QTL methods to detect epistasis have been notoriously poor.

5.2. Fine Mapping of a QTL

5.2.1. Strategies for Fine Mapping

The introgressed region in congenic mice will usually span 10 to 40 cM. This region is too large for a candidate gene approach and needs to be refined. The next stage in the gene identification of a QTL is fine-mapping. Several strategies are available for fine-mapping of a QTL, including selective phenotyping of large F2 or backcross populations, recombinant progeny testing, recombinant inbred segregation testing, and construction of subinterval-specific congenic strains (SISCS) ***(21,34)***. All of these strategies are based on the principle of "genetic chromosome dissection" pioneered in *Drosophila* ***(35–37)***. Except for the construction of SISCS, these methods rely on randomly segregating populations, so each recombinant is unique. This is again a problem if a technically complex trait is measured, if HSC from more than one mouse are required for phenotyping, or when competitive repopulation capacity is investigated.

Theoretically, the best approach to fine-mapping of a hematopoietic trait is the construction of SISCS, where one small segment of the interval of interest, of donor origin in the original congenics, is replaced by a segment derived from the acceptor strain *(34)*. A set of SISCS that covers the interval of interest thus allows fine-mapping of a QTL with a 1 to 2-cM resolution. SISCS are again homozygous inbred mice that can be propagated and used in competitive repopulation studies.

5.2.2. Generation and Analysis of Subinterval-Specific Congenic Strains

With congenic mice in hand where, except for a 10 to 40 cM of introgressed genome, the whole genome is of background origin, SISCS covering this interval can be produced in four generations, and this only requires a limited set of markers to be tested to obtain a 2-cM resolution. The principle, using C57BL/6 and DBA/2 mice as progenitors in this example is as follows (**Fig. 3**). The congenic mice (B6.D2-chromsome no. in **Fig. 3**) are backcrossed with the C57BL/6 parental strain, and then intercrossed to obtain F2 mice. A subset of these mice will have recombinations within the introgressed DBA/2-derived chromosome segment. All other recombination events are irrelevant because the background of the congenics is the same as the parental strain. A set of recombinants is then chosen so that they cover the interval of interest. These are backcrossed with C57BL/6 mice, and appropriate heterozygous offspring in which there is no further recombination within the desired DBA/2-derived segment are inbred to yield the homozygous SISCS. In a total of nine generations, congenic mice and a set of SISCS can be generated that will allow fine mapping of a trait with a 1 to 2-cM resolution, and that can be propagated indefinitely. A critical question in the evaluation of the feasibility of this approach is how many mice need to be genotyped in the F2 generation (**step 2** in the production of SISCS) to assure the detection of at least one recombinant per given cM interval. Darvasi calculated that to find ten recombinants (covering a 10-cM region at 1-cM intervals or a 20-cM region at 2-cM intervals), approx 150 F2 animals (a feasible number) have to be genotyped *(34)*.

If the trait under study is reproduced in one of the SISCS, then fine mapping to a 1 to 2-cM resolution has been achieved. However, this is not necessarily the case. If a trait cannot be reproduced in any of the SISCS, then it is likely that several epistatic or interacting loci are present on the introgressed chromosome segment. Since genes that are functional in similar pathways are sometimes clustered together, this possibility cannot be dismissed. Separating interacting QTL in SISCS can thus abolish the phenotype. Intercrossing SISCS to recreate larger segments of the introgressed chromosome segment may then be envisaged.

5.3. Gene Identification of a QTL

5.3.1. Selection of Candidate Genes

Once a mapping resolution of 1 to 2 cM or less is obtained, the candidate gene approach can be taken. The progress of the Mouse Genome Project makes this approach feasible *(38)*. One cM contains on average (assuming a genome of 1700 cM, with 34,000 genes) 20 genes. If there are too many candidate genes in the mapped interval, then the number of candidate genes can be reduced by further fine-mapping.

The next question is which candidate genes to choose. The presence or absence of sequence polymorphisms in a coding region is not a useful criterion because SNPs occur on average every 1 kB and expression of a gene may be regulated by sequences that are multiple kB away, or that are located in introns ***(9–11,35–37)***. However, genetic variation in the HSC compartment is at least in part caused by cell intrinsic mechanisms ***(3–5)***. Therefore, genes that are not expressed in HSC can initially be discarded, for traits that are thought be intrinsic to the HSC. Mouse strain-dependent differential expression of a gene that maps to the fine-mapped interval is very compelling, especially if differential expression is limited to HSC. However, many genes in a given genomic region may be differentially expressed between congenic and background mouse strains, as has recently been shown for a region of chromosome 11 where a QTL regulating cycling activity of progenitors is located ***(39)***. This could be due to a polymorphism that affects chromatin structure in that region. It is likely that only one or a few of these genes will contribute to the quantitative trait under study.

5.3.2. Confirmation of Candidate Genes

The next step is to prove that a particular gene is involved in the quantitative trait under study. This is done by complementation of a QTL, which can be achieved in several ways ***(9–11,40)***. In principle, transgenic complementation is the most straightforward. This approach has been used successfully to demonstrate that Pla2g2a was the correct candidate gene for Mom1, a modifier of the apc^{min} allele that causes adenomatous polyposis coli ***(41)***. A second example is the spontaneously hypertensive rat, a model for essential hypertension, hyperlipidemia, and human insulin-resistance syndromes including type 2 diabetes (collectively known as syndrome X or metabolic overlap syndrome), where QTL were identified on rat chromosome 4 and 12. Subsequent efforts at gene identification of the QTL on chromsome 4 using strategies that included the construction of congenics, yielded Cd36, a fatty acid translocase, as a causative gene contributing to the metabolic phenotype ***(42)***. Transgenic complementation of Cd36 in spontaneously hypertensive rats reversed insulin resistance ***(43)***.

Transgenic complementation is difficult to achieve rapidly, especially on a C57BL/6 background, and if several candidate genes are to be tested. A trait intrinsic to HSC offers a unique opportunity to pursue this approach. In HSC, the equivalent of transgenic complementation and overexpression can be achieved by retroviral expression of the appropriate candidate gene and analysis of the behavior of the transduced HSC after reconstitution of a lethally irradiated recipient. Overexpression of the gene under study in HSC should affect the hematopoietic phenotype of the mice congenic for the “low” allele of the fine-mapped locus. This would be acceptable evidence that a particular gene is indeed responsible for the quantitative trait. Further confirmation of the QTL can be achieved by quantitative complementation, where the effect of a QTL is assessed in the context of a deficient allele of a candidate gene on the same genetic background.

Gene identification of QTL should be distinguished from identification of the quantitative trait nucleotide (QTN). The latter is a daunting task, since SNPs are so frequent. Final proof for a QTN in mice would require placing a genomic segment containing the putative QTN from a donor mouse strain on the background of another strain using homologous recombination and reproducing the phenotype of the donor strain.

References

1. Morrison, S. J. and Weissman, I. L. (1995) The biology of hematopoietic stem cells. *Ann. Rev. Cell Dev. Biol.* **11,** 35–71
2. Weissman, I. L., Anderson, D. J., and Gage, F. (2001) Stem and progenitor cells: origins, phenotypes, lineage commitments, and transdifferentiations. *Annu. Rev. Cell Dev. Biol.* **17,** 387–403.
3. Van Zant, G., Eldridge, P. W., Behringer, R. R., and Dewey, M. J. (1983) Genetic control of hematopoietic kinetics revealed by analysis of allophenic mice and stem cell suicide. *Cell* **35,** 639–641
4. Van Zant, G., Holland, B. P., Eldridge, P. W., and Chen, J. J. (1990) Genotype-restricted growth and aging patterns in hematopoietic stem cell populations of allophenic mice. *J. Exp. Med.* **171,** 1547–1565.
5. de Haan, G. and Van Zant, G. (1997) Intrinsic and extrinsic control of hematopoietic stem cell numbers: mapping of a stem cell gene. *J. Exp. Med.* **186,** 529–536.
6. Henckaerts, E., Geiger, H., Langer, J. C., Rebollo, P. Van Zant, G., and Snoeck, H. W. (2002) Genetically determined variation in the number of phenotypically defined hematopoietic progenitor and stem cells and in their response to early-acting cytokines. *Blood* **99,** 3947–3954.
7. Morrison, S. J., Qian, D., Jerabek, L., Thiel, B. A., Park, I. K., Ford, P. S., et al. (2002) A genetic determinant that specifically regulates the frequency of hematopoietic stem cells. *J. Immunol.* **168,** 635–642.
8. Muller-Sieberg, C. E. and Riblet, R. (1996) Genetic control of the frequency of hematopoietic stem cells in mice: mapping of a candidate locus to chromosome 1. *J. Exp. Med.* **171,** 1141–1150.
9. Mackay, T. F. C. (2001) The genetic architecture of quantitative traits. *Annu. Rev. Genet.* **35,** 303–339.
10. Moore, K. J. and Nagle D. L. (2000) Complex trait analysis in the mouse: the strengths, the limitations and the promises yet to come. *Annu. Rev. Genet.* **34,** 653–686.
11. Flint, J. and Mott, R. (2001) Finding the molecular basis of quantitative traits: successes and pitfalls. *Nat. Rev. Genet.* **2,** 437–445.
12. Chen, J., Astle, C. M., and Harrison, D. E. (2000) Genetic regulation of primitive hematopoietic stem cell senescence. *Exp. Hematol.* **28,** 442–450.
13. Spangrude, G. J., Brooks, D. M., and Tumas, D. B. (1995) Long-term repopulation of irradiated mice with limiting numbers of purified hematopoietic stem cells: in vivo expansion of stem cell phenotype but not function. *Blood* **85,** 1006–1016.
14. Geiger, H., True, J. M., de Haan, G., and Van Zant, G. (2001) Age- and stage-specific regulation patterns in the hematopoietic stem cell hierarchy. *Blood* **98,** 2966–2972.
15. de Haan, G. and Van Zant, G. (1999) Dynamic changes in mouse hematopoietic stem cell numbers during aging. *Blood* **93,** 3294–3301.
16. De Haan, G. and Van Zant, G. (1999) Genetic analysis of hemopoietic cell cycling in mice suggests its involvement in organismal life span. *FASEB J.* **13,** 707–713.
17. Hasegawa, M., Baldwin, T. M., Metcalf, D., and Foote, S. J. (2000) Progenitor cell mobilization by granulocyte colony-stimulating factor controlled by loci on chromosomes 2 and 11. *Blood* **95,** 1872–1874.
18. Morahan, G., Huang, D., Ymer, S. I., Cancilla, M. R., Stephen, K., Dabadghao, P., et al. (2001) Linkage disequilibrium of a type 1 diabetes susceptibility locus with a regulatory IL12B allele. *Nat. Genet.* **27,** 218–221.

19. Tsao, B. P., Cantor, R. M., Kalunian, K. C., Chen, C. J., Badsha, H., Singh, R., et al. (1997) Evidence for linkage of a candidate chromosome 1 region to human systemic lupus erythematosus. *J. Clin. Invest.* **99,** 725–731.
20. Darvasi, A. (1998) Experimental strategies for the genetic dissection of complex traits in animal models. *Nat. Genet.* **18,** 19–24.
21. Justice, M. J., Jenkins, N. A., and Copeland, N. G. (1992) Recombinant inbred mouse strains: models for disease study. *Trends Biotechnol.* **10,** 120–126.
22. Taylor, B. A. (1978) Recombinant inbred strains: use in gene mapping, in *Origins of Inbred Mice* (Morse H. C., ed), Academic Press, New York, pp. 423–438.
23. Silver, L. M. (1995) *Mouse Genetics. Concepts and Applications.* Oxford University Press, Oxford.
24. Nadeau, J. H., Singer, J. B., Matinm A., and Lander, E. S. (2000) Analysing complex genetic traits with chromosome substitution strains. *Nat. Genet.* **24,** 221–225.
25. Spangrude, G. J. and Brooks, D. M. (1993) Mouse strain variability in the expression of the hematopoietic stem cell antigen Ly-6A/E by bone marrow cells. *Blood* **82,** 3327–3332.
26. Doerge, R. W. (2001) Mapping and analysis of quantitative trait loci in experimental populations. *Nat. Rev. Genet.* **3,** 43–52.
27. Manly, K. F. and Olson, J. M. (1999). Overview of QTL mapping software and introduction to map manager QT. *Mammalian Genome* **10,** 327–334.
28. Williams, R. W., Gu J. , Qi S., and Lu L. (2001) The genetic structure of recombinant inbred mice. High-resolution consensus maps for complex trait analysis. Release 1, January 15, 2001 at www.nervenet.org/papers/bxn.html or mickey.utmem.edu/papers/bxn.html.
29. Lander, E. and Kruglyak, L. (1995) Genetic dissection of complex traits: guidelines for interpreting and reporting linkage results. *Nat. Genet.* **11,** 241–247.
30. Churchill, G. A. and Doerge, R. W. (1994) Empirical threshold values for quantitative trait mapping. *Genetics* **138,** 963–971.
31. Markel, P., Shu, P., Ebeling, C., Carlson, G. A., Nagle, D. L., Smutko, J. S., et al. (1997) Theoretical and empirical issues for marker-assisted breeding of congenic mouse strains. *Nat. Genet.* **17,** 280–284.
32. Wakeland, E., Morel, L., Achey, K., Yui, M., and Longmate, J. (1997) Speed congenics: a classic technique in the fast lane (relatively speaking). *Immunol. Today* **18,** 472–477.
33. Harrison, D. E. (1992) Evaluating functional abilities of primitive hematopoietic stem cell populations. *Curr. Topics Microbiol. Immunol.* **177,** 13–23.
34. Darvasi, A. (1997) Interval-specific congenic strains (ISCS): an experimental design for mapping QTL into a 1-centimorgan interval. *Mamm. Genome.* **8,** 163–167.
35. Mackay, T. F. C. (2001) Quantitative trait loci in Drosophila. *Nat. Rev. Genet.* **2,** 11–20.
36. Mackay, T. F. C. and Langley, C. H. (1990) Molecular and phenotypic variation in the achaete-scute region of Drosophila melanogaster. *Nature* **348,** 64–66.
37. Long, A. D., Lyman, R. F., Morgan, A. H., Langley, C. H., and Mackay, T. F. C. (2000) Both naturally occuring insertions of transposable elements and intermediate frequency polymorphisms at the achaete-scute complex are associated with variation in bristle number in Drosophila melanogaster. *Genetics* **154,** 1255–1269.
38. de Haan, G., Bystrykh, L. V., Weersing, E., Dontje, B., Geiger, H., Ivanova, N., et al. (2002) A genetic and genomic analysis identifies a cluster of genes associated with hematopoietic cell turnover. *Blood* **100,** 2056–2062.
39. Korstanjen R. and Paigen, B. (2002). From QTL to gene: the harvest begins. *Nat. Genet.* **31,** 235–236.

40. Glazier, A. M., Naduau, J. H., and Aitman, T. J. (2002) Finding genes that underlie complex traits. *Science* **298,** 2345–2349.
41. Cormier, R. T., Hong, K. H., Halberg, R. B., Hawkins, T. L., Richardson, P., Mulherkar, R., et al. (1997) Secretory phospholipase Pla2g2a confers resistance to intestinal tumorigenesis. *Nat. Genet.* **17,** 88–91.
42. Aitman, T. J., Glazier, A. M., Wallace, C. A., Cooper, L. D., Norsworthy, P. J., Wahid, F. N., et al. (1999) Identification of Cd36 (Fat) as an insulin-resistance gene causing defective fatty acid and glucose metabolism in hypertensive rats. *Nat. Genet.* **21,** 76–83.
43. Pravenec, M., Landa, V., Zidek, V., Musilova, A., Kren, V., Kazdova, L., et al. (2001) Transgenic rescue of defective Cd36 ameliorates insulin resistance in spontaneously hypertensive rats. *Nat Genet.* **27,** 156–158.

II

Analysis of Cell Fate Outcomes in Transplantation Models

4

Flow Cytometric Analysis of Hematopoietic Development

Edward F. Srour and Mervin C. Yoder

Summary

More than 30 yr ago, a collection of cells isolated from the bone marrow were first demonstrated to repopulate hematopoiesis in a radioablated animal. These cells self-renewed while producing all of the blood products and were named hematopoietic stem cells (HSCs). Since then, HSCs have been a tremendous boon to both basic science in understanding cell biology and as therapy in a cancer transplant setting. More recent work has shown that the HSCs, and possibly populations of cells residing in other tissues, have the properties of stem cells and the ability to repopulate nonrelated organs and tissues. This promiscuous repopulation has been termed plasticity and is the center of much research and even more debate. Our laboratory has recently proven that the HSCs meet the requirements of a stem cell by self-renewing and producing all of the blood lineages while concurrently demonstrating their ability to produce nonhematopoietic endothelial cells of blood vessels. This plasticity of the HSCs demonstrates hemangioblast activity, proven by both single cell and serial HSC transplants, and is the focus of this chapter.

Key Words: Murine; stem cells; progenitor cell; hematopoiesis; flow cytometry.

1. Introduction

The hematopoietic system is established early during mammalian embryonic development and continues to evolve throughout fetal and adult life while emanating from several different anatomical sites. Ontologically, the hematopoietic system goes through several developmental stages. During both murine and human development, blood cells first appear in the yolk sac (YS), then progenitor cells emerge from the intra-embryonic region of the para-aortic splanchnopleura (P-Sp)/aorta–gonad–mesonephros region before seeding the fetal liver and finally settling in the bone marrow (BM) shortly before birth. These developmental stages are controlled by programs that dictate both the functional capacity of predominant progenitor cells at every stage and the phenotypic and molecular fingerprint of these cells and of hematopoietic stem cells (HSCs). Primitive hematopoiesis, which is the first detected hematopoietic activity in the developing embryo, takes place extraembryonically in the yolk sac as early

From: *Methods in Molecular Medicine, Vol. 105: Developmental Hematopoiesis: Methods and Protocols.*
Edited by: M. H. Baron © Humana Press Inc., Totowa, NJ

as embryonic d 7.0 (E7.0) in the mouse and produces largely nucleated primitive erythroblasts expressing fetal hemoglobin *(1,2)*. Intraembryonic hematopoietic stem cells that can repopulate hematopoiesis in irradiated adult hosts autonomously appear in the aorta–gonad–mesonephros *(3)* at E10.0, although long-term repopulating cells continue to be detected at this and later stages of embryonic development in the yolk sac *(4)*. Genes involved in the ontogenesis of the hematopoietic system can also be compartmentalized into those that affect both primitive and definitive hematopoiesis and those that affect definitive hematopoiesis only (reviewed in Godin and Cumano: **ref.** ***5***). Functional and molecular characteristics and differences of hematopoietic cells expressed at different stages of development are the subjects of other chapters and will not be discussed here. Instead, this chapter will focus on the flow cytometric characterization and identification of progenitor and stem cells that can be recognized in and isolated from hematopoietic tissues at various stages during ontogeny of the hematopoietic system.

1.1. Development-Associated Phenotypic Changes in Stem Cells

Given that hematopoietic stem cells are better characterized in the murine system, this section will describe murine development-associated phenotypic changes, and a more limited discussion of the human system will be presented in Chapter 27. Although the phenotypic makeup of putative HSCs in adult tissues can be defined with exquisite specificity that allows extensive enrichment and successful establishment of hematopoiesis from a limited number *(6)* or even one *(7,8)* transplanted HSC in a lethally irradiated recipient, identification of stem cells in fetal tissues is more complex and inefficient. These differences arise from several factors, key among them being that most, if not all, monoclonal antibodies used to identify specific antigens expressed on the surface of candidate HSC were raised against adult cells. This is why, for example, one of the most commonly used markers, stem cell antigen (Sca)-1 (also known as Ly-6A/E), is strongly expressed on adult cells but only weakly on fetal tissues *(9)*. Developmental changes result in differential expression of antigens between fetal and adult stem cells. Although some antigens, such as MAC1, are expressed on embryonic HSCs *(10)*, expression of these same antigens on adult hematopoietic cells is associated with lineage commitment and as such, these cells would no longer be considered part of the HSC pool. A very interesting change in antigen expression between fetal, newborn, and adult murine HSC is that of CD38. Recent evidence from Higuchi, Zeng, and Ogawa *(11)* demonstrates that although fetal and adult HSC express CD38, those isolated from newborn and juvenile mice are CD38-. In addition, harvesting of hematopoietic tissues at very early stages of development yields a very limited number of cells that, in most cases, precludes immunostaining and cell sorting and hinders extensive analysis of the phenotype of candidate stem cells. Moreover, at these early stages of ontogeny, most hematopoietic stem cell preparations are highly enriched for stem cell activity *(12,13)* and therefore further purification of these cells is not warranted. This brief and partial review of our present knowledge of the phenotype of embryonic, neonatal and adult HSC highlights the phenotypic heterogeneity of these cells and underscores the need to properly identify stem cells at different stages of development in order to ensure adequate and correct assessment of hematopoietic function of repopulating cells through ontogeny. This chapter will describe the phenotypic makeup of HSC isolated from different hematopoietic sites at multiple stages of development. Emphasis will be given to the murine system, and where possible, reference to human HSC and their identification will be made. Since the physical isolation of these cells is covered elsewhere, this chapter will focus on immunostaining protocols and the selection of monoclonal antibodies and dyes required for the isolation of populations of cells enriched for stem cell activity.

2. Materials

1. Materials required for the isolation of HSC by flow cytometric cell sorting consist primarily of monoclonal antibodies, purified or conjugated to different fluorochromes, and occasionally metabolic or DNA dyes that are used to further subfractionate a phenotypically defined group of cells based on their metabolic activity or cell cycle status. These reagents and their sources are listed in **Table 1**. Many of the reagents in **Table 1** can be obtained from sources other than the three listed. These three sources were listed because of the familiarity of the authors with the reagents those companies provide and the established specificity and quality of these reagents.
2. The list of markers presented in **Table 1** is incomplete because more and more antigens expressed on HSC at different stages of development are described on a regular basis. However, this list encompasses the majority, if not all, of the common and widely used antigens that can assist in identifying and isolating HSC from different ontologic stages. As will be noted, some of these antigens are also useful in identifying and isolating differentiating or lineage restricted progenitor cells that developmentally appear to be derived from more immature HSC in the developmental hierarchy of stem cells. It is well recognized that mature or lineage committed progenitors also differ from primitive stem cells in their molecular fingerprint. However, these differences will not be covered here.

3. Methods

3.1. Immunostaining

All immunostaining of hematopoietic cells destined to be used for flow cytometric cell sorting begins by preparing a single cell suspension from target tissues or organs. Preparation of single-cell suspensions from different hematopoietic tissues and organs is covered elsewhere and will not be discussed in this chapter. Immunostaining will be described in a rather generic manner, given the large number of staining combinations that result from both examining cells from multiple sources and choosing a particular combination of monoclonal antibodies that applies to the cells being examined, as detailed in **Table 2**.

It is always advisable to prepare single color control samples (in addition to appropriate isotype control tubes) especially when multiple color analysis is involved (*see* **Note 1**). These controls ensure that adequate and correct compensation is applied to avoid the generation of false positive or false negative events and to confirm that percentages of positive cells for each marker obtained in the multi-color analysis sample match those obtained from the single color controls. An example of the required control samples for multicolor analysis is given in the legend of **Fig. 1**.

Table 1
Monoclonal Antibodies and Dyes Used for the Identification and Isolation of Murine Hematopoietic Stem and Progenitor Cells

CD antigens and dyes	Common name	Clone(s)	Source[a]
	Sca-1, Ly–6A/E	IOT-6A.2 D7, E13-161.7	Bec.Coulter Pharmingen
CD11a	LFA-1, Integrin α_L chain	121/7 2D7	Bec.Coulter Pharmingen
CD11b	MAC-1	M1/70	Bec.Coulter Pharmingen
CD24		M1/69	Pharmingen
CD27			
CD34		RAM34	Pharmingen
CD38		90	Pharmingen
CD41	Integrin α_{IIb}	MWReg30	Pharmingen
CD43	Ly-48, Leukosialin	S7	Pharmingen
CD49d	Integrin α_4 chain (VLA4)	9C10 (MFR4.B)	Pharmingen
CD49e	Integrin α_5 chain (VLA5)	5H10-27	Pharmingen
CD62L	L-selectin	MEL-14	Bec.Coulter Pharmingen
CD90	Thy-1	IOT-TH1, OX7 G7	Bec.Coulter Pharmingen
CD117	c-Kit	2B8	Bec.Coulter Pharmingen
AA4.1			Unavailable
CD32/16	FcγR, Low affinity Fc receptor	IOT-17.1+IOT-17.2 Ms	Bec.Coulter Pharmingen
CD127	IL-7 Receptor α chain	SB/199 or SB/14	Pharmingen
MDR	P-gp		
Antigens used collectively to designate "lineage" (incomplete)			
CD3e	T cell ε chain	145-2C11	Pharmingen
CD11b	Integrin α_M chain	M1/70	Pharmingen
CD45R	B220	RA3-6B2	Pharmingen
	Gr-1	RB6-8C5	Pharmingen
	TER-119	TER-119	Pharmingen
Metabolic and DNA dyes			
Hoechst 33342			Molecular Probes
Rhodamine 123			Molecular Probes

[a] Further information for sources of reagents: Bec.Coulter: Beckman Coulter, Inc. 11800 S.W. 147 Avenue, P.O. Box. 169015, Miami, FL 33116-9015, Phone: 800-526-3821. Web: www.beckmancoulter. com/CellAnalysisReg; Pharmingen: BD Biosciences, Pharmingen, 10975 Torreyana Road, San Diego, CA 92121-1106. Phone: 877-232-8995, Web: www.bdbiosciences.com; Molecular Probes: Molecular Probes, Inc. 4849 Pitchford Avenue, Eugene, OR 97402-9165. Phone: 800-438-2209. Web: www. molecularprobes.com.

Table 2
Phenotypes of Candidate Murine Hematopoietic Stem and Progenitor Cells

	Hematopoietic stem cells from						Lineage committed multipotential progenitors from				
	Prenatal				Postnatal		Fetal liver		Adult bone marrow		
Antigens and dyes	YS	AGM	FL	FBM	NBM [a]	ABM [b]	B/M	B/T/M	CLP	B	CMP
Sca-1	–	+	+	+	+	+	+		lo	+	–
CD11a						–					
CD11b		+				–	–				
CD24						+				+	
CD27 (1)						–					
CD31						+					
CD34 (2)	+	+	+	+	+	–/+					+
CD38	+				–	+					
CD41	+					–					
CD43						+				+	
CD45R			+			–	–			–	
CD49d						lo					
CD49e						+					
CD62L						–					
CD90			lo			lo			–	–	
CD117	+	+	+			+			lo	lo	+
CD127						–			+		–
AA4.1	+		+			–	+	+		+	
CD32/16						–		+			lo
MDR						+					
Hst (3)						lo					
R123					(4)	lo					
Lineage (5)	–		–			–				–	–
References	*(14–16)*	*(10,17,18)*	*(19,20)*	*(21)*	*(11)*	*(11,17,22–43)*	*(44)*	*(45)*	*(46)*	*(47)*	*(48)*

Reactivity of each antigen with a given class of progenitors is indicated by "+" sign. The use of "–"sign indicates that cells in question do not express that particular antigen. The designation "lo" indicates low or dim reactivity with a given marker. Empty boxes indicate lack of information regarding the expression of a given antigen on a class of stem/progenitor cells. Abbreviations used in this table are: YS yolk sac; AGM aorta gonad mesonephros; FL fetal liver; FBM, fetal bone marrow; NBM, neonatal bone marrow; ABM, adult bone marrow; B/M, common B-cell and macrophage progenitors; B/T/M: common B-cell, T-cell and macrophage progenitors; CLP, common lymphoid progenitors; CMP, common myeloid progenitors; Hst, Hoechst 33342; R123, Rhodamine 123.

[a] Neonatal bone marrow as defined by Higuchi et al. ***(11)*** is that collected from mice younger than 5 wk old.

[b] The phenotype of adult BM HSC described in **Table 2** was compiled from multiple references. Therefore, collectively, this is a theoretical phenotype of adult BM HSC and cells displaying this phenotype have not been isolated and/or functionally examined.

Specific foot notes to entries in **Table 2** (designated as a number between parentheses next to the entry).

1. Expression of CD27 on HSC is described by Wiesmann et al. ***(36)***. CD27+ cells are enriched for colony forming cells while CD27–cells contain clonal long-term repopulating cells.
2. CD34 is developmentally and functionally regulated ***(31,35)***. Expression of CD34 through ontogeny as shown in **Table 2** is based on the studies of Ito et al. ***(31)***. Approximately 20% of adult BM HSC are CD34+. Long-term repopulating stem cells lacking the expression of CD34 have also been described ***(8)***, and therefore CD34-HSC should be considered as putative adult BM stem cells.
3. Hoechst 33342 has been used for the isolation of primitive HSC by virtue of their ability to efflux the dye and appear as a side population (SP) when the blue versus red emission of Hoechst 33342 is examined ***(49,50)***. However, since hematopoietic cells with SP properties can be visualized without the need for further phenotypic characterization, the use of Hoechst 33342 to isolate SP cells was not included in **Table 2**. It is important to stress however, that phenotypically defined cells can also be stained with Hoechst 33342 and analyzed for their SP cell content thus allowing for further enrichment of HSC.
4. Rhodamine 123 efflux in newborn mouse BM cells is a function of mitochondrial activation rather than MDR activity and efflux properties ***(51)***.
5. Lineage designation as used here should be considered with extreme caution. It is clear that some CD markers included in a common "lineage cocktail" used for the isolation of adult BM HSC are expressed on fetal HSC and, therefore designation of lineage markers when fetal cells are analyzed would be different from that used for adult tissues. Clear examples of such antigens are CD11b and CD4 ***(24)***.

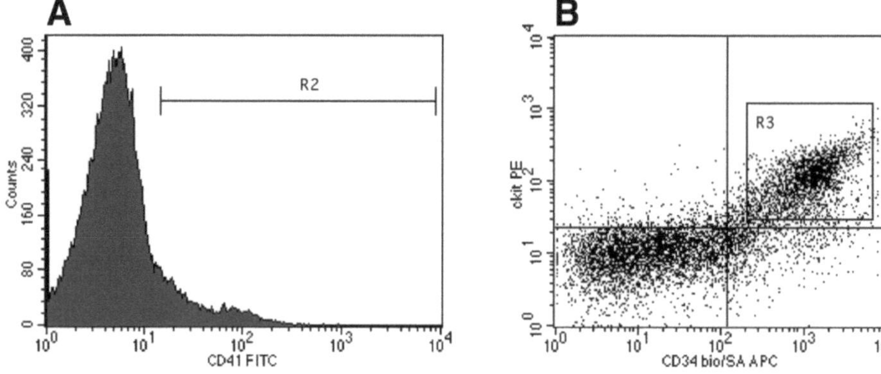

Fig. 1. Cell sorting of murine YS Sca-1+CD34+c-kit+ cells. YS cells were stained with FITC-conjugated CD41, PE-conjugated CD117 (c-kit), and biotinylated CD34 that was developed with APC-conjugated streptavidin. Cells were sorted on a FACS vantage cell sorter using the following gating procedure. Expression of CD41 on cells contained within the small cell population as determined by their light scatter properties (light scatter gate not shown) was determined and a gate defining CD41+ cells was established (R2 in **[A]**). Next, CD41+ cells were analyzed for their expression of CD34 and c-kit along the *x*- and *y*-axes, respectively **(B)**. A distinct population of CD41+CD34+CD117+ cells can be identified in the upper right hand corner of **B**, contained within the sort window R3. In this particular example, CD41+ cells represent 10.3% of analyzed cells (based on light scatter properties) while CD41+CD34+ CD117+ cells represent 30.6% of all the CD41+ cells or 3.2% of total cells.

The staining protocol describes staining of yolk sac cells with CD34, CD117, and CD41 and is used as an example only. Flow cytometric analysis of these cells to isolate D34+CD117+ CD41+ cells is shown in **Fig. 1**. Permutations and changes can be applied as needed.

1. Dispense approx 2.5×10^5 YS cells in all control tubes (remainder of the cells are dedicated to the "sort" tube) and add 2 to 3 mL of a wash buffer to each tube (*see* **Note 2**). Wash buffers can be prepared by adding 1 to 2% bovine calf serum or bovine albumin to phosphate-buffered saline and sterilizing the solution by filtration. Cells in the "sort" tube can be washed with a larger volume.
2. Spin all tubes at 300*g* for 5 min at 4°C. Discard the supernatant and add 100 μL of Fc Block conditioned medium (cultured from the hybridoma 2.4G2) to resuspend the cells. A larger volume of Fc Block should be added to the "sort" tube proportionate to the number of cells contained in this tube.
3. Isotype control samples are prepared by adding 100 μL of Fc Block conditioned medium to YS cells and labeling with isotype-matched antibodies conjugated to the same fluorochromes as those used on primary antibodies. Isotype control tubes are prepared the same way and at the same time single color control and the "sort" tubes are prepared. Additional isotype control tubes specific for a given sort strategy are also required to ensure correct interpretation of dot plots (*see* **Note 4**).

4. Add the appropriate concentration of primary antibodies, usually 1 μg per million cells in a small volume (between 1 and 20 μL). In the example shown in **Fig. 1**, the antibodies to be added are phycoerythrin (PE)-conjugated CD117 (c-Kit), Biotin-conjugated CD34, and fluorescein isothiocyanate (FITC)-conjugated CD41. Each one of these is added to the single color control tube, and all three are added to the "sort" tube simultaneously. Vortex all tubes and incubate on ice in the dark for 30 min. Vortex the tubes at least twice during the 30-min time period.
5. All tubes are washed with 4 mL of wash buffer (300 g) and the supernatant is discarded, leaving approx 100 μL for the secondary labeling.
6. Streptavidin–allophycocyanin (APC) is added to the tubes containing biotinylated isotype or CD34 to deliver also 1 μg of protein per million cells. The cells are vortexed and incubated as is **step 4** on ice.
7. Cells are given a final wash at 300*g* and are resuspended in 200 μL wash buffer for the control tubes (since they contain fewer cells), and in an appropriate volume of wash buffer for the "sort" tube keeping the cell concentration between 5 and 10 × 10^6 cells per mL.

For other staining protocols (such as that for data shown in **Fig. 2**), the same general principles apply. If secondary antibodies are used to develop primary antibodies (*see* **Note 3**), care should be taken that secondary antibodies specifically interact with their intended targets to avoid inadvertent staining of similar primary antibodies. To ensure this, subclass specific secondary antibodies that have been absorbed against other crossreacting classes of antibodies should be used when possible. It is important to note that isotype control tubes should contain all the reagents used in the "sort" sample as isotype-matched, fluorochrome-conjugated non-specific antibodies. When dyes are used in combination with antibodies, staining with dyes that require incubation at 37°C should be completed first. After that, cells should be washed and chilled to 4°C and the staining with antibodies continued as usual.

3.2. Cell Sorting

Again, given the large number of permutations for cell sorting described in **Table 2**, it is difficult to describe a sorting procedure that encompasses all possibilities. Instead, two examples, one for the staining of YS cells, (*see* **Fig. 1**), and another from adult BM cells are presented in **Figs. 1** and **2**, respectively. Figure legends describe in detail the set up used for these examples and the specifics that pertain to these two situations that can be applied to other similar staining and sorting protocols. For comments about plotting the data, *see* **Note 4**.

When designing a four-color sort as shown in **Fig. 2**, many control tubes should be prepared to ensure appropriate and correct adjustments of instrument settings used for analysis and sorting. In this particular example, six control tubes are warranted. First, an isotype control tube to determine the background fluorescence of all four fluorochromes used in the staining protocol. Second, a set of four single-color samples should be prepared to use in adjusting compensation and to establish the values of percent positive cells expected in the "sort" sample. Third, because the first gating sequence (other than light scatter) involves lineage and Thy1 fluorescence (FITC and PE-Cy7), a sample stained with lineage markers and Thy1 in addition to the appropriate PE and APC isotype controls is needed. This sample can then be used to establish PE and APC background fluorescence from gated Lin-Thy1lo events similar to what is shown in

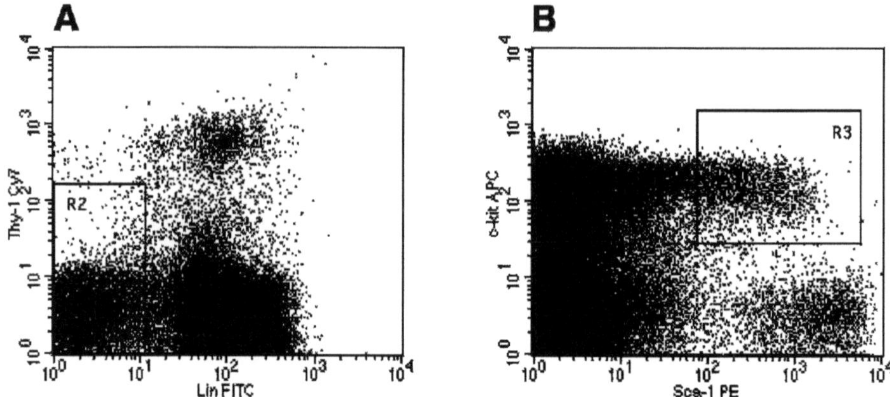

Fig. 2. Cell sorting of adult murine BM Lin-Thy1loSca-1+c-kit+ cells. Low-density BM cells were stained with a cocktail of FITC-conjugated lineage markers, PE-conjugated Sca-1, APC-conjugated c-kit, and biotinylated Thy1 that was developed with PE-Cy7-conjugated streptavidin. Cells were sorted on a FACS vantage cell sorter using the following gating procedure. First, cells were analyzed for light scatter properties and only cells with low side and forward scatter were selected for further analysis (light scatter gate not shown). Gated cells were then analyzed for expression of lineage markers and Thy1 as shown along the *x*- and *y*-axes of panel **A**, respectively. Gate R2 (**A**) was constructed to contain lineage negative (Lin-) cells lacking the expression or expressing low levels of Thy1 and these cells were then analyzed for the expression of Sca-1 and c-kit along the *x*-and *y*-axes, respectively, of panel **B**. In this gating scheme, Lin-Thy1loSac-1+c-kit+ cells can be easily recognized in the upper right hand quadrant of panel **B**. These cells are shown within a sorting window, R3 in (**B**). In this particular example, Lin-Thy1lo cells (gate R2 in [**A**]) represented 20.5% of total cells analyzed (based on light scatter properties). Cells contained in R3 (Lin-Thy1loSca-1+c-kit-) represented 1.1% of those in R2 or approx 0.2% of low-density BM cells.

Fig. 2A. PE and APC events in the "sort" tube displaying more than 97% fluorescence over and above that of the isotype control would then be considered positive.

3.3. Phenotypes of HSC at Different Stages of Development

Phenotypes of hematopoietic stem and progenitor cells recognized at multiple stages of murine ontogeny are presented in a tabular form in **Table 2**. These data were compiled from studies performed over a considerable period of time by a large number of investigators. Undoubtedly, many markers used for the identification of HSC may not appear here. These markers and the studies that reported them were not intentionally ignored, but instead, an effort was made to describe the most commonly used markers and approaches used for the identification of HSC.

3.4. Phenotypic Makeup of Human HSC Through Ontogeny

Obviously, characterization of human hematopoietic stem cells through ontogeny is more problematic than that of murine cells, given the controversy surrounding the use of human fetal tissues in research. Nevertheless, sufficient research with fetal tissues has been conducted to allow for the assembly of enough information to describe the phenotypic makeup of HSC isolated from fetal liver, bone marrow and peripheral blood (*see* other chapters for more detailed analysis of developmental changes of HSC during human ontogeny). CD34 expression has long been considered a hallmark of human HSC definition ***(52)***. This marker is expressed on human HSC at all stages of development although CD34-NOD/SCID repopulating cells have been described ***(53)***. Since then, other reports describing CD34-human stem cells have been published ***(54,55)*** and as in the murine system ***(35)***, the reversibility of expression of CD34 on human repopulating stem cells has also been described ***(56)***. In addition to CD34 and similar to murine cells, other surface antigens have been described on human HSC. However, most of these characterizations have been performed with adult BM cells or with mobilized peripheral blood, and to lesser extent with umbilical cord blood cells. Further purification of adult human HSC has been accomplished by selection of HLA-DR- cells from within the CD34+cell population ***(57,58)***. However, umbilical cord blood CD34+HLA-DR+ cells were found to be more primitive than CD34+HLA-DR-cells when assayed in vitro ***(59)*** and similar findings were later described for human fetal liver CD34+ cells ***(60)***. Absence of another marker on CD34+ cells, namely CD38, is also widely used as means for enrichment of human HSC ***(61)***. More recently, markers other than CD34 were identified on the surface of candidate human HSC including AC133 (CD133) ***(62,63)*** and the vascular endothelial growth factor receptor 2 (VEGFR2), also known as KDR ***(64)***. Recently, the expression of CXCR4 on human HSCs was reported ***(65,66)***, although other reports indicate that both populations of CXCR4+ and CXCR4-human CD34+ cells engraft in NOD/SCID mice ***(67)***.

An interesting parameter with which human hematopoietic cells can be characterized is their position in cell cycle at the time of isolation. Viable cells can be assessed for their cell cycle status and isolated for further functional assays using Hoechst 33342 and Pyronin Y ***(68)***. Unfortunately, the combination of Hoechst 33342 and Pyronin Y is toxic to murine cells (Srour, E. F., unpublished observations) and cannot, therefore, be used to isolate viable murine hematopoietic cells fractionated based on their position in the cell cycle. Cell cycle status of human stem cells capable of engraftment in NOD/SCID mice is one of very few parameters documented to change considerably during ontogeny. While adult human HSCs from BM and mobilized peripheral blood reside predominantly in the G_0 phase of cell cycle ***(69)***, CD34+ cells from cord blood ***(70)***, fetal liver, fetal BM, and fetal peripheral blood ***(71)*** in all phases of cell cycle are capable of engrafting in NOD/SCID mice. The biologic significance of this difference between fetal/neonatal and adult sources of human HSC is not well established. However, it is possible that the ability of cycling fetal cells to engraft in a transplantation model suggests that as these cells migrate from one anatomical hematopoietic site to another during fetal development, they retain the potential to seed and colonize new hematopoietic tissues, thus ensuring continued and uninterrupted hematopoiesis in the fetus.

Finally, as has been described in the mouse system, human multilymphoid progenitor cells devoid of any myeloid differentiation potential were recently described in cord blood ***(72)***. Similar to their murine counterparts, these human common lymphoid progenitors express low levels of CD117 and also express the T-cell marker CD7 ***(72)***.

Because of apparent obstacles in performing in vivo studies with human stem and progenitor cells, hematopoietic lineage commitment and characterization of the phenotypic makeup of classes of human progenitors are not exquisitely developed and defined as in the murine system. A recent review by Payne and Crooks *(73)* summarizes our current knowledge of this area of human hematopoietic stem and progenitor cell research.

4. Notes

1. When cell numbers are limiting, it is advisable to use the smallest cell number possible when single-color and other control tubes are prepared, thus allowing for maximal utilization of the remaining cells for sorting. The smallest cell number possible to use depends on the flow cytometer used and how many times the sample might be analyzed. In general, 5×10^4 or 10^5 cells will be enough and in some cases only 2.5×10^4 cells would be sufficient.
2. When sorting large numbers of cells, a large volume of wash buffer is required to resuspend all available cells. In such a case, it is better to split the sample into several tubes (1–1.5 mL per tube) and keep these on ice and in the dark while one is being sorted.
3. If secondary antibodies or developing reagents are used to visualize unconjugated primary antibodies, care must be taken to prepare adequate isotype controls to establish background fluorescence. These controls should be stained with an isotype-matched nonspecific antibody or a biotinylated isotype-matched nonspecific antibody if the primary antibody used in the staining scheme is biotinylated. These antibodies are then developed the same way as the primary antibodies with a secondary antibody or with a Streptavidin conjugated fluorochrome. It is also advisable that these staining steps be performed simultaneously with staining steps involving specific primary antibodies.
4. In the staining examples given in this chapter, it is recommended that sorting be performed from a two-color dot plot rather than from a single color histogram. The advantage of such an approach is that better visualization of the relationship of one population to another can be seen and isolation of groups of cells with positive and/or negative expression of 2 markers can be achieved. To do this, cells gated on one color (in the example shown in **Fig. 1**, gating is first done on CD41+ cells) are displayed in a dot plot, in this case CD34 versus CD117 emitting APC and PE signals, respectively. For accurate assessment of PE- and APC-positive events, an isotype control should be prepared as follows. Cells are stained with CD41 FITC and a PE-conjugated isotype matched (to CD117) nonspecific antibody and a biotinylated isotype matched (to CD34) nonspecific antibody. The biotinylated antibody is then developed with streptavidin–APC. From this tube, CD41+ events can be gated and used to generate a dot plot displaying the background fluorescence of PE and APC that can be used to identify positive events in these channels generated by specific staining with CD117 and CD34, respectively.

References

1. Russel, E. (1979) Hereditary anemias of the mouse: a review for geneticists. *Adv. Genet.* **20,** 357–366.
2. Keller, G., Lacaud, G., and Robertson, S. (1999) Development of the hematopoietic system in the mouse. *Exp. Hematol.* **27,** 777–787.
3. Medvinsky, A. and Dzierzak, E. (1996) Definitive hematopoiesis is autonomously initiated by the AGM region. *Cell* **86,** 897–906.
4. Kumaravelu, P., Hook, L., Morrison, A. M., Ure, J., Zhao, S., Zuyev, S., et al. (2002) Quantitative developmental anatomy of definitive haematopoietic stem cells/long-term

repopulating units (HSC/RUs): role of the aorta-gonad-mesonephros (AGM) region and the yolk sac in colonisation of the mouse embryonic liver. *Development* **129,** 4891–4899.

5. Godin, I. and Cumano, A. (2002) The hare and the tortoise: an embryonic haematopoietic race. *Nat. Rev.* **2,** 593–604.
6. Spangrude, G., Brooks, D., and Tumas, D. (1995) Long-term repopulation of irradiated mice with limiting numbers of purified hematopoietic stem cells: In vivo expansion of stem cell phenotype but not function. *Blood* **85,** 1006–1016.
7. Jones, R. J., Wagner, J. E., Celano, P., Zicha, M. S., and Sharkis, S. J. (1990) Separation of pluripotent haematopoietic stem cells from spleen colony-forming units. *Nature* **347,** 188–189.
8. Osawa, M., Hanada, K., Hamada, H., and Nakauchi, H. (1996) Long-term lymphohematopoietic reconstitution by a single CD34-low/negative hematopoietic stem cell. *Science* **273,** 242–245.
9. de Bruijn, M. F., Ma, X., Robin, C., Ottersbach, K., Sanchesz, M. J., and Dzierzak, E. (2002) Hematopoietic stem cells localize to the endothelial cell layer in the midgestation mouse aorta. *Immunity* **16,** 673–683.
10. Sanchez, M.-J., Holmes, A., Miles, C., and Dzierzak, E. (1996) Characterization of the first definitive hematopoietic stem cells in the AGM and liver of the mouse embryo. *Immunity* **5,** 513–525.
11. Higuchi, Y., Zeng, H., and Ogawa, M. (2003) CD38 expression by hematopoietic stem cells of newborn and juvenile mice. *Leukemia* **17,** 171–174.
12. Godin, I., Dieterlen-Lievre, F., and Cumano, A. (1995) Emergence of multipotent hematopoietic cells in the yolk sac and paraaortic splanchnopleura in mouse embryos, beginning at 8.5 days postcoitus. *Proc. Natl. Acad. Sci. USA* **92,** 773–777.
13. Godin, I., Garcia-Porrero, J. A., Dieterlen-Lievre, F., and Cumano, A. (1999) Stem cell emergence and hemopoietic activity are incompatible in mouse intraembryonic sites. *J. Exp. Med.* **190,** 43–52.
14. Dagher, R., Hiatt, K., Traycoff, C., Srour, E. F., and Yoder, M. (1998) c-Kit and CD38 are expressed by long-term reconstituting hematopoietic cells present in the murine yolk sac. *Biol. Blood Marrow Transplant.* **4,** 69–74.
15. Yoder, M., Hiatt, K., Dutt, P., Mukherjee, P., Bodine, D., and Orlic, D. (1997) Characterization of definitive lymphohematopoietic stem cells in the day 9 murine yolk sac. *Immunity* **7,** 335–344.
16. Huang, H. and Auerbach, R. (1993) Identifiction and characterization of hematopoietic stem cells from the yolk sac of the early mouse embryo. *Proc. Natl. Acad. Sci. USA* **90,** 10,110–10,114.
17. Oostendorp, R. A. J., Harvey, K. N., Kusadasi, N., de Bruijn, M. F. T. R., Saris, C., Ploemacher, R. E., et al. (2002) Stromal cell lines from mouse aorta-gonads-mesonephros subregions are potent supporters of hematopoietic stem cell activity. *Blood* **99,** 1183–1189.
18. Takeuchi, M., Sekiguchi, T., Hara, T., Kinoshita, T., and Miyajima, A. (2002) Cultivation of aorta-gonad-mesonephros-derived hematopoietic stem cells in the fetal liver microenvironment amplifies long-term repopulating activity and enhances engraftment to the bone marrow. *Blood* **99,** 1190–1196.
19. Ikuta, K., Kina.T., MacNeil, I., Uchida, N., Peault, B., Chien, Y., and Weissman, I. L. (1990) A developmental switch in thymic lymphocyte maturation potential occurs at the level of hematopoietic stem cells. *Cell* **62,** 863–874.
20. Jordan, C. T., McKearn, J. P., and Lemischka, I. R. (1990) Cellular and developmental properties of fetal hematopoietic stem cells. *Cell* **61,** 953–963.

21. Wolber, F. M., Leonard, E., Michael, S., Orschell-Traycoff, C. M., Yoder, M. C., and Srour, E. F. (2002) Roles of spleen and liver in development of the murine hematopoietic system. *Exp. Hematol.* **30,** 1010–1019.
22. Spangrude, G., Heimfeld, S., and Weissman, I. (1988) Purification and characterization of mouse hematopoietic stem cells. *Science* **241,** 58–62.
23. Baum, C. M., Weissman, I. L., Tsukamoto, A. S., Buckle, A., and Peault, B. (1992) Isolation of a candidate human hematopoietic stem-cell population. *Proc. Natl. Acad. Sci. USA* **89,** 2804–2808.
24. Morrison, S. J. and Weissman, I. L. (1994) The long-term repopulating subset of hematopoietic stem cells is deterministic and isolatable by phenotype. *Immunity* **1,** 661–673.
25. Randall, T. D., Lund, F. E., Howard, M. C., and Weissman, I. L. (1996) Expression of murine CD38 defines a population of long-term reconstituting hematopoietic stem cells. *Blood* **87,** 4057–4067.
26. Uchida, N., Friera, A. M., He, D., Reitsma, M. J., Tsukamoto, A. S., and Weissman, I. L. (1997) Hydroxyurea can be used to increase mouse c-kit+ Thy-1.1lo Lin-/lo Sca-1+ hematopoietic cell number and frequency in cell cycle in vivo. *Blood* **90,** 4354–4362.
27. Habibian, H. K., Peters, S. O., Hsieh, C. C., Wuu, J., Vergilis, K., Grimaldi, C. I., et al. (1998) The fluctuating phenotype of the lymphohematopoietic stem cell with cell cycle transit. *J. Exp. Med.* **188,** 393–398.
28. Prem Veer Reddy, G., Tiarks, C. Y., Pang, L., Wuu, J., Hsieh, C. C., and Quesenberry, P. J. (1997) Cell cycle analysis and synchronization of pluripotent hematopoietic progenitor stem cells. *Blood* **90,** 2293–2299.
29. Becker, P. S., Nilsson, S. K., Li, Z., Berrios, V. M., Dooner, M. S., Cooper, C. L., Hsieh, C., et al. (1999) Adhesion receptor expression by hematopoietic cell lines and murine progenitors: Modulation by cytokine and cell cycle status. *Exp. Hematol.* **27,** 533–541.
30. Hirayama, F. and Ogawa, M. (1994) CD43 expression by murine lymphohemopoietic progenitors. *Int. J. Hematol.* **60,** 191–196.
31. Ito, T., Tajima, F., and Ogawa, M. (2000) Developmental changes of CD34 expression by murine hematopoietic stem cells. *Exp. Hematol.* **28,** 1269–1273.
32. Ogawa, M., Matsuzaki, Y., Nishikawa, S., Hayashi, S. I., Kunisada, T., Sudo, T., et al. (1991) Expression and function of c-kit in hemopoietic progenitor cells. *J. Exp. Med.* **174,** 63–71.
33. Ogawa, M., Nishikawa, S., Yoshinaga, K., Hayashi, S., Kunisada, T., Nakao, J., et al. (1993) Expression and function of c-Kit in fetal hemopoietic progenitor cells: transition from the early c-Kit-independent to the late c-Kit-dependent wave of hemopoiesis in the murine embryo. *Development* **117,** 1089–1098.
34. Tajima, F., Deguchi, T., Laver, J. H., Zeng, H., and Ogawa, M. (2001) Reciprocal expression of CD38 and CD34 by adult murine hematopoietic stem cells. *Blood* **97,** 2618–2624.
35. Sato, T., Laver, J. H., and Ogawa, M. (1999) Reversible expression of CD34 by murine hematopoietic stem cells. *Blood* **94,** 2548–2554.
36. Wiesmann, A., Phillips, R. L., Mojica, M., Pierce, L. J., Searles, A. E., Spangrude, G. J., et al. (2000) Expression of CD27 on murine hematopoietic stem and progenitor cells. *Immunity* **12,** 193–199.
37. Spangrude, G. and Brooks, D. (1993) Mouse strain variability in the expression of the hematopoietic stem cell antigen Ly-6A/E by bone marrow. *Blood* **82,** 3327–3332.
38. Spangrude, G. J. and Brooks, D. M. (1992) Phenotypic analysis of mouse hematopoietic stem cells shows a Thy-1- negative subset. *Blood* **80,** 1957–64.

39. Orschell-Traycoff, C. M., Hiatt, K., Dagher, R. N., Rice, S., Yoder, M., and Srour, E. F. (2000) Homing and engraftment potential of Sca-1+lin- cells fractionated on the basis of adhesion molecule expression and position in cell cycle. *Blood* **96,** 1380–1387.
40. Wolf, N. S., Kone, A., Priestley, G. V., and Bartelmez, S. H. (1993) In vivo and in vitro characterization of long-term repopulating primitive hematopoietic cells isolated by sequential Hoechst 33342-rhodamine 123 FACS selection. *Exp. Hematol.* **21,** 614–622.
41. Leemhuis, T., Yoder, M. C., Grigsby, S., Aguero, B., Eder, P., and Srour, E. (1996) Isolation of primitive human bone marrow hematopoietic progenitor cells using Hoechst 33342 and Rhodamine 123. *Exp. Hematol.* **24,** 1215–1224.
42. Moore, T., Huang, S., Terstappen, L. W., Bennett, M., and Kumar, V. (1994) Expression of CD43 on murine and human pluripotent hematopoietic stem cells. *J. Immunol.* **153,** 4978–4987.
43. van der Loo, J. C. M., Xiao, X. L., McMillin, D., Hashino, K., Kato, I., and Williams, D. A. (1998) VLA-5 is expressed by mouse and human long-term repopulating hematopoietic cells and mediates adhesion to extracellular matrix protein fibronectin. *J. Clin. Invest.* **102,** 1051–1061.
44. Cumano, A., Palge, C., Isscove, N. N., and Brady, G. (1992) Bipotential precursor of B and macrophages in murine fetal liver. *Nature* **356,** 612–615.
45. Lacaud, G., Carlsson, L., and Keller, G. (1998) Identification of a fetal hematopoietic precursor with B cell, T cell and macrophage potential. *Immunity* **9,** 827–838.
46. Kondo, M., Weissman, I. L., and Akashi, K. (1997) Identification of clonogenic common lymphoid progenitors in mouse bone marrow. *Cell* **91,** 661–672.
47. Mojica, M. P., Perry, S. S., Searles, A. E., Elenitoba-Johnson, K. S. J., Pierce, L. J., Wiesmann, A., et al. (2001) Phenotypic distinction and functional characterization of pro-B cells in adult mouse bone marrow. *J. Immunol.* **166,** 3042–3051.
48. Akashi, K., Traver, D., Miyamoto, T., and Weissman, I. L. (2000) A clonogenic common myeloid progenitor that gives rise to all myeloid lineages. *Nature* **404,** 193–197.
49. Goodell, M. A., K., B., Paradis, G., Stewart Conner, A., and Mulligan, R.C. (1996) Isolation and functional properties of murine hematopoietic stem cells that are replicating in vivo. *J. Exp. Med.* **183,** 1797–1806.
50. Goodell, M. A., Rosenzweig, M., Kim, H., Marks, D. F., DeMaria, M., Paradis, G., et al. (1997) Dye efflux studies suggest that hematopoietic stem cells expressing low or undetectable levels of CD34 antigen exist in multiple species. *Nat. Med.* **3,** 1337–1345.
51. Kim, M., Cooper, D. D., Hayes, S. F., and Spangrude, G. J. (1998) Rhodamine-123 staining in hematopoietic stem cells of young mice indicates mitochondrial activation rather than dye efflux. *Blood* **91,** 4106–4117.
52. Civin, C., Banguenigo, M., Strauss, L., and Loken, M. (1987) Antigenic analysis of hematopoiesis. VI. Flow cytometric characterization of My-10-positive progenitor cells in normal human bone marrow.*Exp. Hematol.* **15,** 10–17.
53. Bhatia, M., Bonnet, D., Murdoch, B., Gan, O. I., and Dick, J. E. (1998) A newly discovered class of human hematopoietic cells with SCID-repopulating activity. *Nat. Med.* **4,** 1038–1045.
54. Zanjani, E. D., Almeida-Porada, G., Livingston, A. G., Flake, A. W., and Ogawa, M. (1998) Human bone marrow CD34- cells engraft in vivo and undergo multilineage expression that includes giving rise to CD34- cells. *Exp. Hematol.* **26,** 353–360.
55. Verfaillie, C. M., Almeida-Porada, G., Wissink, S., and Zanjani, E. D. (2000) Kinetics of engraftment of CD34(– and CD34(+) cells from mobilized blood differs from that of CD34(–) and CD34(+) cells from bone marrow. *Exp. Hematol.* **28,** 1071–1079.

56. Dao, M. A., Arevalo, J., and Nolta, J. A. (2003) Reversibility of CD34 expression on human hematopoietic stem cells that retain the capacity for secondary reconstitution. *Blood* **101,** 112–118.
57. Brandt, J. E., Baird, N., Lu, L., Srour, E., and Hoffman, R. (1988) Characterization of a human hematopoietic progenitor cell capable of forming blast cell containing colonies in vitro. *J. Clin. Invest.* **82,** 1017–1027.
58. Srour, E. F., Brandt, J. E., Briddell, R. A., Leemhuis, T., van Besien, K., and Hoffman, R. (1991) Human CD34+ HLA-DR- bone marrow cells contain progenitor cells capable of self-renewal, multilineage differentiation, and long-term in vitro hematopoiesis. *Blood Cells* **17,** 287–295.
59. Traycoff, C., Abboud, M. R., Laver, J., Hoffman, R., Brandt, J. E., Leemhuis, T., et al. (1992) Differences in the behavior of purified umbilical cord blood and adult bone marrow hematopoietic progenitor cells in stromal cell-free long-term cultures. *Blood* **80,** 13a.
60. Roy, V., Miller, J. S. and Verfaillie, C. M. (1997) Phenotypic and functional characterization of committed and primitive myeloid and lymphoid hematopoietic precurssors in human fetal liver. *Exp. Hematol.* **25,** 387–394.
61. Terstappen, L. W., Huang, S., Safford, D. M., Lansdrop, P. M., and Loken, M. R. (1991) Sequential generations of hematopoietic colonies derived from single nonlineage committed $CD34^+$ $CD38^-$ progenitor cells. *Blood* **77,** 1218–1227.
62. Yin, A. H., Miraglia, S., Zanjani, E. D., Almeida-Porada, G., Ogawa, M., Leary, A. G., et al. (1997) AC**133,** a novel marker for human hematopoietic stem and progenitor cells. *Blood* **90,** 5002–5012.
63. Gallacher, L., Murdoch, B., Wu, D. M., Karanu, F. N., Keeney, M., and Bhatia, M. (2000) Isolation and characterization of human CD34-Lin- and CD34+Lin- hematopoietic stem cells using cell surface markers AC133 and CD7. *Blood* **95,** 2813–2820.
64. Ziegler, B. L., Valtieri, M., G. Almeida, P., De Maria, R., Muller, R., Masella, B., et al. (1999) KDR receptor: A key marker defining hematopoietic stem cells. *Science* **285,** 1553–1558.
65. Peled, A., Petit, I., Kollet, O., Magid, M., Ponomaryov, T., Byk, T., et al. (1999) Dependence of human stem cell engraftment and repopulation of NOD/SCID mice on CXCR4. *Science* **283,** 845–848.
66. Kollet, O., Spiegel, A., Peled, A., Petit, I., Byk, T., Hershkoviz, R., et al. (2001) Rapid and efficient homing of human CD34+CD38-/lowCXCR4+ stem and progenitor cells to the bone marrow and spleen of NOD/SCID and NOD/SCID/B2mnull mice. *Blood* **97,** 3283–3291.
67. Rosu-Myles, M., Gallacher, L., Murdoch, B., Hess, D. A., Keeney, M., Kelvin, D., et al. (2000) The human hematopoietic stem cell compartment is heterogeneous for CXCR4 expression. *Proc. Natl. Acad. Sci. USA* **97,** 14,626–14,631.
68. Ladd, A. C., Pyatt, R., Gothot, A., Rice, S., J., M., Traycoff, C. M., and Srour, E. F. (1997) Orderly process of sequential cytokine stimulation is required for activation and maximal proliferation of primitive human bone marrow CD34+ hematopoietic progenitor cells residing in G0. *Blood* **90,** 658–668.
69. Gothot, A., van der Loo, J. C. M., Clapp, D. W., and Srour, E. F. (1998) Cell cycle-related changes in repopulating capacity of human mobilized peripheral blood CD34+ cells in non-obese diabetic/severe combined immune-deficient mice. *Blood* **92,** 2641–2649.
70. Wilpshaar, J., Falkenburg, J. H. F., Tong, X., Noort, W. A., Breese, R., Heilman, D., et al. (2000) Similar repopulating capacity of mitotically active and resting umbilical cord blood CD34+ cells in NOD/SCID mice. *Blood* **96,** 2100–2107.

71. Wilpshaar, J., Bhatia, M., Kanhai, H. H. H., Breese, R., Heilman, D. K., Johnson, C. S., et al. (2002) Engraftment potential of human fetal hematopoietic cells in NOD/SCID mice is not restricted to mitotically quiescent cells. *Blood* **100,** 120–127.
72. Hao, Q. L., Zhu, J., Price, M. A., Payne, K. J., Barsky, L. W., and Crooks, G. M. (2001) Identification of a novel, human multilymphoid progenitor in cord blood. *Blood* **15,** 3683–3690.
73. Payne, K. J. and Crooks, G. M. (2002) Human hematopoieitc lineage commitment. *Immunol. Rev.* **187,** 48–64.

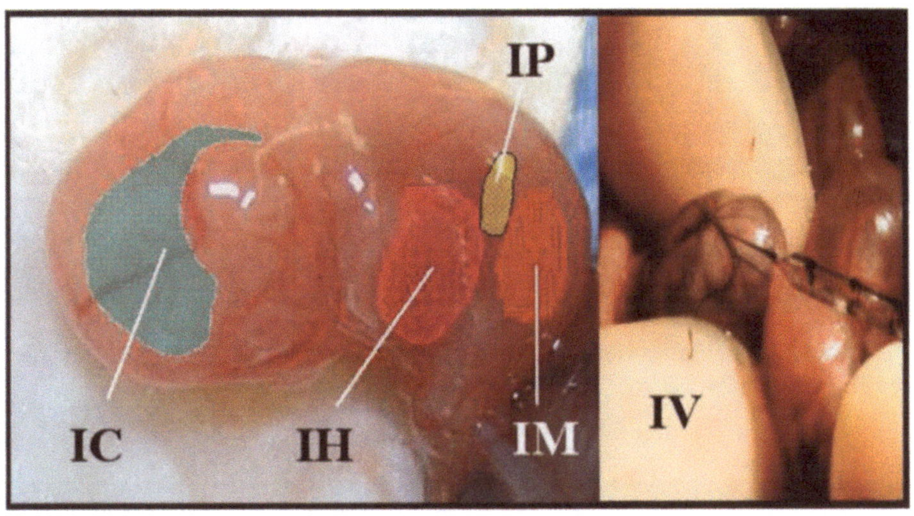

Color Plate 1, Fig. 5. A schematic demonstrating of the various routes of IUHCT. (*See* full caption on p. 88, Chapter 5.)

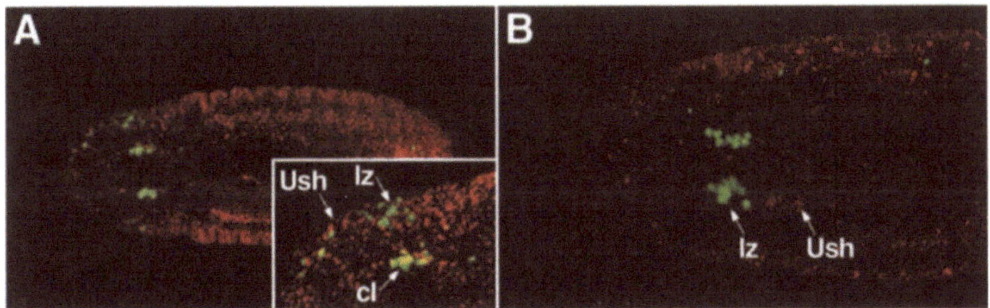

Color Plate 2, Fig. 3. Immunolocalization of lozenge and U-shaped in *Drosophila* blood cells using confocal microscopy. (*See* full caption on p. 119, Chapter 7.)

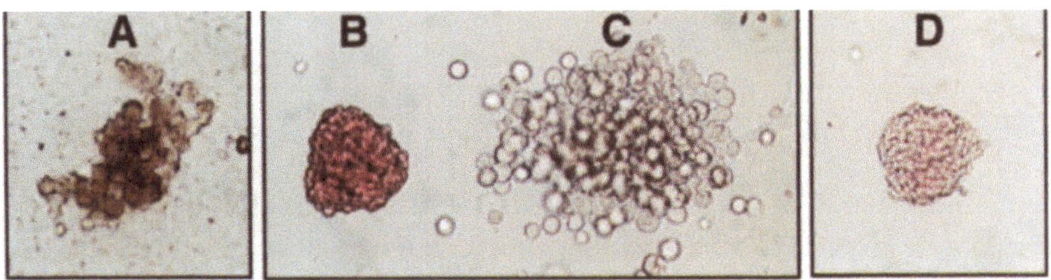

Color Plate 3, Fig. 2. Examples of murine hematopoietic colonies. (*See* full caption on p. 297, Chapter 18.)

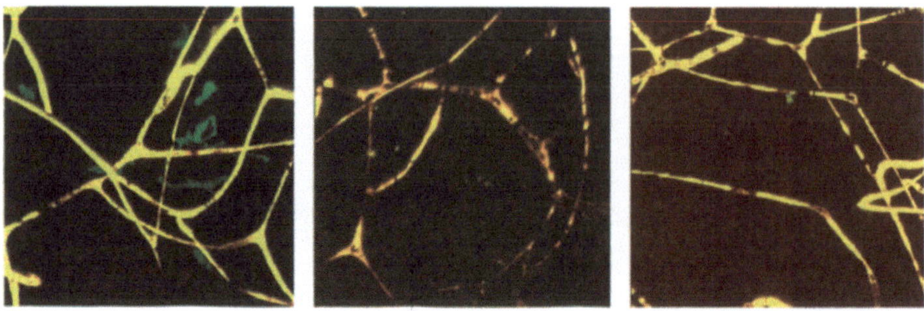

Color Plate 4, Fig. 4. Areas of neovascularization in the retina. (*See* full caption on p. 377, Chapter 24.)

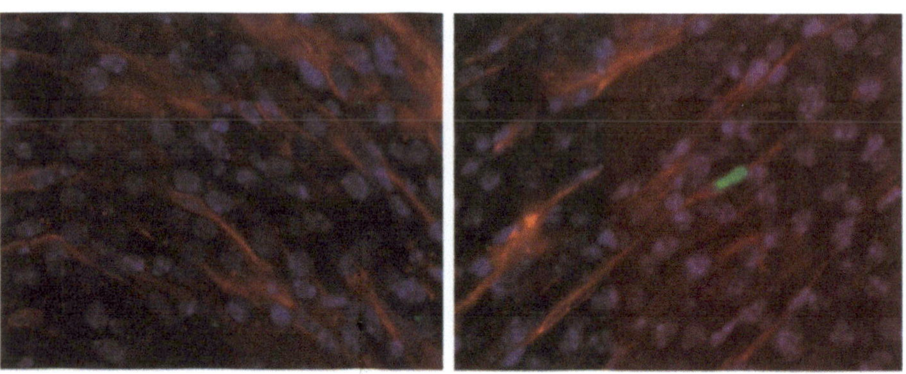

Color Plate 5, Fig. 5. Immunohistochemistry of kidney tissue sections. (*See* full caption on p. 377, Chapter 24.)

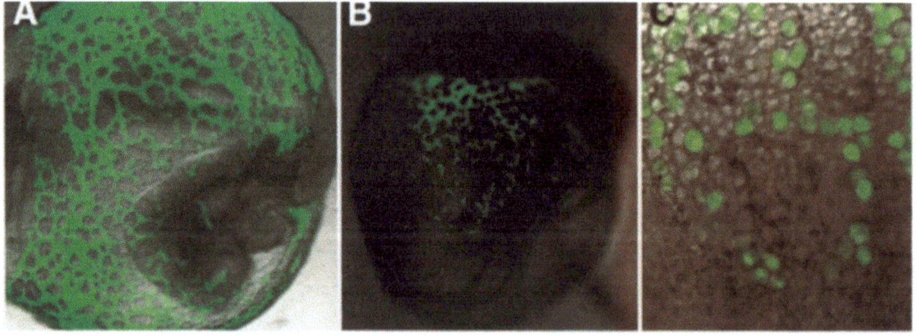

Color Plate 6, Fig. 5. Expression of GFP in Primitive Erythroblasts. (*See* full caption on p. 389, Chapter 25.)

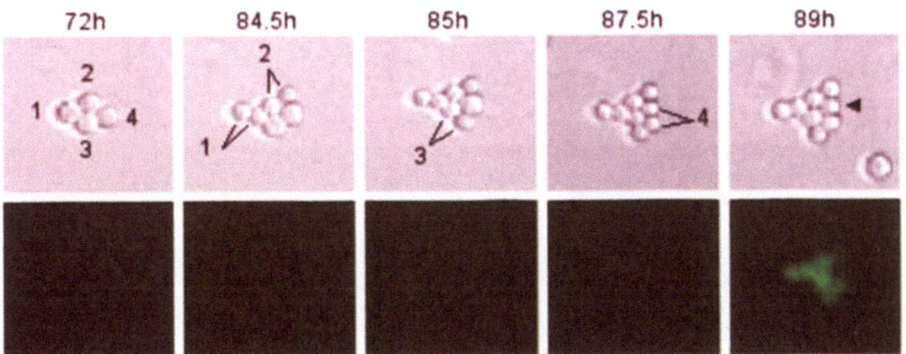

Color Plate 7, Fig. 2. Differentiation of myeloid progenitors visualized by fluorescence time-lapse microscopy. (*See* full caption on p. 398, Chapter 26.)

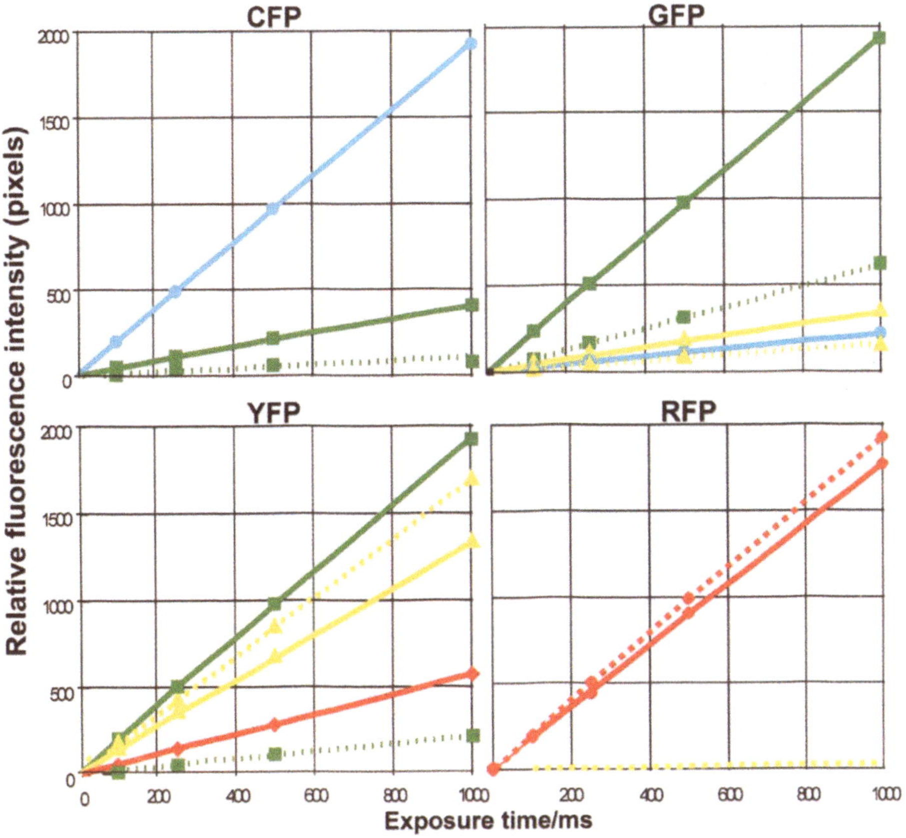

Color Plate 8, Fig. 6. Fluorescent intensities of three GFP variants and of RFP determined with the different filters. (*See* full caption on p. 403, Chapter 26.)

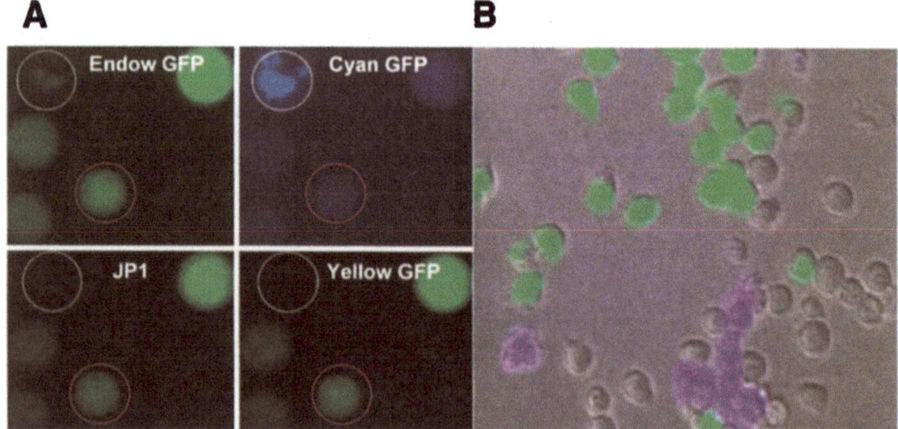

Color Plate 9, Fig. 7. CFP and GFP can be separated using the Yellow GFP filter. (*See* full caption on p. 406, Chapter 26.)

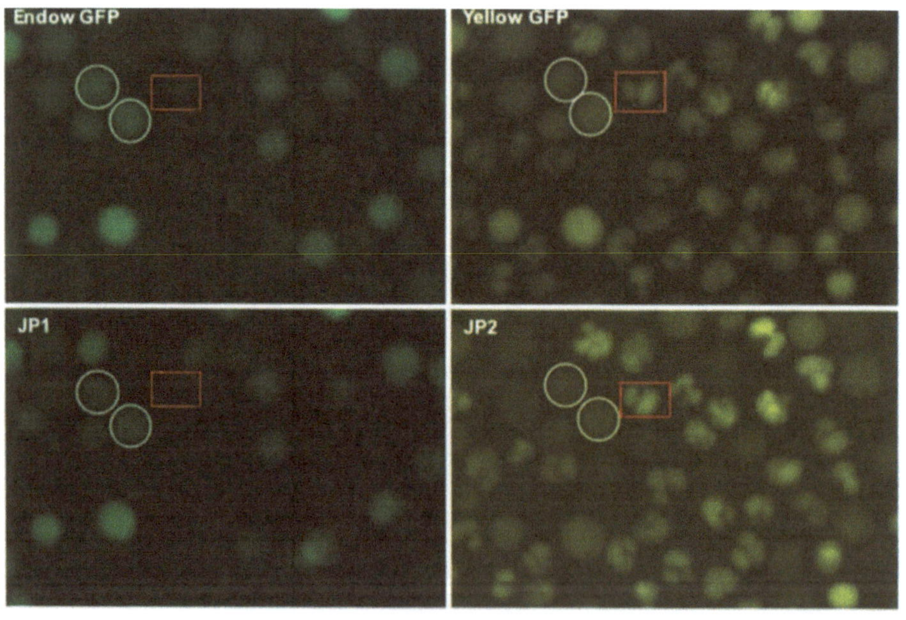

Color Plate 10, Fig. 8. The JP1/JP2 filter combination facilitates separation of GFP and YFP. (*See* full caption on p. 407, Chapter 26.)

5

Reconstitution of Hematopoiesis Following Intrauterine Transplantation of Stem Cells

Elisabeth H. Javazon, Aziz M. Merchant, Enrico Danzer, and Alan W. Flake

Summary

In utero hematopoietic stem cell transplantation is an entirely nonmyeloablative approach to achieve mixed hematopoietic chimerism and associated donor-specific tolerance. This chapter provides the rationale and methodologic detail for the administration of stem cells to the "preimmune" mouse fetus by a variety of routes. The development of murine model systems for *in utero* transplantation has accelerated progress in the field of *in utero* hematopoietic stem cell transplantation. Creative use of these models should also have experimental application to the fields of fetal gene therapy, stem cell biology, and developmental biology.

Key Words: *In utero* transplantation; mouse; fetal therapy; bone marrow transplantation; immunologic tolerance.

1. Introduction

In utero hematopoietic cell transplantation (IUHCT) is a potential therapeutic approach for a wide variety of congenital hematologic disorders that can be diagnosed early in gestation. There are three plausible clinical strategies using IUHCT that have been considered *(1)*. First, and most obvious, is the use of IUHCT as a direct approach for reconstitution of hematopoietic abnormalities that can be successfully treated by postnatal bone marrow transplantation. Second, and perhaps most important, is the use of IUHCT for prenatal tolerance induction to facilitate postnatal cellular or organ transplantation. Third, is the use of IUHCT to facilitate hematopoietic stem cell (HSC)-targeted gene therapy.

The rationale for IUHCT is based on biological advantages for transplantation that are present in the course of normal hematopoietic and immunologic ontogeny. The early gestational environment is unique in many ways that may theoretically facilitate

From: *Methods in Molecular Medicine, Vol. 105: Developmental Hematopoiesis: Methods and Protocols.*
Edited by: M. H. Baron © Humana Press Inc., Totowa, NJ

cellular therapy. First, it is highly proliferative, with exponential expansion of cellular compartments. Second, it is the only stage in life when large-scale migrations of stem cells occur to seed anatomic compartments for development of differentiated tissues. Third, the fetus is extremely small, weighing less than 75 g prior to 13-wk gestation, allowing the transplantation of much larger cell doses on a per kilogram basis than can be achieved after birth. Perhaps the most important potential advantage, however, is the phenomenon of fetal tolerance ***(2)***. The early gestational immune system undergoes a process of self-education. This occurs primarily in the fetal thymus and consists of two components, the positive selection of pre-lymphocytes for recognition of "self" major histocompatibility complex antigen (MHC) and a negative selection (deletion) of prelymphocytes that have high-affinity recognition of self-antigen in association with self-MHC ***(3–5)***. This leaves a repertoire of lymphocytes that recognize foreign antigen in association with self-MHC. Thus, introduction of foreign cells that are capable of appropriate antigen presentation in the thymus prior to completion of this process should result in donor-specific immune tolerance. Taken together, the normal biology of the fetus allows the potential for a therapeutic recapitulation of ontogeny, with engraftment, migration, differentiation and expansion of stem cells in various recipient cellular compartments.

There is now considerable experimental evidence supporting the rationale for IUHCT. The most successful animal model has historically been the sheep. Early gestational transplantation of allogeneic fetal liver-derived HSC into normal sheep fetuses results in a high rate of sustained multilineage hematopoietic chimerism, which persists for many years ***(6,7)*** and is typically in the range of 10 to 15% bone marrow (BM) and peripheral blood donor cell expression. The fetal sheep model is also permissive for widely disparate xenogeneic engraftment. Multilineage hematopoietic chimerism has been well documented after human fetal liver-derived HSC transplantation ***(8,9)*** and after transplantation of a variety of adult populations derived from humans ***(10–12)***. In addition, we have shown that chimerism in the human sheep model is caused by the engraftment of pluripotent HSC by documentation of long-term repopulation by donor cells on retransplantation into second-generation fetal lamb recipients ***(8)***. Despite the success of the sheep model, engraftment in other models has been difficult to achieve. Until recently, the sheep was the only model in which engraftment greater than "microchimerism" was accomplished. The likely barriers to engraftment in most species, including humans, were recently reviewed ***(13)*** and can be categorized as a lack of available space, host cell competition, and undefined immunologic barriers. To systematically examine the relative importance of these barriers and develop strategies to overcome them, the development of the murine model was critical. The available inbred and transgenic strains, defined immunology, large litter size, minimal cost, and short gestation of the mouse allows studies to be performed that simply cannot be considered in other species. In addition, the mouse is, stage for stage, very similar to the human with respect to hematopoietic and immunologic ontogeny. *In utero* cellular transplants can be performed early in gestation (11–15 d), during a time when hematopoiesis is confined to the fetal liver and prior to completion of thymic processing and the appearance of mature lymphocytes in the peripheral circulation. Finally, the normal mouse has proven very difficult to engraft, making it a legitimate model for investigation of barriers to engraftment. For many years, we and others were able to achieve microchimerism only in hematopoietically competitive strains ***(14–19)***. To assess the reason for failure, we performed a kinetic study of homing and engraftment after *in utero* transplantation ***(20)***. The study clearly demonstrated that engraftment efficiency was no better in the fetal recipient than in the adult and that one reason for inability to achieve measurable levels of chimerism was the inability to engraft an adequate number of stem cells. In response to this study, we improved our cell preparations and performed a dose escalation study to investigate the effect of increasing cell doses. With improved delivery of higher numbers of HSC we have been able to achieve macrochimerism in multiple allogeneic strain combinations ***(21,22)***.

Although IUHCT has thus far had only limited clinical success ***(23–25)***, significant experimental progress is being made in animal models and there is reason to be optimistic regarding the future of IUHCT. In addition to IUHCT, the characterization of other, nonhematopoietic stem cell populations allows consideration of prenatal strategies for the treatment of nonhematologic disorders. Finally, *in utero* transplantation may have future experimental applications for stem cell biologists interested in explorations of normal and disease induced stem cell "plasticity" ***(26)***. The purpose of this chapter is to discuss current experimental progress in IUHCT, and describe a murine model system that has proven extremely valuable in achieving this progress.

2. The Murine Model of *In Utero* Stem Cell Transplantation

To systematically investigate the barriers to engraftment after IUHCT, as well as to investigate the efficacy of IUHCT in murine models that closely mimic human diseases, we have focused our efforts on developing the murine model of IUHCT. We will describe the materials and surgical methods required to perform murine *in utero* cellular transplantation.

2.1. Materials for Micropipet Production

1. Micropipet puller (Sutter Instrument Co.; model P-30; **Fig. 1**).
2. Micropipet beveller (Sutter Instrument Co.; model Bv-10; **Fig. 2**) and micropipets (Fisher Scientific, Pittsburgh, PA; *see* **Note 1**).
3. Microinjector or tubing with an attachment for the micropipet (**Fig. 3**; *see* **Note 2**).
4. Microscope reticule (0.5-mm range, with 0.01 minor delineations and 0.05 major delineations is ideal for measuring the external diameter of the micropipets).
5. Stage micrometer (to ensure that the reticle delineations are correct).

2.2. Pipet Design

The production of a sharp, smooth micropipet is crucial to obtaining accurate injections and fetal survival. A micropipet with too large an opening or uneven, sharp borders will increase fetal mortality. Additionally, a micropipet with too small an opening may damage the cells or become occluded. For hematopoietic cell injection we generally aim for an outer diameter between 70 and 90 μm. The heat and height at which the micropipets are pulled will vary according to the external diameter of the micropipets and the model of machine. In our laboratory, settings for a micropipet puller read 910 units for heat and 850 U for pull (**Fig. 4**).

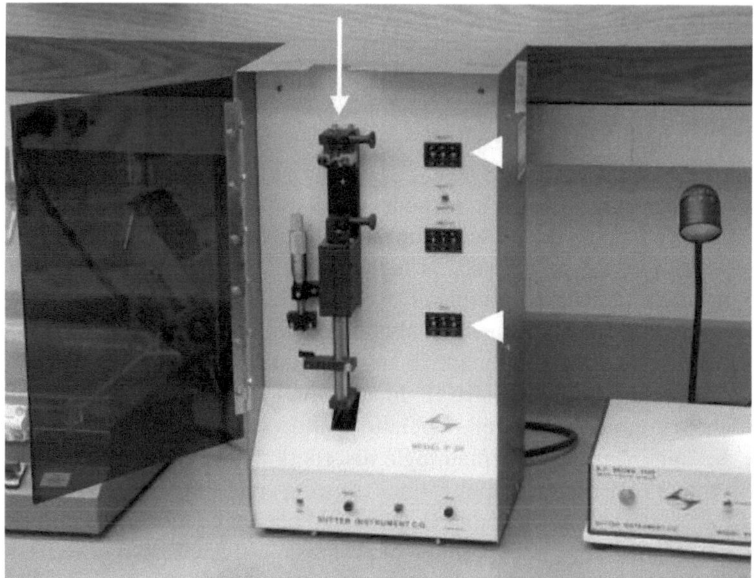

Fig. 1. A model P-30 micropipet puller acquired from the Sutter Instrument Company. The arrow points toward the micropipet holder and weight mechanism. The arrowheads indicate the temperature and weight settings.

1. Place the micropipet into the micropipet puller.
2. After the micropipet has been pulled, use a razor blade to cut approx 1 to 2 mm off the tip of the micropipet.
3. Place the micropipet onto the micropipet beveller. The angle of the micropipet beveller is set between 15 and 20°. The tip of the micropipet is placed onto the grinding stone so that it just barely touches the surface. As the stone spins, a sharp, smooth, surface is created at the micropipet tip. Once the beveling process has begun, the micropipet is checked every 5 min (to ensure the tip of the micropipet is continually touching the surface of the grinding stone). The entire process requires approx 20 to 30 min.
4. Place the beveled micropipet under the microscope containing the reticle to examine the tip (*see* **Note 3**).
5. Draw the volume demarcations onto the micropipet (*see* **Note 4**).

2.3. Animal Husbandry

Accurate time-dated pregnant mice are crucial for efficient and effective IUHCT.

1. From the time of weaning (3–4 wk after birth) or 2 wk before mating, all male mice are housed separately. Female mice are housed three to four per cage.
2. At the time of mating, one or two female mice are placed into a cage containing one male mouse.
3. The following morning, the female mice are examined for vaginal plugs. Female mice with vaginal plugs are separated from the male mice. Female mice that do not have vaginal plugs remain housed with the male mice.

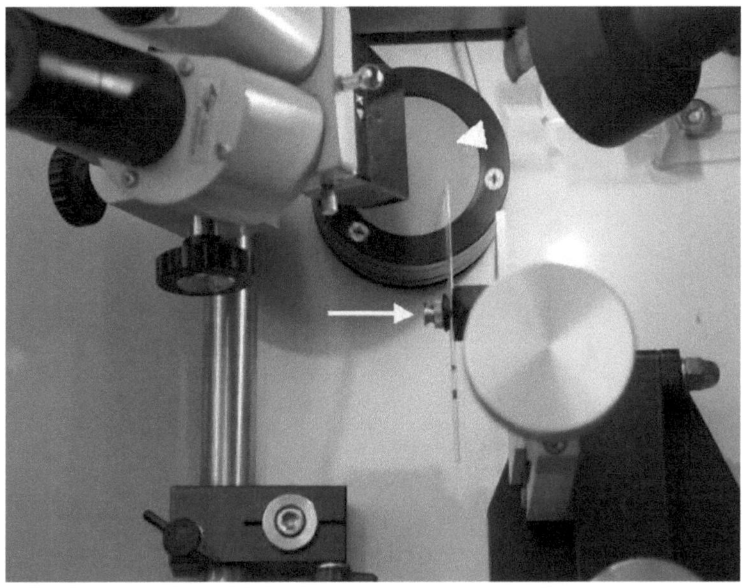

Fig. 2. A model Bv-10 micropipet beveller acquired from Sutter Instrument Company. The arrow points toward the micropipet holder. The arrowhead indicates the grinding stone.

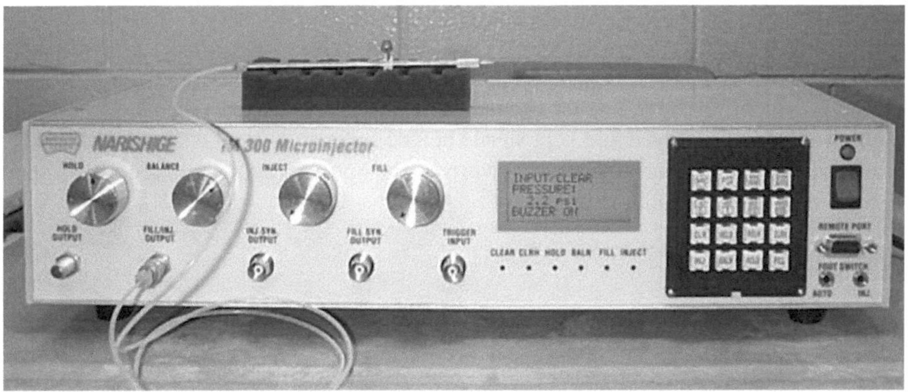

Fig. 3. An IM 300 programmable microinjector (MicroData Instrument, Inc.).

4. The unplugged female mice from the previous day are examined for vaginal plugs again the next morning (36–48 h after the initial mating). Female mice with vaginal plugs are removed. Female mice without vaginal plugs and male mice are separated and returned to the colony for future matings.
5. The day of plugging is defined as gestational d 0.

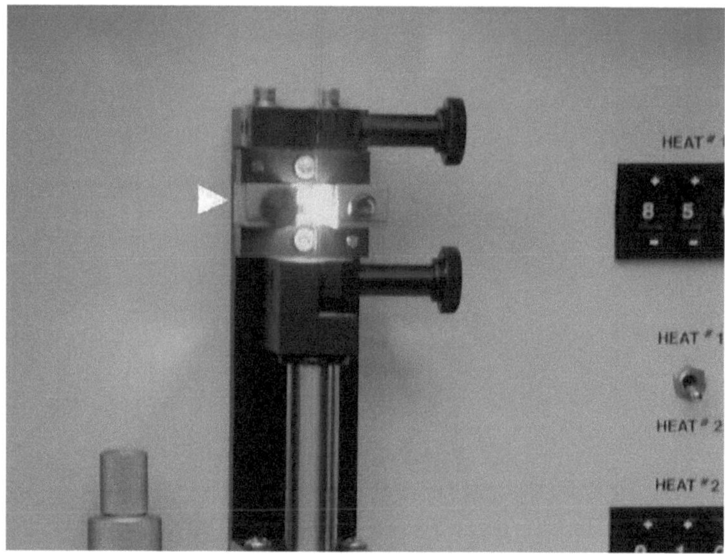

Fig. 4. Once the micropipet is inserted and stabilized into the micropipet puller, the filament (indicated by the arrowhead) becomes hot. As the glass micropipet begins to melt, the weight, pulling downward on the glass, elongates and narrows the micropipet. Eventually the weight causes the micropipet to break apart, forming a small tip, which can then be placed on the beveller to grind into a sharp smooth point.

2.4. Surgical Supplies for IUHCT

A key aspect to IUHCT is clean surgical technique. All instruments, swabs, and drapes must be autoclaved and kept sterile before surgery. During surgery, clean technique is used, that is, sterile gloves are worn by the operator and instruments are wiped with alcohol between mice.

1. Sterile scissors, forceps, needle driver.
2. Sterile cotton swabs.
3. Sterile drapes.
4. Alcohol pads.
5. 5-O Vicryl sutures (C-3 cutting).
6. Surgical tape (3M transpore).
7. Surgical board.
8. Surgical gloves.
9. N_2 gas for the microinjector.
10. Anesthesia.
11. Warm phosphate-buffered saline (PBS).
12. 1-mL and 10-mL syringes.
13. Clean cages.
14. Heating lamp or blanket.
15. 70% ETOH.

2.5. Anesthesia

There are multiple types of anesthesia available for mice. A solution of ketamine and xylazine sustains an anesthetized mouse for 30 min to 2 h; however, once the mice are anesthetized, a salve must be placed onto their eyes to prevent drying and blindness. A vaporizer releasing isoflurane results in rapid sedation and recovery and is an excellent anesthesia method for IUHCT in mice. Without an isoflurane vaporizer, it is difficult to control the dose of isoflurane and it is easy to overdose the mouse. Methoxyflurane is expensive and difficult to obtain; however, a vaporizer is not required and both sedation and recovery are rapid. When choosing an anesthetic technique, keep in mind that the IUHCT procedure, once mastered, is rapid and can be performed in less than 15 min.

Before the surgery begins, make sure to check the level of anesthesia. Perform a sharp tail pinch and foot pinch while examining the mouse's respiratory rate and movement. Increased respiratory rate upon painful stimuli, even in the absence of movement, indicates that the mouse is not completely anesthetized. Wait a few minutes and perform the task again. Breathing of an anesthetized mouse is slow and consistent. Gasping is a result of too much anesthesia and the anesthesia should be removed or decreased until slow, regular respirations are resumed.

2.6. In Utero *Transplantation (IUHCT)*

Visual determination of the pregnancy status of female mice can be obvious or indistinguishable from non-pregnant mice depending on the strain, age, and number of fetuses a mouse may be carrying. The ideal time for *in utero* injections is 14–16 d following the identification of a vaginal plug. There are different types of *in utero* injections: intravenous (iv), intraperitoneal (i.p.), intrahepatic (i.h.), intramuscular (i.m.), and intracranial (i.c.; **Fig. 5**).

1. Once the mouse is anesthetized, place her supine onto a surgical board.
   Using surgical tape, secure the hindlimbs and the forelimbs to the surgical board. Placing the tape too tightly over the upper torso, when securing the forelimbs, can inhibit respiration.
2. Using alcohol pads, clean the abdominal region (*see* **Note 5**).
3. Cut an opening in the center of a sterile drape (small enough to just cover the lower torso of the female mouse) and place it over the abdominal area.
4. Perform a midline laparotomy by incising the skin vertically over approx 2 cm of the lower abdomen.
5. Using fine forceps and scissors lift the fascia of the abdomen in the midline and cut a small opening, taking care not to injure underlying viscera. Extend the fascial incision by placing one blade of the scissors through the opening and incising in both directions.
6. Exteriorize the uterus through the wound using moist sterile cotton swabs (*see* **Note 6**).
7. Determine the number of fetuses available for injection. Using a 10-mL syringe, apply warm (37°C) PBS to the exposed uterus every few minutes to prevent dessication.
8. Aspirate the cells into the micropipet (*see* **Note 7**).
9. Apply PBS to the fingertips of the hand that will be used to maneuver the fetuses. Gently hold the uterus containing a single fetus between the forefinger and thumb. Using slight pressure and movement, guide the fetus into the necessary position for injection (**Fig. 6**).
   a. I.M. injections typically target the hindlimb muscles. For i.p. injections, the micropipet is inserted into the abdomen into a small space that can be visualized between the

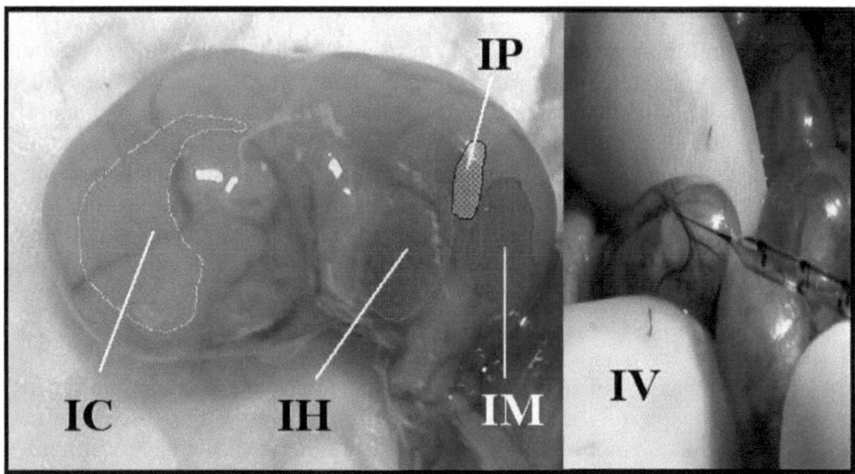

Fig. 5. A schematic demonstrating the various routes of IUHCT. The left panel diagrams i.c., i.h., i.p., and i.m. injections by highlighting the corresponding target areas. The right panel demonstrates iv injections using Trypan blue dye. As the dye enters the vasculature of the fetus, all of the vessels become dark blue. *See* color insert following p. 80.

hindlimb and the liver. Micropipets are inserted directly into the liver for i.h. injections.

b. The vitelline veins are the targets for iv injections. These veins are relatively fixed within the membrane of the visceral yolk sac proximal to their convergence and empty directly into the portal circulation of the fetus. The veins can be differentiated from other vessels within the membranes by their course into the umbilical stalk and their minimal movement when the uterus is manipulated. The tip of the micropipet is inserted, bevel down, into the uterus and through the vessel wall. Once a backflash of blood is seen entering the micropipet, the stem cells are injected (*see* **Note 8**). After an injection, the micropipet is withdrawn and the next fetus is injected. We typically inject the entire litter; however, selected fetuses can be injected.

10. Gently return the fetuses into the peritoneal cavity using the moist cotton swabs. If intestines were exposed, place them into the peritoneal cavity prior to replacing the uterus.
11. Using absorbable sutures (5-O Vicryl C-3 cutting), close the wound in two layers. Just before completely closing the first layer, inject 1 mL of warm PBS into the maternal peritoneal cavity.

2.7. Postoperative Protocol

Female mice undergoing a laparotomy quickly recover. Following the laparotomy, keep the mouse under a warming light until the mouse is dry and mobile. Place the mouse into a clean cage with extra bedding (squares used for the mice to make birthing beds). If a mouse does not become mobile within the allotted time for that specified anesthesia, sacrifice immediately.

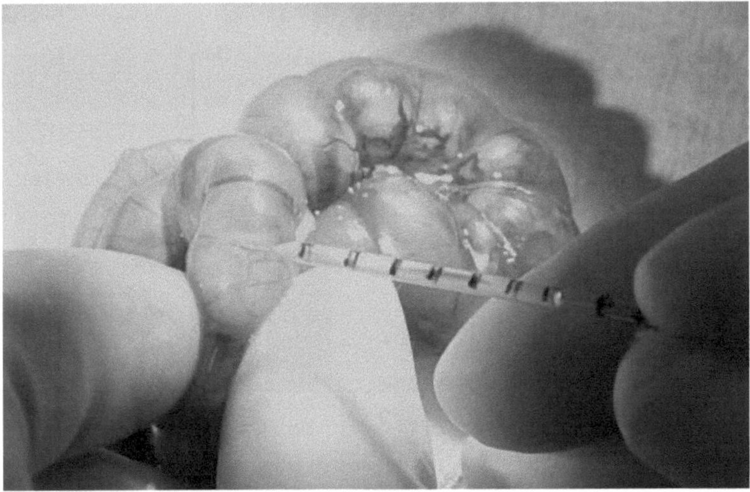

Fig. 6. Demonstrating the correct holding position for IUHCT. By carefully grasping the fetus between the thumb and forefinger, the fetus becomes immobile for visualization and injection of the desired target area.

3. Hematopoietic Engraftment in Normal and Defective Mouse Strains

3.1. Hematopoietic Engraftment in Normal Mouse Strains

The most difficult mice to engraft have been strains with a "normal" hematopoietic system, that is, animals in which there is not a competitive advantage for normal cells. Within normal mouse strains, the engraftment that can be achieved is dependent upon multiple variables, including cell dose, cell source, and the specific strain combination. Representative levels of engraftment that we have achieved after varying each of these parameters are presented in **Fig. 7**. Fetal liver derived donor cells are far more efficient than adult BM-derived cells in all strain combinations tested. There are many potential reasons for this but the most likely is that they compete better after engraftment with the host fetal liver (FL) cells. Levels of engraftment increase with increasing doses of cells transplanted. However, it should be noted that the doses required to achieve even low-level engraftment are much higher on a per kilogram basis than in adult transplantation. Finally, strain combination is critical. There are significant differences in engraftment between strains that have yet to be understood. In general, congenic cells do not engraft better than allogeneic cells ***(22,27)***, so it does not appear to be purely a matter of MHC matching. More likely, it has to do with class I MHC recognition and natural killer (NK) cell-mediated resistance to engraftment, analogous to well documented "hybrid resistance" ***(28,29)***. It is clear that tolerance by a mechanism of clonal deletion can be achieved by IUHCT ***(21)***, but there are abundant NK cells present in FL at 14 d gestation that are functionally active. The role of the innate immune system in resistance to engraftment after IUHCT remains to be defined.

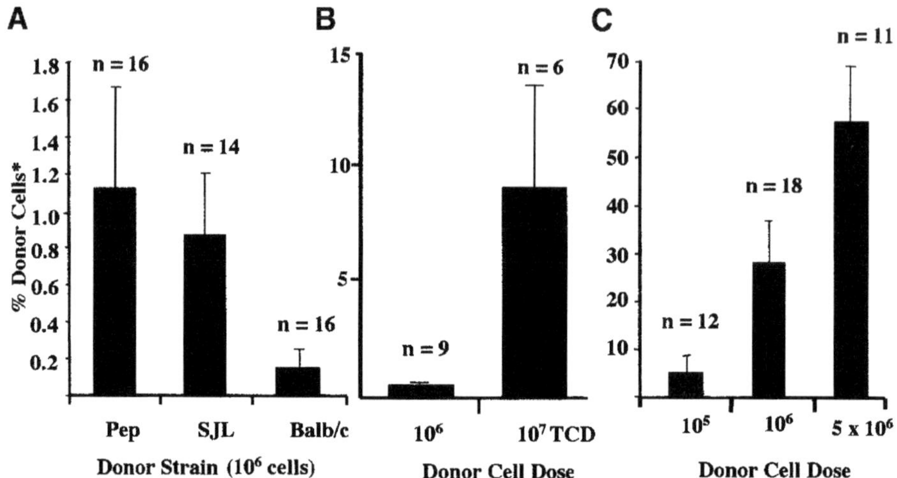

Fig. 7. The effect of strain combination, dose, and cell source on donor cell engraftment after IUHCT. (**A**) PB chimerism in B6 recipients of adult BM from three different strain donors. (**B**) PB chimerism of Balb/c recipients of B6 BM at low and high doses. (**C**) PB chimerism in B6 recipients of various doses of SJL FL demonstrating the dramatically higher levels of dose dependent engraftment achieved with FL derived donor cells (all levels measured at 6 mo of age). Note the difference in scale of the *y*-axis for the three figures. PB, peripheral blood; FL, fetal liver; TCD, T-cell depleted; B6, C57BL6; Pep,C57BL/6; Ly5.1:Pep3B.

Tolerance after IUHCT is related to the level of engraftment. We have found that tolerance by criteria of skin graft survival for greater than 8 wk is variably present in animals with "microchimerism" (levels of engraftment detectable by polymerase chain reaction) and that the presence of tolerance is associated with at least partial deletion of alloreactive T-cells ***(17,18)***. In contrast, all animals with levels of chimerism greater than 2 to 3% have associated tolerance with a high degree of clonal deletion ***(21,22,30)***.

3.2. Hematopoietic Engraftment in Defective Mouse Models

In contrast to normal animal models, it is clear that when a competitive advantage for normal cells exists, high levels of donor cell engraftment can be expected. This was first demonstrated by Fleishman and Mintz ***(31)*** in studies in W mutant anemic mouse strains, that have a stem cell deficiency based on the absence of c-kit. *In utero* transplantation of normal allogeneic FL cells by transplacental injection at 11 d gestation resulted in rescue of severely anemic mice and complete replacement by donor hematopoiesis. The degree of erythroid replacement correlated with the degree of underlying anemia, with complete early replacement by donor erythroid cells in the lethally anemic W/W homozygotes, and partial but progressively increasing replacement by donor erythroid cells in the sublethally anemic W^v/W^v homozygotes. Similarly, in the mouse severe combined immunodeficiency disease model, in which there is early arrest of T- and B-cell development, lymphoid reconstitution occurs following IUHCT

(32,33). In reconstituted animals, T and B lymphocytes were entirely of donor origin. Although donor myeloid and erythroid elements could not be consistently detected, the engraftment of donor HSC in the marrow was clearly documented by retransplantation experiments. Thus, in the presence of a lineage deficiency, IUHCT can selectively reconstitute the defective lineage, but it appears that competitive pressure from the normal host lineages prevents high-level multilineage donor cell expression. More recent studies in the nonobese diabetic-severe combined immunodeficient mouse confirm these observations *(34)*. In this model, the defect in T- and B-cell development is the same as for the SCID mouse, but in addition there are known defects in NK cells and antigen presentation. IUHCT in nonobese diabetic-severe combined immunodeficient recipients results in multilineage engraftment, with increasing donor cell expression over time. The success in these model systems supports the conjecture that the primary barrier to engraftment in the fetus is host cell competition, but does not exclude potential immune-based mechanisms as an additional barrier in specific circumstances.

4. Notes

1. The external diameter of the micropipet can vary depending on the type of injection to be performed. For injections that require volumes of 5 μL or more, use soda-lime glass micropipets with a 1.9- to 2.0-mm external diameter (100-μL volume; Fisher Scientific, Pittsburgh, PA; cat. no. 71900-100). For injections that require volumes of less than 5 μL, use 15 cm of borosilicate glass micropipets with an external diameter of 1.0 mm and an internal diameter of 0.5 mm (Fisher Scientific, Pittsburgh, PA; cat. no. BF100-50-15). Intracranial injections typically use the smaller micropipets because the total injection volume per fetus is 1 μL.
2. A short length of tubing with a small attachment at the end for the micropipet is suitable for IUHCT. However, this method requires two people (one person to aspirate and inject the cells using a 1- to 3-mL syringe for pressure while the other person manipulates and injects the fetuses). A microinjector permits one person to perform the injections and, more importantly, standardizes the procedure so that each injection maintains the same volume, pressure, and duration of injection.
3. A microscope fitted with a reticle is used to examine the smoothness, sharpness, and the external diameter of the micropipets. After pulling and grinding, 2-mm micropipets have an external diameter of between 80 and 100 μm and 1.0-mm micropipets have an external diameter between 40 and 60 μm. By changing the length of the tip, the final external diameter of the tip can be altered to accommodate different stem cell concentrations.
4. To standardize the injections, the micropipets are labeled with accurate volume delineations. The equation to determine the length on a micropipet that is equal to a given volume is: $h = v/\pi r^2$; where h = height, v = volume, and r = radius. Once the internal diameter of the micropipet is known, the height for a given volume is calculated. A graph consisting of a horizontal line with demarcations corresponding to the calculated height is created, printed, and then used as a template to mark the volume demarcations onto the micropipets.
5. Always move in a downward motion from the upper abdominal area down to the vaginal and anal areas. This will ensure that any urine or feces will not be present near your incision and will not infect the area.
6. Before beginning the surgery, place two sterile cotton swabs into preheated (37°C) PBS. These swabs will be used to remove the fetuses from and replace into the maternal body cavity.

7. Stem cells are prepared in a sterile environment and resuspended at 2×10^5 cells/mL or 1×10^6 cells/mL in 0.5-mL microcentrifuge tubes. The tubes are placed on ice until the cells are needed for injections. Immediately prior to aspirating into the micropipet, the cells are resuspended using a vortex.
8. IUHCT iv is the most difficult type of injection to perform. In addition to a dissecting microscope, iv injections require extreme dexterity. Penetration through the entire vessel, which results in bleeding between the membranes and into the amniotic sac, is common when performing iv injections. This blood loss does not necessarily result in fetal death, but that particular vein can no longer be used for injections and visualization of other veins may be compromised. Gestational age is critical for successful IUHCT iv. The transparency of the uterine wall varies with gestational age. The vitelline veins of fetuses younger than embryonic d 14 (E14) or older than E16 are difficult to visualize owing to the opacity of the uterus. The uterus becomes less opaque and more transparent between E14 and E16. A dissecting scope is not required for i.p., i.h., i.m., and i.c. injections, although surgical magnifying loupes (Designs for Vision, 3.5X) are recommended.

References

1. Flake, A. W. and Zanjani, E. D. (1999) In utero hematopoietic stem cell transplantation: Ontogenic opportunities and biologic barriers. *Blood* **94,** 2179–2191.
2. Billingham, R., Brent, L., and Medawar, P. B. (1953) Actively acquired tolerance of foreign cells. *Nature* **172,** 603–607.
3. Sha, W. C. and Nelson, C. A. (1988) Positive and negative selection of an antigen receptor on T-cells in transgenic mice. *Nature* **336,** 73–76.
4. Schwartz, R. (1989) Acquisition of Immunologic Self Tolerance. *Cell* **57,** 1073–1081.
5. Blackman, M., Kappler, J., and Marrack, P. (1990) The role of the T-cell receptor in positive and negative selection of developing T-cells. *Science* **248,** 1335–1342.
6. Flake, A. W., Harrison, M. R., Adzick, N. S., and Zanjani, E. D. (1986) Transplantation of fetal hematopoietic stem cells in utero: the creation of hematopoietic chimeras. *Science* **233,** 776–778.
7. Zanjani, E. D., Ascensao, J. L., Flake, A. W., Harrison, M. R., and Tavassoli, M. (1992) The fetus as an optimal donor and recipient of hemopoietic stem cells. *Bone Marrow Transplant.* **10(Suppl. 1),** 107–114.
8. Zanjani, E. D., Flake, A. W., Rice, H., Hedrick, M., and Tavassoli, M. (1994) Long-term repopulating ability of xenogeneic transplanted human fetal liver hematopoietic stem cells in sheep. *J. Clin. Invest.* **93,** 1051–1065.
9. Zanjani, E. D., Pallavicini, M. G., Flake, A. W., Ascensao, J. L., Langlois, R. G., Reitsma, M., et al. (1992) Engraftment and long-term expression of human fetal hemopoietic stem cells in sheep following transplantation in utero. *J. Clin. Invest.* **89,** 1178–1188.
10. Srour, E. F., Zanjani, E. D., Brandt, J. E., Leemhuis, T., Briddell, R. A., Heerema, N. A., et al. (1992) Sustained human hematopoiesis in sheep transplanted in utero during early gestation with fractionated adult human bone marrow cells. *Blood* **79,** 1404–1412.
11. Civin, C. J., Lee, M. J., Hedrick, M., Rice, H., and Zanjani, E. D. (1993) Purified CD34+/lineage-/38- cells contain hematopoeitic stem cells. *Blood* **82(Suppl. 1),** 180a (abstract 707).
12. Zanjani, E. D., Almeida-Porada, G., Livingston, A. G., Flake, A. W., and Ogawa, M. (1998) Human bone marrow CD34- cells engraft in vivo and undergo multilineage expression that includes giving rise to CD34+ cells. *Exp. Hematol.* **26,** 353–360.
13. Almeida-Porada, G., Flake, A. W., Glimp, H. A., and Zanjani, E. D. (1999) Co-transplantation of stroma results in enhancement of engraftment and early expression of donor hematopoietic stem cell in utero. *Exp. Hematol.* **27,** 1569–1575.

14. Carrier, E., Lee, T. H., Busch, M. P., and Cowan, M. J. (1995) Induction of tolerance in nondefective mice after in utero transplantation of major histocompatibility complex-mismatched fetal hematopoietic stem cells. *Blood* **86,** 4681–4690.
15. Carrier, E., Gilpin, E., Lee, T. H., Busch, M. P., and Zanetti, M. (2000) Microchimerism does not induce tolerance after in utero transplantation and may lead to the development of alloreactivity. *J. Lab. Clin. Med.* **136,** 224–235.
16. Blazar, B. R., Taylor, P. A., and Vallera, D. A. (1995) Adult bone marrow-derived pluripotent hematopoietic stem cells are engraftable when transferred in utero into moderately anemic fetal recipients. *Blood* **85,** 833–841.
17. Kim, H. B., Shaaban, A. F., Yang, E. Y., Liechty, K. W., and Flake, A. W. (1998) Microchimerism and tolerance after in utero bone marrow transplantation in mice. *J. Surg. Res.* **77,** 1–5.
18. Kim, H. B., Shaaban, A. F., Milner, R., Fichter, C., and Flake, A. W. (1999) In utero bone marrow transplantation induces tolerance by a combination of clonal deletion and anergy. *J. Pediatr. Surg.* **34,** 726–730.
19. Pallavicini, M. G., Flake, A. W., Madden, D., Bethel, C., Duncan, B., Gonzalgo, M. L., et al. (1992) Hemopoietic chimerism in rodents transplanted in utero with fetal human hemopoietic cells. *Transplant. Proc.* **24,** 542–543.
20. Shaaban, A. F., Kim, H. B., Milner, R., and Flake, A. W. (1999) A kinetic model for homing and migration of prenatally transplanted marrow. *Blood* **94,** 3251–3257.
21. Hayashi, S., Peranteau, W. H., Shaaban, A. F., and Flake, A. W. (2002) Complete allogeneic hematopoietic chimerism achieved by a combined strategy of in utero hematopoietic stem cell transplantation and postnatal donor lymphocyte infusion. *Blood* **100,** 804–812.
22. Peranteau, W. F., Hayashi, S., Hsieh, M., Shaaban, A. F., and Flake, A. W. (2002) High level allogeneic chimerism achieved by prenatal tolerance induction and postnatal nonmyeloablative bone marrow transplantation. *Blood* **100,** 2225–2234.
23. Flake, A., Roncarolo, M.-G., Puck, J., Almeida-Porada, G., Evans, M., Johnson, M., et al. (1996) Treatment of X-linked severe combined immunodeficiency by in utero transplantation of paternal bone marrow. *N. Engl. J. Med.* **335,** 1806–1810.
24. Wengler, G., Lanfranchi, A., Frusca, T., Verardi, R., Neva, A., Brugnoni, D., et al. (1996) In-utero transplantation of parental CD34 haematopoietic progenitor cells in a patient with X-linked severe combined immunodeficiency (SCIDX1). *Lancet* **348,** 1484–1487.
25. Westgren, M., Ringden, O., Bartmann, P., Bui, T. H., Lindton, B., Mattsson, J., et al. (2002) Prenatal T-cell reconstitution after in utero transplantation with fetal liver cells in a patient with X-linked severe combined immunodeficiency. Am. J. Obstet. Gynecol. **187,** 475–482.
26. Liechty, K. W., MacKenzie, T. C., Shaaban, A. F., Radu, A., Moseley, A. M., Deans, R., et al. (2000) Human mesenchymal stem cells engraft and demonstrate site-specific differentiation after in utero transplantation in sheep. *Nat. Med.* **6,** 1282–1286.
27. Milner, R., Shaaban, A., Kim, H. B., Fichter, C., and Flake, A. W. (1999) Postnatal booster injections increase engraftment after in utero stem cell transplantation. *J. Surg. Res.* **83,** 44–47.
28. Bennett, M. (1987) Biology and genetics of hybrid resistance. *Adv. Immunol.* **41,** 333–345.
29. Daley, J. P. and Nakamura, I. (1984) Natural resistance of lethally irradiated F1 hybrid mice to parental marrow grafts is a function of H-2/Hh-restricted effectors. *J. Exp. Med.* **159,** 1132–1148.
30. Hayashi, S., Abdulmalik, O., Peranteau, W. H., Ashizuka, S., Campagnoli, C., Chen, Q., et al. (2003) Mixed chimerism following in utero hematopoietic stem cell transplantation in murine models of hemoglobinopathy. *Exp. Hematol.* **31,** 176–184.

31. Fleischman, R. and Mintz, B. (1979) Prevention of genetic anemias in mice by microinjection of normal hematopoietic cells into the fetal placenta. *Proc. Natl. Acad. Sci. USA* **76,** 5736–5740.
32. Blazar, B. R., Taylor, P. A., and Vallera, D. A. (1995) In utero transfer of adult bone marrow cells into recipients with severe combined immunodeficiency disorder yields lymphoid progeny with T- and B-cell functional capabilities. *Blood* **86,** 4353–4366.
33. Blazer, B. R., Taylor, P. A., McElmurry, R., Tian, L., Panoskaltsis-Mortari, A., Lam, S., et al. (1998) Engraftment of severe combined immune deficient mice receiving allogeneic bone marrow via in utero or postnatal transfer. *Blood* **92,** 3949–3959.
34. Archer, D. R., Turner, C. W., Yeager, A. M., and Fleming, W. H. (1997) Sustained multilineage engraftment of allogeneic hematopoietic stem cells in NOD/SCID mice after in utero transplantation. *Blood* **90,** 3222–3229.

6

Reconstitution of Hematopoiesis Following Transplantation Into Neonatal Mice

Scott A. Johnson and Mervin C. Yoder

Summary

The primary sites of hematopoiesis change during murine ontogeny. The first blood cells emerge in two waves in the yolk sac; primitive erythroblasts, megakaryocytes, and macrophages emerge on embryonic d (E) 7.0, whereas definitive progenitor cells appear as clusters within the yolk sac vasculature on E8.25. Of interest, yolk sac cells isolated prior to d 10.5 fail to engraft in myeloablated adult recipient mice and do not reconstitute hematopoiesis. We describe a method of sublethally myeloablating newborn mice in which E9.0 yolk sac cells engraft and repopulate all lineages of the hematopoietic system for up to 12 mo in primary recipients and up to 6 mo in secondary recipients. The exact mechanisms that permit yolk sac engraftment in the conditioned newborn mice remain elusive, but this method has been used by a number of investigators to pursue transplantation studies using embryo- or fetal-derived donor cells.

Key Words: Newborn; mouse; yolksac; hematopoiesis; embryo.

1. Introduction

Hematopoiesis is developmentally regulated and tissue-specific. The primary sites of hematopoiesis change during murine ontogeny *(1)* The first blood cells to emerge in the embryo can be found in the yolk sac (YS) on embryonic d 7.0 (E7.0) and are composed primarily of primitive erythroblasts *(2)*. These red blood cells are large, nucleated cells filled with embryonic and some adult-type hemoglobins. Some embryonic macrophages and megakaryocytes can also be found in the YS by E7.5 *(2,3)*. These cells express properties that are unique to this stage of development. On E8.25, definitive progenitors that give rise to red blood cells (expressing only adult-type hemoglobins), granulocytes, macrophages, megakaryocytes, and mast cells appear in the YS *(2)*. Multipotent high proliferative potential colony-forming cells also are first detectable on E8.25 *(4)*. Definitive progenitors subsequently appear in the circulation, embryo proper, and liver. Of interest, the definitive progenitors formed in the YS do not appear to differentiate in the YS or in the circulation. The temporal appearance of maturing blood cells in the

From: *Methods in Molecular Medicine, Vol. 105: Developmental Hematopoiesis: Methods and Protocols.*
Edited by: M. H. Baron © Humana Press Inc., Totowa, NJ

liver within hours of progenitor cell seeding from the blood suggests that YS-derived progenitors must seed the liver and serve as the source of the mature blood elements differentiating in the liver.

The site of hematopoietic stem cell (HSC) emergence has been controversial. Compelling evidence supports autonomous in vitro emergence of HSCs in explanted E8.0 paraaortic splanchnopleure tissue, with direct isolation of HSCs from dorsal aortic endothelium or subendothelial mesenchymal cells in the aorta–gonad–mesonephros region in the E10 embryo ***(5–7)***. HSCs from these sites engraft and repopulate hematopoietic lineages in lethally irradiated mice. In contrast, adult repopulating HSCs have also been isolated from the precirculation YS and embryo proper after a brief in vitro coculture with an aorta–gonad–mesonephros-derived stromal cell line ***(8)***. Infection of the precirculation YS and embryonic stem cell-derived hematopoietic cells with a retrovirus encoding the transcription factor HOXB4 also results in multilineage repopulation of the peripheral blood of lethally irradiated adult mice upon transplantation of the transduced cells ***(9)***. These results contrast with multiple studies documenting the inability of <E11.0 YS-derived hematopoietic cells to engraft and repopulate lethally irradiated mice. In sum, one questions whether HSC emerge in the early YS.

We have previously reported that E9.0 YS cells engraft and repopulate hematopoiesis in sublethally myeloablated newborn mice for 6 to 11 mo and repopulate lethally irradiated adult recipient mice in secondary transplant assays ***(10–12)***. Our rationale for performing these studies centered on the knowledge that the fetal liver remains an active hematopoietic organ for several wk postnatally and, thus, could serve as a site for transplanted cell seeding. We were also aware that transplantation of YS cells into recipient embryos *in utero* had been successfully accomplished, although high-level engraftment was frequently difficult to achieve ***(13,14)***. We hypothesized that newborn mice conditioned in utero should be effective recipients for transplantation of cells postnatally and that <E11.0 YS-derived cells would engraft.

Busulfan is a chemotherapeutic agent used to condition human and murine hosts for transplantation. We performed preliminary studies to determine an in utero dose of busulfan that would myeloablate and condition the newborn mouse for transplantation at an acceptable level of morbidity ***(15)***. We determined that 15.5 mg/kg administered intraperitoneally in two doses to pregnant dams (E17 and E18) transiently suppressed hematopoiesis in newborn pups, with the majority of pups surviving. Growth was normal in the pups exposed to a single dose but was stunted in animals exposed to two in utero doses of busulfan. Similar levels of conditioning could be achieved using either a single dose of busulfan (administered to the dam on E18) followed by irradiation of the pup with 250 cGy of irradiation, or by two doses of irradiation within the first 24 h of postnatal life. Higher doses of either agent were associated with high mortality or severe growth restriction. As noted above, subsequent studies demonstrated engraftment of E9.0 YS and paraaortic splanchnopleure cells in the sublethally irradiated newborn mice.

The primary objective of the methods section to follow is to provide the investigator with the necessary information to perform transplantation of hematopoietic cells into newborn recipient mice. We also describe two methods for evaluating donor cell chimerism in recipient mice: a flow cytometric analysis of differential CD45 isoform expression or glucose phosphate isomerase-1 (Gpi-1) expression.

2. Materials

2.1. Dissection

1. IMDM 5:2: Iscove's modified Dulbecco's medium (IMDM, Invitrogen; cat. no. 12440-053) supplemented with 5% fetal bovine serum (FBS, Bio-Whitaker; cat. no. 14-501f) and 2% penicillin (10,000 U/mL)/streptomycin (10,000 μg/mL, Invitrogen; cat. no. 15140-122).
2. Phosphate-buffered saline, pH 7.2 (PBS, Invitrogen; cat. no. 20012-027).
3. Dissecting scissors: surgical scissors (Fine Science Tools; cat. no. 14002-12) and 12-cm straight Noyes spring scissors (Fine Science Tools; cat. no. 15012-12).
4. Dissecting forceps: one pair of Biologie tip Dumoxel no. 5 dissecting forceps (Fine Science Tools; cat. no. 11252-30).
5. Dissection microscope: Leica WILD M8 dissecting microscope with a magnification range from 6×–50×.

2.2. Digestion/Cell Dissociation

1. Hank's balanced salt solution (HBSS, Invitrogen; cat. no. 14170-112).
2. Liberase Blendzyme-3 (Roche; cat. no. 1814176): prepared as recommended by adding 2 mL of sterile water to 7 mg to make a solution of 14 collagenase Wünsch U/mL. This solution is aliquoted into 50-μL volumes and frozen at –20°C for up to 4 mo. Aliquots are frozen and thawed no more than two times and then discarded.
3. Dounce with pestle "A" large clearance (Kimble-Kontes; cat. no. 885300-0007).
4. 70-μm Cell strainers (BD Biosciences Discovery Labware; cat. no. 352350).

2.3. Injection

1. Busulfan: 50 mg busulfan (Sigma; cat. no. B-2635) dissolved in 1 mL of warm (55°C) dimethyl sulfoxide (DMSO, Sigma; cat. no. D-8779) diluted into 49 mL of warm (55°C) PBS to make a 1 mg/mL solution. This solution is made fresh and should be kept warm throughout all injections, and discarded and remade if a precipitate is noticed. Busulfan powder should be purchased fresh every 6 mo and kept in the dark.
2. Irradiation: standard mouse radiation pie (Dan-Kar Corp., MPC) and C^{137} Gamma Irradiator (Nordion, Kanata, Canada).
3. Injection medium: HBSS supplemented with 12% FBS.
4. Syringe: 100-μL Hamilton glass syringe (Fisher Scientific; cat. no. 81020) fitted with a 30G 1/2-inch needle (Becton Dickinson and Company; cat. no. 305106).

2.4. Analysis of Peripheral Blood of Transplanted Mice

2.4.1. Fluorescence-Activated Cell Sorting (FACS) Analysis

1. Tail vein injector (Dan-Kar Corp, MTI).
2. Grafco Silver Nitrate Applicator (Graham-Field; cat. no. 012165-000).
3. Blood collection medium (BCM): Dulbecco's modified Eagle medium, high glucose (Invitrogen; cat. no. 11965-092) supplemented with 5% FBS, 2% penicillin (10,000 U/mL)/streptomycin (10,000 μg/mL), and 2% heparin sodium (20 U/mL, American Pharmaceutical Partners, Inc.; cat. no. 63323-0544-01).
4. Red blood cell lysing buffer (Sigma; cat. no. R-7757).
5. Fc block medium: conditioned media harvested from hybridoma 2.4G2 (ATCC, HB-197), cultured in serum free media, supplemented with 1% penicillin (10,000 U/mL)/streptomycin (10,000 μg/mL) after harvesting. This media can be stored for several months at 4°C.

6. Antibodies: CD45.1 fluorescein isothiocyanate (FITC) (553775), CD45.2 FITC (553772), and an appropriate IgG2a isotype control antibody (FITC), all purchased from BD Biosciences Pharmingen.

2.4.2. Gpi-1 Analysis

2.4.2.1. Buffers

The following buffers are needed: 25 m*M* Tris-HCl, pH 8.7, 200 m*M* glycine in 1 L of water for use as a soaking buffer and 100 m*M* Tris-HCl, pH 8.5, 750 m*M* glycine in 1 L of water for use as a running buffer.

2.4.2.2. Stain Reagents

1. Phenazine methosulfate (Sigma; cat. no. P-9625): 0.5 mg/mL in distilled water.
2. β-Nicotinamide adenine dinucleotide phosphate sodium salt (NADP, Sigma; cat. no. N-0505): 10 mg/mL in distilled water.
3. Thiazolyl Blue Tetrazolium Bromide (MTT, Sigma; cat. no. M-2128): 10 mg/mL in distilled water.
4. D-Fructose 6-phosphate disodium salt dihydrate (Fructose, Sigma; cat. no. F-3627): 100 mg/mL in distilled water.
5. Glucose-6-phosphate dehydrogenase from torula yeast (Glucose, Sigma; cat. no. G-8289): 140 U/mL in distilled water.
6. Magnesium acetate tetrahydrate (Mg acetate, Sigma; cat. no. M0631): 42.9 mg/mL in distilled water.
7. Tris-HCl, pH 8.
8. 2% Agar (Fisher Scientific, BP2641-100): 2 g dissolved in 100 mL of boiling distilled water.

2.4.2.3. Electrophoresis Equipment

Zip Zone Chamber (1283), Zip Zone Chamber Wicks (5081), Titan III cellulose acetate plates (3023), and Super Z applicator kit (4088) all purchased from Helena Laboratories.

Finally, glacial acetic acid (Fisher Scientific; cat. no. A38-500) diluted (7 mL) with distilled water (93 mL) should be acquired to make a 7% solution.

3. Methods

3.1. Dissection

1. Embryonic tissue is obtained by mating sexually mature GPI-1^a/Gpi-1^a/CD45.1/CD45.1 (GB) female mice with males in the late afternoon. The next morning, the presence of a vaginal plug indicates that mating has occurred, and this is considered embryonic d (E) 0.5.
2. Females at E9.5 are euthanized by CO_2 inhalation followed by cervical dislocation. The abdominal hair is wetted with 70% ethanol. The hair and skin is removed from pelvis to sternum. An incision is made through the abdominal muscles with scissors to expose the gravid uterus and then the uterine horns are freed by snipping connecting tissues at the cervix and fallopian tubes. Embryos are placed into IMDM 5:2 (IMDM with 5% FBS and 2% penicillin/streptomycin) on ice for transport back to the laboratory.

3. Viewed under a dissecting microscope at 6× magnification in Petri dishes containing IMDM 5:2, after washing in PBS, the embryos and surrounding uterine deciduas are separated by cutting between individual embryos using spring scissors. Forceps are then inserted between the uterine musculature/decidua and the YS, using a tearing motion to expose the intact YS surrounding the embryo.
4. The YS is penetrated and gently peeled away from the embryo using dissecting forceps by severing the vitelline and umbilical vessels. The somites of the exposed embryo are counted and the YS placed into a 15-mL tube containing IMDM 5:2.

3.2. Digestion/Dissociation

1. The intact YS membranes are centrifuged at 300*g* for 5 min at 4°C, the supernatant is discarded, and 500 μL of HBSS is added. The YS is resuspended by pipeting up and down several times to disperse the pelleted membranes.
2. Liberase Blendzyme-3 is added (*see* **Note 1**), 1 μL per YS. The YS are then gently triturated and placed in an incubator at 37°C. During the incubation, the YS are triturated several times every 5 min. The total digestion time varies from 2 to 3 min for E8.5 YS to up to 30 min for E12.5 YS.
3. When the YS are thoroughly disrupted and only a stringy mass of extracellular matrix is left undigested, 5 mL of IMDM 5:2 is added to stop further protease activity. The cells are filtered through a 70-μm cell strainer into a 50-mL tube.
4. An additional 30 mL (in 5- to 10-mL aliquots) of IMDM 5:2 is used to wash cellular contents from the 15-mL tube into the 50-mL tube. While medium is being filtered through the cell strainer, the tip of the pipet is gently rubbed across the mesh to help push cells through. Alternatively, the plunger from a 3- or 5-mL syringe can be rubbed across the mesh.

3.3. Injection

3.3.1. Busulfan Administration to Pregnant Dams (see **Notes 2–4**)

1. Timed pregnant C57Bl6/J (CD45.2 expressing) mice are bred to give birth at approx midnight before the day of anticipated transplantation studies. We find that our colony of C57BL6/J mice give birth 19.5 d after coitus and thus plan on performing the transplant on d 20 after coitus.
2. On the morning of d E17 and E18, the pregnant dam is given an intraperitoneal injection of 15.5 mg/kg of busulfan (*see* **Note 3**). Each dose is delivered by injecting the mother in the middle of an imaginary square formed by the last two pairs of mammary glands using a 30G 1/2 in. needle.
3. The pups are born and injected the same d (*see* **Subheading 3.3.3.**).

3.3.2. Irradiation of Recipient Newborns (see **Note 2**)

1. C57BL6/J (CD45.2 expressing) dams are bred to give birth at midnight of the d of anticipated transplantation studies.
2. On the morning of birth, pups are placed into a standard plexiglas radiation animal holder (pie shaped device with movable lid to insert animals into individual compartments).
3. The pups are exposed to 200 cGy using a C^{137} Gamma Irradiator and are returned to their mother's cage. After 4 h, the pups are again placed in the "pie" and receive another 200-cGy total body irradiation.
4. The pups are then injected the next d (*see* **Subheading 3.3.3.**).

5. If both busulfan and irradiation conditioning are desired, then the pregnant dam receives an intraperitoneal injection of 15.5 mg/mL of busulfan (*see* **Subheading 3.3.1.**) on E18 and the newborn pups receive 200 cGy the morning of birth (*see* **Subheading 3.3.2.**). Pups can then be injected with donor hematopoietic cells on the same d (*see* **Subheading 3.3.3.**).

3.3.3. Facial Vein Injection of Newborn Pups

1. The single-cell YS cell suspension is centrifuged at 300*g*, the supernatant discarded, and the cells resuspended in HBSS + 12% FBS for transplantation. The cells are warmed to room temperature prior to the injection.
2. Each pup receives the desired number of cells (or embryo equivalents) in 25 μL of final injection volume.
3. To prepare for the injection, thoroughly mix the YS cells and, using a pipet, add 25 μL of directly inside the hub of a 30G 1/2-in. needle. With the Hamilton syringe plunger pulled back to the 20-μL mark, slowly screw the needle onto the syringe. As fluid forms at the tip of the syringe, continue drawing back on the plunger to draw up the fluid. Once the needle is firmly set, it is ready for injection.
4. To inject the facial vein, the pup is held so that its body is pinned between the thumb and middle finger of the left hand. The index finger is placed on the pup's chin or nose so that the head can be tilted to the side to expose the face and neck vessels. The needle is inserted into the facial vein and the cells injected toward the heart (**Fig. 1**). If the fluid does not inject smoothly or the vein is missed, the needle can be reinserted further down the facial vein nearer the jugular vein to try again (*see* **Note 5**).
5. The plunger is depressed until it reaches the starting mark (20 μL), and great care is taken to avoid the injection of air. The needle is withdrawn as the last of the cells are injected. After the needle is withdrawn, a piece of gauze or cotton is used to quickly staunch the flow of blood caused by the injection (*see* **Note 6**). Any blood on the pup is cleaned off to prevent the mother from later killing it (*see* **Note 7**).
6. After injection, we recommend leaving the mother and pups undisturbed for several d. After the first wk, the mother is less likely to kill the pups, and they can be examined. We typically wait to examine the peripheral blood of the recipient mice for evidence of donor cell chimerism for at least 1 mo.

3.4. Analysis of Peripheral Blood of Transplanted Mice

3.4.1. FACS Analysis

1. The mouse to be bled is placed into the restraining compartment of the tail vein injector with its tail accessible. Scissors are used to snip 1–2 mm off of the tip of the tail and the tail is then "milked" to extract the desired number of drops of blood (as few as 7–9 can be used for monthly bleeds). The blood is collected into 1 mL of BCM and placed on ice and the mouse's tail is cauterized with a silver nitrate applicator.
2. The blood is centrifuged at 300*g* for 5 min at 4°C, supernatant is removed, and 1 mL of red blood cell lysing buffer is added, disrupting the pellet. After 5 min, the cells are washed with BCM and centrifuged again at 300*g* for 5 min at 4°C.
3. The supernatant is removed, and 205 μL of Fc block medium is added. An isotype control sample is prepared by adding 5 μL of the blood cells to 95 μL of Fc block medium and labeling with appropriate fluorochrome conjugated isotype antibodies.
4. The remaining blood is equally aliquoted into two tubes, one tube receiving 1 μL of CD45.1 FITC antibody (donor type cells) and the other tube receiving 1 μL of CD45.2 FITC antibody (recipient type cells) per million peripheral blood cells.

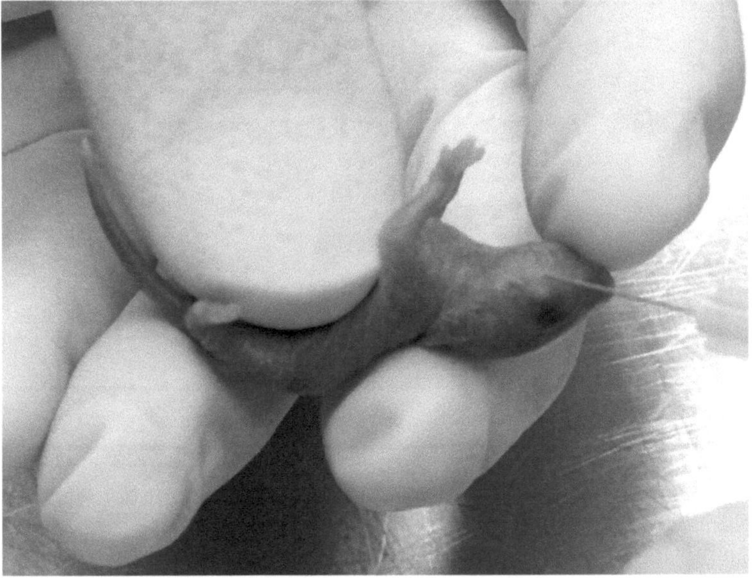

Fig. 1. Holding of newborn pups for injection. This photograph (of an older 6-d newborn) depicts a method of holding the newborn pup with the left hand and thereby allows for injection of donor cells via the Hamilton syringe held in the right hand. Care must be taken to turn the pup's head away from the side of injection to visualize and permit access to the facial vessel.

5. The cells are then placed on ice and kept in the dark (wrapped in foil). Tubes are gently shaken every 10 to 15 min for 1 h.
6. After the 1-h incubation, 4 mL of BCM is added and the cells are centrifuged at 300*g* for 5 min at 4°C. The supernatant is discarded and the cells are resuspended in 200 μL of BCM to be analyzed.
7. The isotype labeled peripheral blood cells are used to set the Forward and Side Scatter dot plot to identify the population of interest. Next the non-specific binding of the fluorophore-conjugated isotype antibody to the peripheral blood cells is measured. Gates are set so that no more than 1% nonspecific binding is accepted as positive.
8. The labeled cells are then analyzed for both CD45.1 FITC (donor cells) and CD45.2 FITC (recipient cells) expressing populations (**Fig. 2**).
9. Monthly analysis is performed to determine the percent of the peripheral blood of the recipient mice that comprises donor-derived cells (*see* **Note 8**).

3.4.2. Gpi-1 Analysis

1. At the same time that blood is collected for FACS analysis (*see* **Subheading 3.5.1.**), an additional four to five drops of blood are collected into 100 μL of distilled water. The blood is then frozen and thawed several times to lyse both red and white blood cells.
2. Soak Titan III cellulose acetate plates in soaking buffer (coated side down). When placing the plates into the buffer, don't trap any bubbles under the plate or the cellulose acetate will peal away and the plate will have to be discarded. Let the plates soak for at least 30 min.

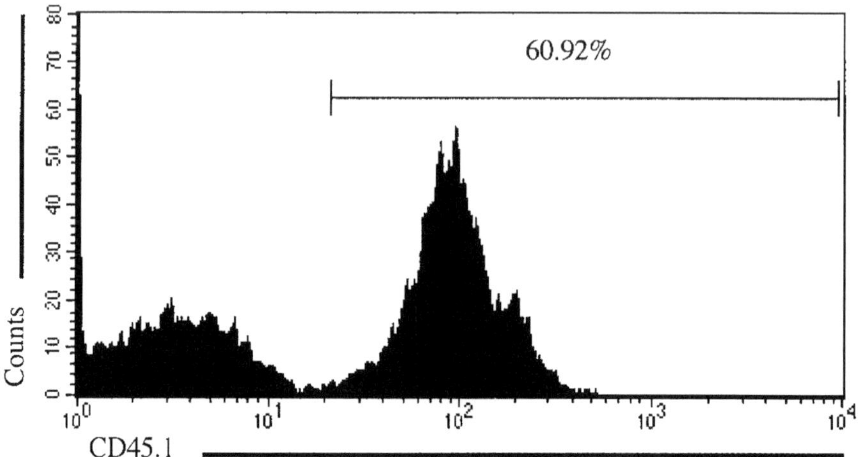

Fig. 2. Donor hematopoietic cells expressing the CD45.1 antigen can be readily identified in the peripheral blood of the host animal using flow cytometry. CD45.1 expressing cells that represent nearly 61% of all of the peripheral blood cells of the host animal are readily identified in this histogram.

3. Set up the electrophoresis chamber by filling the outer chambers with running buffer and placing Zip Zone Chamber Wicks over the internal tray edges, making sure that they are in contact with the running buffer.
4. Remove the cellulose acetate plates one at a time from the buffer. Blot excess moisture with towels dampened with soaking buffer. It is important not to allow the plates to dry or the proteins will not migrate appropriately.
5. Load 10 μL of the lysed blood sample per well of the eight-well applicator tray. Load Gpi-1^a- and Gpi-1^b-positive controls for each plate into wells 1 and 2, respectively, with the remaining six wells for samples of individual recipient mice. Then, using the aligning base and the eight-well applicator, apply the samples onto the plate. The samples should be applied at least three times to assure that a sufficient volume was loaded.
6. Place the cellulose acetate plates across the wicks, coated side down. A glass slide should be placed on top of the plate to keep it in contact with the wick. Apply the electrical current at 150 to 160 volts for 30 min. The Gpi-1 proteins migrate towards the negative pole, though the "red" hemoglobin will migrate towards the positive pole, occasionally running off the plate.
7. After the plates have been run, prepare the detection stain by mixing the following reagents in a single tube. Use the following volumes for each plate: 2 mL of warm Tris-HCl, 0.1 mL of Mg acetate, 0.1 mL of fructose, 0.1 mL of MTT, 0.005 mL of glucose, 0.1 mL of phenazine methosulfate , 2 mL of warm 2% Agar, and 0.1 mL of NADP. Add the NADP last because the addition of this enzyme initiates the cascade of enzymatic reactions leading to reduction of the MTT and emergence of the deep blue/purple color. Pour the reagents over the plate, paying particular attention to avoid bubbles and provide a homogenous overlay of agar and constituent reagents.
8. Place the agar-coated plate in the dark for 5 to 15 min or until the deep blue/purple bands are clearly visible. Quench the staining by immersing the plate into 7% acetic acid.

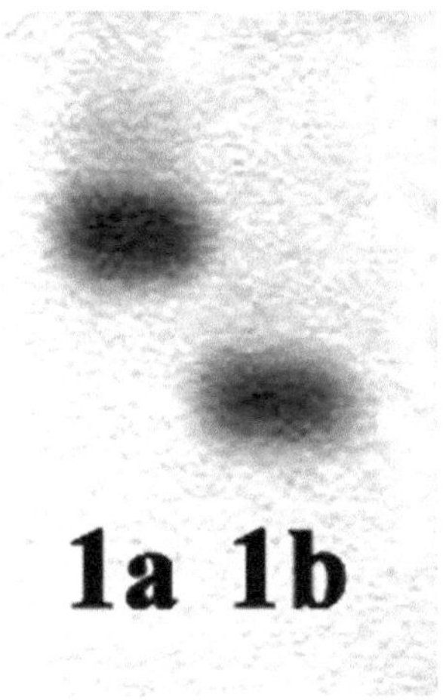

Fig. 3. Gpi-1 isoforms differentially migrate during electrophoresis. The Gpi-1^a isoform in the first lane migrates more slowly than the Gpi-1^b isoform in the second lane.

9. The plate can now be photographed, or the agar can be slid off of the plate onto an absorbent material (such as Whatman's paper) and allowed to dry. The Gpi-1^b isoform (expressed by the C57BL6/J strain) migrates faster than the 1^a (expressed by the GB "donor" mice), forming distinct bands (**Fig. 3**).

4. Notes

1. The type of enzyme used to digest the YS is very important. Liberase Blendzyme-3 works very well for E9.5 and older YS. Additionally, a very weak trypsin (Worthington Biochemical Corporation; cat. no. LS003667) solution can be used. The trypsin is prepared as a 0.25% solution in PBS with 1 m*M* ethylenediamine tetraacetic acid and then used at a 1 to 30 dilution (1 mL for every 5 YS). Earlier YS (E7.5–8.5), however, require a much gentler digestion protocol. For these early tissues we prepare a 1 mg/mL solution of collagenase/dispase (Roche; cat. no. 1097113) in PBS with 20% FBS. Using 1 mL per YS, we digest the YS for 1–2 h at 37°C, triturating the cells gently every 30 min. Because of the fragile nature of these early cells, we also tried using two matrix metalloproteinases (MMPs), MMP-7 (Matrilysin, Calbiochem, 444270) and MMP-9 (Gelatinase B, Oncogene, PF024) to digest the YS. MMP-7 was used at a concentration of approx 150 U per YS, whereas MMP-9 was used at a concentration of 0.05 μg per YS in the presence of either 150 or 75 U of MMP-7. Although digestion with these enzymes seemed comparable to either Liberase or trypsin digestion, the number of progenitor colonies was reduced by 50%, and therefore the use of these enzymes was abandoned. We recommend testing each new batch of enzyme to screen for those that permit digestion of the tissues with retention of progenitor and stem cell function at each stage of development.
2. Both the irradiation and the Busulfan treatments are sublethal, though stunting of the growth of treated mice does occur. Both irradiation and Busulfan result in the same amount of growth stunting, as measured by weight (at 1 mo after birth) and physical appearance (throughout the life of the animal).

3. The largest amount of Busulfan tolerated by the pups should be used to maximize myeloablation. We have determined that with C57Bl6/J mice, more than 15.5 mg/kg in two doses is fatal to the pups, resulting in stillbirths.
4. The Busulfan solution must be kept warm. Make sure that the DMSO and PBS are initially warmed to 55°C so that they don't cool too much. Busulfan is notoriously difficult to keep in solution and rapidly precipitates even in the presence of the DMSO if the solution comes to room temperature for a few minutes.
5. If the initial injection of the pup fails, several more attempts can be made. For this reason, it is best to start the injections at the periphery of the vein, working in towards the jugular vessel of the animal with subsequent attempts. It is possible to inject an animal on subsequent days. An excellent primer on facial vein injections has been published recently ***(16)***.
6. If there is excessive blood loss during injection because of increased fluid volume, the injection volume can be decreased to 22 μL.
7. Despite the small volume injected, this infusate causes a rapid expansion of the blood volume in the injected pups. Many of the pups will become cyanotic (turn blue) and appear to gasp. This behavior usually passes after a few minutes and color returns to normal.
8. At any point in following the transplanted recipients, one may choose to perform a multilineage analysis of donor cell chimerism. This is readily accomplished by following the protocol in **Subheading 3.4.1.** and staining recipient animal peripheral blood cells for the donor CD45.1 FITC along with antibodies to lineage antigens to determine the percent of T and B lymphocytes and granulocytes derived from donor cells. In our protocol, each of the following antibodies is conjugated to biotin, including the T lymphocyte antigens CD4 (553045) and CD8a (553029), the B lymphocyte marker CD45R/B220 (553086), and the granulocyte marker Ly-6G (Gr-1) (553125). These lineage antigens are all secondarily labeled with streptaviden–allophycocyanin (554067). Isotype controls include IgG1, IgG2a, and IgG2b (all biotinylated), and all are purchased from BD Biosciences Pharmingen.

References

1. Palis, J. and Yoder, M. (2001) Yolk sac hematopoiesis-the first blood cells of mouse and man. *Exp. Hematol.* **29,** 927–936.
2. Palis, J., Robertson, S., Kennedy, M., Wall, C., and Keller, G. (1999) Development of erythroid and myeloid progenitors in the yolk sac and embryo proper of the mouse. *Development* **126,** 5073–5081.
3. Xu, M.-J., Matsuoka, S., Yang, F.-C., Ebihara, Y., Manabe, A., Tanaka, R., et al. (2001) Evidence for the presence of murine primitive megakaryocytopoiesis in the early yolk sac. *Blood* **97,** 2016–2022.
4. Palis, J., Chan, R., Koniski, A., Patel, R., Starr, M., and Yoder, M. (2001) Spatial and temporal emergence of high proliferative potential hematopoietic precursors during murine embryogenesis. *Proc. Natl. Acad. Sci. USA* **98,** 4528–4533.
5. Cumano, A., Ferraz, J., Klaine, M., Di Santo, J., and Godin, I. (2001) Intraembryonic, but not yolk sac hematopoietic precursors, isolated before circulation, provide long-term multilineage reconstitution. *Immunity* **15,** 477–485.
6. de Bruijn, M., Ma, X., Robin, C., Ottersbach, K., Sanchez, M.-J., and Dzierzak, E. (2002) Hematopoietic stem cells localize to the endothelial cell layer in the midgestation mouse aorta. *Immunity* **16,** 673–683.

7. North, T., de Bruijn, M., Stacy, T., Talebian, L., Lind, E., Robin, C., et al. (2002) Runx1 expression marks long-term repopulating hematopoietic stem cells in the midgestation mouse embryo. *Immunity* **16,** 661–672.
8. Matsuoka, S., Tsuji, K., Hisakawa, H., Xu, M.-J., Ebihara, Y., Ishii, T., et al. (2001) Generation of definitive hematopoietic stem cells from murine early yolk sac and paraaortic splanchnopleura by aorta-gonad-mesonephros region-derived stromal cells. *Blood* **98,** 6–12.
9. Kyba, M., Perlingeiro, R., and Daley, G. Q. (2002) HoxB4 confers definitive lymphoid-myeloid engraftment potential on embryonic stem cell and yolk sac hematopoietic progenitors. *Cell* **109,** 29–37.
10. Yoder, M. and Hiatt, K. (1997) Engraftment of embryonic hematopoietic cells in conditioned newborn recipients. *Blood* **89,** 2176–2183.
11. Yoder, M., Hiatt, K., and Mukherjee, P. (1997) In vivo repopulating hematopoietic stem cells are present in the murine yolk sac at day 9.0 postcoitus. *Proc. Natl. Acad. Sci. USA* **94,** 6776–6780.
12. Yoder, M. C., Hiatt, K., Dutt, P., Mukherjee, P., Bodine, D. M., and Orlic, D. (1997) Characterization of definitive lymphohematopoietic stem cells in the day 9 murine yolk sac. *Immunity* **7,** 335–344.
13. Weissman, I., Papaioannou, V., and Gardner, R. (1978) Fetal hematopoietic origins of the adult hematolymphoid system, in *Differentiation of Normal and Neoplastic Hematopoietic Cells* (Clarkson, B., Marks, P. A., Till, J. E., eds.), Cold Spring Harbor Laboratory, Cold Spring Harbor, NY, pp. 33–47.
14. Toles, J. F., Chui, D. H. K., Belbeck, L. W., Starr, E., and Barker, J. E. (1989) Hemopoietic stem cells in murine embryonic yolk sac and peripheral blood. *Proc. Natl. Acad. Sci. USA* **86,** 7456–7459.
15. Yoder, M., Cumming, J., Hiatt, K., Mukherjee, P., and Williams, D. (1996) A novel method of myeloablation to enhance engraftment of adult bone marrow cells in newborn mice. *Biol. Blood Marrow Transplant.* **2,** 59–67.
16. Sands, M. and Barker, J. E. (1999) Percutaneous intravenous injection in neonatal mice. *Lab. Ani. Sci.* **49,** 328–330.

III

Animal Models

7

Hemocyte Development During *Drosophila* Embryogenesis

Robert A. Schulz and Nancy Fossett

Summary

The model genetic organism *Drosophila melanogaster* has a rudimentary hematopoietic system with two embryonic blood cell types, crystal cells, and plasmatocytes. These distinct lineages provide the animal with an innate immune response and a means to remove apoptotic cells. Genetic analyses of *Drosophila* hematopoiesis have identified specific genes that function in blood cell formation. Complimentary deoxyribonucleic acid and antibody probes for these hematopoietic factors serve as important reagents to follow hemocyte lineage commitment and differentiation during embryogenesis. This is possible through methods described in this chapter on messenger ribonucleic acid localization by *in situ* hybridization and protein localization by immunohistochemical staining within hemocyte precursors and mature blood cells.

Key Words: Blood cells; confocal microscopy; *Drosophila melanogaster*; hematopoiesis; lozenge; mRNA *in situ* hybridization; protein immunolocalization; serpent; U-shaped.

1. Introduction

Hematopoiesis in the fruit fly *Drosophila melanogaster* occurs in distinct phases during development within specialized primordia and tissues. In the embryo, two blood cell lineages arise from a common hemocyte precursor within the cephalic mesoderm *(1–5)*. Crystal cells, named for their crystalline inclusion bodies, represent 5% of circulating hemocytes and function in wound healing and encapsulation of small foreign invaders. Plasmatocytes constitute the remaining 95% of embryonic blood cells and closely resemble the vertebrate monocyte/macrophage cell type. This hemocyte population synthesizes anti-microbial peptides and differentiates into macrophage-like cells that phagocytize microbes and apoptotic particles. For later stages of life, the lymph glands serve as the site of blood cell production *(1–6)*. Both crystal cells and plasmatocytes, along with a third class of hemocyte, called the lamellocyte, are generated during larval development. Lamellocytes differentiate from hemocyte precursors that also produce the crystal cells and plasmatocytes, with lamellocytes induced upon parasitic invasion *(6)*. The function of this class of hemocyte is to encapsulate large size

From: *Methods in Molecular Medicine, Vol. 105: Developmental Hematopoiesis: Methods and Protocols.*
Edited by: M. H. Baron © Humana Press Inc., Totowa, NJ

invaders that are beyond the phagocytic capacity of plasmatocytes. Thus, *Drosophila* blood cells are functionally analogous to certain vertebrate hemocytes, providing the organism with an innate immune response and a means to remove apoptotic cells. During metamorphosis, the larval lymph glands histolyze and only the plasmatocyte population persists into the adult fly.

Elucidating the genetic basis of *Drosophila* hemocyte production, differentiation, and function has been a research area of intense interest in recent years. These studies have shown that transcription factors of the GATA, Friend of GATA, and Runt homology domain families ***(4,7–9)*** and proteins of the Notch signal transduction pathway are essential players in this complex developmental process ***(10,11)***. Specialized molecular and immunological reagents have been developed for these regulators and such reagents can be used as markers to assess the normal or abnormal proceedings of hematopoiesis. Herein, we focus on materials and techniques used to study hemocyte development during *Drosophila* embryogenesis.

2. Materials

1. Flies: ordered online from the Stock Centers listed on flybase (http://flybase.bio.indiana.edu/) or obtained from *Drosophila* workers.
2. Fly food: *see* Ashburner ***(12)***.
3. Bottles and plugs (Fisher; cat. no. AS-355 and 14-127-40E, respectively).
4. Grape plates: *see* Ashburner ***(12)***.
5. Petri plates (Fisher; cat. no. 08-757-100B).
6. Collection chambers: holes punched in polypropylene beakers (Fisher; cat. no. 02-593-50B).
7. Rubber bands.
8. Yeast paste.
9. Collection baskets: cut the 5-mL end off of a 50-mL Falcon 2070 tube; cut a hole in the conical end and cover the hole with Nitex nylon mesh.
10. Small paintbrushes.
11. 50% Household bleach.
12. 20-mL vol scintillation vials.
13. Methanol.
14. Heptane.
15. Rotary shaker.
16. 1.5-mL Eppendorf tubes.
17. Nutator.
18. 4% Paraformaldehyde in phosphate-buffered saline (PBS): use within 2 to 3 d, storing at 4°C.
19. Dry ice.
20. Hemocyte-expressed gene complimentary deoxyribonucleic acid (cDNA) cloned into a plasmid adjacent to a T7 or a SP6 promoter.
21. 5 *M* NH_4OAC.
22. Phenol:chloroform:isoamyl alcohol (25:24:1).
23. Chloroform.
24. Ethanol.
25. Diethyl pyrocarbonate (DEPC)-treated water.
26. Rnasin (Roche).
27. TE: 10 m*M* Tris-HCl, pH 8.0; 1 m*M* ethylenediamine tetraacetic acid with Rnase-free ddH_2O. Autoclave entire TE buffer.

28. Dig ribonucleic acid (RNA) labeling (SP6/T7) kit (Roche; cat. no. 1 175 025).
29. 4 *M* LiCl.
30. 0.2 *M* Ethylenediamine tetraacetic acid.
31. 20 mg/mL tRNA.
32. Hybridization buffer: deionized formamide, 50%; standard saline citrate, 5X (3 *M* NaCl, 300 m*M* tri-sodium citrate, pH 6.0, with 1 *M* citric acid); tRNA, 100 μg/mL; heparin, 50 μg/mL; Tween-20, 0.1%.
33. NTMT: 100 m*M* NaCl, 50 m*M* $MgCl_2$, 100 m*M* Tris-Cl, pH 9.5, 0.1% Tween-20, (made the d of use).
34. PBS: 130 m*M* NaCl, 7 m*M* Na_2HPO_4, 3 m*M* NaH_2PO_4.
35. PTW: PBS, 0.1% Tween.
36. Proteinase K: 20 mg/mL proteinase K, 50% glycerol, 10 m*M* Tris-HCl, pH 7.8.
37. Blocking solution: PBS; 0.1% Tween-20, Roche blocking reagent (Roche; cat. no. 1096 176), 2 mg/mL.
38. Anti-digoxigenin alkaline phosphatase Fab fragments (Roche; cat. no. 1093274).
39. 5-Bromo-4-chloro-3-indolyl-phosphate, 50 mg/mL in 70% dimethyl formamide (DMF).
40. 4-Nitro blue tetrazolium chloride, 50 mg/mL in 70% dimethyl formamide.
41. PEM: PIPES, 100 m*M* pH 6.9, 1 m*M* $MgCl_2$, 1 m*M* ethylenebis(oxyethylenenitrilo)tetra-acetic acid.
42. 37.7% Formaldehyde.
43. PBT: PBS, 0.1% Trition X-100, 2 mg/mL Roche blocking reagent.
44. PBTN: 100 μL of normal goat serum added to 2 mL of PBT (made the day of use).
45. Vectastain ABC kit: (Vector; cat. no. PK-6100) ABC reagent: 5 mL of PBT; two drops (approx 100 μL) reagent A; two drops (approx 100 μL) reagent B.
46. DAB Peroxidase Substrate kit: (Vector; cat. no. SK-4100) light brown stain: 2.5 mL of ddH_2O; one drop stock buffer; two drops DAB; one drop of H_2O_2; add one drop NiCl for black stain (*see* **Note 1**).
47. Dissecting microscope with light source.
48. CO_2 supply.
49. CO_2 staging (Lab Scientific; cat. no. BGSU-7).
50. Dissecting dishes.
51. Straight probe.
52. Compound microscope with camera.
53. Confocal microscope with computerized data capture.
54. Slides and cover slips.
55. 50% Glycerol.
56. Prolong anti-fade kit (Molecular Probes; cat. no. P-7481).
57. Nail polish.

3. Methods

3.1. Drosophila *Strains and Maintenance*

3.1.1. Selected Strains

A variety of *Drosophila* strains have been used to assign hematopoietic gene functions. Stocks carrying genetic mutations are used in loss-of-function analyses. Examples of these are *srp*^{3}*/TM3, Sb*^{1} *Ser*^{1}; *ush*^{1}*/SM6, Roi, eve-lacZ*; and *lz*^{s}*/w*^{1} *sn*^{1} *oc*^{1} *ptg*^{1} ***(4,7,8)***.

Gain-of-function studies are conducted using the UAS/Gal4 binary system developed by Brand and Perrimon ***(13)***. With this approach, one transgenic fly line carries the yeast Gal4 protein cDNA under the control of a tissue-specific genomic enhancer element, the Gal4 driver. A second line carries a cDNA for the gene of interest under the control of the Gal4 recognition site, the upstream activating sequence (UAS). When animals from the two strains are mated, the resulting progeny present a gain-of-function phenotype because of the forced expression of the gene of interest under the control of the cell-specific transcriptional enhancer.

Because the mesodermal determinant gene *twist* (*twi*) is expressed throughout the early embryonic mesoderm ***(14)***, the *twi-Gal4* strain can be used to drive cDNA expression in the hematopoietic primordia. In contrast, the *lozenge* (*lz*) *lz-Gal4* strain can be used to selectively induce expression in the crystal cell lineage ***(4)***. Examples of *UAS-cDNA* strains that produce hematopoietic phenotypes are *UAS-SrpC*, *UAS-SrpNC*, *UAS-Lz*, *UAS-Gcm*, *UAS-Ush*, and *UAS-*$N^{\Delta E}$ ***(4,8,9,15)***.

3.1.2. Drosophila *Maintenance*

1. A detailed discussion of fly maintenance can be found in Ashburner ***(12)***. Stocks are usually maintained at room temperature or 18°C.
2. Flies should be transferred to fresh food every 14 to 17 d for those kept at room temperature or every 25 to 28 d for those incubated at 18°C.

3.2. Drosophila *Embryo Collection*

1. Embryos can be collected from matings ongoing in stock bottles or from designed interstrain crosses. To set up a specific cross, virgin females must be collected from one strain and mated to males from another. Details regarding *Drosophila* genetics can be found in Greenspan ***(16)***.
2. Adult flies from either stocks or crosses should be anesthetized with CO_2 and placed in polypropylene beaker collection chambers (*see* **Notes 2** and **3**).
3. A small dollop of yeast paste is placed on the grape plate. The plate fits snugly on top of the collection chamber, is held in place with a rubber band, and then the egg collection chamber/grape plate combination is inverted.
4. Grape plates containing laid eggs should be changed twice daily, once in the morning and again in the evening. Embryos are preferentially collected in the morning. Embryo plates recovered at the end of the day can be placed at 18°C overnight for egg harvesting the next morning.
5. Embryos are washed off the plate with distilled water and brushed into the collection basket with a paintbrush.
6. The basket is immersed in 50% household bleach for 3 min to dechorionate the embryos.

3.3. *Preparing* Drosophila *Embryos for Hemocyte Gene Expression Analyses*

3.3.1. *Embryos to be Used for Determining mRNA Localization by* In Situ *Hybridization*

1. Using a paintbrush, transfer the dechorionated embryos to a scintillation vial containing 5 mL of 4% paraformaldehyde in PBS and 5 mL of heptane.
2. Attach the vials to a rotary shaker and shake at 200 rpm for 20 min at room temperature.
3. The embryos should be at the aqueous/organic interface. Remove as much of the aqueous layer as possible, while leaving the embryos in the scintillation vial.
4. Add 5 mL of –70°C methanol, place the vials on dry ice, and agitate for 10 min.

5. Remove the vials from the dry ice and allow the embryos to settle for about 10 min.
6. Using a pasture pipet, remove the heptane layer, and add 5 mL of methanol that has been kept at room temperature.
7. Allow the embryos to settle, remove most of the methanol, and wash with 5 mL of methanol.
8. After the embryos have settled to the bottom of the vial, transfer the embryos to a 1.5-mL Eppendorf tube.
9. Remove methanol and rehydrate the embryos with the following methanol:PBS-graded series: 70:30; 50:50; 30:70; 0:100. The methanol:PBS wash is added to the Eppendorf tube and the embryos are rotated on a nutator for 10 min for each wash.
10. When the final wash is complete, remove the PBS and fix the embryos in 4% paraformaldehyde in PBS for 20 min with nutation.
11. Wash the embryos one time with PBS for 10 min with nutation.
12. Dehydrate the embryos with a series of 10-min washes, in which the ethanol concentration is increased in 30%, 50%, and 70% increments, and the embryos are rotated on a nutator.
13. After the embryos are dehydrated, remove the 70% ethanol wash and store in 70% ethanol at –20°C until use. It is advisable to collect at least 100 μL of embryos because of losses that occur during processing. Embryos collected on successive days can be combined for staining ***(17)***.

3.3.2. Embryos to be Used for Determining Protein Localization by Immunohistochemical Staining

1. Using a paintbrush, transfer dechorionated embryos (*see* **Subheading 3.2.**) to scintillation vials containing 4.5 mL of PEM buffer and 0.5 mL of 37.7% formaldehyde.
2. Add 5 mL of heptane.
3. Attach the vials to a rotary shaker and shake at 200 rpm for 20 min at room temperature.
4. The embryos will be at the aqueous/organic interface. Remove most of the aqueous layer, leaving the embryos in the scintillation vial.
5. Add 5 mL of methanol and shake at 200 rpm for 2 to 3 min.
6. Remove the heptane layer and add 5 mL of methanol.
7. Allow embryos to settle, remove most of the methanol and wash with 5 mL of methanol.
8. After the embryos have settled, transfer them to a 1.5-mL Eppendorf tube and add 1 mL of methanol.
9. Store at –20°C until use. Overnight storage helps to eliminate any nonspecific background signal ***(17)***.

3.3.3. Embryos to be Used for Determining Protein Localization by Confocal Microscopy

Embryos to be used for protein localization by confocal microscopy are collected in the same manner as those for immunohistochemical staining.

3.4. mRNA Localization by* In Situ *Hybridization

3.4.1. mRNAs That Serve as Markers for Hemocyte Precursors and Crystal Cells

The *serpent* gene is expressed in the hematopoietic mesoderm and hemocyte precursors ***(7,9,18)***. During embryogenesis, *prophenol oxidase A1* is expressed specifically in developing crystal cells ***(19)***. cDNAs for hematopoietic marker genes should be cloned into plasmids that contain either a T7 or SP6 promoter. The gene must be cloned upstream of the promoter in order to transcribe an antisense cRNA for mRNA detection.

3.4.2. Preparation of Digoxigenin-Labeled Antisense RNA Probes

Care must be taken to prevent contamination of RNA probes with RNases. Use only DEPC-treated water for synthesis and storage of the probe. In addition, RNase inhibitor should be added, the probe aliquoted, and subsequently stored at –20°C. Prior to probe synthesis, the DNA template must be linearized at a restriction enzyme recognition site located downstream of the final cRNA product.

1. To avoid transcription of undesirable sequences, use a restriction enzyme that leaves 5'-overhangs or blunt ends.
2. Digest 10 to 25 µg of DNA.
3. Add TE to a final volume of 20 µL.
4. Add 2 µl of 2 mg/mL proteinase K and incubate at 37°C for 1 h. From this point on, the template should be treated as an RNase-free solution.
5. Add 5 µL of 5 *M* NH_4OAc and 28 µL of DEPC-treated water.
6. Extract the solution twice with 50 µL of phenol:chloroform:isoamyl alcohol and once with chloroform.
7. Precipitate the DNA with 120 µL of 95% ethanol, wash once with 80% ethanol, resuspend in 10 µL of TE, and store at –20°C.
8. The probe should be synthesized in a sterile, RNase-free microfuge tube, using the components from the Roche Dig RNA Labeling Kit. Add 1 µg of linearized DNA template, 2 µL of NTP labeling mixture, 2 µL of transcription buffer, 1 µL of RNase inhibitor, DEPC-treated water to a final volume of 18 µL, and 2 µL of RNA polymerase (either SP6 or T7), depending on the promoter site.
9. Incubate the mixture for 2 h at 37°C.
10. The DNA template can be removed by adding 2 µL of DNase I (RNase-free).
11. To stop the reaction, add 2 µL of EDTA.
12. The RNA transcript should be analyzed for size and intactness using agarose gel electrophoresis.
13. Add 2.5 µL of 4 *M* LiCl and 75 µL of cold 100% ethanol. Store at least 2 h at –20°C.
14. Centrifuge for 15 min at 12,000*g* and wash the pellet with 50 µL of 70% cold ethanol.
15. Dry the pellet briefly and dissolve in 10 µL of DEPC-treated water with 1 µL of RNase inhibitor.
16. Store in 2-µL aliquots at –20°C ***(17)***.

3.4.3. Prehybridization of Embryos

1. Because of losses during processing, we recommend using 50 to 100 µL of dehydrated embryos for *in situ* hybridization.
2. Rehydrate the embryos with a series of 10-min ethanol washes, in which the concentration is decreased by 70%, 50%, and 30% increments. Follow the ethanol washes with two PTW washes for 3 min each.
3. Treatment of embryos with proteinase K may be necessary and should be titrated. Begin with a final concentration of 50 µg/mL proteinase K and treat for 3 min at room temperature. If the embryos aggregate, then decrease the proteinase K concentration and/or the duration of treatment.

4. Wash the embryos immediately with PTW three times for 1 min.
5. Fix the embryos with 4% paraformaldehyde in PBS for 5 min.
6. After fixation, wash the embryos with PTW five times for 1 min.
7. Remove the PTW and rinse the embryos with 1 ml hybridization solution.
8. Remove the rinse, add 1 ml hybridization solution, and incubate at 60 to 70°C (*see* **Note 4**) for at least 4 h *(17)*.

3.4.4. Hybridization of Embryos

1. Preparation of the *in situ* hybridization probe is described in **Subheading 3.2.4.** Dilute the probe in hybridization solution. Dilutions can range from 1:20 to 1:100, depending on the probe.
2. Remove the hybridization solution and add 1 μL of diluted probe. Incubate at 60 to 70°C (*see* **Note 4**) overnight *(17)*.

3.4.5. Washing Embryos

1. Remove the hybridization solution containing the probe.
2. Add 1 mL of fresh hybridization solution and incubate at 60 to 70°C for 20 min.
3. Remove hybridization solution, add 1 mL of a 1:1 dilution of hybridization solution:PTW, and incubate at 60 to 70°C for 20 min.
4. Remove the hybridization solution/PTW mix and follow with five 20-min washes with PTW *(17)*.

3.4.6. Staining Embryos

1. To reduce the background staining, embryos should be incubated in blocking solution for 1 h at room temperature.
2. When blocking is complete, remove the blocking solution.
3. Dilute the α-digoxigenin antibody 1:2000 in PTW and add 1 mL to embryos.
4. Incubate for 1 h at room temperature with nutation (*see* **Note 5**).
5. Remove the antibody solution and wash the embryos with PTW for 20 min, four times.
6. Rinse the embryos with 1 mL of NTMT.
7. Remove the rinse and add 1 mL of fresh NTMT, 3.5 μL of 5-bromo-4-chloro-3-indolyl-phosphate, and 4.5 μL of 4-Nitro blue tetrazolium chloride.
8. Place the embryos on a nutator and shield from the light. The cover of a black slide box works well for this purpose.
9. Monitor staining intermittently using a dissecting microscope. The stained tissues should be dark purple *(17)*.

3.4.7. Analysis and Photography of Embryos

1. Staining quality should be determined using a dissecting microscope. Place embryos in a dissecting dish and inspect the degree of staining.
2. Sort embryos to be photographed using a straight probe.
3. Using a pipet, place embryos to be photographed in a pool of 50% glycerol.
4. To produce embryo whole mounts, place two drops of glycerol on a microscope slide about 20 to 30 mm apart.
5. Place cover slips over the drops of glycerol.
6. Remove one embryo from the 50% glycerol and position it between the cover slips.
7. Add a drop of glycerol and cover with a cover slip.

Serpent gene transcripts are detected in the hematopoietic mesoderm around stage 5 (**Fig. 1A**) and in hemocyte precursors until stage 11 *(7,9,18)*. *Serpent* hematopoietic

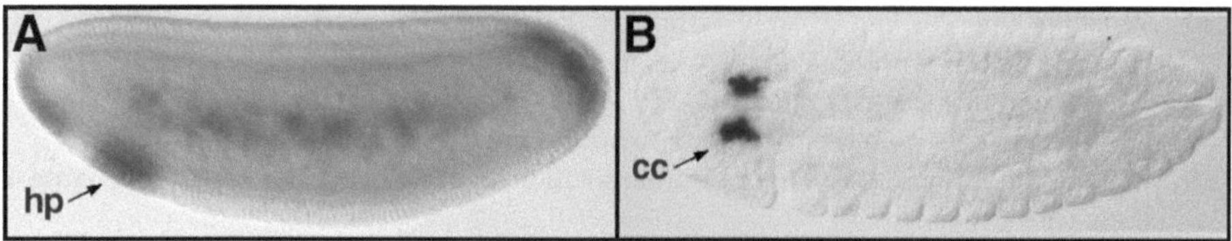

Fig. 1. mRNA localization during hemocyte development using an *in situ* hybridization technique. **(A)** Lateral view of a stage 5 embryo showing serpent expression in ventrally located hemocyte primordia (hp). **(B)** Dorsal view of a stage 13 embryo showing pro-phenol oxidase A1 gene expression in anterior clusters of crystal cells (cc).

expression is best photographed from a lateral or ventral view. *Prophenol oxidase A1* gene transcripts are detected in bi-lateral clusters of crystal cells (**Fig. 1B**), with expression in the crystal cell lineage throughout embryogenesis ***(19)***. This expression is best viewed and photographed either laterally or dorsally.

3.5. Protein Localization by Immunohistochemical Staining

3.5.1. U-Shaped Protein as a Marker of Hemocyte Precursors and Plasmatocytes

U-shaped protein is detected in hemocyte precursors around stage 8 (**Fig. 2A**). By stage 13, U-shaped expressing plasmatocytes can be seen migrating throughout the head mesoderm (**Fig. 2B**). Later in embryogenesis, U-shaped expressing plasmatocytes are circulating throughout the embryo ***(8)***.

3.5.2. Antibody Reagents

A U-shaped peptide antibody was raised in rabbits ***(8)***. A biotin conjugated goat anti-rabbit secondary antibody (Vector) is used to recognize the U-shaped protein–antibody complex.

3.5.3. Prewash and Blocking of Embryos

1. At least 30 µL and up to 50 µL of embryos should be used for immunohistochemical staining.
2. Remove methanol from embryos.
3. Wash with 1 mL PBT for at least 30 min at room temperature with nutation.
4. Remove the PBT, add 100 µL of PBTN and allow embryos to sit at room temperature for 30 min ***(20)***.

3.5.4. Primary Antibody Staining

1. Dilute the primary antibody in PBTN to twice the recommended final concentration.
2. Add 100 µL of diluted antibody to the embryos in PBTN.
3. Shake on a nutator overnight at 4°C ***(20)***.

3.5.5. Wash and Reblocking of Embryos

1. Remove the antibody solution (*see* **Note 6**) and perform four 20-min washes with 1 mL of PBT.

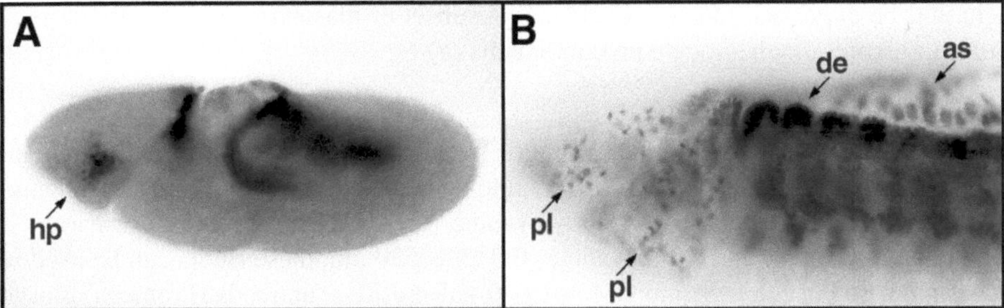

Fig. 2. U-shaped protein localization during hemocyte development by immunohistochemical detection. **(A)** Lateral view of a stage 8 embryo showing U-shaped accumulation in hemocyte precursors (hp). **(B)** Lateral view of a stage 13 embryo showing U-shaped expression in plasmatocytes (pl), as well as cells of the amnioserosa (as) and dorsal ectoderm (de).

2. Remove PBT, add 100 μL of PBTN, and allow embryos to sit at room temperature for 30 min *(20)*.

3.5.6. Secondary Antibody Staining

1. Dilute the secondary antibody in PBTN to twice the recommended final concentration.
2. Add 100 μL of the diluted antibody to the embryos in PBTN.
3. Shake on nutator for 1 h at room temperature *(20)*.

3.5.7. Wash and Colorimetric Staining of Embryos

1. Remove the antibody solution and wash four times for 20 min each with 1 mL of PBT.
2. The Vectastain ABC reagent should be made 30 min prior to finishing the washes.
3. Remove the PBT and add 0.5 mL of the ABC reagent to the embryos.
4. Incubate with nutation for 15 min at room temperature.
5. Wash the embryos at least five times for 5 min with PBT at room temperature with nutation.
6. Immediately prior to use, mix the Vectastain staining solution.
7. Remove PBT, add 0.5 mL of staining solution, and rotate the embryos on a nutator for 3 min in the dark. The cover of a black slide box works well for this purpose.
8. Wash immediately with PBT at least five times *(20)*.

3.5.8. Analysis and Photography Methods

Embryos are mounted as described in **Subheading 3.4.7.** U-shaped hematopoietic expression is best viewed and photographed laterally or ventrally.

3.6. Localization of a Single Protein, or Co-Localization of Proteins, in Hemocytes by Confocal Microscopy

3.6.1. Using the Gal4/UAS System to Direct Lozenge Expression in Crystal Cells

The UAS/Gal4 system and the *lz-Gal4* strain are described in **Subheading 3.1.1.** *lz-Gal4* virgins are mated to *UAS-lacZ* males. There are a variety of *UAS-lacZ* stocks with insertions on either the second or third chromosomes. The β-galactosidase protein will be expressed in crystal cells and a subset of plasmatocytes that are derived from Lz-expressing hemocyte precursor cells *(4)*.

3.6.2. Antibody Reagents

For colocalization studies, the excitation peaks of the two secondary antibody conjugate fluors must be sufficiently different to be detected as separate signals. Because the peak of fluorescence of indocarbocyanine (Cy3; Jackson Immuno Research) is 570 nm and fluorescein isothiocyanate (FITC) is 520 nm, these fluors can be used to determine protein colocalization. Mouse α-β-galactosidase antibody (Promega) is used to detect *lz-Gal4:UAS-lacZ* expression (**Fig. 3A**). Cy3 conjugated anti-mouse IgG (Jackson Immuno Research) is used to detect the α-β-galactosidase antibody. The rabbit α-U-shaped antibody and the Alexa fluor (FITC) conjugated anti-rabbit IgG (Molecular Probes) are used in the colocalization studies (**Fig. 3B**).

3.6.3. PreWash and Blocking of Embryos (see **Subheading 3.5.3.**)

3.6.4. Primary Antibody Staining (see **Subheading 3.5.4.**)

3.6.5. Wash and ReBlocking of Embryos (see **Subheading 3.5.5.**)

3.6.6. Secondary Antibody Staining

1. Because the fluors are subject to photobleaching, embryos should be transferred to an opaque tube or a tube wrapped in aluminum foil.
2. Dilute the secondary antibody in PBTN and incubate as described in **Subheading 3.5.6.**

3.6.7. Embryo Washing and Stain Monitoring

1. Wash embryos as described in **Subheading 3.5.3.**, being careful to limit the exposure of antibody bound embryos to light (*see* **Note 7**).
2. After washing is complete, monitor staining using fluorescent microscopy.
3. If staining is satisfactory, proceed to mounting (*see* **Subheading 3.6.9.**) or double antibody staining (*see* **Subheading 3.6.8.**).
4. If staining is unsatisfactory, consider titrating the secondary antibody. It is usually best to test a series of dilutions between 1:200 and 1:1000.

3.6.8. Double Antibody Staining for Studies of Co-Localization of Two Proteins

1. During the following steps, limit the exposure of the antibody bound embryos to light (*see* **Note 7**).
2. Remove the PBT, block, stain with the second primary antibody, and wash and stain with the second secondary antibody as described in **Subheadings 3.6.3.–3.6.7.**

3.6.9. Embryo Mounting

1. Embryos are mounted in an antifade compound to protect the fluorescent signal from photobleaching. We use Prolong antifade from Molecular Probes.
2. The antifade compound comes in two tubes that are mixed just prior to using. The mixed compound should be used within an hour after preparation.
3. Embryos whole mounts are made as described in **Subheading 3.4.7.**, except that the antifade compound is used in place of glycerol.
4. The embryos should be shielded from light until the compound has hardened.
5. The slides can be sealed with nail polish after the compound hardens.

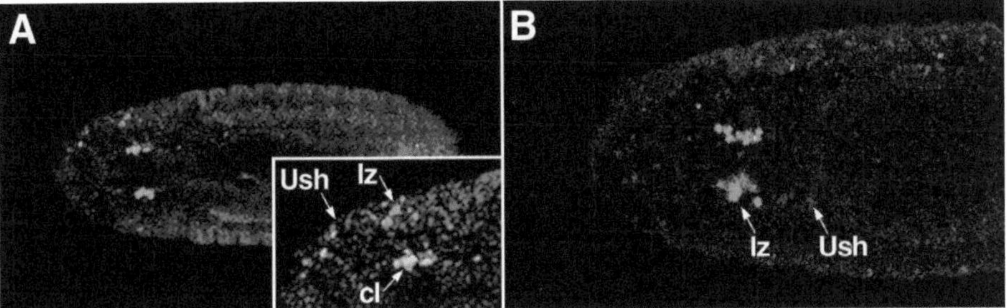

Fig. 3. Immunolocalization of lozenge and U-shaped in *Drosophila* blood cells using confocal microscopy. **(A)** Stage 13 embryo in which lz-Gal4:UAS-lacZ results in β-galactosidase activity (green) in crystal cells, whereas U-shaped protein (red) is more widely expressed. The inset demonstrates the colocalization (cl) of lozenge enhancer activity (lz) with U-shaped protein (Ush) in crystal cells (yellow). **(B)** Noncoincident expression of lozenge and U-shaped in a stage 15 embryo caused by the downregulation of U-shaped expression in crystal cells at this stage. *See* color insert following p. 80.

3.6.10. Analysis and Imaging Methods

It is advisable to work with someone who is experienced with confocal microscopy. The image can be digitally captured and manipulated. Using the appropriate lasers and filters, the staining pattern from each fluorescent probe can be visualized and photographed separately, then merged digitally to monitor colocalization.

4. Notes

1. Protein localization by immunohistochemistry: wash and colorimetric staining of embryos. The black stain is recommended to visualize plasmatocytes.
2. Embryo collection for *in situ* hybridization. It is advisable to start with large numbers of adult flies (100 to 200 pairs) to obtain a sufficient number of embryos to compensate for the potential loss of animals during embryo processing.
3. Embryo collection for protein localization by immunohistochemistry. In general, only 20 to 30 adult pairs are required to collect a sufficient number of embryos for immunochemical staining. However, larger numbers of adults will yield more embryos, reducing the number of collections.
4. mRNA localization by *in situ* hybridization: prehybridization and hybridization of embryos. Embryos should be placed in boiling resistant Eppendorf tubes to prevent them from opening during incubation at 60 to 70°C.
5. mRNA localization by *in situ* hybridization: staining of embryos. Complete staining of embryos can take from 1 h to overnight. For convenient monitoring of a prolonged staining reaction, antibody bound embryos ready for staining can be stored overnight at 4°C, with the staining reaction started the next morning.
6. Protein localization by immunohistochemistry: washing and reblocking of embryos. The antibody solution can be saved, stored at 4°C, and later reused.
7. Double antibody staining for colocalization of two proteins. We recommend checking the quality of the fluorescent double antibody staining prior to mounting embryos for confocal microscopy. Care should be taken to keep embryos shielded from light as much as

possible. Because photobleaching can occur during fluorescent microscopy, it is recommended that embryos be checked quickly and then placed back in the dark.

Acknowledgments

The authors thank L. McCord for assistance with the figures. This research was supported by National Institutes of Health grants HL059151 and HL071540 (to R. A. Schulz) and American Heart Association grants 0150007N (to R. A. Schulz) and 0230020N (to N. Fossett).

References

1. Rizki, T. M. (1978) The circulatory system and associated cells and tissues, in *The Genetics and Biology of Drosophila, Vol. 2B.* (Ashburner, M. and Wright, T. R. F., eds.), Academic Press, New York, pp. 397–452.
2. Tepass, U., Fessler, L. I., Aziz, A., and Hartenstein, V. (1994) Embryonic origin of hemocytes and their relationship to cell death in *Drosophila. Development* **120,** 1829–1837.
3. Dearolf, C. R. (1998) Fruit fly leukemia. *Biochim. Biophys. Acta* **1377,** M13–M23.
4. Lebestky, T., Chang, T., Hartenstein, V., and Banerjee, U. (2000) Specification of *Drosophila* hematopoietic lineage by conserved transcription factors. *Science* **288,** 146–149.
5. Fossett, N. and Schulz, R. A. (2001) Functional conservation of hematopoietic factors in *Drosophila* and vertebrates. *Differentiation* **69,** 83–90.
6. Lanot, R., Zachary, D., Holder, F., and Meister, M. (2001) Postembryonic hematopoiesis in *Drosophila. Dev. Biol.* **230,** 243–257.
7. Rehorn, K. P., Thelen, H., Michelson, A. M., and Reuter, R. (1996) A molecular aspect of hematopoiesis and endoderm development common to vertebrates and *Drosophila. Development* **122,** 4023–4031.
8. Fossett, N., Tevosian, S. G., Gajewski, K., Zhang, Q., Orkin, S. H., and Schulz, R. A. (2001) The Friend of GATA proteins U-shaped, FOG-1, and FOG-2 function as negative regulators of blood, heart, and eye development in *Drosophila. Proc. Natl. Acad. Sci. USA* **98,** 7342–7347.
9. Waltzer, L., Bataille, L., Peyrefitte, S., and Haenlin, M. (2002) Two isoforms of Serpent containing either one or two GATA zinc fingers have different roles in *Drosophila* haematopoiesis. *EMBO J.* **21,** 5477–5486.
10. Duvic, B., Hoffmann, J. A., Meister, M., and Royet, J. (2002) Notch signaling controls lineage specification during *Drosophila* larval hematopoiesis. *Curr. Biol.* **12,** 1923–1927.
11. Lebestky, T., Jung, S.-H., and Banerjee, U. (2003). A Serrate-expressing signaling center controls *Drosophila* hematopoiesis. *Genes Dev.* **17,** 348–353.
12. Ashburner, M. (1989) *Drosophila: A Laboratory Handbook.* Cold Spring Laboratory Press, Cold Spring Harbor, NY.
13. Brand, A. H. and Perrimon, N. (1993) Targeted gene expression as a means of altering cell fates and generating dominant phenotypes. *Development* **118,** 401–415.
14. Baylies, M. K. and Bate, M. (1996) *Twist*: a myogenic switch in *Drosophila. Science* **272,** 1481–1484.
15. Fossett, N., Hyman, K., Gajewski, K., Orkin, S. H., and Schulz, R. A. (2003) Combinatorial interactions of Serpent, Lozenge, and U-shaped regulate crystal cell lineage commitment during *Drosophila* hematopoiesis. *Proc. Natl. Acad. Sci. USA* **100,** 11,451–11,456.
16. Greenspan, M. (1989) *Fly Pushing: The Theory and Practice of Drosophila Genetics.* Cold Spring Laboratory Press, Cold Spring Harbor, NY.

17. Ingham, P. and Jowlett, T. (1997) *The Molecular Biology of Insect Disease Vectors: A Methods Manual.* Chapman and Hall, London, UK.
18. Sam, S., Leise, W., and Hoshizaki, D. K. (1996) The *serpent* gene is necessary for progression through the early stages of fat body development. *Mech. Dev.* **60,** 197–205.
19. Rizki, T. M., Rizki, R. M., and Bellotti, R. A. (1985) Genetics of a *Drosophila* phenoloxidase. *Mol. Gen. Genet.* **201,** 7–13.
20. Patel, N., Snow, P. M., and Goodman, C. S. (1987) Characterization and cloning of fasciclin III: a glycoprotein expressed on a subset of neurons and axon pathways in *Drosophila. Cell* **48,** 975–988.

8

Tracking and Programming Early Hematopoietic Cells in *Xenopus* Embryos

Maggie Walmsley, Aldo Ciau-Uitz, and Roger Patient

Summary

The fates of lineage labeled hematopoietic precursor populations in *Xenopus* embryos are followed by use of *in situ* hybridization, looking for overlap between lineage labeled cells and *in situ* probes specific for known cell populations or states of differentiation. By coinjection of dominant interfering constructs, it also is possible to define the environmental cues or signals required for specification and/or maintenance of the hematopoietic program at different times and locations in the early embryo. As a lineage trace, we use β-galactosidase, which is injected as in vitro synthesized ribonucleic acid (RNA) in to *Xenopus* embryos at early cleavage stages. Because the interfering constructs we use also are in the form of injected RNA, the use of β-galactosidase RNA as a lineage trace assures accurate determination of the cells expressing the dominant negative construct. Embryos are cultured to desired developmental stages, fixed briefly and processed for the β-galactosidase reaction. Embryos are then analyzed by whole mount *in situ* hybridization, embedded in wax, and sectioned. Alternatively, after the β-galactosidase reaction, embryos can be fixed long term in paraformaldehyde, mounted in wax, sectioned, and probed by *in situ* hybridization directly on sections.

Key Words: Hematopoiesis; blood; endothelium; lineage labeling; *Xenopus*; cell fate; β-galactosidase; hematopoietic/endothelial precursors; embryonic signaling.

1. Introduction

The *Xenopus* embryo is an ideal system for experiments designed to follow early precursor cell populations during developmental time. The embryos are large (1 mm in diameter) and thus are easily visualized and manipulated at low magnification. They are laid externally in large numbers and are therefore accessible from the earliest times of development. In vitro fertilization allows for the synchronous development of embryos at experimentally suitable times. The speed of development is dependent on temperature and thus can be manipulated to suit experimental needs or design. The first six cleavage divisions are easy to follow under the microscope because they occur

From: *Methods in Molecular Medicine, Vol. 105: Developmental Hematopoiesis: Methods and Protocols.*
Edited by: M. H. Baron © Humana Press Inc., Totowa, NJ

relatively synchronously at approx 30-min intervals (at 23°C). In a small percentage of embryos, the cleavage planes are perfectly regular and fulfill the idealized portrayal of *Xenopus* cleavage stage embryos depicted by early fate mappers (**Fig. 1E**; *see* **refs.** ***1*** and ***2***) with readily identifiable rows and tiers of cells (at these stages called blastomeres). Using such 'regular cleavers,' it is possible to label and/or manipulate, by injection, defined populations of precursor cells and to follow their journey through the embryo and their developmental fate.

A number of fate maps of the early *Xenopus* embryo were performed in the last century ***(1–7)*** and some valuable major revisions have been made very recently (for an excellent review, *see* **ref.** ***8***). Importantly, solid evidence in favor of redefining the major axes in the *Xenopus* embryo has been presented ***(8,9)*** and in the new terminology the dorsal/ventral axis becomes the rostral/caudal axis. We shall adopt this new terminology wherever appropriate. In the case of blood, recent evidence has led to a complete revision of earlier fate maps ***(9–11)***. The embryonic blood in the ventral blood islands derives from two regions on opposite sides of the 32-cell stage embryo. The anterior blood island derives from blastomeres C1 and D1 on the rostral (formerly dorsal) side of the embryo whereas the posterior blood island derives mainly from D4 ***(11)*** or from the C4/D4 boundary ***(9)*** on the caudal (formerly ventral) side. Transplantation studies have established that the precursors of adult blood are located in the dorsal lateral plate of neurula-stage embryos ***(12–14)***, and this region is derived from blastomere C3 ***(11)***. With a knowledge of the blood fate map, early targeting of lineage label along with dominant interfering molecules or constructs to well defined regions of the embryo allows us to investigate the environmental requirements for the specification and establishment of both embryonic and adult blood.

Fig. 1. *(opposite)* Diagram of cleavage stage embryos between 4 and 32 cells. **(A)** Animal view of four-cell stage embryo showing rostral/caudal patterning. Note that the caudal blastomeres are larger and more pigmented than the rostral ones. **(B)** Lateral view of a four-cell stage embryo showing two lightly pigmented rostral blastomeres and one darkly pigmented caudal blastomere (the second caudal blastomere is hidden behind the plane of the paper). **(C)** Animal view of an eight-cell stage embryo showing two caudal and two rostral blastomeres pinched off by the third cleavage plane, which has formed around the circumference of the embryo near the animal pole (AP). Irregularly cleaving embryos at this stage commonly form cleavage planes in an animal vegetal direction. **(D)** Lateral view of eight-cell stage embryo depicted in **(C)**. **(E)** A regularly cleaving embryo at the 16-cell stage. Note that the newly formed cleavage planes form in an animal to vegetal direction and meet at the centre of the vegetal pole (VP). **(F)** An irregularly cleaving embryo very common at the 16-cell stage. Note that the new cleavage planes do not bisect the eight-cell blastomeres and do not meet at the vegetal pole. As a result blastomeres AB3, AB2, CD3, and CD2 take over territory that belongs to AB4, AB1, CD4, and CD1 in the regularly cleaving embryo. **(G)** A regularly cleaving embryo at the 32-cell stage. **(H)** An irregularly cleaving embryo at the 32-cell stage. With respect to blood origins note that 1) the C3 blastomere, which gives rise to adult blood in a regularly cleaving embryo, is greatly enlarged and the C4 and D4 blastomeres are correspondingly reduced in size and 2) that regions of blastomeres C1, D1, and D4, which give rise to embryonic blood in a regularly cleaving embryo, now, in the irregularly cleaving embryo become incorporated into neighboring blastomeres C2, D2, and D3. Thus, C2, D2, and D3 contribute to blood in the irregular embryo **(H)** but not in the regular embryo **(G)**.

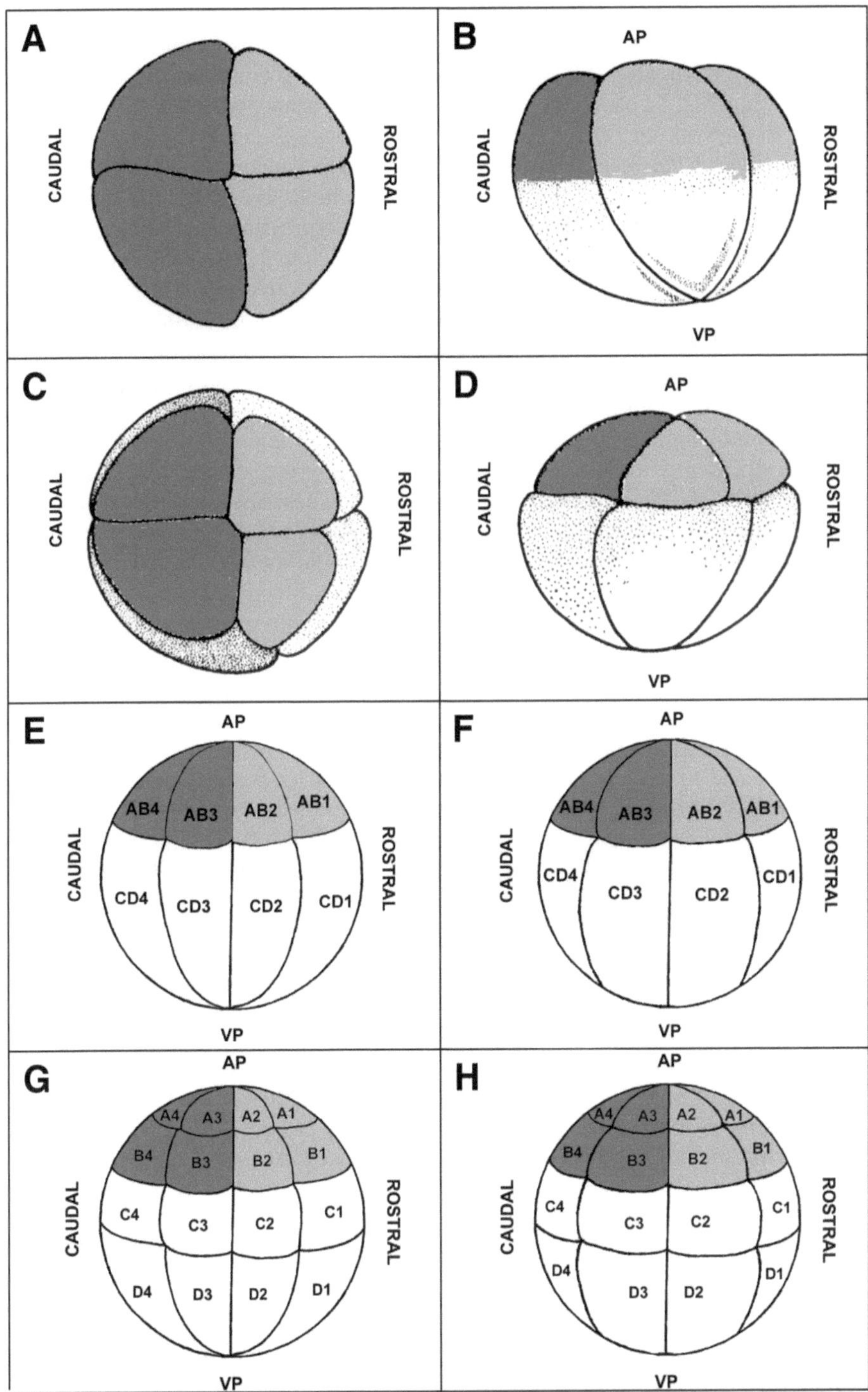
A
CAUDAL
ROSTRAL
B
AP
CAUDAL
ROSTRAL
VP
C
CAUDAL
ROSTRAL
D
AP
CAUDAL
ROSTRAL
VP
E
AP
AB4
AB3
AB2
AB1
CAUDAL
ROSTRAL
CD4
CD3
CD2
CD1
VP
F
AP
AB4
AB3
AB2
AB1
CAUDAL
ROSTRAL
CD4
CD3
CD2
CD1
VP
G
AP
A4
A3
A2
A1
B4
B3
B2
B1
CAUDAL
ROSTRAL
C4
C3
C2
C1
D4
D3
D2
D1
VP
H
AP
A4
A3
A2
A1
B4
B3
B2
B1
CAUDAL
ROSTRAL
C4
C3
C2
C1
D4
D3
D2
D1
VP

Embryonic blood and vascular endothelium develop in close association from early developmental stages in the vertebrate yolk sac, and they represent the first differentiated cell types to form after mesoderm induction ***(15)***. This close association of blood and endothelium also is observed in the ventral blood island, which is the amphibian equivalent of the yolk sac ***(16)***. Recent evidence in *Xenopus* embryos suggests a similar close association between definitive or adult blood and endothelial lineages ***(11,16)***. A common cellular precursor, the hemangioblast, which gives rise to both lineages, has long been proposed ***(17)***. Precursor populations expressing markers for both lineages have been described in several species, and knockout mouse and zebrafish studies of single genes affecting both lineages have been reported ***(15,18,19)***. Also, blast colonies derived from embryonic stem cells can give rise to both lineages ***(20)***, and similar transient bipotential colonies have been detected in cultures of mouse embryonic tissues ***(21,22)***. Thus, studies of the early development of either lineage should yield information on both.

Using a combination of lineage tracing to follow cell migration (*see* **Note 1**) and *in situ* hybridization with tissue/stage-specific marker probes to identify differentiating or differentiated cell populations, we have started to describe the earliest location of blood and endothelial precursors in the *Xenopus* embryo ***(11,16)***. Furthermore, using dominant-negative constructs, we have begun to look at the signals required for the correct specification and fate within the embryo of early blood and endothelial precursors. The methods used for such a study are described in this chapter.

2. Materials

1. Message Machine kit (Ambion).
2. 1X Modified Barth's saline (MBS): to 900 mL distilled water, add 40 mL of solution A, mix, then add 40 mL of solution B, mix, then add 1 mL of pen/strep stock. Make up to 1 L with distilled water. Solution A: to 900 mL of distilled water, add sequentially with stirring the following ingredients, assuring that each is dissolved before addition of the next: 128 g of NaCl, 2 g of KCl, 5g of $NaHCO_3$,, 89 g of HEPES (adjust to pH 7.6 with 1 *M* NaOH). Make up to 1 L with distilled water and store in fridge. Solution B: to 900 mL of distilled water, add sequentially with stirring the following ingredients, assuring that each is dissolved before addition of the next: 1.9 g of $CaNO_3 \cdot 4H_2O$, 2.25 g of $CaCl_2 \cdot 6H_2O$, 5 g of $MgSO_4 \cdot 7H_2O$. Make up to 1 L with distilled water and store in fridge. Pen/strep stock: (Sigma; cat. no. P0781). Prepare 5-mL aliquots and store at –20°C. Have a thawed aliquot ready for use in the fridge.
3. 0.1X MBS: Dilute 100 mL of 1X MBS to 1 L and add 1 mL of pen/strep stock.
4. 2% Cysteine: dissolve 4 g of L-cysteine HCl (Sigma) in 200 mL of 1X MBS while stirring. Add approx 1.2 g of NaOH pellets to bring the pH to 7.8–8.1. Complete the pH adjustment with a 1 *M* NaOH solution if needed. Make fresh.
5. 1X MBS + 3% Ficoll: dissolve 3 g of Ficoll (Sigma; cat. no. F9378) in 100 mL of 1X MBS and store at 14°C.
6. MEMFA: 0.1 *M* MOPS, pH 7.4; 2 m*M* ethylenebis(oxyethylenenitrilo)tetraacetic acid, pH 8.0, 1 m*M* $MgSO_4$; 3.7 % formaldehyde PBS-Tween: Phosphate-buffered saline (PBS) containing 0.1% Tween-20: 50 μL of 10X PBS (Gibco), 2.5 mL of 20% Tween-20 (Sigma; cat. no. P1379), and water to 500 mL.
8. Buffer A: to 20 mL 1X PBS, add 20 μL of 1 *M* $MgCl_2$,, 0.115 g of $K_3Fe(CN)_6$, 0.148 g of $K_4Fe(CN)_6$. Store as frozen aliquots at –20°C.

9. X-Gal stock: X-gal is from Sigma. Stock is 20 mg/mL in dimethyl formamide. Store protected from light at –20°C.
10. 4% Paraformaldehyde: In a 50-mL Falcon tube, place 2 g of paraformaldehyde (use a mask!), 40 mL of distilled water, 20 mL of 1 *M* NaOH. Heat in 75°C oven to dissolve, then add 5 mL of 10X PBS. Make up to 50 mL with water.
11. Hybridization buffer (whole mounts): 50% formamide, 5X standard saline citrate (SSC) pH 7.0, 1 mg/mL yeast ribonucleic acid (RNA), 100 μg/mL heparin, 1X Denharts, 0.1% Tween-20, and 5 m*M* ethylenediamine tetraacetic acid, pH 8.0.
12. Antibodies, anti-DIG-AP Fab Fragments, and anti-fluorescein-AP Fab fragments conjugated with alkaline phosphatase are purchased from Roche.
13. TEA: 0.1 *M* triethanolamine adjusted to pH 7.9 with HCl.
14. Acetic anhydride, BDH, cat. no. 100022M.
15. Bleach, H_2O_2 solution approx 30%, BDH, cat no. 101284N.
16. Formamide is from Sigma, cat. no. F7508. Aliquot on arrival and stored at –20°C. Note that the formamide solutions used in hybridization and wash down steps are labile. Solutions more than 2-mo-old result in whole mounts showing nonspecific background staining. 20X SSC: 88.2 g of sodium citrate and 175.3 g of NaCl. Adjust to pH 7.0 (for whole mounts) or pH 4.5 (for sections) with citric acid. Dissolve in 1 L of distilled water and autoclave.
18. MAb: 100 m*M* maleic acid and 150 m*M* NaCl; adjust to pH 7.5 with NaOH.
19. Blocking reagent, Boehringer, cat. no. 1096176.
20. AP buffer: 0.1 *M* Tris-HCl, pH 9.5; 50 m*M* $MgCl_2$, 0.1 *M* NaCl, 10.1% Tween-20.
21. AP buffer + PVA. Add 2.5 g of polyvinyl alcohol (MW 30,000–70,000, Sigma, cat. no. P8136) to 50 mL AP buffer. Dissolve carefully in a microwave.
22. BM-purple, Boehringer, cat. no. 1442074.
23. 5-Bromo-4-chloro-3-indolyl-phosphate (BCIP, Boehringer; cat. no. 1383221).
24. 5X Transcription buffer and 100 m*M* dithiothreitol are supplied with SP6, T7, and T3 polymerases (Promega).
25. Fibrowax™, pastillated (BDH).
26. Glycerol, 80% in water.
27. Polysine-coated slides, BDH, cat. no. 406/0178/00.
28. Glutaraldehyde, Sigma, cat. no. 104H5015.
29. Hybridization mix (*in situ* on sections): 50% formamide, 5X SSC, pH 4.5, 50 mg/mL yeast RNA (torula), 1% sodium dodecyl sulfate, 50 mg/mL heparin.
30. Solution I: 50% formamide, 5X SSC, pH 4.5, 1% sodium dodecyl sulfate.
31. Solution II: 50% formamide, 2X SSC, pH 4.5.
32. Proteinase K stock solution, 20 mg/mL.
33. Glycine, 2 mg/mL in PBS/Tween.

3. Methods

The methods described give details of 1) preparation of in vitro synthesized RNA for injection; 2) generation, selection, and culture of regularly cleaving embryos; 3) embryo injection procedure; 4) β-galactosidase reaction; 5) fixation methods; 6) whole-mount *in situ* hybridization; 7) embedding and sectioning embryos; and 8) *in situ* on sections.

3.1. Preparation of In Vitro Synthesized RNA for Injection

3.1.1. Template for RNA Synthesis

Prepare by linearizing an appropriate complimentary deoxyribonucleic acid (cDNA) plasmid construct with a suitable restriction enzyme. Template is purified by phenol:chloroform:isoamyl alchohol (25:24:1) then chloroform:isoamyl alchohol

(24:1) treatments (twice each) followed by EtOH precipitation. Template is then taken up in RNase-free water at a concentration of 500 ng/μL and stored at –20°C until use. The construct for β-galactosidase contains a nuclear localization signal-nuc β-galactosidase *(23)*. This results in a more concentrated and therefore stronger signal from the enzymatic reaction compared with the cytoplasmic version.

3.1.2. RNA for Injection

RNA is synthesized using a Message Machine kit according to the manufacturer's instructions, except that RNA is precipitated twice with isopropanol to remove toxic excess unincorporated nucleotides. Note that this also increases the accuracy of estimation of RNA concentration using a spectrophotometer because unincorporated nucleotides contribute to the O.D. 260 reading. Finally, the RNA pellet is taken up in 100 μL of RNase-free water (supplied in kit), divided into five equal aliquots, and stored at –80°C until use.

3.2. Generation, Selection, and Culture of Regularly Cleaving Embryos

All procedures are conducted on the bench at approx 19°C unless otherwise stated. Plasticware is used throughout. Selection of embryos from the 4- to 32-cell stages is described.

1. Prime 2 or 3 female frogs with 600 to 750 U Chorulon (Intervet U.K. Ltd.).
2. The next morning, squeeze eggs from female frog onto a 9-cm Petri dish.
3. Macerate a piece of testis (approx 2 mm^3) in 1-2 mL of 0.1X MBS, pour over eggs and, disperse eggs to a monolayer using blunt watchmakers forceps. Leave for 5 min.
4. Wash off sperm by filling dish with 0.1X MBS. Decant then refill dish with 0.1X MBS. Leave eggs to develop to first cleavage (approx 1.5 h; *see* **Note 2**).
5. Remove jelly coat as follows (*see* **Note 3**). Pour off 0.1X MBS and replace with approx 30 mL of 2% cysteine. Using blunt forceps, release eggs from Petri dish and pour into a 50-mL Falcon tube. Invert gently several times until jelly coat has dissolved (*see* **Note 4**).
6. Decant cysteine and wash embryos with 4 × 50 mL of 1X MBS. Resuspend in a final 50 mL of 1X MBS and transfer to Petri dishes, allowing for no more than 200 to 300 eggs per dish (*see* **Note 5**).
7. When the embryos reach the four-cell stage start to select regular cleavers. Choose embryos with distinct rostral (formerly dorsal) and caudal (formerly ventral) blastomeres (*see* **Note 6**). If embryos are to be injected at this stage, transfer embryos to an injection dish containing 1X MBS + 3% Ficoll chilled to 14°C (*see* **Note 7**).
8. Using blunt forceps or a pipet tip mounted on forceps, gently orient the embryos in the nylon grid with vegetal side down and rostral or caudal blastomeres (as appropriate) on the side of the injection needle. Wait for at least 25 min until cleavage planes are externally complete and well formed to avoid leakage of injected material between blastomeres and then inject (*see* **Note 8**).
9. At the eight-cell stage, select embryos that have pinched off two dark and two light blastomeres at the top/animal pole (*see* **Fig. 1B**). Transfer embryos to an injection dish containing chilled 1X MBS + 3% Ficoll, orient the embryos appropriately, and inject if this stage is required.
10. With the embryos already oriented on the injection grid, wait for the next cleavage to the 16-cell stage, watching carefully. Eliminate any embryos that cleave irregularly (*see* **Note 9**).
11. Observe the next cleavage to the 32-cell stage. This normally occurs in two stages. The animal pole cleavage furrow forms first, pinching off the A row blastomeres followed by

the vegetal pole furrow separating off the D row of blastomeres (**Fig. 1G**). Eliminate irregular cleavers (*see* **Note 10**). Wait until the vegetal pole furrow is complete before injection.

12. Transfer injected embryos to a fresh dish containing 1X MBS + 3% Ficoll. Cultivate for at least 2 h before replacing buffer with 0.1X MBS. Place embryos in a 16°C incubator overnight (*see* **Note 11**). Next morning replace buffer with fresh 0.1X MBS and grow embryos to the appropriate stages on the bench at 19°C.

3.3. Embryo Injection

Injection needles are pulled using a Flaming/Brown micropipet puller model P-97 supplied by Sutter Instrument Co. Injections are performed using a PLI-100 injection rig manufactured by Medical Systems Corp. (Greenvale, NY) supplied by Digitimer Ltd. in the U.K.

1. With the needle mounted in the injection rig, cut off the sealed end of the needle using fine watchmakers forceps.
2. Fill the needle with water and, with the foot pedal, eject a bubble of water, which is held at the end of the needle. Quantitate the volume of the water bubble using a micrometer scale set within the eyepiece of the microscope. By adjusting injection time or by re-cutting the end of the needle, set the rig to inject 0.5 nL (for 16- and 32-cell blastomeres) or 4 nL (for four- and eight-cell blastomeres) of water during a period of 30 to 40 ms (*see* **Note 12**). Eject water and fill needle with the appropriate RNA(s) for injection. Coinject the lineage trace RNA (approx 200 pg) and the RNA for the interfering molecule (amounts vary) as a mix.
3. With the embryo oriented in an injection dish filled with 1X MBS + 3% Ficoll, inject RNA in to the centre of the blastomere (*see* **Note 13**).

3.4. β-Galactosidase Reaction

At the appropriate stage of development transfer 10 to 20 embryos to a 1.5-mL Eppendorf tube, remove all buffer, and fix embryos in 1 mL of MEMFA at room temperature for 1 h (*see* **Note 14**).

1. Wash embryos with gentle rocking in 1mL of PBS/Tween four to five times for 10 min each.
2. Replace PBS/Tween with 1 mL of Buffer A for 10 min.
3. Replace with Buffer A containing 40 μL X-gal stock/mL (X-gal stock is 20 mg/mL).
4. Incubate for 1 to 1.5 h at 37°C, inverting Eppendorf tube gently every 15 min. The embryos should turn blue and this can be monitored by eye or under a binocular microscope (*see* **Note 15**).
5. Stop reaction by washing three times in 1 mL of PBS/Tween for 5 min.
6. Refix in 1mL of MEMFA for 20 min.
7. Replace with 1 mL of methanol for 10 min twice.
8. Replace with final 1mL methanol and store at –20°C until *in situ* procedure.

3.5. Fixation Methods

The method of fixation used depends on which *in situ* procedure is used. For whole-mount *in situ* use the MEMFA fixation procedure described in **Subheading 3.4.** For *in situ* on sections, follow the procedure outlined in **Subheading 3.4.** up to **step 5**. Then wash embryos for 5 min in 4% paraformaldehyde. Replace with fresh 4%

paraformaldehyde and store at 4°C for at least 1 wk. Embryos can be stored in paraformaldehyde for months with no deterioration in β-galactosidase signal and indeed long-term storage enhances subsequent morphology of sectioned embryos.

3.6. *Whole-Mount* In Situ *Hybridization*

1. For gastrula-stage embryos, leave the vitelline membranes intact, but remove membranes from midtailbud-stage embryos and allow embryos to straighten out for 5 to 10 min before fixation.
2. Fix in MEMFA for 1 h at room temperature 10 to 20 embryos in 1 mL of MEMFA in 1.5-mL Eppendorf tubes laid on their sides. All subsequent washes are in 1 mL unless otherwise stated.
3. Dehydrate with three washes in menthanol. At this point embryos can be stored for several months at –20°C.
4. Rehydrate embryos through a decreasing methanol:PBS/Tween series (75%, 50%, 25% methanol:PBS/Tween then PBS/Tween) 5 min each wash.
5. Bleach embryos in freshly made 5% formamide, 0.5% SSC, 10% H_2O_2 on a light box for 3 to 5 min (*see* **Note 16**).
6. Wash three times in PBS/Tween 5 min each.
7. Wash in 0.1 *M* TEA for 5 min, replace with 0.1 *M* TEA plus 2.5 μL of acetic anhydride/mL for 5 min then with 0.1 *M* TEA plus 5 μL of acetic anhydride/mL for 5 min.
8. Wash twice in PBS/Tween 5 min each.
9. Wash with 0.5 mL of hybridization buffer for whole-mount *in situ* hybridization for 10 min.
10. Replace with fresh 0.5 mL of hybridization buffer and prehybridize for at least 6 h at 65°C in a heating block with tubes lying on their sides.
11. Replace with 0.5 mL of hybridization buffer containing digoxigenin (DIG) and/or fluorescein (FL) riboprobes (*see* **Note 17**). Incubate at 65°C overnight.
12. The next morning, remove probe mix from embryos and save for future use, storing probes at –20°C.
13. Wash embryos sequentially with the following: 50% formamide/5X SSC (65°C, 10 min); 25% formamide/2X SSC (65°C, 10 min); 12.5% formamide/2X SSC (65°C, 10 min); 2X SSC/0.1% Tween (65°C, 10 min); 0.2X SSC/0.1% Tween (65°C, 30 min); PBS/Tween (room temperature, 3 × 5 min); MAb (room temperature, 10 min).
14. Block for 4 to 5 h at room temperature in MAb + 2% Boehringer block reagent (*see* **Note 18**).
15. Replace block solution with fresh block solution containing 1/2000 dilution of anti-DIG or anti-FL antibody conjugated to alkaline phosphatase, depending on which probe has been used (single *in situ* experiments) or which probe is to be stained first (double *in situ* experiments). Incubate overnight with tubes lying on their sides at 4°C with rocking.
16. Wash in MAb five times for 1 h per wash at room temperature, tubes lying on sides and with gentle rocking.
17. Wash twice for 5 min in AP buffer.
18. For probing of a single gene by *in situ* hybridization, replace AP buffer with BM purple diluted 1:3 (v/v) with AP buffer. Develop stain (*see* **Note 19**).
19. When probing for two genes by *in situ* hybridization ('double *in situ*'), set up first stain using 1 mL of AP buffer containing 5-50 μL of BCIP (*see* **Note 20**) and incubate at room temperature for color development. When satisfied with staining, wash three times in PBS/Tween, 5 min (*see* **Note 21**).

20. For double *in situ*, now fix in MEMFA for 30 min. Transfer embryos to fresh tubes and wash twice in methanol for 30 min.
21. Wash in MAb 5 min then twice in MAB+0.1% Tween for 5 min.
22. Reblock in MAb-block solution for 1 h minimum then replace with fresh solution containing 1/2000 dilution of the second antibody.
23. Repeat **steps 16** and **17**.
24. Replace AP buffer with BM-purple:AP buffer (1:3 v/v) and develop stain.
25. When staining is complete, fix in MEMFA for 1 h, wash three times in methanol for 30 min and store in methanol at –20°C until photography.

3.7. Preparation of In Situ Hybridization Probes

Templates for *in situ* probes are prepared exactly as for in vitro RNA synthesis (*see* **Subheading 3.1.**).

1. Prepare 2.5 m*M* DIG- or FL-NTP mix. For 40 μL: 10 μL of 10 m*M* ribo-ATP, CTP, GTP mix, 6.5 μL of 10 m*M* UTP, 3.5 μL of 10 m*M* DIG- or FL-UTP, 20 μL of RNase free water (*see* **Note 22**). Prepare probe synthesis mix. Add in order at room temperature: 10 μL of 5X transcription buffer, 10 μL of DIG- or FL-NTP mix, 15.5 μL of RNase-free water, 5 μL of 100 m*M* dithiothreitol, 0.5 μL of RNAsin, 4-μL template DNA (2 ng), 5 μL of polymerase (SP6, T7, or T3). Mix gently, spin briefly to bottom of tube and incubate at 37°C for 2 h (or overnight if convenient).
2. Remove 1 μL from mix and store on ice. Add 5 μL of Rnase-free DNase I to remaining mix and incubate for 15 min at 37°C.
3. Stop reaction by addition of 1 μL of 0.5 *M* ethylenediamine tetraacetic acid, 66 μL of 5 *M* NH_4OAc, 11 μL of RNase free water, 335 μL of EtOH. Incubate on dry ice 10 min. Centrifuge for 10 min at 17,000*g*, 4°C, wash pellet with 70% EtOH , dry, and take up in 100 μL hybridization mix.
4. Remove 1 μL and run on an agarose gel alongside previous sample to check for yield of product and that template has been removed.

3.8. Embedding and Sectioning Embryos

1. Remove paraformaldehyde-fixed embryos from fridge and wash in PBS/Tween at 4°C for 30 min; 70% EtOH (2X) at room temperature (RT) for 15 min; 85% EtOH at RT for 30 min; 95% EtOH at RT for 30 min; and 100%EtOH at RT for 30 min.
2. Wash in 100% EtOH, 30 min, RT twice. (You may stop at this point and store in fridge overnight.)
3. Wash in 100% xylene, 30 min, twice at RT (all xylene steps are done in a fume hood).
4. Wash in 1:1 xylene/paraffin for 45 min at 70°C.
5. Wash in 100% paraffin for 30 min at 70°C three times. (You may stop at this point leaving embryos in wax overnight.)
6. Place 100% paraffin (kept at 70°C in an oven) in a plastic embedding container.
7. Place and orient embryos in hot wax using hot forceps for orientation. Allow wax to solidify overnight at RT.
8. The next day, mount the embedded embryo on a microtome for sectioning. Alternatively embryos can be stored indefinitely in wax until needed for sectioning.
9. Cut 10-mm thin sections using microtome. Place sections on water on a prepared "polysine" slide, allow to dry overnight at 40°C, and then store protected from dust or proceed immediately with *in situ* hybridization on sections.

3.9. In Situ *Hybridization on Sections*

1. Place slides in 50-mL plastic Coplin jars then, in a fume hood, dewax slides in xylene 3 × 5 min (xylene can be used twice).
2. Wash in ethanol 2 × 5 min.
3. Incubate with gentle shaking in 6% H_2O_2 in methanol for 3 h.
4. Rehydrate slides in 75%:50%:25% methanol:PBS:Tween for 5 min each.
5. Wash 3 × 5 min. in PBS/Tween.
6. Wash in 12.5 μg/mL proteinase K in PBS/Tween for 15 min (*see* **Note 23**).
7. Stop reaction by washing with glycine (2 mg/mL in PBS/Tween) 2 × 5 min.
8. Refix in 4% paraformaldehyde and 0.2% glutaraldehyde in PBS for 20 to 30 min.
9. Wash 2 × 5 min in PBS/Tween.
10. Drain slides and dry round edges one at a time then again one at a time (*see* **Note 24**) place in sandwich box lined with wet paper towel, add to each slide 120 μL of hybridization mix and cover with parafilm cut wider than slide (the parafilm will shrink during hybridization at high temperature). Seal sandwich box and incubate at 70°C for 1 or 2 h.
11. One at a time, drain slides, replace hybridization mix with 120 μL of probe mix (5 μL probe/mL hybridization mix) and cover with parafilm. Hybridize overnight at 70°C in sandwich box, assuring that paper towels are well dampened.
12. Make up solutions I and II for next d and incubate overnight in 70°C oven.
13. Transfer slides to Coplin jars and wash twice in solution I for 30 min at 70°C.
14. Wash slides in solution II twice for 30 min at 65°C.
15. Wash in MAb 3 × 5 min at room temperature.
16. Drain slides one at a time, transfer to sandwich boxes and cover each slide with 0.5 mL of 2% Boehringer blocking reagent in MAb for at least 2 h.
17. Drain slides and cover with 0.5 mL of MAb plus block containing 1/2000 dilution of anti-DIG or FL antibody. Incubate at room temperature for 2 h.
18. Transfer slides to Coplin jars and wash three times in MAb + 0.1% Tween for 20 min at room temperature.
19. Wash in AP buffer 3 × 5 min.
20. Transfer to sandwich trays, cover slides with 120 μL of BM-purple (1:4 v/v) in AP buffer containing 5% PVA, and cover with parafilm cut to size of slides.
21. Develop color in the dark (*see* **Note 25**).
22. When satisfied with color development, transfer slides to Coplin jars and wash 3 × 10 min in PBS/Tween.
23. Refix in 4% paraformaldehyde for PBS/Tween 1 h.
24. Wash 2 × 5 min in PBS/Tween.
25. Mount in 80% glycerol, seal slides, and photograph.

4. Notes

1. A number of possible lineage labels have been used in *Xenopus*, particularly in the lipid-soluble fluorescent dextran range of products. We chose to use β-galactosidase RNA for our studies because if the aim of the experiment is not simply to lineage label but to mark a population of cells which have received an interfering molecule in the form of an RNA construct, then the lineage label must also be in the form of RNA to assure equal spread of both molecules within the injected cell. Criticism has been leveled against the use of β-galactosidase as a lineage marker on the grounds that it does not spread as far as dextran compounds ***(24)***. However, in the Lane and Sheets study, biotinylated ruby dextran was detected by an antibody against biotin. A number of laboratories, including ours,

report that biotin use results in excessive non-specific staining in vertebrate embryos *(25–27)*. This raises doubts about the claims of unequal spreading. The advantages of β-galactosidase RNA as a lineage trace are that, as stated previously, the spread is equal to the coinjected RNA molecule whose activity is under investigation, the signal-to-noise ratio is excellent, and the detection of signal has the advantage of being rapid and cheap because it does not involve the use of antibodies.

2. Fertilized eggs will turn within the surrounding jelly coat to present their pigmented animal pole upwards within 30 min. Using macerated testes the rate of fertilization is usually close to 100% provided that the eggs are of good quality. Time to first cleavage varies between individual frogs and is temperature-dependent.
3. It has been suggested that delaying removal of the jelly coat to the four-cell stage enhances the percentage of regularly cleaving embryos. We have not found this to be true. The surest way to get regular cleavers in large numbers is to set aside those female frogs, which lay regularly cleaving embryos and to use eggs from such females whenever possible.
4. The eggs will fall to the bottom of the tube and, if held up to the light, spaces between the pigmented eggs can be seen because the eggs are being kept apart by the jelly coats. When these are dissolved, the eggs will fall more rapidly to the bottom of the tube and will nestle closely together in the v-shaped tube bottom.
5. At this point it is advantageous to split the embryos and incubate batches at different temperatures (16 and 14°C) to stagger development and allow longer for injections. An average squeeze will contain approx 600 eggs.
6. At this stage regular cleavers will have two small light blastomeres (rostral) and two large dark caudal blastomeres (*see* **Fig. 1A**).
7. The injection dish consists of a circle of nylon mesh attached by means of a few drops of chloroform to the lid of a 5-cm Petri dish. The nylon mesh has subdivisions of 5 mm^2. Chilled injection buffer slows down cleavage rates and allows longer injection times.
8. Cleavage furrows start in the less yolky, pigmented animal pole and extend slowly towards the vegetal pole during a period of 30 min or more depending on temperature. To avoid leakage of injection material between blastomeres, inject just as the next cleavage starts.
9. This is a common stage for cleavages to become irregular. A highly frequent problem occurs when the new cleavage planes, which form from animal pole to vegetal pole, do not cleanly bisect the existing blastomeres and fail to meet at the centre of the vegetal pole (**Fig. 1**, compare **C** and **D**). Note that these were the type of embryos used by Lane and Smith in their revised fate map of hematopoietic origins *(9)*. Therefore, theirs is not the fate map of regularly cleaving embryos. For details of how the blood fate map is distorted by use of irregular embryos see the legend to **Fig. 1**.
10. At this stage the most common problem is that the new cleavage planes do not form at right angles to the animal–vegetal cleavage planes. Often this occurs on one side of the embryo only and the blastomere on the regular side can be used for injection. This is feasible because the very first cleavage plane is sagittal and divides the embryo in to two mirror image halves so that one half of the embryo may be labeled by lineage tracer and can be legitimately investigated in isolation from the other half.
11. Ficoll prevents blebbing at the site of injection, which can result in loss of injected material in to the pinched off bleb (this can be visualized when injecting green fluorescent protein RNA). Embryos must be moved in to low salt (0.1X MBS) before the start of gastrulation, which does not occur normally in high salt (1X MBS). Gastrulation is more successful at lower temperatures (however, to avoid developmental defects do not go lower than 14°C).

12. Delivery times of less than 30 ms means that the needle diameter is too large and embryos may be damaged. Needle diameter is approx 10 µm.
13. This requires practice and judgment. The needle should be comfortably under the surface of the embryo but not so deep that you run the risk of penetrating other blastomeres internally.
14. Do not fix for more than 1 h to avoid inactivation of the β-galactosidase activity.
15. Do not overdo this step or you will compromise the *in situ* reaction to follow. Always put uninjected control embryos through the β-galactosidase reaction so that the *in situ* signals in controls and injected samples are comparable.
16. Do not overbleach to avoid embryos falling apart in subsequent hybridization steps. Bleach solution is for a 10 mL mix: 5.67 mL H_2O, 3.33 mL of H_2O_2, 1 mL 50% formamide, and 5X SSC (this last is the first solution used in the post-hybridization wash down). Make up the bleach solution in the previous order because this is a potentially explosive mixture.
17. For first time use of a fresh probe, use 5 µL (of 100-µL total probe suspension) in 1 mL of hybridization buffer. At the end of the procedure, you can judge whether this needs to be decreased or increased next time. Probes can be reused at least three times. We have used probes against highly abundant mRNAs up to six times.
18. The longer the blocking time, the lower the background.
19. Length of time to achieve satisfactory staining varies between probes. For an abundant mRNA, incubate at room temperature for several hours checking reaction regularly. Stop staining when signal is clear and background remains low. For less abundant probes, staining may be carried out overnight at 4°C with gentle rocking then continued next morning at room temperature.
20. The two stains we routinely use are BCIP (turquoise) and BM-purple (purple). BCIP is the weaker stain of the two, so we use this to probe for abundant mRNAs. Use up to 50 µL of BCIP for faster staining. Probe using BCIP first because we have found it difficult to completely wash out BM purple, which will continue to (over) develop during the second staining. Use BM-purple for the second staining of nonabundant mRNAs.
21. At this point, you may take photographs for comparison with the second staining in order to accurately locate regions of overlap in staining.
22. For Rnase-free water, we use low-conductivity doubly distilled water, which has been autoclaved in new storage bottles. These bottles are set aside and used for no other purpose.
23. To avoid sections detaching from the slides, do not overdo this step.
24. Slides are dealt with one at a time, to avoid drying out because this is the commonest cause of background signal.
25. Color development can take place over a period of 2 to 3 wk without danger of background stain developing. However, check every 3 d for drying out of slides. If this looks likely, apply 20 µL of AP buffer to border of parafilm.

References

1. Nakamura, O. and Kishiyama, K. (1971) Prospective fates of the blastomeres at 32 cell stage of *Xenopus laevis* embryos. *Proc. Jpn. Acad.* **47,** 407-412.
2. Dale, L. and Slack, J. (1987) Fate map for the 32-cell stage of *Xenopus laevis. Development* **99,** 527–551.
3. Vogt, W. (1929) Gestaltungsanalyse am Amphibienkeim mit ortlicher Vitalfarburg. II. Teil gastrulation und mesodermbildung bei urodelen und anuren. *Wilhelm Roux's Arch.* **120,** 384–706.

4. Keller, R. E. (1975) Vital dye mapping of the gastrula and neurula of *Xenopus laevis*. I Prospective areas and morphogenetic movements of the superficial layer. *Dev. Biol.* **42,** 222–241.
5. Keller, R. E. (1976) Vital dye mapping of the gastrula and neurula of *Xenopus laevis* II. Prospective areas and morphogenetic movements of the deep layer. *Dev. Biol.* **51,** 118–137.
6. Moody, S. A. (1987) Fates of the blastomeres of the 16-cell stage *Xenopus* embryo. *Dev. Biol.* **119,** 560–578.
7. Moody, S. (1987) Fates of the blastomeres of the 32-cell stage *Xenopus* embryo. *Dev. Biol.* **122,** 300–319.
8. Lane, M. C. and Sheets, M. D. (2002) Rethinking axial patterning in amphibians. *Dev. Dyn.* **225,** 434–447.
9. Lane, M. C. and Smith, W. C. (1999) The origins of primitive blood in *Xenopus*: implications for axial patterning. *Development* **126,** 423–434.
10. Tracey Jr., W. D., Pepling, M. E., Horb, M. E., Thomsen, G. H., and Gergen, J. P. (1998) A *Xenopus* homologue of aml-1 reveals unexpected patterning mechanisms leading to the formation of embryonic blood. *Development* **125,** 1371–1380.
11. Ciau-Uitz, A., Walmsley, M., and Patient, R. (2000) Distinct origins of adult and embryonic blood in *Xenopus*. *Cell* **102,** 787–796.
12. Kau, C. and Turpen, J. B. (1983) Dual contribution of embryonic ventral blood island and dorsal lateral plate mesoderm during ontogeny of hemopoietic cells in *Xenopus laevis*. *J. Immunol.* **131,** 2262–2266.
13. Maeno, M., Tochinai, S., and Katagiri, C. (1985) Differential participation of ventral and dorsolateral mesoderms in the hemopoiesis of *Xenopus*, as revealed in diploid-triploid or interspecific chimeras. *Dev. Biol.* **110,** 503–508.
14. Maeno, M., Todate, A., and Katagiri, C. (1985) The localisation of precursor cells for larval and adult hemopoietic cells of *Xenopus laevis* in two regions of the embryos. *Dev. Growth Diff.* **27,** 137–148.
15. Baron, M. H. (2001) Induction of embryonic haematopoietic and endothelial stem/progenitor cells by hedgehog-mediated signals. *Differentiation* **68,** 175–185.
16. Walmsley, M., Ciau-Uitz, A., and Patient, R. (2002) Adult and embryonic blood and endothelium derive from distinct precursor populations which are differentially programmed by BMP in *Xenopus*. *Development* **129,** 5683–5695.
17. Murray, P. D. F. (1932) The development in vitro of the blood of the early chick embryo. *Proc. Royal Soc. Lond.* **11,** 497–521.
18. Keller, G. (2001) *The Hemangioblast,* Cold Spring Harbor Laboratory Press, Cold Spring Harbor, NY, pp. 329–348.
19. Stainier, D. Y. R., Weinstein, B. M., Detrich, H. W., Zon, L. I., and Fishman, M. C. (1995) cloche, an early acting zebrafish gene, is required by both the endothelial and hematopoietic lineages. *Development* **121,** 3141–3150.
20. Choi, K., Kennedy, M., Kazarov, A., Papadimitriou, J. C., and Keller, G. (1998) A common precursor for hematopoietic and endothelial cells. *Development* **125,** 725–732.
21. Nishikawa, S.-I., Nishikawa, S., Hirashima, M., Matsuyoshi, N., and Kodama, H. (1998) Progressive lineage analysis by cell sorting and culture identifies FLK+VE-cadherin+ cells at a diverging point of endothelial and hemopoietic lineages. *Development* **125,** 1747–1757.
22. Palis, J., Robertson, S., Kennedy, M., Wall, C., and Keller, G. (1999) Development of erythroid and myeloid progenitors in the yolk sac and embryo proper of the mouse. *Development* **126,** 5073–5084.

23. Smith, W. C. and Harland, R. M. (1991) Injected Xwnt-8 RNA acts early in *Xenopus* embryos to promote formation of a vegetal dorsalising centre. *Cell* **67,** 753–765.
24. Lane, M. C. and Sheets, M. D. (2002) Primitive and definitive blood share a common origin in *Xenopus*: A comparison of lineage techniques used to construct fate maps. *Dev. Biol.* **248,** 52–67.
25. Hauptmann, G. (2001) One-, two-, and three-color whole-mount *in situ* hybridization to *Drosophila* embryos. *Methods* **23,** 359–372.
26. Jowett, T. (2001) Double in situ Hybridisation Techniques in Zebrafish. *Methods* **23,** 345–358.
27. Beumer, T. L., Veenstra, G. J. C., Hage, W. J., and Destree, O. H. J. (1995) Whole-mount immunohistochemistry on *Xenopus* embryos using far red fluorescent dyes. *Trends Genet.* **11,** 9.

9

Fate Mapping Hematopoietic Lineages in the *Xenopus* Embryo

Mary Constance Lane and Michael D. Sheets

Summary

Fate maps reveal the normal contribution of various regions of an early embryo to larval and adult structures. This chapter describes the mapping of primitive blood in embryos of the frog *Xenopus laevis* by the technique of lineage tracing with a fluorescent dextran.

Key Words: Fate map; *Xenopus laevis*; lineage tracing; primitive blood; fluorescent dextrans.

1. Introduction

A fundamental tool for embryologists is a fate map. Fate maps are topographic projections of older developmental stages onto younger developmental stages. When fate maps were invented, the intent was to provide a description of the embryo as it underwent morphogenesis. Subsequently, fate maps were exploited experimentally to isolate particular regions of an embryo for specification and commitment testing. Today, they are used routinely to target the expression of proteins of interest and mutated proteins to select regions or tissues in an embryo.

Fate maps are constructed by marking a cell or group of cells at an early stage and assessing the distribution of marked tissues at an older stage. Originally, the tracers were vital dyes, like Nile blue sulfate, that investigators distinguished by the naked eye in a light microscope. In the 1980s, injectable tracers, such as the protein horseradish peroxidase or fluorescent, high-molecular-weight dextrans, were introduced. These tracers remain the tracers of choice for fate mapping because they are more stable than vital dyes. Among the required properties of the tracer are the following: 1) they are small enough to diffuse through the injected cell and label all its descendants; 2) they are too large to pass through gap junctions, and thus are inherited only by descendants of the injected cell; 3) they are readily detectable throughout development; and 4) they do not change the fate of the injected cell. Of the available lineage tracers, fluorescent dextrans have two distinct advantages. First, they can be distinguished in living tissues,

From: *Methods in Molecular Medicine, Vol. 105: Developmental Hematopoiesis: Methods and Protocols.*
Edited by: M. H. Baron © Humana Press Inc., Totowa, NJ

which allows an investigator to examine label at multiple stages in a single embryo. In contrast, tracers such as horseradish peroxidase require the embryo to be fixed at a single time point and stained. Second, only dextrans have been shown to fill the cytoplasm of an injected blastomere *(1)*, which means all of the descendants are labeled. In the last decade, investigators tried several mRNAs, including lacZ and GFP, as lineage tracers in development. Although adequate to trace lineage in some situations, because mRNAs do not fill the cytoplasm of an injected blastomere, they are not suitable for fate mapping. Many progeny are not labeled so the data sets underestimate contributions *(2)*, and the resulting map is incomplete.

As a fate map can be constructed between any two stages, there is no single fate map for an organism. However, some maps find wider use than others, and the maps used most often in the frog *Xenopus laevis* ***(3,4)*** were constructed from early blastula (st. 6, the 32-cell stage) to late tailbud stages (st. 28–30, late tailbud stage, and st. 32–34, late tailbud/early tadpole stages). Although these maps are useful for finding the origins of many embryonic structures, they are less useful in determining the origins of hematopoietic tissues, which are insufficiently differentiated at stages 30 or 34, and thus cannot be mapped.

In this chapter we outline how to map the primitive blood compartment in *Xenopus laevis*, using the fluorescent dextran mini-ruby at the 32-cell stage ***(2,5)***. This protocol could be modified to inject earlier or later, as well as to inject other molecules. As mini-ruby dextran injected at the 32-cell stage continues to label tissues until late stages of development (st. 49+, MCL, unpublished observation), it could also be used to find the sources of definitive blood cells.

2. Materials

2.1. Injection

1. Injection system capable of repeatedly delivering nanoliter volumes (e.g., Picospritzer II, General Valve Corp.).
2. Programmable, horizontal micropipet puller (e.g., Sutter Instruments Model P-97 flaming brown pipet puller, San Rafael, CA; www.sutterinstruments.com).
3. Borosilicate capillary glass, with filament, outer diameter ca. 1.0 mm, inner diameter ca. 0.8 mm (e.g., Sutter catalogue no. BF100-78-15).
4. Micromanipulator with controls in three axes (e.g., Narishige no. 4952).
5. Micromanipulator mount with magnetic base.
6. Injection dish (*see* **Note 1**).
7. Dissecting microscope equipped with epi-fluorescence (e.g., Leitz MZFLIII) and suitable filter cubes (e.g., rhodamine and green fluorescent protein or fluorescein isothiocyanate). This should be mounted on a stage with a steel base to hold the magnetic micromanipulator mount. The scope should be placed on a tabletop that is free of vibrations, and has sufficient working space above and around the stage to place the injection apparatus and the fiber optic light, as well as free space for dishes of embryos.
8. FiberOptic light to illuminate microscope stage.
9. Mineral oil.
10. Sequencing or gel loading pipet tips that fit within the inner diameter of the borosilicate glass capillary tubes (e.g., Bio-Rad; cat. no. 223-9912).
11. Forceps for breaking pipet tips (e.g., Dumont no. 5).

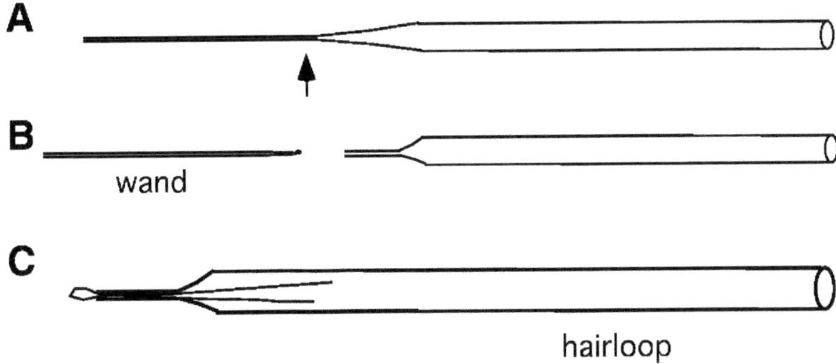

Fig. 1. **(A)** Construction of tools from a 9-in. borosilicate Pasteur pipet. Hold the pipet in the flame of a Bunsen burner, indicated by the arrow. Pull apart quickly as the glass softens. **(B)** Use the smaller piece to fashion a glass wand for vital dye marking with Nile blue sulfate. Position the pulled tip of the smaller piece into the flame until it rounds up. **(C)** Use the larger piece to fashion a hairloop for manipulating embryos in dishes. Break off the tip, insert a human hair and proceed as described in the text.

12. Eyepiece micrometer (Klarmann Rulings; www.reticles.com) mounted in eyepiece of the dissecting microscope used for injections.
13. Stage micrometer.
14. Mini-ruby dextran lineage tracer (*see* **Note 2**).

2.2. Embryos

1. Adult male and female *Xenopus laevis* (Nasco; Ft. Atkinson, WI; www.enasco.com).
2. Human chorionic gonadotropin.
3. Benzocaine.
4. Marc's modified ringers (MMR) and dilutions thereof. Make a sterile 10X stock: 1 *M* NaCl, 20 m*M* KCl, 20 m*M* $CaCl_2$, 10 m*M* $MgCl_2$, 50 m*M* HEPES, pH 7.4. Dilute as required.
5. Syringe and 26 1/2-gage needle.
6. 2% Cysteine hydrochloride in 1/10X MMR, pH 8.1.
7. Polystyrene culture dishes.
8. Nile blue sulfate, 1% in sterile water.
9. 100 m*M* Na_2CO_3 for marking embryos with Nile blue sulfate.
10. Beeswax.
11. Long strands of human toddler hair.
12. Hair loop and fine glass wand (*see* **Fig. 1** and **Note 3**).
13. 3% Ficoll in 1/4 MMR, sterile filtered.
14. Black electrical tape and standard microscope slides to make welled slides for live observation (*see* **Fig. 2** and **Note 4**).
15. Paraformaldehyde (*see* **Note 5**).
16. Fixative: 1X MEMPFA, and wash, 1X MEM, both diluted from sterile 10X MEM stock. 10X stock is 1.0 *M* MOPS, 20 m*M* ethylenebis(oxyethylenenitrilo)tetraacetic acid, 10 m*M* $MgSO_4$, pH 7.4. MEMPFA fix contains 4% paraformaldehyde.
17. Aluminum foil.

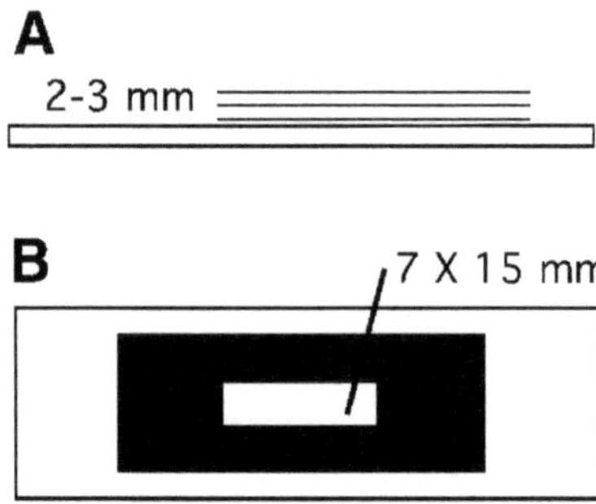

Fig. 2. Make welled slides for observing live tadpoles from black electrical tape by layering multiple (6–10) pieces of tape. **(A)** Side view. **(B)** top view after a well is cut with a razor blade.

18. Slides for observation of fixed, cleared whole-mount embryos (*see* **Note 6**). Construct slides using a Sylgard 184 elastomer kit (Dow Corning) of several depths and once cured, cut wells with a razor blade as described earlier for live observation slides.
19. Methanol.
20. Clearing reagent = 2:1 (v/v) benzyl benzoate/benzyl alcohol. Wear gloves, store in glass and use in fume hood as much as possible.
21. Glass cover slips.

3. Methods

3.1. Injection Rig

1. Commercial microinjection rigs vary between manufacturers. Some operate on house air lines (e.g., PLI-100 Pico-Injector, Medical Systems) whereas others require N_2 tanks (e.g., Picospritzer II, Parker Instrumentation). Following the manufacturer's instructions, set up the microinjection rig.
2. Pull needles from borosilicate glass capillary tubing using a horizontal pipet puller (*see* **Note 7**), following the manufacturer's instructions.
3. Calibrate the eyepiece micrometer to the stage micrometer and construct a chart of injection volume as a function of droplet diameter (*see* **Note 8**).
4. Thaw an aliquot of mini-ruby and centrifuge 2 min at maximum speed in a microfuge. Backload a needle with 2 to 3 μL of mini-ruby dextran using gel sequencing tips and a 20 μL pipetman. Insert the loaded tip into the blunt end of the capillary tube and deliver the solution as far into the capillary tube as possible. Mount the loaded needle on the micromanipulator and observe the tip in the dissecting microscope. Break the tip with Dumont no. 5 forceps such that the tip is approx 5 to 10 μm. Gently submerge the tip below the surface of some mineral oil in a small Petri dish, and push the injection solution into the tip using pressure from the microinjection rig.
5. Each needle must be calibrated immediately before use. Adjust the apparatus to deliver small volumes (i.e., by selecting a very short time pulse; e.g., 30 ms). Inject a small drop into a dish of mineral oil and measure the diameter of the drop using the eyepiece micrometer and the calibration chart. Determine the volume of the droplet. Adjust the delivery time to yield 1 nL (*see* **Note 9**). Leave the tip of the needle submerged in the oil until ready to inject embryos (*see* **Note 10**).

3.2. Generating, Selecting, and Injecting Embryos

The basic concept behind mapping is to follow a "reproducible package" of cytoplasm. Because frog embryos do not undergo determinate cleavage, an investigator must use embryos that cleave in a conventional, stereotypic pattern. This allows different investigators to obtain comparable results. The conventional pattern for the first five divisions is shown in **Fig. 3**. Most embryos do not cleave this way, and in some clutches, fewer then 2% cleave according to the conventional pattern. Thus, many embryos must be generated and regularly cleaving embryos selected whenever one maps. We prefer to use in vitro fertilization over natural matings, as in vitro fertilization yields large numbers of synchronous embryos, which facilities mapping.

1. To fertilize in vitro, inject a female *Xenopus laevis* with 800 U of human chorionic gonadotropin and maintain her at 16 to 18°C until she begins laying eggs (approx 16–18 h).
2. Sacrifice a male by submerging him in 0.02% benzocaine or other suitable anesthetic for about ten minutes. Check reflex reactions before starting surgery to ensure that the male is deeply anesthetized. Surgically remove the testes and store in sterile 1X MMR containing 10 µg/mL gentamycin at 4°C. Testes keep about 1 wk. Eggs are fragile and should be handled gently throughout. Freshly obtained eggs and sperm and must be used within min.
3. The female is gently squeezed, and the extruded eggs collected in 1X MMR.
4. A small piece of testis is cut and either macerated with forceps on the lid of a Petri dish or triturated in a microcap tube with 1X MMR.
5. Remove the excess MMR from the eggs and gently rub the eggs with macerated testis held with forceps, or add the dilute sperm suspension in 1X MMR. Sperm will bind to the egg surface, but not penetrate, in 1X MMR.
6. To trigger synchronous fertilization, gently flood the eggs with 1/4X MMR and swirl. Set the dish on the stage of a dissecting microscope and monitor their progress until they reach the desired stage.
7. At 2 h, begin selecting embryos cleaving by the conventional arrangement (**Fig. 3**). Following cortical rotation in the first cell cycle, one side of the animal hemisphere will be lightly pigmented and the other side darkly pigmented. The light-colored side is the future rostral (anterior) side and the dark-colored side is the prospective caudal (posterior) side (*see* **Fig. 3B** and **Note 11**). Frog embryos undergo two meridional cleavages to yield a four-cell embryo, followed by a third cleavage that is usually equatorial (**Fig. 3E**) to yield an eight-cell embryo.
8. De-jelly the embryos (*see* **Note 12**) when the cleavage furrow from the second division (four-cell stage, **Fig 3D**) reaches the vegetal pole (about 2 h at 21°C) in 2% cysteine HCl for 3.5 to 4 min, wash five to six times in 1/4X MMR.
9. Select those embryos that have a regular appearance at the eight-cell stage (**Fig. 3E**). Transfer the regular eight-cell embryos to a nitex dish filled with 3% Ficoll in 1/4X MMR, orient them with the prime meridian (0^0; formerly called the dorsal midline) facing upwards, and mark both sides of the prime meridian below the equator with a wand coated with Nile blue sulfate (marked with an X in **Fig. 3D,E**; *see* **Note 13**). After 1 to 3 min, transfer the marked embryos to a dish containing 1/4X MMR. When the embryos reach the 32-cell stage (*see* **Note 14**), blue marks will lie in the two C1 blastomeres. These marks allow one to rapidly orient and inject many embryos in a short period of time.
10. Select regularly cleaving, marked embryos again at the 16- and 32-cell stages.
11. At the 32-cell stage, transfer the selected embryos to a nitex injection dish filled with 3% Ficoll +1/4X MMR, orient the embryos such that the desired blastomere is tilted upwards and faces the needle (**Fig. 4**).

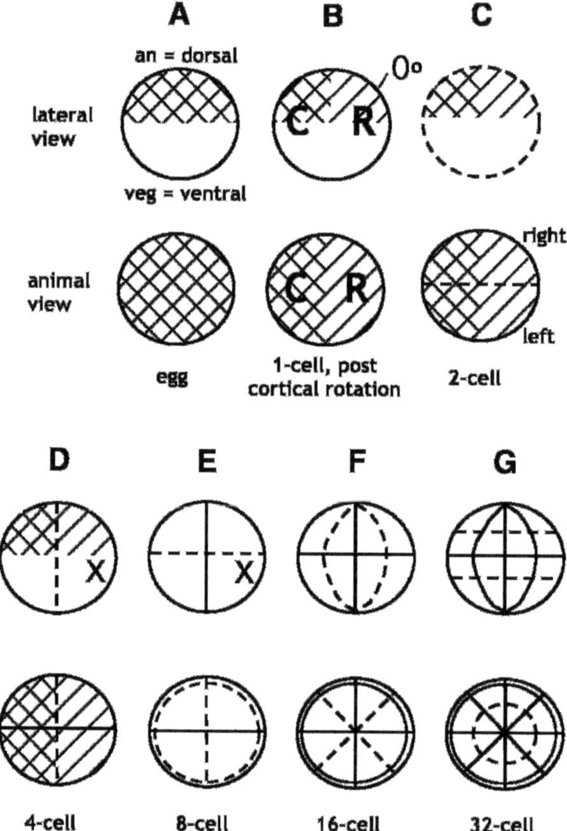

Fig. 3. Conventional cleavage pattern used for mapping in *Xenopus laevis*. Embryos are shown schematically in a lateral view in the top row, and from the animal pole in the bottom row. Throughout this figure, the newest cleavage plane is shown as a dashed line, while older cleavage planes are shown as solid lines. **(A)** In the egg, the animal hemisphere is heavily pigmented, whereas the vegetal hemisphere is relatively nonpigmented. **(B)** As a result of cortical rotation during the first cell cycle, the future rostral (R) end of the embryo is lightly pigmented (hatched) and the future caudal side C is darkly pigmented (crosshatched). The prime meridian is indicated as 0°. **(C)** The first cleavage plane bisects the embryo along the prime meridian into a right and left blastomere. **(D)** The second cleavage plane (dashed line divides the embryo into four equal-sized blastomeres, two of which are lightly pigmented (rostral blastomeres, formerly called dorsal blastomeres), and two of which are darkly pigmented (caudal blastomeres, formerly called ventral blastomeres). "X" indicates the site, which should be marked with Nile blue sulfate in order to mark the C1 blastomere. **(E)** For clarity, we have deleted the hatching and crosshatching representing light and dark pigmentation for the rest of the figures. The orientation is the same as in A–D. The third cleavage plane divides animal from vegetal blastomeres. The animal blastomeres are slightly smaller than the vegetal blastomeres. "X" again indicates the target site for Nile blue marking. **(F)** The fourth cleavage planes result in eight cells in each hemisphere. **(G)** The fifth cleavage planes result in an embryo comprised of four tiers of eight cells.

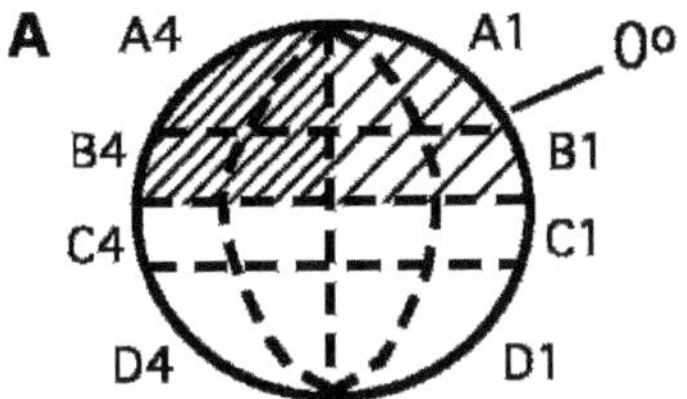

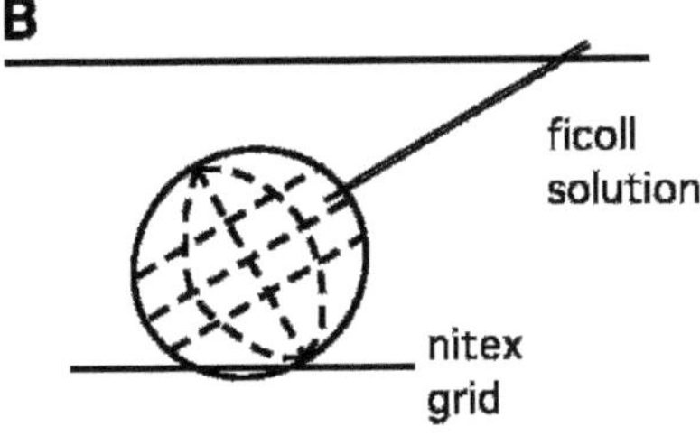

Fig. 4. **(A)** Nomenclature of the blastomeres at the 32-cell stage. **(B)** Lateral view diagram of an embryo undergoing injection into a B-tier blastomere.

12. Inject 1 nL of tracer dye into the appropriate blastomere by moving the needle with the *x*-axis of the micromanipulator. Point the tip of the needle away from the newest membrane (indicated by dashed lines in **Fig. 3**) because it is fragile and prone to leaking. When the needle enters the blastomere, the outer membrane will push inwards towards the tip of the needle. Gently back the needle outwards so that the membrane returns to its original position. Deliver the injection bolus, and gently back the needle out of the cell (*see* **Note 15**). On any given mapping day, inject at least four different embryos in each of at least three different blastomeres (e.g., blastomeres C1, B4 and A3; *see* **Note 16**). Because all 16 of the named blastomeres must be tested, preferably using eggs from at least three different females, it will take many injection days to construct the map.
13. When all of the embryos from a given clutch have been injected for at least 5 min, check the injections using uv-epifluorescence. Only a single blastomere should be labeled, or if the injected cell has subsequently divided, there should be two smaller, adjacent blastomeres labeled that occupy the territory of the injected blastomere. Discard any embryos in which dye has leaked into other blastomeres. Also ascertain the accuracy of the injection. Nile blue sulfate fluoresces faintly in the red channel and marks the two C1 blastomeres. Tracer dye injected into blastomere C2 should fill the blastomere next to C1, dye injected into C3 should be two blastomeres away from a Nile blue mark, dye injected into B1 should mark the blastomere immediately animal of the Nile blue marks, etc. Mis-injected embryos should be discarded.
14. Collect the injected embryos and transfer to labeled dishes filled with Ficoll + 1/4X MMR.
15. The embryos need to be screened once more at early gastrula stage. Culture the embryos at room temperature (22°C) and examine in approx 6.5 h or culture at 14 to 15°C and

examined the next morning. Screen injected embryos when the blastopore lip first appears on the future rostral side of the embryo. The Nile blue sulfate marks should lie on or very near the early lip st. 10. If the marks are not within 15° latitude of the lip, discard the embryo. This final screen ensures that the Nile blue truly marked the prime meridian and C1 blastomeres, from which all of the injections were oriented.

16. Change the solution to 1/4X MMR sometime during gastrulation. Performing these two screens—immediately after injection and at the onset of gastrulation—is additional work, but well worth the effort. The screens allow you to recognize misinjected embryos, which is a major advantage of using a fluorescent dextran to map.Discarding misinjected embryos at the gastrula stage greatly reduces the variability that has plagued some maps.

3.3. Assessing Injected Embryos

From fertilization through early tadpole stages (ca. st. 41), embryos are cultured in 1/10 to 1/4 strength MMR. Older tadpoles (ca. st. 45 onwards) should be cultured in 1/20 strength MMR.

1. The hallmark characteristic of blood is that it circulates through the vasculature. Primitive blood enters the circulation between st. 35 and 42 to 43, whereas definitive blood does not enter the circulation until many days later (after st. 49; **ref. *6***). Either cell type can be scored in live embryos at appropriate stages, although one will not be able to discern primitive from definitive blood merely by observation once definitive blood has entered the circulation.

   To observe circulating primitive blood in live embryos, anesthetize tadpole embryos in 0.01% benzocaine in appropriate strength MMR for 1 to 2 min. Transfer the embryos still in anesthetic to a welled-slide for live observation (*see* **Note 4**). It is difficult to orient the younger stages in any position other than on the embryo's side. Observe both the right and left sides under fluorescence, choose the preferred side, and place a cover slip over the well before observing at high power on either a dissecting or compound microscope equipped with epifluorescence. Primitive blood is easily observed at several locations, including the vitelline veins on the flank, the gill arches, the heart and the major blood vessels in the tail. To observe older tadpoles in which the head has widened significantly in the left/right axis, use a slide with a deeper well. Older embryos tend to orient with either their dorsal or ventral surfaces upward. Blood is easily observed circulating through the heart (both the inflow and outflow tracts) and major blood vessels of the head. Anesthetic should be washed out and embryos returned to appropriate-strength MMR within 10 to 15 min. They should resume swimming within minutes.
2. Fix embryos in MEMPFA for 2 h at room temperature or overnight at 4°C, wash in 1X MEM (two changes for 1 h or more) and post-fix in MeOH at –20°C overnight or longer, changing the MeOH the next day (*see* **Note 16**). Whole-mount observation of intact embryos to assess label distribution (*see* **Notes 17** and **18**), immunostaining or *in situ* hybridization can now be performed on embryos, and once these procedures are complete, re-fix the embryos at 4°C in MEMPFA. Refix for 24 h if the embryos will remain intact, but refix for 1 wk if the embryos will be sectioned for analysis.

4. Notes

1. Construct by placing a disc of nitex nylon mesh (Fisher Scientific; cat. no. 8-760–176) in the bottom of a polystyrene tissue culture dish. Spot weld the mesh by pressing a glass rod heated in a Bunsen burner against the nitex and the dish. They should melt together.

Secure each disc with 4 to 6 spot welds. Soak the dish overnight in several changes of water or before using the first time to remove impurities. Dishes can be used repeatedly. Clean between uses in detergent such as Terg-A-zyme to remove organic material that deposits on the nitex.

2. Many forms of fluorescent dextran are available from Molecular Probes (www.probes.com) and many factors will influence your choice of dextran. Choose either a 10K or 70K molecular weight (both diffuse well but are too large to pass through gap junctions), lysinated form (aldehyde-fixable). Choose a fluor that is compatible with your filter sets. Avoid fluorescein isothiocyanate because it is very sensitive to pH and fades quickly, especially in the clearing reagent used to examine fixed embryos. Other green dyes (e.g., AF 488) that are both brighter and more stable are available. Many dextrans are available with a biotin substitution in addition to the fluor. This is helpful if you will be staining histochemically and examining/documenting in white light rather than fluorescence (e.g., you may want to determine an mRNA expression pattern by *in situ* hybridization, and subsequently stain the progeny of the injected cell with a streptavidin–enzyme conjugate that recognizes the biotinylated dextran. These conjugates are available from Molecular Probes.) The chapter on dextrans available from Molecular Probes (Chapter 14, Section 5 in their catalog, which is also online at www.probes.com/lit/) is indispensable reading before you choose a dextran. In addition, they provide excellent technical assistance. In this chapter, we use mini-ruby dextran, which has rhodamine and biotin substitutions and is aldehyde-fixable. Resuspend in sterile 0.2 *M* KCl or ddH_2O at 33 mg/mL. Sterile filter and divide into 10- to 20-µL aliquots in microcap tubes and store at –20°C. Once thawed for use, store at 4°C in the dark. Over a period of years, stored dextrans can become toxic, and this will be obvious in embryos within a few hours of injection. Labeled cells will not have divided and will have odd pigmentation patterns.
3. Hair loops to manipulate embryos and fine glass wands to mark embryos with vital dye are made from 9-inch borosilicate Pasteur pipets (**Fig. 1**). Hold the pipet in a Bunsen burner flame (shown as an arrow in **Fig. 1**) and pull apart as the glass softens. To make a wand from the small piece, hold the pulled tip in the flame briefly until the glass begins to round up. To make a hairloop from the large piece, break the very end of the pulled tip. Fold a 7- to 10-inch piece of fine human hair (preferably toddler) in half, dip ca. 0.5 cm of the bent section into melted beeswax, and allow to harden, reinforcing the bend. Thread both loose ends through the narrow tip of the pulled pipet, until only the wax-coated, bent loop (ca. 0.2–0.3 cm) remains outside the pipet. Dip the tip in melted beeswax such that both the glass tip and the protruding loop are coated. Allow to cool. Heat a piece of metal (a flat spatula will work) in the burner, set down, cover with a Kim wipe, and touch the loop to the tissue. The heat from the enclosed metal will melt the wax off the hair. Store hairloops and wands in a box to protect them from breakage.
4. Live embryos strongly refract light, which can be reduced by observing them in a "black" well that absorbs refracted light. To construct a black well, place multiple layers of black electrical tape on a standard microscope slide (*see* **Fig. 2**). Cut a well larger then the embryo using a razor blade. The depth of tape layers required depends on the stage being examined and whether you want the embryo to be pinned in place or able to move. Make several slides of different depths and well sizes. These can be rinsed and reused.
5. Paraformaldehyde is toxic and should be mixed and used in a fume hood while wearing gloves and eye protection. Make a 20% stock solution from powder by heating to 65°C and slowly adding solid NaOH pellets until the solution clears. Store as 20-mL aliquots at –20 or –80°C.

6. The clearing reagent (BB:BA) used to view fixed specimens is a dangerous organic mixture that requires a special slide made from Sylgard elastomer. To make these slides, fold a large tray from aluminum foil, line the bottom with standard microscope slides and following the manufacturer's instruction mix, the Sylgard and pour it on the slides. Make slides of different depths. Once cured, cut a well in the Sylgard as you did with the black electrical tape (**Fig. 2**).
7. Pulled needles must be protected. Cut slits in a strip of foam and mount the foam in a box. Place the needles in slits or alternatively, press into artist's modeling clay mounted in the box.
8. The stage micrometer provides an absolute measurement, whereas the eyepiece micrometer provides a relative measurement. Once you assemble the injection apparatus, calibrate distances in the eyepiece micrometer with the stage micrometer at the highest magnification of the dissecting microscope. Use the conversion to make a chart that gives the volume of a droplet as a function of the diameter in your eyepiece micrometer and post it on the injection machine for quick reference. When you are ready to inject embryos, use the eyepiece micrometer and the highest magnification to measure the diameter of the injection droplet. Manufacturers often provide a table that lists volumes by diameter. Alternatively, divide the diameter by two in order to get the radius, and calculate the volume using the equation for the volume of a sphere:

$$V = 4/3\ \pi\ r^2$$

Volumes typically injected into blastomeres at different stages and their corresponding absolute diameters are: 0.5 nL = 100 μm; 1 nL = 127 μm; 2 nL = 165 μm; 5 nL = 214 μm; 10 nL = 268 μm.
9. Injecting too large volumes can affect the fate of frog blastomeres. At the 32-cell stage, the limit is approx 1 nL/blastomere. Larger blastomeres can receive proportionally more, and smaller blastomeres proportionally less.
10. While submerged, the needle should neither take up oil nor expel dye. If this occurs, there is a leak in the pressure system. Check the blunt end of injection needle. It must be even so that it rests flush against the gasket. If it is not, load a new needle, break the tip and recalibrate.
11. Traditionally, the light-colored side was termed dorsal and the dark-colored side ventral. Revisions in a modern fate map *(7)* assigned the rostral/caudal (or anterior/posterior) axis to the old dorsal/ventral axis.
12. De-jellying prior to the completion of the four-cell stage results in embryos undergoing unconventional D-tier cleavage.
13. Coat a fine glass wand (*see* **Note 3**) with Nile blue sulfate as follows. On a plastic or glass surface, mix 1 drop of 1% Nile blue sulfate with 1 drop of 100 m*M* Na_2CO_3. While observing in a dissecting microscope, stir the drops together with a fine glass wand. The Nile blue sulfate will turn a deep red and begin to precipitate. Catch chunks of precipitate on the wand and allow to air dry. Coat several wands as they can be kept for several days.
14. In some batches of embryos, cleavages are less synchronous than depicted in **Fig. 3**. At room temperature, cleavages occur roughly every 30 min, but often animal hemisphere blastomeres finish cleaving before vegetal hemisphere blastomeres, because they are significantly smaller. In these embryos, you will see 16 animal blastomeres (the A- and B-tiers), but for a brief period there will be only eight vegetal blastomeres (the C-and D-tiers have not yet separated by division). You can use these embryos by simply injecting the blastomere when it assumes its "conventional" appearance.

15. There should be neither extruded cytoplasm nor blebbing membrane at the site of injection. There will be a small dark spot, indicative of concentrated pigment at the site. This is a normal aspect of membrane healing. If cytoplasm leaks or membrane protrudes through the vitelline, the needle is too large. Change needles and break off a smaller tip.
16. Inject several different blastomeres every day that you map so that you can compare your results to previous results. Make four or more replicates of each injected blastomere in order to assess reproducibility. For comparison, use Fig. 5 in Dale and Slack's 1987 fate map, which depicts representative examples for each named blastomere at the 32-cell stage. Occasionally, there are batches of embryos in which, for one reason or another, the pigmentation difference observed at the four-cell stage did not correspond well with the embryonic axes. This is easy to determine if you have data for several blastomeres. For instance, the cement gland should not be labeled by blastomere C1 and the notochord should not be labeled by B4. If odd label is observed, discard that day's work.
17. Although circulating blood is easily distinguished in live embryos, it is difficult to unequivocally distinguish blood cells in dead specimens. In sectioned specimens, blood vessels tend to be small, and even in large vessels, it is difficult to clearly distinguish cells that once circulated from cells of the vessels, with the exception of the chambered heart. In intact embryos, the two easiest sites to view blood cells are the gill arches and tail, but depending on the distribution of label in other tissues, it is often difficult to distinguish blood cells at these sites. Fixed embryos should first be dehydrated in MeOH, preferably overnight with several changes, cleared in BB:BA and transferred to a well in a Sylgard slide. Embryos in alcohol or clearing reagent are extremely brittle and should be moved cautiously. They should be manipulated with tools (e.g., forceps, hair knives, or tungsten needles) that are used only with fixed specimens. Observe under epi-fluorescence to orient the embryo and add a coverslip before observing on a compound microscope.
18. Paraformaldehyde must be washed out of the embryos or you will observe high background fluorescence in the specimens. Handle the specimens in a manner consistent with future intentions. For instance, do not clear in BB:BA and view in epifluorescence prior to *in situ* hybridization, which requires that starting materials be RNAse-free. *In situ* hybridization will destroy much of the fluorescence, so if you need to visualize label after *in situ* hybridization, use a biotinylated dextran and stain for biotin with a streptavidin conjugate.

Acknowledgments

Our research is supported by grants from the Pew Charitable Trust, the Beckman Foundation, the James D. and Dorothy Shaw Fund of the Greater Milwaukee Foundation and the Howard Hughes Medical Institute.

References

1. Vodicka, M. A. and Gerhart, J. C. (1995) Blastomere derivation and domains of gene expression in the Spemann organizer of *Xenopus laevis*. *Development* **121,** 3505–3518.
2. Lane, M. C. and Sheets, M. D. (2002) Primitive and definitive blood share a common origin in *Xenopus*: a comparison of lineage techniques used to construct fate maps. *Dev. Biol.* **248,** 52–67.
3. Dale, L. and Slack, J. M. W. (1987) Fate map for the 32-cell stage of *Xenopus laevis*. *Development* **99,** 527–551.
4. Moody, S. A. (1987) Fates of the blastomeres of the 32-cell-stage *Xenopus embryo*. *Dev. Biol.* **122,** 300–319.

5. Lane, M. C. and Smith, W. C. (1999) The origins of primitive blood in *Xenopus*: implications for axial patterning. *Development* **126,** 423–434.
6. Kau, C.-L. and Turpen, J. B. (1983) Dual contribution of embryonic ventral blood island and dorsal lateral plate mesoderm during ontogeny of hematopoietic cells in *Xenopus laevis*. *J. Immunol.* **131,** 2262–2266.
7. Lane, M. C. and Sheets, M. D. (2000) Designation of the anterior/posterior axis in pregastrula *Xenopus laevis*. *Dev. Biol.* **225,** 37–58.

10

Analyses of Immune Responses to Ontogeny-Specific Antigens Using an Inbred Strain of *Xenopus laevis* (J Strain)

Yumi Izutsu and Mitsugu Maéno

Summary

In this chapter, the procedures for specific detection of ontogenic emerging antigens during animal development are described. Anuran metamorphosis has provided us with a good experimental model for investigation of the mechanisms of tissue remodeling. The establishment of a syngeneic strain of *Xenopus laevis* described in this chapter has enabled us to perform a unique experiment to develop antibodies that specifically react to ontogenic antigens by immunizing syngeneic animals. This strategy was successful because the antibody repertoires produced in the adult frog serum were well subtracted by a number of common antigens expressed in syngeneic larvae. Here we show, using results of immunohistochemical and T-cell proliferation analyses that adult frogs exhibit humoral and cell-mediated immune responses to larva- or metamorphosis-specific antigen molecules in epidermal cells.

Key Words: Larval antigens; epidermal cells; skin; metamorphosis; tissue remodeling; transformation; antiserum; antibodies; transplantation; skin graft; immunohistochemistry; T-cell proliferation; immunological recognition; *Xenopus laevis*; strain; immune system; larva; adult; ontogeny; subtraction.

1. Introduction

Metamorphosis of anuran amphibians involves morphological and functional tissue remodeling from larval to adult in various organs for adaptation from aquatic to terrestrial life. For instance, epidermal cells in the larval tail are completely resorbed at metamorphosis, and epidermal cells in the larval head are replaced by adult cells. Metamorphic changes also take place in the immune system. The larval immune system easily becomes tolerant to antigens. The immune system in the adult frog generates strong immune responses to various types of antigens comparable to those of the mammalian immune system. Therefore, we assumed that the adult-type immune system recognizes ontogenic antigens and takes part in the elimination of larval cells *(1)*. Experiments using a major histocompatibility complex-homozygous inbred strain of *Xenopus laevis* were conducted to verify this possibility. This unique strain, named J

From: *Methods in Molecular Medicine, Vol. 105: Developmental Hematopoiesis: Methods and Protocols.*
Edited by: M. H. Baron © Humana Press Inc., Totowa, NJ

strain ("J" for Japan), was established over a period of 30 yr by Drs. Tochinai and Katagiri at Hokkaido University *(2)*. Adult J strain animals are completely histocompatible and do not reject skin grafts from adult animals of the same strain, whereas we have demonstrated that young adults rejected skin grafts from syngeneic larvae *(1)*. The fact that an accelerated secondary response was induced after repeated skin grafts indicates that the rejection of the skin grafts occurred as a result of immunological responses. It has also been shown that these animals produced specific antibodies against larval skin antigens *(3)*. Therefore, the J strain provides us with a unique experimental system to identify development- or metamorphosis-specific tissue antigens. Here we describe the protocols for the transplantation technique and preparation of antiserum to examine immune responses to larva-specific antigens. We also describe the methods used for an adult T-cell proliferation assay to detect larval antigens.

2. Materials

2.1. Animals

The MHC-homozygous J strain of *Xenopus laevis* *(2,4)* was used. The J strain animals used are completely histocompatible, and no rejection of skin grafts occurs among the same strain of adult animals *(1)*. Larvae and adults were reared at 23 ± 1°C. Tadpoles were staged according to the Normal Table of Nieuwkoop and Faber *(5)*.

2.2. Reagents and Equipment

1. Gonadotropic hormones (Teikoku Zoki Co. Ltd., Tokyo, Japan).
2. Mashed green peas (Kagome Co. Ltd., Tokyo, Japan).
3. Fish meal (Oriental Yeast Co. Ltd., Tokyo, Japan).
4. MS222 (3-aminobenzoic acid ethyl ester, cat. no. A-5040, Sigma, St Louis, MO): 1% stock solution is stable for several months if stored in the dark at 4°C.
5. Steinberg's solution: (3.4 g/L NaCl, 0.05 g/L KCl, 0.08 g/L $Ca(NO_3)_2 4H_2O$, 0.1025 g/L $MgSO_4$, 0.56 g/L Tris-HCl, pH 7.5, 10 mg/L phenol red), 10X stock solution is stable for a few months at room temperature. The solution should be stored at 4°C after being supplemented with antibiotics.
6. Penicillin G and streptomycin sulfate mixture (100X solution, cat. no. Gibco 15240-062, Invitrogen Co., Carlsbad, CA).
7. 10-cm Petri dishes (Falcon35-3803, Becton Dickinson and Co., Franklin Lakes, NJ).
8. Forceps (0508-L5-PO, Natsume Seisakusho Co., Tokyo, Japan).
9. Scissors (Napox B-12H, Natsume Seisakusho Co).
10. 70% Ethanol.
11. Needled suture (cat. no. 5-O Nylon-blue color, Azwell, Osaka, Japan).
12. Cotton stick (Johnson and Johnson Co.).
13. 24-Gage needle (Terumo, Co., Tokyo, Japan).
14. 1-mL Syringe (Terumo, Co.).
15. 1.5-mL Centrifuge tube (Asahi Techno Glass Co., Tokyo, Japan).
16. 0.2-μm Pore filter (Millipore Japan, Tokyo, Japan).
17. OCT compound (cat. no. 4583, Sakura Seiki Co., Tokyo, Japan).
18. Tissue Tek (Plastic-Tissue-Tek cryomold, Cat. No. 4565, Miles Inc. Elkhart, IN).
19. Liquid nitrogen.
20. 50-mL Plastic tube (Falcon 35-2070, Becton Dickinson and Co.).
21. Precleaned slide glasses (cat. no. S-2445, Matsunami Glass Ind., Osaka, Japan).

22. Cryostat (Leica CM1850, Leica Instruments, Nussloch, Germany).
23. Dako Pen (Dako Co., Kyoto, Japan).
24. Fetal calf serum (FCS; Gibco, Invitrogen Co.).
25. Phosphate-buffered saline (PBS): 8 g/L NaCl, 0.2 g/L KCl, 1.15 g/L Na_2HPO_4, 0.2 g/L KH_2PO_4, pH 7.2.
26. Bovine serum albumin (BSA; Fraction V, cat. no. A-3311, Sigma).
27. NaN_3 (Wako Pure Chem. Ind., Osaka, Japan).
28. Monoclonal antibody 11D5 (a mouse anti-Xenopus IgY [IgG analog], ***(6)***).
29. Cy3-conjugated secondary antibodies against mouse Ig (cat. no. AP130C, Chemicon International, Temecula, CA).
30. Quinacrine dihydrochloride (cat. no. Q-3251, Sigma).
31. MacIlivain solution: 3.81 g/L citric acid, 23.24 g/L Na_2HPO_4, pH 7.
32. Sucrose (cat. no. 196-00015, Wako Pure Chem. Ind.).
33. Fluorescent microscope (BX51, Olympus Co., Japan).
34. Laminar flow hood.
35. L-15 Medium (Leibovitz's L-15 medium, cat. no. Gibco 11415-064, Invitrogen Co.). The medium mixed with supplements is freshly prepared and store at 4°C.
36. 7.5% $NaHCO_3$ (7.5% sodium bicarbonate solution, cat. no. Gibco 25080-094, Invitrogen Co.).
37. 1 *M* HEPES (cat. no. Gibco 15630-080, Invitrogen Co.).
38. Razor blade (Ophthalmic blade 21BZ0082, Feather Safety Razor Co., Japan).
39. Glass Petri dish (Iwaki glass dish, Asahi Techno Glass Co., Tokyo, Japan).
40. 96-Well U plate culture dish (Falcon cat. no. 35-3077, Becton Dickinson and Co.).
41. 35-mm Plastic petri dishes (Falcon35-3801, Becton Dickinson and Co.).
42. Rubber policeman (cat. no. 125-50-69-21, Tokyo Garasu Kiki Co., Tokyo, Japan).
43. Cell strainer (Falcon 35-2350, Becton Dickinson and Co.).
44. Plastic pipets (5 mL; Falcon 35-7543, Becton Dickinson and Co.).
45. 15-mL Plastic tubes (Falcon 35-2096, Becton Dickinson and Co.).
46. Hemocytometer.
47. 28°C CO_2 Incubator (Benchtop low-temperature CO_2 incubator, 9100, Wakenyaku Co., Kyoto, Japan).
48. 5% CO_2/95% air gas cylinder.
49. 5-Bromo-2'-deoxyuridine (BrdU; cat. no. B-5002, Sigma). The stock solution should be freshly prepared.
50. Pipetman (Gilson Co., USA).
51. Methanol (stored at 4°C).
52. 2 N HCl (mixture of 100 mL of conc. HCl and 465 mL of distilled water).
53. Borate-buffered solution (pH 8.5): prepared by mixing approx 850 mL of 0.2 *M* boric acid and 700 mL of 0.05 *M* sodium borate to make a solution of pH 8.5. This solution is stable for at least one year if stored at room temperature).
54. Anti-BrdU mouse monoclonal antibody (cat. no. 8003; Sanbio, Netherlands).

All reagents should be sterilized prior to use and stored at 4°C.

3. Methods

The following methods outline 1) the operation of transplantation using the J strain of *Xenopus laevis*, 2) preparation of antiserum from immunized adult frogs, 3) immunohistochemistry using antisera, and 4) the proliferation assay for adult T-cells to detect ontogenic antigens.

3.1. Transplantation of Larval Skin Tissues Into Adults

1. Obtain fertilized eggs after ovulation and mating induced by gonadotropic hormones.
2. Rear the larvae at 24 ± 1°C. Feed the tadpoles mashed green peas and commercial fish meal. For tadpoles after stage 58, when the forelimbs have begun to develop, feed fish meal only (same for froglets). Grind the fish meal into small pieces using a food mixer.
3. Keep the adult frogs unfed in clean dechlorinated tap water for 1–2 d before use (*see* **Note 1**).
4. Gently wash the tadpoles (stage 56/57) and 1- to 2-yr-old female frogs with deionized water 10 times.
5. Anesthetize the animals by immersing them in MS222 solution, 0.01% (for tadpoles) or 0.05% (for adults) in sterile Steinberg's solution containing 100 IU/mL penicillin G and 100 μg/mL streptomycin sulfate. The duration of anesthesia should not exceed 10 min for larvae and 30 min for adults. All treatments should be done aseptically.
6. Cut the tails from the tadpoles using forceps and scissors that have been sterilized with 70% ethanol, and transfer the tails into a 10-cm Petri dish containing ice-cold Steinberg's solution supplemented with antibiotics.
7. Isolate skin tissues from five tails in the Petri dish under a dissecting microscope. Keep the Petri dish on ice.
8. Transfer a host frog into the 10-cm Petri dish, pinch a grafting point of the dorsal skin of the frog with forceps, and make a slit of approx 5 mm in width with scissors.
9. Immediately insert the pieces of tail skins through the slit into the subcutaneous space.
10. Sew up the slit at one or two points using needled suture (*see* **Note 2**).
11. Maintain the hosts in Steinberg's solution containing antibiotics for 2–3 d without feeding. The solution should be changed every day. Then rear the animals in clean dechlorinated tap water as mentioned previously (*see* **Notes 3** and **4**).
12. Repeat grafting three times at one-month intervals into different sites of the dorsal skin of host animals.

3.2. Preparation of Antiserum

Antisera are obtained from 1- to-2-yr-old frogs (female) that have received repeated tadpole tissue grafts or injections of larval cells (*see* **Note 2**) three times.

1. One month after the final skin grafting, anesthetize the immunized animals in 0.05% MS222 in Steinberg's solution for 10–20 min.
2. Place each animal on its back in a 10-cm Petri dish with a sheet of clean Kim wipe. Keep the Petri dish on ice. Carefully dissect off a small area of skin around the heart and remove muscle layers to expose the heart. Use a cotton stick to pull up the heart without injury. Then tear off the thin integument membrane of the heart with fine forceps as shown in **Fig. 1**.
3. Pierce the point of the ventricle of the heart directly with a 24-gage needle and a 1-mL syringe and collect clean blood. Pull little by little in accordance with beats of the heart. About 1 to 1.5 mL of blood is usually collected from one adult J strain frog (*see* **Note 5**).
4. Transfer the blood into a 1.5-mL centrifuge tube and keep it over night at 4°C.
5. Centrifuge the tubes at 1000*g* for 15 min at 4°C and transfer the supernatant into a new tube. Spin the supernatant one more time to avoid contamination of the serum by the cell pellet.
6. Incubate the serum at 56°C for 30 min for inactivation of complements. If it is necessary, sterilize the serum by filtration through a 0.2-μm pore filter and then dispense aliquots into 1.5-mL centrifuge tubes and store them at –80°C until use (*see* **Notes 6** and **7**).

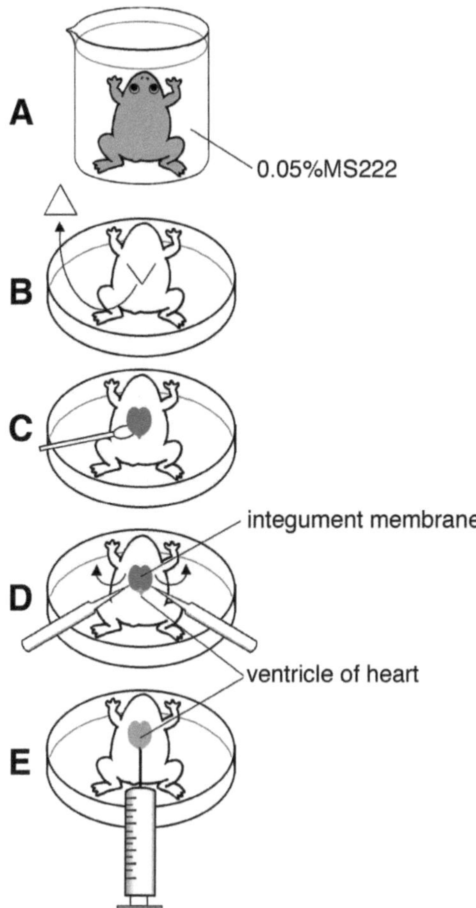

Fig. 1. Flow chart diagrams of bleeding procedure. **(A)** Anesthetize the immunized animals in MS222 solution for 10 to 20 min. **(B)** Place each animal on its back in a 10-cm Petri dish and then dissect off a small area of skin around the heart. **(C)** Pull up the heart using a cotton stick. **(D)** Tear off the thin integument membrane of the heart with fine forceps by pulling on both sides. **(E)** Pierce the point of the ventricle of the heart directly with a needle and syringe.

3.3. Detection of Antibodies by Immunohistochemistry

To estimate the titer of antiserum, we usually employ an immunohistochemical assay *(3,7)*.

1. Anesthetize animals in MS222 solution for 5 to 10 min.
2. Immediately dissect skin tissues, including both the tail and dorsal trunk junction regions, from tadpoles at stage 63, using forceps and scissors.
3. Transfer the tissues into OCT compound in plastic Tissue-Tek specimen molds after one-time wash with a sufficient amount of OCT compound.

4. After gently orientating the tissues with forceps, dip each specimen very slowly into liquid nitrogen. Store the mounted tissues in a 50-mL plastic tube at –80°C until use (*see* **Note 8**).
5. Prepare 4-μm thick frozen sections using a cryostat, transfer sections to precleaned glass slides (*see* **Note 9**), dry them by air blowing for 30 min at room temperature, and store dried, without fixation, in an airtight container at 4°C until use (within 1–2 wk).
6. Using a Dako Pen, trace a circle around the sectioned tissues and dry the slides by air blowing for 5 to 10 min at room temperature.
7. Apply 50 to 100 μL of 10% FCS in PBS to the sections, and incubate the slides for 30 min in a moist chamber at room temperature for blocking.
8. Wipe off the blocking solution, and apply 50 to 100 μL of 10-fold diluted frog serum in 0.1% BSA in PBS with 0.01% NaN_3 onto the sections. Then incubate the slides for 12 h at 4°C in a moist chamber.
9. Wash the sections gently with PBS three times for 5 min each at room temperature.
10. Wipe off the remaining PBS and apply 50 to 100 μL of 200-fold diluted monoclonal antibody 11D5 (a mouse anti-*Xenopus* IgY [IgG analog], *[6]*) in PBS with 0.1% BSA and 0.01% NaN_3 onto each section. Then incubate the slides for 2 h at room temperature in a moist chamber.
11. Wash the sections gently with PBS three times for 5 min each at room temperature.
12. Wipe off the remaining PBS and apply 50 to 100 mL of Cy3-conjugated secondary antibodies against mouse Ig at a 300 to 600-fold dilution in PBS with 0.1% BSA and 0.01% NaN3 onto the sections. Then, incubate the slides for 30 min to 1 h at room temperature in a moist chamber in the dark.
13. Wash the sections gently with PBS for 5 min at room temperature three times.
14. Counterstain the tissues with 0.025% quinacrine dihydrochloride for 8 min and gently wash the slides with distilled water for 4 min by changing the water five to six times. Then, immerse the slides in McIlivein solution for a few minutes.
15. Cover the sections with saturated sucrose solution (*see* **Note 10**).
16. Observe the sections under a fluorescent microscope (*see* **Note 11**).

3.4. T-Cell Proliferation Assay

The T-cells show proliferative responses when they meet "nonself" targets in vitro. We have demonstrated that adult splenocytes were able to proliferate if the larva-specific antigens were added to the culture *(2,8,9)*. We also found that co-culture of adult T-cells with larval tissues, with larval cells, with synthetic peptides derived from larval proteins and even with recombinant products of larval proteins resulted in specific proliferation of adult T-cells. This assay is therefore a powerful tool for detecting ontogenic antigens.

3.4.1. Preparing Larval Skin Tissues for Co-Culture With Adult Splenocytes

1. Feed the larvae every day and keep them at low density in dechlorinated tap water (approx 10 tadpoles in 3 to 4 L of water) for a few days before use. Change the water every day.
2. Wash the tadpoles (stage 56/57) gently with deionized water 10 times.
3. Anesthetize the tadpoles in 0.01% MS222 in Steinberg's solution for 5 min.
4. Pick up each tadpole using forceps and wash the tadpole by pouring ice-cold sterilized distilled water from a water bottle in a laminar flow hood. Dissect the tails from the tadpoles with scissors and transfer the tails to a 10-cm Petri dish containing ice-cold 70%

L-15 medium supplemented with 10 m*M* $NaHCO_3$, 10 m*M* HEPES, 100 IU/mL penicillin G and 100 µg/mL streptomycin sulfate. Keep the Petri dish on ice. After this step, perform all manipulations of the tissues or cells aseptically in a laminar flow hood.

5. Transfer up to 10 tail pieces to a 50-mL tube containing 30 mL of ice-cold 70% L-15 medium (*see* **Note 12**). Keep the tubes on ice for a few seconds. Wait for the tails to settle down to the bottom of the tube.
6. Discard more than half of the supernatant and transfer the tails together with the remaining medium to a 10-cm Petri dish. Then place the tails in 30 mL of ice-cold 70% L-15 medium in a new tube. Wash the tails five times with 70% L-15 medium as same.
7. After washing, the Petri dish containing the tails in 70% L-15 medium should be kept on ice. Excise approx 2 × 2 mm^2 square tissues from the ventral tail fin in a glass Petri dish with a fine blade under a dissecting microscope (*see* **Note 13**).
8. Transfer the tail fin tip to a 96-well U-bottom culture dish containing 100 µL of 60% L-15 medium supplemented with 10% FCS, 10 m*M* $NaHCO_3$, 10 m*M* HEPES, 100 U/mL penicillin G, and 100 µg/mL streptomycin sulfate. FCS is heat-inactivated at 56°C for 30 min before use. Let the tail fin tip settle down to the bottom of each well (*see* **Note 14**).

3.4.2. Preparing Adult Splenocytes

1. Keep 1 to 2-yr-old adult frogs (female) unfed in clean dechlorinated tap water for 3 to 4 d before use. Change the water every day.
2. Anesthetize the frogs in 0.05% MS222 solution.
3. Aseptically remove the spleen from each frog and place in a 35-mm plastic Petri dish containing 70% L-15 medium with antibiotics. Trim any contaminating tissues off the spleen and discard them. Keep the dish on ice during the operation.
4. Wash the spleens in 70% ethanol for 5 s and immediately transfer to 70% L-15 medium. Then wash the spleens three times with 70% L-15 medium in 35-mm plastic Petri dishes.
5. Mash the spleen using a rubber policeman on a cell strainer. While mashing the spleen, occasionally drop ice-cold 70% L-15 medium until most of the isolated cells have fallen to the bottom of a 50-mL plastic tube. Keep the 50-mL tube on ice during the operation.
6. Disrupt any cell clumps by gentle pipetting using a 5-mL plastic pipet. Transfer the cells to a new 15-mL plastic tube.
7. Centrifuge at 400*g* for 10 min at 4°C.
8. Carefully remove the supernatant from the sediment and re-suspend in an appropriate volume (6–8 mL) of 70% L-15 medium by gentle pipetting (*see* **Note 15**).
9. Count the cells using a hemocytometer and prepare a cell suspension at a concentration of 5 × 10^5 splenocytes/100 µL of 60% L-15 medium supplemented with 10% FCS, 10 m*M* $NaHCO_3$, 10 m*M* HEPES, 100 IU/mL penicillin G, and 100 µ/mL streptomycin sulfate. Gently add 100 µL of cell suspension into the cultured fin tissues in a 96-well culture dish.
10. Maintain the culture at 28°C in an incubator humidified atmosphere supplemented with 5% CO_2. Do not exchange the medium during the course of culture until the splenocytes have been harvested.

3.4.3. Harvest

1. Label cells in S phase with 500 µ*M* BrdU for 24 h. Add 20 µL of 10 times stock solution of BrdU to the culture wells 24 h before harvest.
2. Put the culture dish on ice immediately after incubation, resuspend the cultured splenocytes by gentle pipetting, and collect the splenocytes into a 1.5-mL centrifuge tube.

3. Centrifuge at 400g for 10 min at 4°C. Discard the supernatant, and gently resuspend the pellet in 20 μL of ice-cold 70% L-15 medium using a Pipetman.
4. Add 1 mL of ice-cold absolute methanol to the tube, and immediately resuspend the cells thoroughly, 10 to 20 times.
5. Centrifuge at 400g for 10 min at 4°C. Discard the supernatant and suspend the pellet in 20 μL of absolute methanol, and then drop an approx one-third volume of cell suspension on a pre-cleaned slide glass. Fix and then quickly air-dry the smeared cells. Store under a dry condition at 4°C until use (within 1 mo; *see* **Note 16**).

3.4.4. Immunohistochemical Detection of BrdU-Incorporated Cells

1. Treat the smear with 2 N HCl for 30 min at room temperature.
2. Immerse in borate-buffered solution (pH 8.5) twice for 10 min each for neutralization.
3. Apply 50 to 100 μL of 10% FCS in PBS onto the smeared cells, and incubate the cells for 30 min in a moist chamber at room temperature for blocking.
4. Wipe off the blocking solution, and add 50 to 100 μL of 20-fold diluted anti-BrdU mouse monoclonal antibody for 2 h at room temperature or for 12 h at 4°C in a moist chamber.
5. Wash the slide glass with PBS three times for 5 min each at room temperature.
6. Wipe off the remaining PBS, and add 50 to 100 μL of Cy3-conjugated secondary antibodies against mouse Ig at 600-fold dilution in 0.1% BSA in PBS with 0.01% NaN_3 onto the slide. Then incubate for 30 min to 1 h at room temperature in a moist chamber in the dark.
7. Wash the slide with PBS three times for 5 min each at room temperature.
8. After washing, counterstain the cells with 0.025% quinacrine dihydrochloride, and then immerse the slides in McIlivein solution for a few minutes.
9. Cover the smeared cells with a saturated sucrose solution.
10. Examine specimens under a fluorescent microscope. A total of 1000 to 1500 cells should be counted in five to six randomly selected areas of individual specimens prepared from each of the responder splenocytes, which are labeled with a randomized number to avoid possible anticipation. Proliferative responses are represented as percentages of the total number of leukocytes, as shown in the example of **Fig. 2**. Values are means ± SDs obtained from four different experiments.

4. Notes

1. If the animals are fed, they sometimes vomit during the operation.
2. If cells are used as an immunogen instead of tissues, inject the cell suspension (approx 2×10^7 cells) directly through the ventral skin into the peritoneal space.
3. If necessary, histologically examine the tissues excised from the transplanted sites of donor frogs.
4. If the grafted animals are not kept in a clean condition, mold sometimes grows in the wound.
5. If serum is collected from the heart using a needle and a syringe, clear serum can be obtained because red corpuscles seldom break.
6. The titer of frog antiserum will drop after freezing and thawing. Therefore, the minimum volume for an assay (10–50 μL) should be aliquotted into each tube.
7. At least one in two animals produced a high-titer antiserum without non-specific staining.
8. Frozen tissues in OCT compound are stable for at least 1 yr if stored at –80°C. The 50-mL plastic tube should be capped firmly to avoid drying.
9. If necessary, use a commercial silane-coated slide glass.
10. To prepare saturated sucrose, dissolve approx 3 M sucrose solution in hot distilled water in a water bath. Keep the stock solution with 0.1% NaN_3 at room temperature. The stock solution is stable for at least 1 yr.

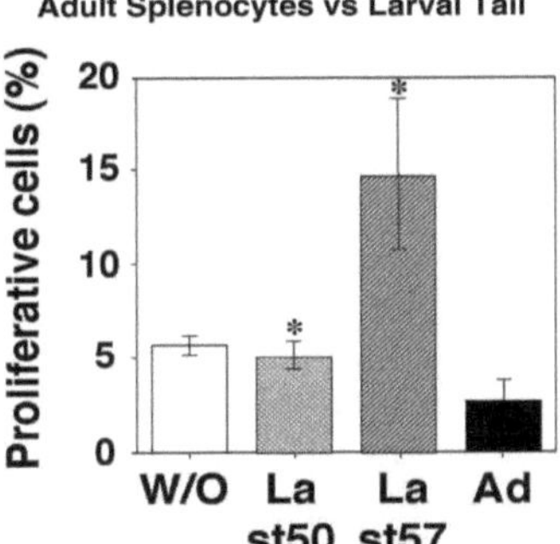

Fig. 2. Specific proliferative response of adult splenocytes. Adult splenocytes were cultured for 5 d with larval tail tissues of stage 50 tadpoles (La st50, hatched column) when the larval antigen was not detected by anti-LS frog antiserum or stage 57 tadpoles (La st57, striped column) expressing the larval antigen at the maximum level (7) or with adult skins (Ad, closed column), or without stimulators (W/O, open column). Larval tissues were prepared from the tail fin, and adult skins were excised from the backs of 2 to 3-mo-old froglets. Proliferative responses are shown as percentages to the total numbers of leukocytes. Values represent means ± SDs obtained from four different experiments. Asterisks at the top of columns indicate a statistically significant difference.

11. Keep the stained sections in the dark at 4°C. Sections are stable for at least 1 wk without decay.
12. In this step, ice-cold Steinberg's solution can be used instead of L-15 medium.
13. Precleaned slide glasses can be used instead of glass Petri dishes. They should be sterilized in an autoclave.
14. If isolated epidermal cells are used as a target instead of tail tip tissues, seed 1.2×10^5 cells/100 µL into a 96-well U bottom culture plate (9).
15. The spleen of a 1- to 2-yr-old frog contains approx 2–3 × 10^7 leukocytes.
16. Before preparing a smear slide, make a circle with a Dako Pen to allow the cells to spread.

Acknowledgments

We thank Mr. Kouki Fujiwara at Niigata University for helping with the preparation of the manuscript.

References

1. Izutsu, Y. and Yoshizato, K. (1993) Metamorphosis-dependent recognition of larval skin as non-self by inbred adult frogs (*Xenopus laevis*). *J. Exp. Zool.* **266,** 163–167.
2. Tochinai, S. and Katagiri, C. (1975) Complete abrogation of immune response to skin allografts and rabbit erythrocytes in the early thymectomized *Xenopus Dev. Growth Differ.* **17,** 383–394.
3. Izutsu, Y., Tochinai, S., Maéno, M., Iwabuchi, K., and Onoé, K. (2002) Larval antigen molecules recognized by adult Immune cells of Inbred *Xenopus laevis*; partial characterization and implication in metamorphosis. *Dev. Growth Differ.* **44,** 477–488.
4. Nakamura, T., Kawahara, H., and Katagiri, C. (1985) Rapid production of a histocompatible colony of *Xenopus laevis* by gynogenetic procedure. *Zool. Sci.* **2,** 71–79.

5. Nieuwkoop, P. D. and Faber, J. (1956) *Normal table of* Xenopus laevis *(Daudin)*, North-Holland, Amsterdam, pp. 162–203.
6. Hsu, E., and Du Pasquier, L. (1984) Studies on *Xenopus* immunoglobulins using monoclonal antibodies. *Mol. Immunol.* **21,** 257–270.
7. Watanabe, M., Ohshima, M., Morohashi, M., Maéno, M., and Izutsu, Y. (2003) Ontogenic emergence and localization of larval skin antigen molecule recognized by adult T cells of *Xenopus laevis*: its regulation by thyroid hormone during metamorphosis. *Dev. Growth Differ.* **45,** 77–84.
8. Izutsu, Y., Yoshizato, K., and Tochinai, S. (1996) Adult-type splenocytes of *Xenopus* induce apoptosis of histocompatible larval tail cells in vitro. *Differentiation* **60,** 277–286.
9. Izutsu, Y., Tochinai, S., Iwabuchi, K., and Onoé, K. (2000) Larval antigen molecules recognized by adult immune cells of inbred *Xenopus laevis*; two pathways for recognition by adult splenic T cells. *Dev. Biol.* **221,** 365–374.

11

Use of Flow Cytometry and Combined DNA Surface Staining for Analysis of Hematopoietic Development in the *Xenopus* Embryo

James B. Turpen

Summary

Xenopus embryos provide a model for studying the earliest stages in the development of the vertebrate hematopoietic system. This chapter provides detailed procedures describing the production of hematopoietic chimeras in *Xenopus* embryos and the analysis of these chimeras using flow cytometry. Protocols for analysis include the determination of deoxyribonucleic acid content of hematopoietic cells, staining of cells with antibodies against cell surface antigens and the combined analysis of deoxyribonucleic content and cell surface phenotype. Examples of data that can be expected are included.

Key Words: *Xenopus*; hematopoiesis; flow cytometry; DNA analysis; blood; embryonic; chimera.

1. Introduction

Understanding the development and differentiation of hematopoietic stem cells presents several unique challenges because of the association of hematopoietic cells with the developing vascular system. Once circulation has been established in the embryo, any developmental relationship between the presence of hematopoietic cells at a particular anatomical site and the origin of hematopoietic cells at that site becomes blurred. Nevertheless, it is now well established that hematopoietic organs such as the liver, bone marrow, spleen and thymus are colonized by hematopoietic stem cells, or lineage restricted stem cells, that originate extrinsically to these organs ***(1,2)***. Moreover, once hematopoiesis or lymphopoiesis is established and the organism develops and matures, the frequency of the most primitive stem cells within a particular organ diminishes as the proliferative and amplification potential of the hematopoietic system is realized ***(3,4)***.

The amphibian embryo provides a useful model to examine the earliest events of hematopoiesis, events that take place prior to the initiation of circulation and the amplification of the committed hematopoietic progenitors ***(5,6)***. The large size of these

From: *Methods in Molecular Medicine, Vol. 105: Developmental Hematopoiesis: Methods and Protocols.*
Edited by: M. H. Baron © Humana Press Inc., Totowa, NJ

embryos, their availability at all developmental stages, and the reliable production of a permanent cytogenetic marker make it possible to identify, isolate, and experimentally manipulate hematopoietic stem cells prior to circulation. In my laboratory, we have taken advantage of these unique developmental features and combined them with flow cytometry in order to analyze the earliest stages of hematopoiesis. This approach can continue to provide insight into the complex process of hematopoiesis. Several basic protocols will be described in this chapter. These protocols will enable interested investigators and students to conduct experiments starting with the construction of embryonic chimeras and carrying through to final analysis using flow cytometry.

2. Materials

2.1. Animals

Adult male and female outbred *Xenopus laevis* (*see* **Note 1**).

2.2. Solutions

1. 10X Amphibian phosphate-buffered saline (10X APBS): dissolve 60 g of NaCl, 2 g of KCl, 3.8 g of KH_2PO_4, and 11.5 g of Na_2HPO_4 in dd H_2O in a 1-L volumetric flask. Sterile filter and store at room temperature (*see* **Note 2**). Dilute this solution 1:10 for use with adult cells. The pH of the 1X solution should be 7.3 to 7.4 without any further adjustment and the osmolarity of the 1X solution should be 220 mOs. Adjust the osmolarity to 200 mOs for use with larval cells. (90 mL of APBS plus 10 mL of ddH_2O).
2. DeBoer's solution (DBS): dissolve 6.42 g of NaCl, 0.96 g of KCl, and 0.588 g of $CaCl_2$-$2H_2O$ in approx 800 mL of ddH_2O. Adjust to pH 7.2 using a 1 *M* solution of $NaHCO_3$. Bring final volume to 1 L, sterile filter (*see* **Note 2**), and store at room temperature. DBS is diluted to either 5% or 10% (v/v) as necessary.
3. Modified Ringers (MMR): dissolve 58.44 g of NaCl, 1.49 g of KCl, 2.46 g of $MgSO_4 \cdot 7H_2O$, 2.94 g of $CaCl_2$, 11.92 g of HEPES buffer and 0.37 g of ethylenediamine tetraacetic acid in 1 L of ddH_2O. pH should be 7.6. Sterile filter (*see* **Note 2**) and store at room temperature.
4. Anesthetic: dissolve 0.02 g of ethyl-m-aminobenzoate methanesulfonate in 100 mL of dechlorinated tap water, 0.1X APBS, or 0.1X MMR. Place larvae in solution and observe for loss of swimming behavior. A higher concentration of anesthetic is advisable (e.g., 0.2 g/100 mL) for euthanasia of adult males.
5. Deionized bovine serum albumin (BSA): dissolve 20 g of BSA (Bovine Albumin Fraction V, Sigma Chemical Co; cat. no. A-4503) in 100 mL of double-distilled H_2O (*see* **Note 3**). Deionized by incubating overnight at 4°C with 2 g of an ion exchange resin (e.g., Amberlite, Serva Feinbiochemica). Provide gentle stirring during this incubation. Dialyze the deionized BSA against 1X APBS for 24 h at 4°C with at least three changes of 1X APBS. Determine the final protein concentration, sterile filter the solution (*see* **Note 4**), aliquot to 15-mL tubes, and store at 4°C.
6. APBS plus BSA (APBS/BSA): add 2.5 mL of 20% BSA to 97.5 mL of APBS to yield a final solution of 0.5% BSA. Sterile filter and store at 4°C.
7. Vindelov's reagent *(7)*: this reagent MUST be prepared in a plastic vessel. Dissolve 0.21 g of Tris-8-hydroxymethylaminomethane (Trizma-base) and 0.29 g of NaCl in 400 mL of ddH_2O. Titrate pH to 7.6 using 1 *N* HCl and bring final volume to 500 mL. Add 700 Kunitz U/L RNAase (Sigma; cat. no. R-5000), 0.0375 g of propidium iodide and 0.5 mL of

Nonidet P-40 or a NP40 substitute, such as Imbentin-N/52 (Sigma; cat. no. 74385). Sterile filter this reagent into another plastic container and store at 4°C. Reagent lasts for 8 to 10 wk.

8. Hoechst 33342 for DNA staining: dissolve Hoechst 33342 (Molecular Probes) in APBS containing 0.625% NP40 to a final concentration of 10 μg/mL.
9. 3% Cysteine: dissolve 30 g of cysteine in 1 L of 0.1X MMR. Add 7.5 g of NaOH, pH should be 7.6. Adjust pH with additional pellets of NaOH if necessary. This solution should be prepared immediately prior to use and discarded after 1 to 2 h.
10. Heparin: add 100 IU heparin to 10 mL of APBS/BSA. Sterile filter and store at 4°C.
11. Primary and secondary antibodies: specific antibodies will depend on the investigator's experimental design. The examples presented in this chapter are based on the use of a primary antibody directed against a common leukocyte antigen (CD45 homologue) found on the surface of *Xenopus* hematopoietic cells.

2.3. Microsurgical Instruments and Supplies

1. Dissecting microscope and a cold light source.
2. Microdissection tools (*see* **Note 5**): watchmaker's forceps (Dumoxel no. 5); extra fine iris scissors; surgical blades (Bard-Parker no. 11); surgical blade handles; glass needle holders: use insect pin holders (Fine Science Tools, cat. no. 26018-17, 26016-12, or 26015-11 according to user preference); glass cover slips, (22 × 22 mm, no. 1 thickness; *see* **Note 6**); Micropipet puller (Kopf Model 750, www.kopfinstruments.com); and glass rods (1 mm o.d. Drummond Scientific Company, www.drummondsci.com).
3. Black agar operating dishes: add 10 g of animal bone black (*see* **Note 7**) to 450 mL of 10% DeBoer's solution in a 1-L beaker. Bring suspension to a gentle boil with constant stirring. Add 9 g of agar, stir gently until all agar is dissolved. Cover the beaker with a sterile mesh (a nylon stocking works well) and pour the black agar into 60-mm plastic Petri dishes. Fill each dish approximately half full. The surface of the agar should not contain any air bubbles. After cooling, store dishes at 4°C.

3. Methods

3.1. Embryos

Sibling embryos from outbred matings of *Xenopus laevis* can be used in all experiments.

1. Induce ovulation by injection of 50 IU human chorionic gonadotropin (HCG, *see* **Note 8**) 72 h prior to the time when ovulation is desired, followed by the injection of 400 IU HCG 8 h prior to ovulation.
2. Terminally anesthetize male frogs in ethyl-m-aminobenzoate methanesulfonate. Open the abdominal cavity, remove the testes, and place in 100% DeBoer's solution (1X DBS). Place testes between the frosted ends of two glass microscope slides and apply gentle pressure with a circular motion until the capsule is ruptured and the organs are flattened. Rinse the sperm into a 15 mL of test tube using 1X DBS. Sperm suspensions are kept on ice and are usable for at least 4 to 6 h.
3. Express eggs into 60-mm plastic Petri dishes. If triploid embryos are to be produced, express another aliquot of eggs into a separate 60-mm Petri dish.
4. Add five drops of sperm suspension sperm directly to the egg mass using a Pasteur pipet. Activate the sperm by adding a 20 fold excess of 5% DBS (e.g., five drops of sperm to 100 drops 5% DBS).

3.2. Triploid Embryos (8)

1. The night before the anticipated fertilization, place 1 L of 10% DBS at 4°C. It is advisable to use a 2-L glass beaker as a container for the DBS. Approximately 1 h prior to fertilization, place the beaker containing the chilled 10% DBS in an ice bucket and pack crushed ice around the outside of the beaker. The temperature should be approx 2°C at the start of the procedure.
2. Twelve minutes after fertilization, immerse the Petri dish containing the zygotes in the chilled 10% DBS for 15 min. At the end of the cold shock, gently rinse the zygotes in room temperature DBS and set aside for further development.
3. Maintain diploid and triploid embryos at 20°C until gastrulation. Gastrula and subsequent staged embryos can be maintained in controlled temperature incubators at 13, 16, and 18°C.
4. Raise control and experimental larvae in aquaria at a density of one larva per three liters of conditioned or dechlorinated H_2O (*see* **Note 9**). Feed with suspensions of Tetra Conditioning Food (fish food for herbivorous species) as required. Larvae should be maintained in environmental rooms at 21°C with a 12-h light cycle. Embryos and larvae are staged according to Nieuwkoop and Faber *(9)*.

3.3. Microsurgery

One of the advantages of using *Xenopus* embryos is that cytogenetically labeled hematopoietic stem cells can be introduced into developing embryos prior to the initiation of circulation *(10)*. Hematopoietic populations derived from these labeled stem cells can then be recovered and analyzed for DNA content and surface phenotype using a variety of approaches. The easiest region of the embryo to manipulate is the ventral blood island, located within the ventral abdominal region of the postgastrulae embryo (**Fig. 1**). The preferable developmental stages for manipulating these embryos are between Niewkoop and Faber stages 15 and 22. All microsurgical procedures require the use of a dissecting microscope and cold light source.

1. Remove jelly coats by placing eggs in approx 300 mL of 3% cysteine (*see* **Note 10**). Gently swirl for 2 min, pour off solution, replace with a second aliquot of cysteine, and swirl for an additional 2 min. Pour off and replace with a third aliquot of cysteine and swirl for 1 min. Rinse with at least five, large volume changes (250 mL) of 0.1X MMR. Remove vitelline membranes in sterile 100% DBS using watchmaker's forceps. Hold a pair of forceps in each hand, grasp the membranes with the tips of the forceps and tear the membrane open as if you were tearing a piece of paper in half.
2. Fill a black agar dish with 100% DBS containing 10% Pen/Strep. Prepare two depressions in the agar by cutting embryo-sized rectangles in the surface of the agar using Bard-Parker a surgical blade no. 11. Place a diploid donor and a triploid host embryo in these depressions in black agar lined operating dishes.
3. Excise ectoderm and underlying VBI mesoderm from a diploid-donor embryo using fine glass needles (**Fig. 1**). The thin ectoderm is highly pigmented, the thicker mesoderm is lightly pigmented and the endoderm is composed of very large, unpigmented cells. Use fine motor control similar to that used for sketching with pencil.
4. Outline and remove a similar sized area from a stage matched triploid host. Transfer the diploid tissue to the triploid hose and hold the graft in place with small pieces of glass coverslips. Healing should be complete in about 30 min.

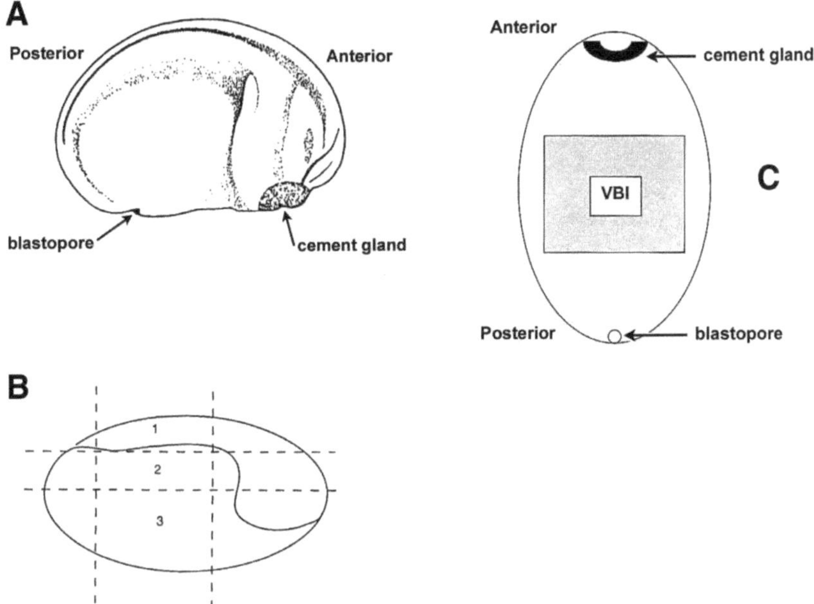

Fig. 1. Diagrammatic representation of the late neurula (stage 18–22) embryo. **(A)** Lateral view showing major landmarks including the cement gland and blastopore. **(B)** Line drawing showing a lateral view of the major hematopoietic compartments. Area indicated by no. 2 is the region of the dorsal lateral plate, the amphibian equivalent of the aortic–gonad–mesonephros region of the mammalian embryo. Area indicated by no. 3 is the ventral blood island (VBI). **(C)** Line drawing showing a ventral view of the VBI. This is the area that is excised and transplanted to construct a hematopoietic chimera as described in this protocol.

5. Transfer embryos to either 0.1X MMR (or dechlorinated tap water) containing 10% antibiotics. Embryos should be removed from antibiotics after control embryos hatch (NF stage 35).
6. Rear embryos to analysis in 0.1X MMR or dechlorinated tap water.

3.4. Cell Harvesting

All procedures involved in cell harvesting are best performed with the aid of a dissecting microscope.

1. Anesthetize larvae with ethyl-m-aminobenzoate methanesulfonate.
2. Collect larval erythrocytes from the ventral aorta (**Fig. 2A,B**). Place larvae ventral side up on a small piece of paper towel or filter paper. Using fine scissors, prepare a "V" shaped incision through the skin in the cardiac region. Retract the flap of skin and flood the cardiac area with APBS/BSA containing 10 IU/mL heparin. Sever one branch of the ventral aorta and immediately place a heparinized microcapillary tube in the path of the blood flow. Keep the microcapillary tube in place with one hand and gently irrigate the area with additional APBS/BSA/Heparin. Transfer aspirated cells to polystyrene tubes (12 × 75) containing 1–2 mL of fresh APBS/BSA and store at 4°C.

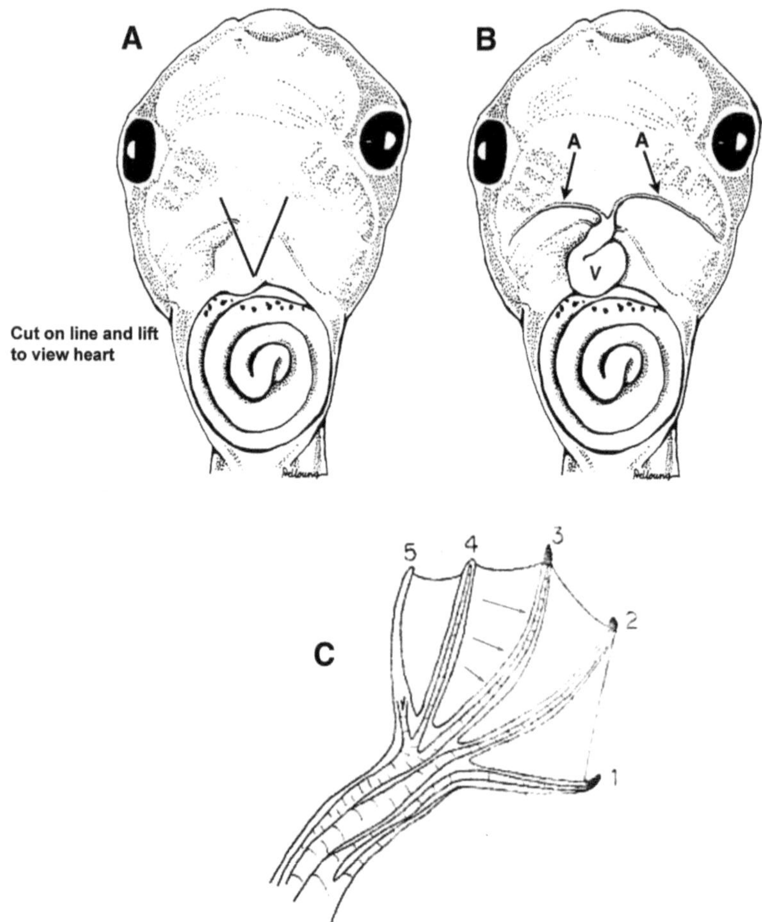

Fig. 2. Exposure of the ventral aorta and tarsal vein for collection of blood samples. **(A)** Ventral view of a larva. The lines indicate the region that should be cut and retracted to expose the heart. **(B)** Ventral view after exposure of the cardiac area. A, ventral aorta; V, ventricle. Only sever one of the ventral aortas. **(C)** View of the foot of an adult *Xenopus*. A large vein runs along each digit. The veins associated with digits 3 and 4 are easiest to expose and sever.

3. Collect adult erythrocytes from one of the tarsal veins lying along the digits of the hind foot (**Fig. 2C**). Prepare a small incision through the overlying skin using a sharp scalpel blade, exposing the underlying vessel. Sever the vessel and irrigate the region with APBS/BSA/Heparin. Collect blood cells using heparinized microcapillary tubes and transfer these cells to polystyrene tubes (12 × 75) containing 1 to 2 mL of APBS/BSA.
4. Bilateral thymic lobes or individual spleens can also be easily analyzed. The thymus is easily recognizable as a darkly pigmented organ located on dorsal surface of the head, posterior to the eye.

a. Make an incision through the transparent skin and retract this tissue to expose the underlying thymus.
b. Remove the thymus by cutting through the surrounding gill tissue using fine scissors. Include some gill tissue as a means of holding on to the thymus during subsequent manipulations.
c. The spleen is a small, red, oval-shaped organ located in the mesentery of the abdominal cavity near the junction of the duodenum and the stomach. Place the larvae ventral side up. Open the abdominal cavity using fine scissors. The spleen can be removed by grasping the surrounding mesentery with forceps. Use fine scissors to cut through the mesentery and free the spleen.
d. Once the organs are dissected, use watchmaker's forceps to transfer them to depression slides containing 0.4 mL of APBS/BSA.
e. Dissociate cells by disrupting the capsule and gentle teasing of the tissue with watchmaker's forceps. Remove any large clumps of remaining tissue such as remnants of gill or mesentery. Transfer cell suspensions to 12 × 75 tube containing 1 mL of APBS/BSA.
f. Wash all cell suspensions in a tabletop centrifuge at 500 rpm for 5 min. Resuspend in 1 mL of APBS/BSA and stored at 4°C.

3.5. DNA Staining (10)

Staining with Vindelov's reagent provides a quick and convenient method for determining the DNA content of cells harvested from either circulation or from individual hematopoietic organs such as the thymus or the spleen.

1. Wash cells in APBS/BSA. Resuspend cell pellet in 0.5 mL of Vindelov's reagent by gentle pipetting or vortexing. Incubate cell suspension from 10 min to 2 h.
2. Analyze cells using a flow cytometer. Excitation wavelength should be at 488 n*M* and emissions collected through a 630/20-bp filter. Acquire data using a linear scale. Use adult erythrocytes as a DNA standard. These cells provide a reference for diploid, non-synthetic cells. Typical DNA profiles are shown in **Fig. 3**.

3.6. Surface Staining (11)

1. Harvest cells from either circulation or specific hematopoietic organs. Wash in APBS/BSA containing 0.05% sodium azide (ABA). Carry out all staining reactions and washings at 4°C.
2. Resuspend cells in 0.1 mL of ABA. Incubate cells in the appropriate dilution (*see* **Note 11**) of the primary antibody for 45 min to 1 h at 4°C. Wash cells 2X in ABA. All experiments should include the use of an isotype control antibody in place of the primary antibody.
3. Incubate with secondary antibody conjugated to a fluorochrome such as fluorescein isothiocyanate for 30 min. Wash cells 2X at 4°C. Directly labeled antibodies can also be used to allow for multicolor analyses.
4. Flow cytometer configurations will depend on the fluorochrome being used. Acquire data using a log amplified scale. **Figure 4** shows a typical one-color fluorescence profile.

3.7. Combined Surface/DNA Staining

We have used two approaches for combined DNA and surface staining *(12,13)*. The difference in the approaches is based on differences in the emission spectra of the dye used for DNA staining and the range of fluorochromes that can be used for surface staining.

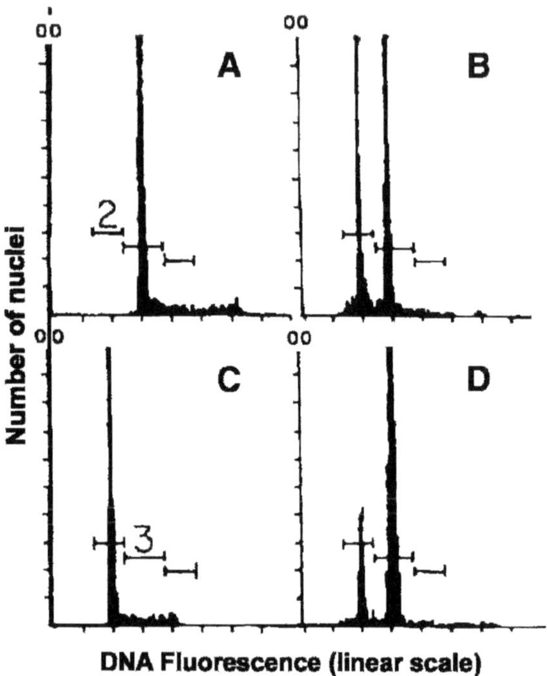

Fig. 3. Typical cytogram showing the results of staining with Vindelov's reagent. Fluorescence intensity is shown on the x-axis and the number of events is shown on the y-axis. Triploid and diploid control samples are shown in **(A)** and **(C)**. Examples of mixed populations found in hematopoietic chimeras are shown in **(B)** and **(D)**. (Modified from data published in **ref. *10*.**)

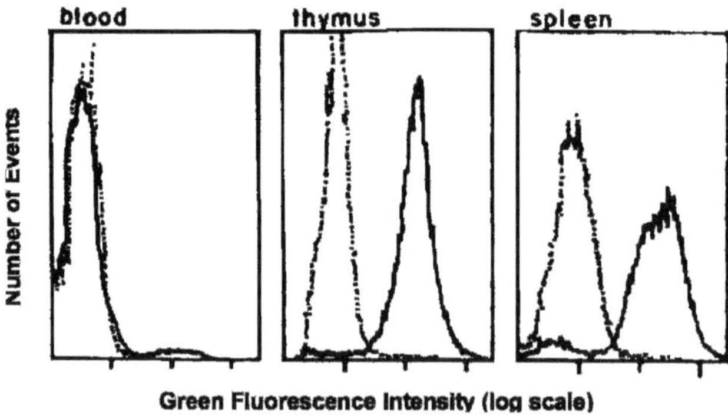

Fig. 4. Single-color fluorescence using a single primary antibody. These examples show fluorescence patterns when the monoclonal antibody CL21 was used to stain the blood, thymus and spleen. CL21 recognizes a CD45 homolog that is present of all white blood cells but is absent from erythrocytes. The dotted lines represent fluorescence patterns when the cells were stained using an isotype control in place of CL21. (Modified from data published in **ref. *11*.**)

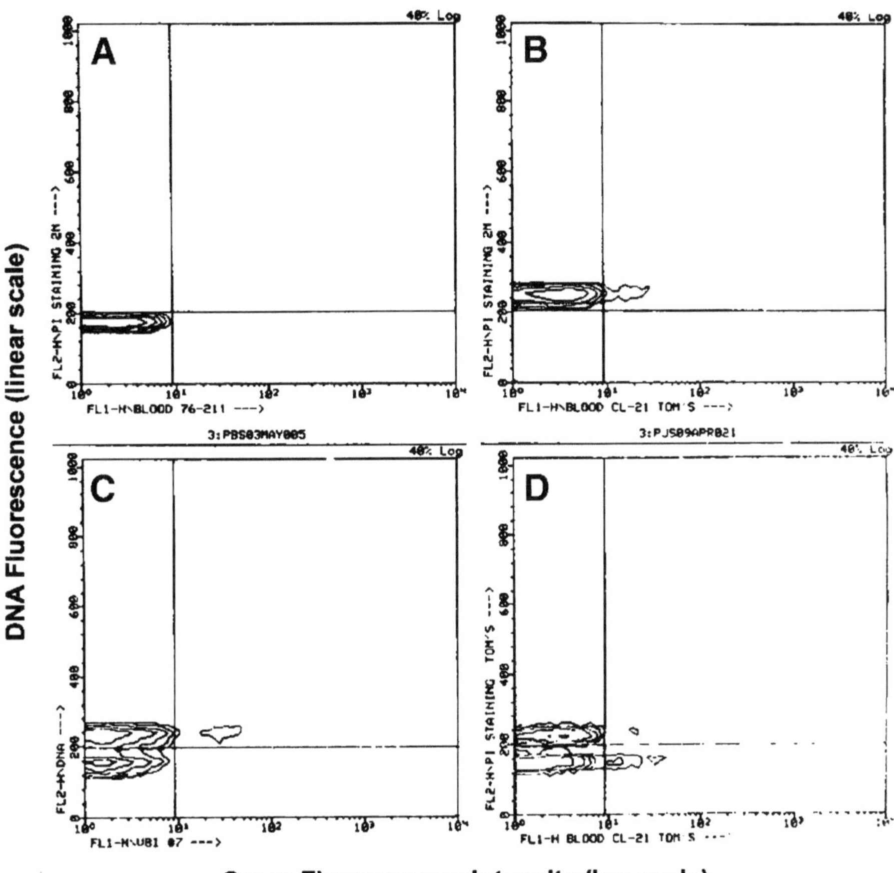

Fig. 5. Combined DNA and surface staining using Vindelov's reagent. DNA staining is shown on the *y*-axis and surface staining is shown on the *x*-axis. **(A)** Diploid cells harvested from larval circulation were stained with the isotype control antibody. **(B)** Triploid cells harvested from circulation and stained with the monoclonal antibody CL21. **(C,D)** Circulating cells from hematopoietic chimeras stained with CL21. These examples show that a small population in circulation stains with the antibody. (Modified from data published in **ref. *12*.**)

3.7.1. Surface Staining Combined With Vindlov's Reagent (12)

1. Collect cells and stain with specific antibodies using the protocol (*see* **Note 12**) described in **Subheading 3.6.**
2. Resuspend cells in 0.75 mL of APBS and add 0.25 mL of 2% paraformaldehyde drop wise with constant gentle agitation using a vortex. Cell handling at this step of the procedure is critical. Incubate the cells for 1 h at 4°C.
3. Wash cells in APBS/BSA, and resuspend in Vindelov's reagent. Incubate for at least 30 min.
4. Analyze cells using an excitation of 488 nm and emission filters of 525/30 bp (green, log scale) and 630/20 bp (red, linear scale). A typical cytogram is shown in **Fig. 5**.

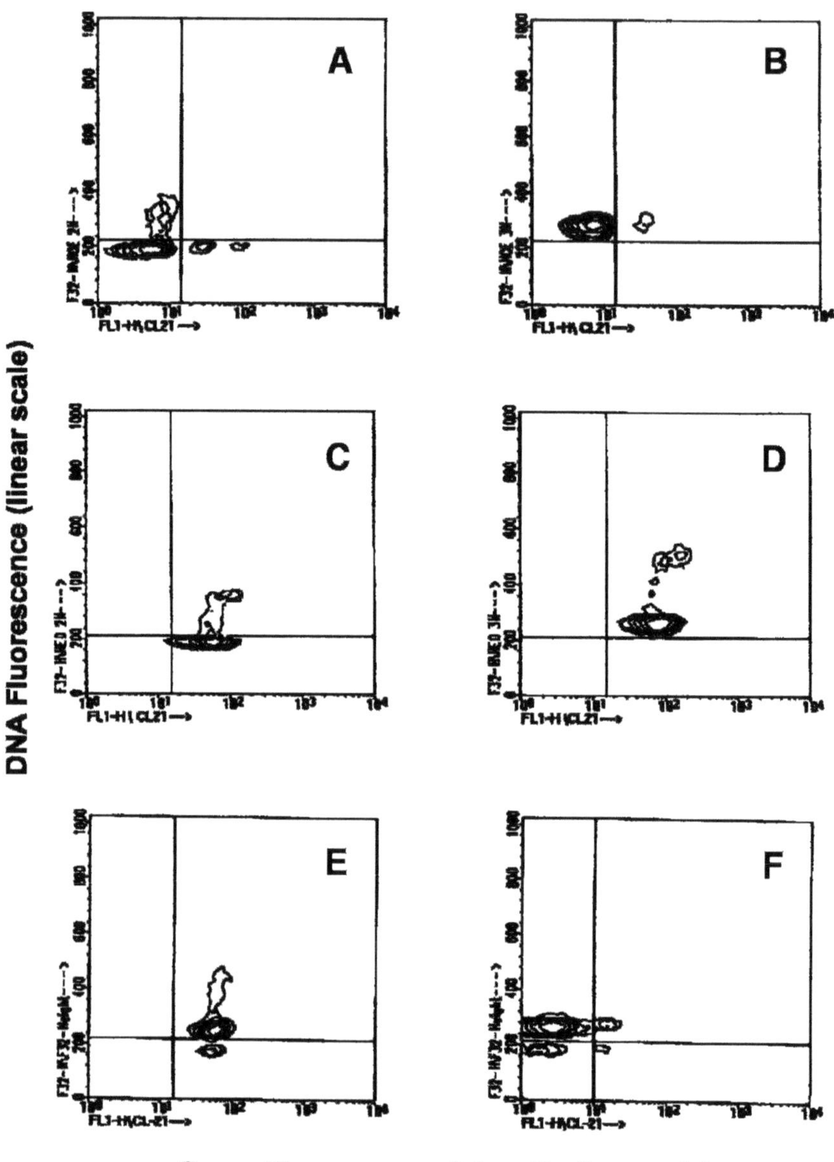

Fig. 6. Combined DNA and surface staining using Hoechst 33342. DNA staining is shown on the *y*-axis and surface staining on the *x*-axis. (**A**) and (**B**) Control diploid and triploid cells from peripheral blood contain a small population of CL21 positive leukocytes. (**C,D**) Control diploid and triploid cells from thymus are all CL21 positive. (**E**) Both diploid and triploid thymocytes from a hematopoietic chimera are positives for CL21. (**F**) Diploid and triploid cells from the peripheral blood of a hematopoietic chimera contain both CL21 positive and CL21 negative populations. (Modified from data published in **ref. *13***).

3.7.2. Surface Staining Combined With Hoechst 33342 ***(13)***

1. Collect and surface stain cells.
2. Resuspend cells in 0.5 mL of APBS/BSA. Gently add 0.5 mL of 4% paraformaldehyde dropwise. Incubate cells overnight at 4°C.
3. Add 110 mL of 10 mg/mL Hoechst 33342 with 0.625% NP40 to each fixed cell suspension, (final concentrations will be 1 μg/mL Hoechst and 0.0625% NP40). Incubate overnight at 4°C.
4. Analyze cell suspensions using a dual laser flow cytometer. Examine surface staining using excitation and detection wavelengths appropriate for the fluorochromes being used (e.g., 488 nm excitation and detection at 525 nm and 577 nm for green and red, respectively). Examine DNA content with a second, UV laser with excitation at 360 nm and emission detected at 485 nm. Acquire these data using a linear scale. A typical cytogram is shown in **Fig. 6**.

4. Notes

1. It is preferable to use proven breeders that can be purchased from several commercial suppliers. We have found NASCO (www.enasco.com/prod/Home) and XENOPUS I (www.xenopusone.com/) to be reliable sources.
2. Salt solutions that do not contain protein can be autoclaved.
3. This is best accomplished by sprinkling the BSA on top of the H_2O, letting the protein slowly enter solution without stirring. This can require 2 to 3 h.
4. Filtration of 20% BSA is slow but can be speeded up by pre-filtering with large pore sized membranes.
5. Fine Science Tools (www.finescience.com) provides a wide variety of microdissection instruments.
6. Glass cover slips are washed in 70% EtOH, air dried, and broken into small pieces for use with the embryos.
7. Do not use Norit or activated charcoal.
8. Sigma Chemical, St. Louis, MO, is one source of HCG. If access to a university pharmacy is available, an injectable solution prepared for human use works well.
9. Water quality will vary depending on the municipal water supply. Depending on the municipality, some tap water can be successfully treated by adding dechlorination drops available at local pet stores.
10. It is best to wait until after first cleavage before dejellying embryos.
11. Optimal dilution for each specific antibody must be determined experimentally. If the primary antibody is in a culture supernatant, the supernatant should be adjusted to amphibian osmolarity and then used without further dilution. If the source of a primary antibody is an ascites, a series of dilutions should be tested. For most of our ascites, dilutions of 1:800 have been used. Concentrations of secondary antibody are usually 2 to 20 μg/mL.
12. When using this protocol, it is preferable to use a secondary antibody that is conjugated to fluorescein isothiocyanate, providing a green signal for surface staining and a red signal for DNA. This approach limits the investigator to the use of a single antibody for surface staining. If directly conjugated primary antibodies are available, their use can expand the number of surface molecules that can be analyzed in conjunction with Vindelov's reagent.

References

1. Boggs, S. S. (1999) The hematopoietic microenvironment: phylogeny and ontogeny of the hematopoietic microenvironment. *Hematology* **4,** 31–44.

2. Galloway, J. L. and Zon L. I. (2003) Ontogeny of hematopoiesis: examining the emergence of hematopoietic cells in the vertebrate embryo. *Curr. Top Dev. Biol.* **53,** 139–158.
3. Cumano, A. and Godin, I. (2001) Pluripotent hematopoietic stem cell development during embrygenesis. *Immunology* **13,** 166–171.
4. Godin, I. and Cumnao, A. (2002) The hare and the tortoise: an embryonic haematopoietic race. *Immunology* **2,** 593–604.
5. Turpen, J. B. (1998) Induction and early development of the hematopoietic and immune systems in *Xenopus. Dev. Comp. Immunol.* **2,** 265–278.
6. Turpen, J. B., Kelley, C. M., Mead, P. E., and Zon, L. I. (1997) Bipotential primitive-definitive hematopoietic progenitors in the vertebrate embryo. *Immunity* **7,** 325–334.
7. Vindelov, L. L. (1977) Flow microflurometric analysis of nuclear DNA in cells from solid tumors and cell suspensions. *Virchows Arch. B.* **24,** 227–242.
8. Kawahara, H. (1978) Production of triploid and gynogenetic diploid *Xenopus* by cold treatment. *Dev. Growth Differ.* **20,** 227–236.
9. Nieuwkoop, P. D. and Faber, J. (1994) *Normal Table of Xenopus Laevis (Daudin)*, Garland Publishing, New York, NY, London, UK.
10. Smith, P. B., Flajnik, M. F., and Turpen J. B. (1989) Experimental analysis of ventral blood island hematopoiesis in *Xenopus* embryonic chimeras. *Dev. Biol.* **131,** 302–312.
11. Smith, P. B. and Turpen, J. B. (1991) Expression of a leukocyte-specific antigen during ontogeny in *Xenopus laevis. Dev. Immunol.* **1,** 295–307.
12. Bechtold T. E., Smith P. B., and Turpen, J. B. (1992) Differential stem cell contributions to thymocyte succession during development of *Xenopus laevis. J. Immunol.* **148,** 2975–2982.
13. Chen, X. and Turpen, J. B. (1995) Intraembryonic origin of hepatic hematopoiesis in *Xenopus laevis. J. Immunol.* **154,** 2557–2567.

12

Analysis of Hematopoietic Development in the Zebrafish

Noëlle N. Paffett-Lugassy and Leonard I. Zon

Summary

The zebrafish (*Danio rerio*) has emerged as a powerful vertebrate genetic and developmental model that is particularly amenable to the study of hematopoiesis. The zebrafish embryo develops externally and its optical clarity allows the number and morphology of circulating blood cells to be visualized using a dissecting microscope. Both the morphology of the blood lineages and the expression of critical blood genes are highly conserved between zebrafish and mammals. The high fecundity and short generation time of zebrafish facilitate genetic analysis, and a number of large-scale mutagenesis screens have identified mutations in genes affecting blood development. The discovery of novel hematopoietic genes, as well as the cloning of zebrafish homologs of known hematopoietic genes, necessitates the use of efficacious and reliable methods for complete gene characterization. In this chapter, we illustrate frequently used techniques that are essential for evaluating hematopoiesis in the zebrafish, including whole-mount *in situ* hybridization, the detection of erythrocytes by *o*-dianisidine staining, and a description of the microinjection procedure, which has various applications, including overexpression of messenger ribonucleic acid, gene 'knockdown' by antisense technology, and the creation of transgenic zebrafish. Also included is an explanation of the use of flow cytometry to separate hematopoietic lineages from the adult kidney and to isolate relatively pure populations of cell types from transgenic embryos based on the expression of fluorescent markers.

Key Words: Zebrafish hematopoiesis; zebrafish blood mutants; whole-mount *in situ* hybridization; *o*-dianisidine staining; microinjection; morpholino-mediated knockdown; zebrafish transgenics; hematopoietic lineage separation.

1. Introduction

Zebrafish have characteristics typically restricted to invertebrate model systems, such as small size, large number of progeny, and short generation time. The rapid and synchronous development of the embryos and larvae facilitates phenotypic analysis and large-scale experimental approaches, while the transparency, accessibility and robustness of the zebrafish embryos make them well suited to micromanipulation and

From: *Methods in Molecular Medicine, Vol. 105: Developmental Hematopoiesis: Methods and Protocols.*
Edited by: M. H. Baron © Humana Press Inc., Totowa, NJ

in vivo observation. Overall, the zebrafish is an attractive system for studying vertebrate hematopoiesis *(1–7)*. One of the advantages of using the zebrafish lies in the ability to easily modulate gene expression in vivo by microinjection of nucleic acids. Furthermore, gene function can be rapidly assayed by the microinjection of antisense morpholino nucleotide analogues that specifically block messenger ribonucleic acid (mRNA) translation of the target or alter transcriptional processing *(8,9)*. The results of these manipulations are most commonly evaluated by examining alterations in gene expression by whole-mount *in situ* hybridization (WISH) and by assessing blood levels with *o*-dianisidine staining. In addition to these more traditional approaches, the use of transgenic technology is on the rise and is most frequently used to generate fish that express a fluorescent reporter under the regulatory elements of blood specific genes. In addition, recent advancements in our laboratory have surprisingly revealed that adult zebrafish blood can be separated into distinct populations by light scatter characteristics, thus enabling purification of erythroid, myeloid, lymphoid, and precursor lineages without relying on antibodies.

1.1. Zebrafish Hematopoiesis

As in other vertebrates, the formation of hematopoietic cells in zebrafish proceeds in successive waves of primitive and definitive steps that occur in distinct anatomical sites. Primitive blood cells originate from bilateral stripes in the posterior lateral plate mesoderm and migrate medially to form the intermediate cell mass, which contains both vascular and hematopoietic precursors and is the zebrafish equivalent to the mammalian yolk sac blood islands *(10–12)*. Primitive erythroid cells migrate from the intermediate cell mass along the tail to enter circulation in a path over the yolk sac concomitant with the onset of heart contractions at 24 hpf *(11)*. Embryonic circulation comprises of primitive erythroblasts, which express embryonic globins, macrophages, and neutrophils *(12–15)*. As development progresses, there is a transition to definitive hematopoiesis, which is evident by the appearance of hematopoietic cells in the kidney primordium (the mammalian bone marrow equivalent) as early as d 4 of development. Definitive hematopoiesis in the adult zebrafish produces cells of the erythroid, myeloid, lymphoid, and megakaryocytic lineages; these cells arise primarily from hematopoietic tissue in the kidney *(12)* and morphologically resemble their mammalian counterparts with the exceptions that erythrocytes remain nucleated and thrombocytes perform the clotting functions of platelets *(16–18)*.

1.2. WISH

Zebrafish orthologs of genes required for both primitive and definitive hematopoiesis, including *scl*, *lmo2*, *gata 1-3*, *c-myb*, *runx-1*, *pu.1*, *ikaros*, *rag*, and *globins*, have been isolated and are functionally analogous to their mammalian equivalents (R. A. Wingert and L. I. Zon, submitted). The expression of these genes and others has been used to ascertain the sites of hematopoiesis during ontogeny by WISH. WISH is an inexpensive, rapid, and robust technique frequently used by zebrafish researchers to examine the temporal and spatial localization of blood genes in wild-type, mutant, or genetically altered zebrafish embryos. This method involves the preparation of an epitope-tagged RNA probe complementary to the gene of interest, which is then hybridized to the embryo and subsequently visualized using an antibody conjugated to a fluorophore or chromogenic enzyme. There are various ways to non-radioactively label and detect antisense RNA probes, though digoxigenin or fluorescein are frequently used to label the probes, and an alkaline phosphatase-conjugated antibody is often used to visualize the hybridized probe by creating a colored, insoluble precipitate *(19)*. The small size of the zebrafish embryos enables hybridization and detection in the whole mount, facilitating three-dimensional analysis of transcript expression.

1.3. Staining Erythroid Cells With O-Dianisidine

It is often of interest to ascertain whether an alteration in gene expression, by nucleic acid injection or in a mutant embryo, has an effect on the level of circulating erythrocytes. Erythroid levels can be readily evaluated using *o*-dianisidine staining in which hemoglobin catalyzes the oxidation of *o*-dianisidine by hydrogen peroxide. Living embryos are incubated in a solution containing *o*-dianisidine and hydrogen peroxide, resulting in the formation of a rust-colored precipitate specifically in erythroid cells.

1.4. Overexpression of mRNA, Gene Knockdown by Morpholino, and Creation of Transgenics

The bulk of our understanding of hematopoiesis in the zebrafish is a result of evaluating novel genes and zebrafish homologs of known blood genes by overexpression analysis, knockdown studies and, more recently, the direct observation of hematopoietic cells in fluorescent transgenic lines. The introduction of nucleic acids and nucleic acid analogues is achieved by microinjection, which remains the fastest and most efficient means to modulate gene expression. The applications of mRNA overexpression and morpholino-mediated loss-of-function experiments in wild-type and mutant embryos are enumerable and are a necessity for studying hematopoiesis in the zebrafish embryo. The increasing number of hematopoietic mutants that have been isolated provide yet another requirement for the introduction of nucleic acids as it is important to be able to rescue mutant phenotypes by mRNA or candidate complimentary deoxyribonucleic acid (cDNA) injection. Furthermore, the introduction and expression of recombinant DNA constructs enables transient protein expression during development and the production of transgenic lines that express a particular construct in subsequent generations. Transgene constructs that express markers such as green fluorescent protein (GFP) under the control of tissue-specific enhancers facilitate the identification of distinct cell types in vivo and also can be used to identify *cis*-acting sequences and trans-activating factors that regulate tissue-specific expression. Recent developments in the creation of quickly folding and brightly fluorescent proteins has led to the production of various transgenic zebrafish lines, some with fluorescent markers under the control of different regulatory elements, enabling both a direct observation of hematopoiesis during development, as well as the ability to isolate relatively pure cell populations by flow cytometry. Given the lack of reagents for isolating distinct blood populations in the zebrafish, this transgenic technology provides an invaluable tool for studying embryonic and adult hematopoiesis. The ability to cross mutant lines to transgenics maintaining expression of fluorescent markers in blood greatly facilitates the analysis of hematopoiesis in a given mutant and is becoming routine.

1.5. Purification of Hematopoietic Cells by Flow Cytometry

One of the limitations in the zebrafish hematopoietic field has been the lack of reagents for purifying cell populations. Recent developments in our laboratory have addressed this deficiency and have led to the discovery that adult blood lineages can be isolated to relative purity on the basis of light scatter characteristics alone. Flow cytometry is also invaluable for sorting fluorescently labeled cells from adult and embryonic transgenic zebrafish.

The aim of this chapter is to describe methods frequently used in our laboratory to study hematopoiesis in the zebrafish. Both *in situ* hybridization and microinjection of zebrafish embryos have been previously illustrated but this chapter will cover recent advances in these standard protocols. Also included is a description of the morpholino knockdown technique, the methods used in the creation of transgenic zebrafish lines, and the isolation of hematopoietic cells from adult kidneys and transgenic zebrafish by flow cytometry.

The Zebrafish International Resource Center is an invaluable source of information *(20)* and can be accessed on the Internet at www.zfin.org. For excellent reference books, consult *The Zebrafish Book: A Guide for the Laboratory Use of the Zebrafish (Danio rerio)* and *Zebrafish* in the Practical Approach Textbook Series *(21,22)*.

2. Materials

2.1. General Embryo Preparation

1. E3 embryo medium: 5 m*M* NaCl, 0.17 m*M* KCl, 0.33 m*M* $CaCl_2$, 0.33 m*M* $MgSO_4$, 10^{-5}% Methylene blue (Sigma; *see* **Note 1**).
2. Methylene blue: 1000X stock; store at 4°C or room temperature.
3. Glass vials: i.e., 5.5 mL (Fisher).
4. Pipets: glass pulled and plastic pipets for transferring embryos.
5. Embryo manipulator: wire/loop holder with 24-gage wire; an eyelash or fine loop of nylon immobilized on a pipet tip with Parafilm works well for delicate embryos.
6. Watchmaker's forceps (Roboz, Dumont).
7. Incubator (28.5°C).

2.2. WISH

2.2.1. Embryo Dechorionation and Fixation

1. Phosphate-buffered saline (PBS): 0.14 *M* NaCl, 0.003 *M* KCl, 0.002 *M* KH_2PO_4, 0.01 *M* Na_2HPO_4, pH 7.2.
2. Paraformaldehyde (PFA): 4% PFA in PBS. PFA is extremely toxic, use gloves, prepare in fume hood and handle with care (*see* **Note 2**).
3. Watchmaker's forceps with fine, sharp point.
4. Pronase: 50 mg/mL in E3, store at –20°C.

2.2.2. Embryo Pigment Removal

1. 1-Phenyl-2-thiourea (PTU): 0.2 m*M* in E3. PTU is toxic; use gloves and prepare in fume hood, store at room temperature. PTU is stable for 2 wk.
2. Bleach solution: 0.8% KOH, 0.9% H_2O_2, 0.1% Tween-20 in deionized H_2O, prepared fresh.

2.2.3. Hybridization and Detection

2.2.3.1. Rehydration and Permeability Enhancement

1. Water bath or hybridization oven (60–70°C).
2. PBST: 1X PBS plus 0.1% Tween-20.
3. 50% Methanol (MeOH)/PBST.
4. Proteinase K (Boehringer Mannheim): 10 µg/mL in PBST, store in aliquots at –20°C.
5. 4% PFA (**Subheading 2.2.1.**).

2.2.3.2. Hybridization

1. Heparin: 100 mg/mL in sterile deionized H_2O; store in aliquots at –20°C.
2. Yeast tRNA: 50 mg/mL in sterile deionized H_2O. The yeast tRNA should be cleaned thoroughly by phenol-chloroform extraction prior to use, store in aliquots at –20°C (Sigma).
3. Deionized formamide: formamide is toxic and should be handled with care; store in aliquots at –20°C.
4. Saline sodium citrate (SSC): 20X: 3 *M* NaCl, 300 m*M* trisodium citrate, pH 6.0.
5. SSCT: 1X SSC plus 0.1% Tween-20.
6. HYB^-: 50% formamide, 5X SSC, 0.1% Tween-20, 9.2 m*M* citric acid, pH 6.0; store at 4°C.
7. HYB^+: 50% formamide, 5X SSC, 0.1% Tween-20, 9.2 m*M* citric acid, pH 6.0, 500 µg/mL yeast tRNA, 50 µg/mL heparin; store at 4°C.
8. Probe: dilute 1 µL of probe (**Subheading 2.2.5.**) in 100 µL of HYB^+; can be used up to five times. Store at –20°C.

2.2.3.3. Probe Removal and Detection

1. Maelic acid buffer (MAB): 100 m*M* maleic acid, 150 m*M* NaCl, pH 7.5.
2. MABT: 1X MAB with 0.1% Tween-20.
3. Blocking buffer: MABT with 2% blocking reagent (Roche) or 2% bovine serum albumin and 2% heat inactivated fetal calf serum.
4. Anti-digoxigenin or anti-fluorescein alkaline phosphatase (AP) Fab fragments (Roche).
5. Staining Buffer: 100 m*M* Tris-HCl, pH 9.5, 50 m*M* $MgCl_2$, 100 m*M* NaCl, 0.1% Tween-20, prepared fresh (*see* **Notes 3** and **4**).

2.2.3.4. Chromogenic Substrates

1. 4-Nitroblue tetrazolium chloride (NBT): NBT is toxic. Prepare 75 mg/mL in 70% dimethylformamide Store at –20°C (Boehringer Mannheim).
2. 5-Bromo-4-chloro-3-indolyl-phosphate or X-phosphate 4-toluidine salt (BCIP): BCIP is toxic. Prepare 50 mg/mL in dimethylformamide; store at –20°C (Boehringer Mannheim).
3. Staining buffer with NBT and BCIP: add 135 µL of NBT and 105 µL of BCIP to 30 mL of staining buffer (*see* **Note 5**).

2.2.4. Double WISH

In addition to the materials for **Subheading 2.2.3.**, include the following items:

1. AP inactivation buffer: 100 m*M* glycine-hydrochloride, 0.1% Tween-20, pH 2.2.
2. Fast Red tablets: each tablet contains 0.5 mg of naphthol substrate, 2 mg of Fast Red chromogen, and 0.4 mg of levamisole; wear gloves and handle tablets with forceps. Dissolve one tablet in 2 mL of 100 m*M* Tris-HCl, pH 8.2, and use within 30 min. Store tablets at –20°C (Boehringer Mannheim or Sigma).
3. Vector Red: mix stock solutions immediately before use as described in kit; store at 4°C (Vector Labs).

2.2.5. Probe Generation

1. Template cDNA in an appropriate transcription vector (i.e., pBluescript, or pCS2$^+$) containing RNA polymerase promoter sequence (T3, T7, or SP6) at both ends.
2. Linearize template at a suitable site (polylinker at 5' end for antisense), purify by phenol-chloroform extraction and ethanol precipitation. Polymerase chain reaction (PCR) fragments containing RNA polymerase promoter sequences can also act as templates for transcription and should be purified by gel electrophoresis prior to transcription.
3. DIG or fluorescein RNA labeling kit (Roche) including: DIG-11-UTP NTP or fluorescein-12-UTP NTP Mix, 5X Transcription buffer, SP6/T3/T7 polymerase, RNase inhibitor, RNase-free DNase, RNase-DNase-free dH_2O.

2.3. Hemoglobin Staining With O-Dianisidine

1. 2,3-Diphosphoglyceric acid fast blue B, free base (*o*-dianisidine), i.e., Sigma.
2. *O*-dianisidine solution: dissolve 100 mg of *o*-dianisidine in 70 mL of 100% ethanol. This solution is light sensitive and will generally last for 4 to 8 wk at 4°C in the dark. The solution is still fully functional after it turns a brownish–yellow color, but do not use if the solution forms a considerable amount of precipitate.
3. Sodium acetate (NaOAc): 0.1 *M* NaOAc, pH 4.5.
4. Hydrogen peroxide (H_2O_2): 30% solution.

2.4. Observation and Photography

1. Watchmaker's forceps with fine point (Roboz or Dumont).
2. Glycerol 30%, 60%, 90% in PBST.
3. Glass slides.
4. Glass cover slips 22 × 22 mm.
5. Modeling clay.
6. Microscope: to take advantage of the optical transparency of zebrafish transgenics, we advise investing in microscopy equipment that will enable clear observation and accurate depiction in still photographs or movies. We have had good success using an inverted Leica with a Hamamatsu camera and Open Lab software.

2.5. Microinjection

A typical setup includes a dissecting microscope, a micromanipulator immobilized by a magnetic clamp and a pneumatic microinjector, complete with air compressor. Microinjection needles are pulled using a needle/pipet puller and are held by a microelectrode holder, which is attached to the pneumatic injector with Teflon tubing, and is maneuvered by the micromanipulator.

1. Dissecting microscope or stereomicroscope: a large working distance is recommended when using a micromanipulator, Nikon and Zeiss have various suitable models.
2. Micromanipulator: this devise is used to maneuver the injection needle in three-dimensions. Commonly used micromanipulators are supplied by Leitz (M type) and Narishige (MN-151 or MN-152).
3. Microinjector: an automatic injection system is used to control the pressure and duration of the injection and should have fine pressure control in the range of 0–100 psi, i.e., PV820, PV830; World Precision Instruments or PLI-188; Nikon.
4. Microinjection capillaries: borosilicate capillaries (outer diameter 1.0 mm, inner diameter 0.5 mm, 10 cm long) with an inner filament. The filament allows the needle to be

back-filled, by capillary action, from the back-end to the needle tip (i.e., Narishige, World Precision Instruments, or Sutter Instruments).

5. Micropipet/needle puller: DMZ-Universal; Zeitz Instruments, or P-80/PC Flaming/Brown; Sutter Instruments.
6. Teflon tubing: CT-1; Narishige.
7. Microloader pipet tips: these tips are designed for loading sequencing gels and can be used for back-loading microinjection needles, i.e., Eppendorf.

2.5.1. Injection Molds

1. 24 × 50 mm Cover slips.
2. Cyanoacrylate adhesive (e.g., "Crazy Glue").
3. 150 × 15 mm Petri dishes.
4. 1% Molten agarose solution in E3 embryo medium (**Subheading 2.1.**).

2.6. RNA Overexpression

2.6.1. Preparation of RNA

In vitro transcribed mRNA should contain a 5'-methyguanosyl cap and a poly-A tail to ensure efficient translation upon injection. Vectors for in vitro transcription should have promoters for two RNA polymerases, such as SP6, T3, or T7, separated by a multiple cloning site to facilitate insertion of cDNA sequences, allowing transcription of both the sense and antisense strand. The plasmid should be linearized downstream of the insert (in the polylinker after the poly-A) to ensure that the polymerase creates a uniform transcript. The linearized DNA should be cleaned by phenol–chloroform extraction to remove residual RNases, and then transcribed using a commercially available kit in the presence of a cap analog.

1. Multipurpose expression vector: we recommend $pCS2^+$.
2. Commercially available kit: we recommend the m*M*ESSAGE m*M*ACHINE™ High Yield Capped RNA Transcription kit (Ambion).
3. RNase-free water (*see* **Note 6**).

2.7. Morpholino-Mediated Knockdown

1. 30X Danieau's solution: 58 m*M* NaCl, 0.7 m*M* KCl, 0.4 m*M* $MgSO_4$, 0.6 m*M* $Ca(NO_3)_2$ 5 m*M* *N*-2-hydroxyethylpiperazine-*N*'-ethenesulfonic acid (HEPES). HEPES changes pH after dilution, so pH to 7.6 after diluting Danieau's to 1X working concentration.
2. Morpholino oligonucleotides can be ordered from Gene Tools LLC (www.gene-tools.com).

2.8. Creation of Transgenic Fish

2.8.1. Preparation of DNA

Prepare plasmid DNA using a Qiagen kit or other plasmid preparation kit, as directed by the manufacturer.

2.8.2. Screening Embryos for Transgene Expression by PCR

1. Extraction buffer: 1X PCR buffer (10 m*M* Tris-HCl, pH 8.3; 50 m*M* KCl), 0.3% Nonidet P40 (NP40), 0.3% Tween-20, detergent should be PCR-grade.
2. Proteinase K: 10 mg/mL, PCR-grade.

3. Zebrafish primers: i.e., ef1α (470 base pair product) and GFP (267 base pair product).
   ef1α (sense) 5' TACGCCTGGGTGTTGGACAAA 3'
   ef1α (antisense) 5' TCTTCTTGATGTATCCGCTGAC 3'
   GFP (sense) 5' AATGTATCAATCATGGCAGAC 3'
   GFP (antisense) 5' TGTATAGTTCATCCATGCCATGTG 3'

2.9. Flow Cytometry of Adult and Embryonic Hematopoietic Cells

2.9.1. Preparation of Adult Kidneys for Flow Cytometry

1. 3-Amino benzoic acidethylester (Tricaine): for lethal anesthetic dose, prepare a 0.2% solution in water, dilute to pH 7.0. Tricaine is an anesthetic, handle appropriately (Sigma).
2. Microdissecting forceps: fine tip, i.e., Roboz or Dumont.
3. Microdissecting scissors: for kidney removal, we suggest a "blunt-sharp" blade tip, i.e., Roboz or Dumont.
4. Pipet fitted with a 1000-μL tip.
5. Nylon cell strainer: 40 μm (Becton Dickinson Labware).
6. Syringe: 1 mL (Becton Dickinson Labware).
7. 0.9X PBS/FCS: 0.9X PBS with 5% heat inactivated, 0.2-μm filtered fetal calf serum, store at 4°C, monitor for bacterial contamination.
8. Propidium iodide (PI): 500 μg/mL from Roche or Sigma, keep the solution tightly closed and protected from light, store at 4°C. PI is a carcinogen, use gloves when handling. PI intercalates into double-stranded nucleic acids and is excluded by viable cells but can penetrate cell membranes of dying or dead cells. PI's peak excitation wavelength is 536 nm and its emission peak is 620 nm.

2.9.2. Preparation of Embryos for Flow Cytometry

In addition to the materials listed for **Subheading 2.6.1.** include tissue grinder and a sterile polypropylene pellet pestle with matching 1.5-mL microfuge tubes, i.e., Kimble/Kontes.

2.9.3. Flow Cytometry

1. FACS tubes: 5-mL polystyrene round bottom tube 12 × 75 mm style, nonpyrogenic (Falcon).
2. Flow cytometer, i.e. FACS Vantage flow cytometer (Beckton Dickinson).

3. Methods

Outlined next are methods to: 1) analyze expression of blood markers by WISH; 2) detect hemoglobinized red blood cells with *o*-dianisidine; 3) microinject zebrafish embryos for the purpose of mRNA overexpression, morpholino-mediated knockdown, and the creation of transgenics; and 4) use flow cytometry to isolate hematopoietic cells from adult kidneys by light scatter characteristics and from transgenic zebrafish expressing fluorescent markers in specific cell types.

3.2. WISH

WISH is frequently used to evaluate the spatiotemporal expression patterns of hematopoietic genes during ontogeny, and is the basis of our understanding of blood development. Furthermore, WISH is essential for evaluating the effects of perturbing gene expression by overexpression and morpholino-mediated knockdown. More recently, WISH has been implemented as screening criteria to uncover deficiencies in early stem cell specification and definitive hematopoiesis, including the lymphoid and myeloid lineages ***(13,14,23–25)*** and have yielded mutants that fail to specify early larval lymphoid and myeloid populations.

Included here is a basic protocol that is used in our laboratory and has been adapted from Jowett and Lettice ***(23)***. All steps are at room temperature unless otherwise noted (*see* **Note 7**).

3.2.1. Embryo Dechorionation and Fixation (see **Note 8**)

3.2.1.1. Embryo Dechorionation and Fixation: Less Than 20 Somites

Fix embryos in 4% PFA/PBS overnight at 4°C, rinse 1X PBST 3 × 5 min, dechorionate with a pair of sharp forceps using a dissecting microscope. After fixation, the yolk will appear dark and opaque under a dissecting microscope, this is normal and will not affect results.

3.2.1.2. Embryo Dechorionation and Fixation: Greater Than 20 Somites

1. Remove all E3, tilt Petri dish to collect embryos at one side of the dish, add enough pronase (at 50 mg/mL) to cover the embryos, incubate for several minutes. Embryos will fall apart if exposed to pronase for too long or if roughly manipulated (*see* **Note 9**).
2. Wash extensively with E3.
3. Fix in 4% PFA/PBS overnight at 4°C.

3.2.1.3. Dehydration

1. After fixation, rinse 1X PBST 3 × 5 min at room temperature (*see* **Note 10**).
2. Rinse once with MeOH and store in MeOH at –20°C. If using the embryos immediately for *in situ* hybridization, keep the embryos in MeOH at –20°C for at least 20 min prior to use for sufficient dehydration.

3.2.2. Embryo Pigment Removal

One of the main advantages of using zebrafish lies in the transparency of the embryos, yet this optical clarity becomes restricted around 24 h postfertilization (hpf) when melanization begins to obstruct observation. The melanization process can be inhibited by treating embryos with PTU, which works effectively when applied no later than 24 hpf, yet this also causes a mild developmental delay and sometimes edema after 5 d postfertilization (dpf). If this is a concern, a popular alternative is to bleach embryos after fixation, but prior to *in situ* hybridization, to remove pigmentation. Bleaching eliminates any risk of obscuring results owing to developmental delay caused by blocking melanization with PTU and may even enhance probe accessibility in older embryos. As a guideline, embryos between 24 hpf and 48 hpf are not significantly inhibited by PTU treatment, but bleaching is recommended for embryos older than 4 dpf. Please note that the bleaching procedure affects tissue integrity and subsequent proteinase K treatments should be adjusted to account for the delicate tissue. For *in situ* hybridization, bleaching can be performed after fixation and before or after dehydration in methanol. Bleaching can also be performed after color development and some argue that this gives better signal intensity, yet it is sometimes better to observe color development unhindered by ectodermal pigment. For hemoglobin staining with *o*-dianisidine, embryos should be bleached after staining and fixation.

3.2.2.1. Embryo PTU Treatment

1. After 18 somites and before 24 hpf, remove E3 and add PTU/E3. PTU/E3 should be changed once daily for optimal results.

3.2.2.2. Embryo Bleaching

1. After fixing and/or dehydrating embryos, wash 1X PBST 2 × 5 min.
2. Incubate the embryos in bleach solution for approx 10 min at room temperature and observe pigment removal. This may take as long as 30 to 40 min for older embryos. Embryos will be fragile after bleaching, so handle with care.
3. Remove the bleach solution and wash 1X PBST for 2 × 5 min; the bleach makes the embryos sticky so it is best to use a glass pipet.
4. Fix for at least 1 h at room temperature with 4% PFA or overnight at 4°C.

For *in situ* hybridization, transfer to methanol for dehydration for at least 30 min at –20°C. If bleaching after dehydration, embryos can be used directly in the *in situ* hybridization procedure. For long-term storage, transfer to methanol and keep at –20°C.

3.2.3. Hybridization and Detection

3.2.3.1. Rehydration and Permeability Enhancement

1. 50% MeOH/PBST 5 min.
2. PBST 3 × 5 min.
3. Fix 4% PFA/PBS 20 min at room temperature (save PFA on ice for subsequent steps).
4. PBST 2 × 5 min.

3.2.3.2. Proteinase Digestion and PostFixation

1. Digest with proteinase K at room temperature (10 μg/mL: 1–10 hpf 60 s, 10–24 hpf 75 s, 48 hpf 20 min; 20 μg/mL: 3–4 dpf 30 min, 5–6 dpf 40 min). These times are a rough guideline and may vary depending on the batch of pronase used and some adjustments may be necessary (*see* **Note 11**).
2. Rinse immediately in PBST 2 × 5 min.
3. Fix 4% PFA/PBS 20 min at room temperature (use saved PFA).
4. PBST 2 × 5 min.

3.2.3.3. Prehybridization

1. Incubate HYB^- 5 min at 60–70°C.
2. Incubate HYB^+ for at least 60 min at 60–70°C.
3. Replace HYB^+ with HYB^+ with probe (0.1–0.5 μg/μL), incubate overnight at 65°C (*see* **Note 12**).

3.2.3.4. Probe Removal and Detection

1. Prepare the following wash solutions and heat to 60 to 70°C prior to use: 1) 50% formamide/2X SSCT/0.1% Tween-20; 2) 55% formamide/1XSSCT/0.1% Tween-20; 3) 1XSSCT/0.1% Tween-20; 4) 0.5X SSCT/0.1% Tween-20; and 5) 0.2X SSCT/0.1% Tween-20.
2. Remove probe and store at –20°C; probe can be used up to five times.
3. Incubate embryos in washes 1 to 5 for 20 to 30 min each at 60 to 70°C.

Subsequent steps at room temperature:

4. MABT 2 × 5 min.
5. Incubate in blocking solution for at least 1 h (*see* **Note 13**).
6. Replace blocking solution with a 1:5000 dilution (0.15 U/mL) of anti-digoxigenin AP Fab fragments in blocking solution, incubate rocking overnight at 4°C.

3.2.3.5. Detection Continued

1. Rinse embryos in MABT for 6 × 30 min (*see* **Note 14**).
2. Wash 2 × 5 min in freshly made staining buffer. Transfer the embryos to 6-well culture dishes to facilitate observation as the staining procedure progresses.
3. Incubate in staining buffer containing NBT and BCIP. This reaction is light sensitive and must be covered. Monitor the reaction as it proceeds to prevent high background staining.
4. Remove staining solution and rinse extensively in PBST to stop the reaction, it is easiest to do this in glass vials.
5. Incubate in 100% MeOH for 30 min to clear background staining, can be left overnight.
6. Fix in 4% PFA/PBS for at least 1 h at room temperature, or 4°C overnight.
7. Prior to observation/photography rinse two times in PBST, transfer to 30%, 60%, 90% glycerol (glycerol has increased viscosity and will facilitate photography).
8. Photograph (*see* **Subheading 3.4.**), rinse well with PBST, store in MeOH, PFA, or PBST pH 4.0.

3.2.4. Double WISH

For double-labeled *in situ* hybridization, two probes with different antigenic labels should be used, we recommend using digoxigenin- and fluorescein-labeled antisense probes, which are both detected by antibodies that are conjugated to alkaline phosphatase ***(26)***. It is most convenient to mix the probes for simultaneous hybridization. The unhybridized probes are then washed off and the tissues incubated in blocking solution to prevent nonspecific binding of antibodies. The signals are then visualized separately by staining with an enzymatic substrate for alkaline phosphatase that produces a colored, insoluble precipitate. In general, fluorescein-labeled probes are less stable than those labeled with digoxigenin and should be visualized first. After visualizing the signal of the fluorescein probe, the antibody must be inactivated by heat or low pH treatment, depending on the substrate, to prevent false co-localization of signal. Before attempting double *in situ* hybridization, you should know where each transcript is expressed and the relative strength of the signal to guide the design of the experiment. Commonly used alkaline phosphatase substrate combinations are NBT/BCIP and a Fast Red. The NBT/BCIP is more sensitive and should be used for the weaker signal. There are several commercially available Fast Red substrate kits that differ slightly in their sensitivity and the background that they produce.

Vector Red (Vector Laboratories) is supplied as a kit containing three solutions that are stored at 4°C and must be mixed immediately before use. Staining is rapid, within a few minutes or several hours, and prolonged incubation does not significantly intensify the signal. The yolk stains yellow, but the background remains low. The red precipitate is heat stable and so the alkaline phosphatase can be inactivated by heating to 65°C for 30 min.

Fast Red (Boehringer Mannheim or Sigma) is supplied in tablet form and can be stored at –20°C for prolonged periods. The tablet is dissolved in Tris-HCL, pH 8.2, immediately prior to use and the solution yields a precipitate after prolonged incubation. The reaction takes longer than Vector Red but yields a more intense signal. The background is orange in both the yolk and the embryo, but can be reduced by adding PVA in the staining reaction. The precipitate is heat labile and so the alkaline phosphatase should be inactivated by incubating in 100 m*M* glycine-hydrochloride, pH 2.2 for 30 min.

If a combination of NBT/BCIP and Fast Red is to be used, the fluorescein-labeled probe must be visualized first with Fast Red to identify the more abundant, stronger transcript. The second staining reaction, to visualize the weaker signal, should be monitored carefully to ensure that the second, blue signal does not mask the initial, red signal.

Follow steps from **Subheading 3.2.3.** through **step 15**, with the following exception:

1. Add appropriate amounts of both probes in HYB$^+$ to the embryos (*see* **Note 15**).

Then continue:

2. Remove unhybridized probes and block for at least 1 h at room temperature.
3. Replace blocking solution with a 1:5000 dilution of anti-fluorescein AP Fab fragments in blocking solution, incubate rocking overnight at 4°C.
4. Rinse embryos in MABT for 6 × 30 min.
5. Wash 2 × 5 min in freshly made staining buffer. Transfer the embryos to six-well culture dishes to facilitate observation as the staining procedure progresses.
6. Incubate in staining buffer containing Fast Red (or Vector Red). This reaction is light sensitive and must be covered. Monitor the reaction as it proceeds to prevent high background staining.
7. Remove staining solution and rinse 3 × 5 min in PBST, it is easiest to do this in glass vials.
8. Inactivate alkaline phosphatase by incubating in alkaline phosphatase inactivation buffer for 30 min (or if using Vector Red, heat to 65°C for 30 min).
9. Fix in PFA for 20 min at room temperature.
10. Rinse with MABT 3 × 5 min.
11. Block in blocking solution for at least 1 h.
12. Replace blocking solution with a 1:5000 dilution of anti-digoxigenin AP Fab fragments in blocking solution, incubate rocking overnight at 4°C.
13. Follow **Subheading 3.2.3.5., steps 1–6**, for detection of NBT/BCIP.

3.2.5. Making a Probe

The probe is made using an in vitro transcription kit that incorporates digoxigenin- or fluorescein-conjugated UTP into the antisense RNA. It is possible to make probe from a variety of vectors as long as the template can be linearized opposite from a T3, T7, or SP6 RNA polymerase site. Probes are typically 1-kilobase pairs in length, though larger and smaller probes can elicit a robust signal depending on the abundance of message present. A complete clone is not required as a partial clone can yield a strong signal and the elimination of repeat sequences can decrease non-specific staining. Partial PCR products or partial clones from cDNA libraries can also be used as a template.

RNA probes are to be prepared according to the manufacturers instructions (Roche).

1. Linearize template DNA, purify, and resuspend in water at 1 μg/μL (*see* **Note 16**).
2. Approximately 2 μg of linearized, cleaned template are required in the reaction, balance to 20 μL total with deionized H_2O, 2 μL of nucleotides, 0.5 μL of RNase inhibitor, 2.0 μL

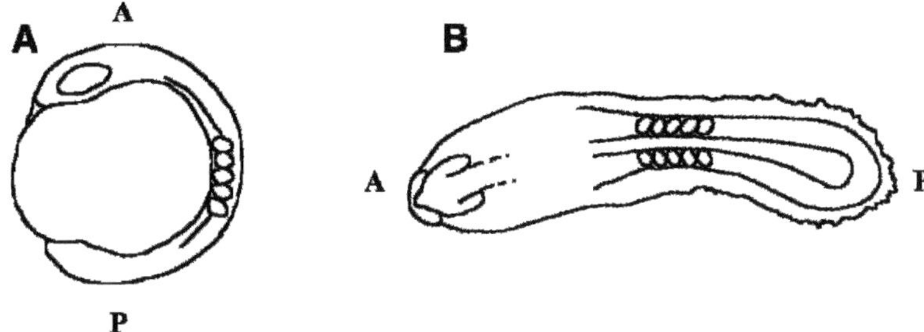

Fig. 1. **(A)** A 5-somite embryo prior to flat-mounting. **(B)** A 5-somite embryo after yolk removal and flat-mounting. A, anterior; P, posterior.

of buffer (warmed to 37°C and mixed well), 2 µL of T7 polymerase. Assemble the reaction mix at room temperature and incubate at 37°C for 2 h.

3. Treat with RNase-free DNase for 20 min at 37°C in appropriate DNase buffer, check on a gel to make sure the template has been digested (*see* **Note 17**).
4. Precipitate probe with 3 *M* NaOAc and 100% EtOH at –20°C for at least 30 min, wash with 70% EtOH, resuspend in 10 µL of sterile, deionized H_2O. Resuspend purified template at 1 µg/µL in RNase-free water (*see* **Note 18**).

3.3. Hemoglobin Staining With O-Dianisidine

1. Prepare the following solution: 2 mL of *o*-dianisidine solution; 500 µL of 0.1 *M* NaOAc, pH 4.5; 2 mL of deionized H_2O; 100 µL of H_2O_2. We recommend adding the components in this order.
2. Add 500 µL to live, dechorionated embryos (**Subheading 3.2.1.**) in glass vials after removing as much of the E3 as possible.
3. Incubate in the dark for 15 to 45 min. The samples can be examined under a dissecting microscope to monitor the reaction; it is not necessary to remove samples from the glass vials.
4. Once staining is complete, wash three times with deionized H_2O. Embryos are very sticky; therefore, it is best to use a glass pipet.
5. Fix stained samples in 4% PFA for at least 1 h at room temperature.
6. If embryos are pigmented, rinse in PBST and then bleach (**Subheading 3.2.2.**).
7. Store embryos in PBST at 4°C or in MeOH at –20°C (*see* **Note 19**).

3.4. Observation and Photography

1. Transfer embryos from 1X PBST into 30%, 60%, and 90% glycerol/PBST.
2. For embryos older than 18 somites, it is easiest to photograph directly using a depression slide to keep embryos in the desired orientation. For embryos between 3 and 15 somites, we recommend flat-mounting to obtain representative photographs (**Fig. 1**).
3. Flat mounting embryos for photography.
   a. Using sharp forceps, carefully remove the yolk from the embryo, leaving the embryo proper intact.
   b. Using a pipet, transfer the embryo to a glass slide in a drop of glycerol, avoid placing the embryo directly in the middle of the slide.
   c. Using an eyelash or fine nylon loop, carefully maneuver the embryo to the edge of the glycerol droplet such that the embryo is oriented with the dorsal side facing upwards,

drag the embryo towards the middle of the slide to an area that is void of glycerol; this should help prevent the embryo from curling on itself.

d. Apply a very small amount of modeling clay to the four corners of a square cover slip by swiping the cover slip gently into the clay to scoop out a small portion.
e. Use the cover slip to gently press the embryo flat, but do not apply too much pressure, only enough to keep the embryo from curling up.
f. After the cover slip is in place, pipet a very small amount of glycerol to the edge of the coverslip to surround the embryo with glycerol. Adjust the amount of clay, the amount of glycerol, and the pressure applied until the embryo is correctly oriented and completely stationary. This process requires extensive practice and a steady hand, but in the end the results are well worth the effort.

3.5. Microinjection

Microinjection is the most widely used technique for introducing nucleic acids and nucleic acid analogues into zebrafish embryos. The technique for these experiments is identical, though the timing of injection is slightly different and will be detailed in each of the subsequent sections (**Subheadings 3.6.–3.8.**). Microinjection of freshly fertilized eggs has a high survival rate, is relatively nonintrusive, yields reproducible results, and with practice, it is possible to inject hundreds of embryos within an hour. Although the specific equipment used can vary, the basic requirements for microinjection are as follows: a needle puller, capillary needles, a pneumatic microinjector to modulate the amount of pressure within the needle for delivering the injection solution, a micromanipulator for controlling the injection needle, and a mold to immobilize the embryos. Injection is facilitated by temporarily immobilizing embryos in agarose molds. Various immobilization techniques are available and have been described adequately in other sources *(21,22)*. Here, we will detail one recently developed approach that makes use of glass slides to create a simple agarose ledge that holds embryos in a specific orientation with respect to the injection needle. Very little agarose is used to create the mold, permitting clear observation of the needle, the embryos, and the subsequent injection.

3.5.1. The Ledge Mold

Simple glass cover slips are used to create an agarose ledge that will immobilize embryos in the correct orientation (*see* **Note 20**).

1. To create a cover slip mold, glue three to four coverslips together to create a "unit," and then glue one unit to another, leaving a thin recess approx 2 mm in width along the length of the unit, as shown in **Fig. 2**. Make two to four cover slip molds.
2. Place two molds in a Petri dish as shown in **Fig. 2** such that the recess faces up and is closest to the top of the Petri dish.
3. Using a transfer pipet, carefully add 1% molten agarose to cover only the recess of the cover slip mold and the surrounding area, as shown in gray in **Fig. 2**. Only a small amount of agarose is needed as most of the recess will fill by capillary action.
4. After the agarose has cooled, carefully cut along the edge of the recess with a fresh razor blade, separating the agarose from the glass cover slip mold. Extract the cover slip mold from the agarose with the aid of blunt forceps, leaving behind a delicate ledge of agarose.
5. Fill the dish with E3 containing Methylene blue and store at 4°C (*see* **Note 21**).

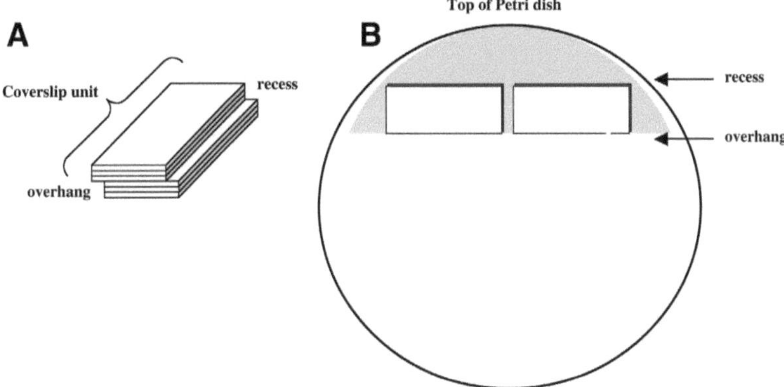

Fig. 2. (**A**) A cover slip unit assembled by gluing two sets of three to four cover slips together, forming a recess that will be filled with molten agarose/E3 as shown in (**B**) to create a ledge for immobilizing embryos.

3.5.2. Needle Preparation

1. Using a suitable pipet/needle puller, pull needles that narrow quickly to a tip. Microinjection needles should be thick enough to easily penetrate the chorion but not so thick as to damage the embryo. Needles that are pulled too long and fine will bend when in contact with the chorion and are more prone to blockages.
2. Break the tip of the needle with fine forceps creating an oblique angle to facilitate penetration. For reproducible results, use a microscope equipped with a micrometer. A large opening will damage embryos, while a small opening is more likely to become blocked. If the needle becomes blocked, use the forceps to re-open the needle by removing the very tip to enlarge the needle. Adjustment of injection pressure or time may be required to maintain a constant volume.
3. Load the needle using a pipet fitted with a microloader pipet tip. Place the tip as far into the back of the capillary as possible and slowly expel the solution as the tip is withdrawn. The filaments facilitate flow of the solution towards the needle tip. Several hundred embryos can be injected with 2 μL of solution. Insert the needle into the microelectrode; the fit should be snug (*see* **Note 22**).

3.5.3. Embryo Collection and Microinjection

Postinjection survival rate is influenced by the quality of zebrafish embryos obtained. Adult fish can be kept together overnight, or they can be kept separate and put together in the morning, in which case it usually takes around 10 min for mating to occur. Immediately after collection, it is difficult to ascertain whether eggs are unfertilized or of low-quality. Therefore some researchers prefer to mix clutches prior to injection, ensuring that not too much time is wasted on injecting embryos that will not develop.

1. Carefully align the embryos under the ledge as shown in **Fig. 3** such that the cell is facing outwards, we recommend using a 24-gage wire that has been lightly filed to remove sharp edges. The chorion should remain intact with gentle pressure as it is quite durable.

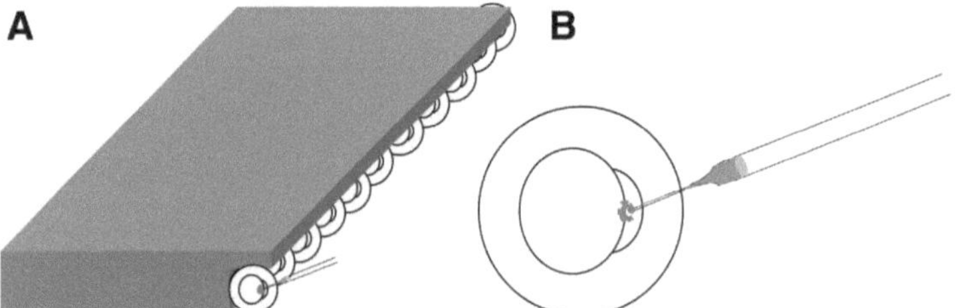

Fig. 3. (**A**) Embryos are gently pushed under an agarose ledge for injection, which accommodates almost 50 embryos. (**B**) The microinjection needle glides through the chorion, the blastomere, and the injection solution is expelled into the cell, right at the margin of yolk and cytoplasm in a volume approx one-fifth the volume of the cell.

2. After the embryos are aligned, set up the micromanipulator so that the needle is in line with the embryos in the center of the microscope stage. It helps to orient the needle at an angle (around 45°) with respect to the cell.
3. Using a single fluid motion, drive the needle through the chorion and into the cytoplasm of the embryo, expel the injection solution, extract the needle, and repeat. When using the ledge mold it is possible to see the injection location and volume without the aid of a dye, but at first it might be helpful to use Phenol Red as a marker for the solution (*see* **Note 23**; **Fig. 3**).
4. The injection volume should be one fifth that of the embryo, which is approx 1 nL at the one-cell stage. The injection pressure and injection time should be adjusted accordingly to maintain a consistent injection volume. To calibrate the volume, inject into a drop of mineral oil, measuring the diameter of the resulting droplets and convert to volume; adjust injection time, pressure, and needle diameter accordingly; *see* **Note 24**).

3.5.4. Postinjection Care

1. After all embryos have been injected, carefully remove the embryos from the mold using gentle pressure from the 24-gage wire; embryos with punctured chorions are very fragile, so exercise caution. The chorions will recover within a few hours.
2. After 4 to 5 h have passed, remove any embryos that are unfertilized, necrotic, or irreparably damaged, transfer to a new dish with fresh E3, and allow development to progress. The survival of resulting embryos is increased by maintaining sanitary conditions *(21,22)*. Embryos that will be raised in a fish facility should be carefully monitored over the course of their development into juveniles and adults.

3.6. RNA Overexpression

Injection of in vitro transcribed mRNA is a quick way to gain insight into the in vivo activity of novel cDNAs and is widely used to misexpress protein in zebrafish embryos. Injections of mRNA are most frequently performed to assay gene function by overexpression, to rescue or evaluate a mutant, or to test specificity of morpholino-mediated knockdown results. Expression of functional protein from an injected mRNA is extremely rapid and can be detected as early as the 256-cell stage, preceding the initiation of zygotic transcription at the mid-blastula transition. Thus, one advantage of using mRNA injection lies in the ability to address early developmental events.

However, mRNA is also quickly diluted and/or degraded, leading to a rapid reduction in expression. Therefore, it is less useful for studying events that occur later in development. Furthermore, expression from injected mRNA is nearly ubiquitous, indicating that most cells receive and translate the message. This is beneficial if you want uniform expression and a low degree of mosaicism, but problematic if you are interested in expressing a gene in specific cell types.

The process of injecting mRNA is more forgiving with respect to overall incorporation than the injection of DNA, which is limited by accessibility of DNA to the cell nucleus and subsequent transcription. Immediately upon fertilization, embryos undergo cytoplasmic streaming in which the egg cytoplasm separates from the yolk and migrates to the forming cell. This process is evident as thin, parallel threads within the yolk and is capable of transporting large molecules such as high molecular weight dyes or mRNAs from the yolk into the cytoplasm. It is therefore possible to inject mRNA into vegetal positions within the yolk and still have robust incorporation of message in every blastomere. The membrane separating the yolk cell from the blastomeres does not form until the 16-cell stage, and so it is possible to detect ectopic protein expression in almost every cell, even when mRNA is injected into the yolk of an 8-cell stage embryo. Injection into the yolk is thus advisable for mRNA or morpholinos prior to the formation of the first blastomere and thereafter.

3.6.1. Preparation of RNA

1. Linearize 5 μg of plasmid by digestion with the appropriate restriction enzyme (in polylinker 5' of cDNA) for 2 h.
2. Phenol–chloroform extract, ethanol precipitate, resuspend in diethyl pyrocarbonate (DEPC)–H_2O.
3. mMESSAGE mMACHINE™ High Yield Capped RNA transcription kit (Ambion). Follow manufacturers instructions for in vitro RNA production. Add 1 μg of linearized sample to 10 μL of 2X ribonucleotide mix, 2 μL of 10X reaction buffer, and 2 μL of 10X enzyme mix, balance to 20 μL with DEPC–H_2O, incubate at 37°C for 2 h to allow transcription.
4. Treat with RNase-free DNase for 15 min at 37°C to remove the template, extract with phenol-chloroform, and precipitate with ammonium acetate/isopropanol.
5. Dilute RNA in 10 μL of sterile, deionized H_2O, creating a stock concentration for making working dilutions for injections, store at –80°C. The optimal concentration is dependent on the nature of the encoded protein, for example, embryos have a low tolerance of ectopically expressed transcription factors and can have varied responses to a range of signaling molecule concentrations. To begin, inject several dilutions within a 1:10 to 1:100 range of the stock.

3.7. Morpholino-Mediated Knockdown

The characteristics of zebrafish make this system well tailored to the execution of large-scale forward genetic screens in which mutants with interesting phenotypes are isolated, and then the genes underlying the phenotypes are identified and analyzed at the molecular level. The converse reverse genetic approach entails an analysis of gene function by mutating or deleting the gene of interest and then evaluating the resulting phenotype. The absence of a reverse genetics approach was a severe limitation of the zebrafish system until the advent of an antisense knockdown technology that makes use of synthetic DNA analogues, or morpholinos *(8,9)*. Morpholinos are chemically modified oligonucleotides that bind and inactivate selected mRNA sequences by blocking translation and can be used to quickly and easily study gene function. These DNA analogs are assembled from four different morpholino subunits, each of which contains one of the four genetic bases linked to a six-membered morpholine ring, which are joined in a specific order using non-ionic phosphorodiamidate intersubunit linkages. Unlike nucleic acids, morpholinos are uncharged, stable in vivo, and can be injected at high concentrations. The morpholino reverse genetic approach complements the forward genetic approach, and can ameliorate some shortcomings of genetic screens, such as redundancy, in which case morpholinos of redundant genes can be injected into mutant embryos. Morpholinos can also be used to confirm or rule out candidate genes thought to underlie mutant phenotypes.

Despite these advantages, the use of morpholinos can be frustrating because of the frequent observation of non-specific toxicity, including widespread cell death (dark, necrotic cells), defects in epiboly, neural degeneration, and a shortened or curved body axis. It is unclear if the observed toxicity is a result of unexpected complementarity to other genes or other nonspecific effects of the morpholinos *(8,9)*. Morpholinos are most often used to eliminate the functions of genes important early in development, including maternally localized messages, and display a phenotypic series when a range of concentrations is injected. The potential for variability in the penetrance of a morpholino is an important consideration when interpreting results. A gradation of phenotypes may be similar to an allelic series in some cases and would thus be beneficial for functional analysis, yet a phenotypic series also makes it difficult to distinguish real results from nonspecific toxicity, especially when investigating the function of a novel gene. It may take several failed morpholino designs before a morpholino will specifically knockdown a target and stringent controls are critical to support the results of any morpholino experiment. To test for specificity, one simple option is to rescue by microinjecting mRNA of the target, yet if the injected mRNA is complementary to the morpholino, it will hybridize to the morpholino and directly compete for binding with the endogenous message. A better alternative is to use an mRNA that either lacks the 5' UTR recognized by the morpholino, or an mRNA that has silent mutations such that the protein encoded by the message remains unchanged, yet the mRNA is not complementary to the morpholino. Unfortunately, such rescue experiments are often confounded by incorrect distribution and activity of the injected mRNA. It is advisable to inject two unique morpholinos directed against the same target to determine if both yield the same phenotype.

Morpholino oligos are not susceptible to enzymatic degradation and therefore have a high biological stability, yet morpholinos eventually lose effectiveness by dilution *(27)*. For evaluating genes early in hematopoiesis, this is not a concern; however, it may be challenging to assay the function of genes that are important for definitive hematopoiesis. The duration of the loss-of-function effect of an injected morpholino depends on the transcription and translation characteristics of the targeted mRNA, as well as the dose of the morpholino, and needs to be determined for each morpholino. The variables underlying the activity of morpholinos remain unknown, and so numerous morpholinos might need to be tested before finding a functionally specific morpholino. This may be cost prohibitive for some research groups.

1. We recommend designing 18- to 25-mer morpholinos complementary to sequence between the 5' UTR through the first 25 bases 3' of the AUG start site; design subsequent morpholinos to span exon/intron boundaries to inhibit message processing. Consult the Gene Tools LLC web site for assistance (www.gene-tools.com).
2. Dissolve lyophilized morpholino powder into 1X Danieau's solution to a final concentration of 10 m*M*. Typical injection concentrations range from 10 μ*M* to 5 m*M* and a wide range of injection concentrations should be assayed when working with a morpholino for the first time as it is likely that a range of concentration will yield results from no-effect to nonspecific toxicity.
3. Store stock solutions at –20°C or –80°C and keep working dilutions at 4°C. Before injecting working dilutions, heat to 65°C for 5 min, spin quickly, and allow the solution to cool.
4. Morpholinos, like mRNA, can be injected prior to the one-cell stage and thereafter. Injection after the eight-cell stage is not recommended (follow guidelines presented in **Subheading 3.6.**; *see* **Note 25**).

3.8. Creation of Transgenic Fish

The use of transgenic technology has become more prominent among researchers in the zebrafish hematopoietic field. There are myriad reasons for creating a transgenic line, and while transgenics are most frequently created to label a distinct cell type with a fluorescent marker, transgenics are also used to investigate gene interactions and to drive conditional expression ubiquitously or within a certain subset of cells. For example, in the event of RNA toxicity, as is the case with *gata-1* mRNA, it is possible to circumvent the toxicity issue by driving *gata-1* expression under a blood specific promoter such as *lmo2*.

The first blood specific transgenic line was reported by S. Lin et al. ***(28)***, who generated a line of fish expressing GFP under the regulatory elements of the erythroid specific *gata-1* promoter (*gata-1*^{GFP}). Other blood-specific GFP lines have been created, including *rag-2*^{GFP} and *lck*^{GFP}, which label early lymphocytes (**ref. *29***; D. M. Langenau et al., submitted), *lmo2*^{GFP}, which marks hematopoietic and vascular cells (H. Zhu and L. I. Zon, unpublished results), *pu.1*^{GFP}, which labels the myeloid lineage (K. E. Hsu and A. T. Look, submitted for publication), and *CD41*^{GFP}, which labels thrombocytes (H.F. Lin et al., unpublished observations). In addition to GFP, the red fluorescent marker dsRED can also be used to label specific blood lineages, enabling the generation of multicolored zebrafish expressing a different marker for different cell types. These transgenic animals are not only useful for tracking populations in vivo, but can also be used to isolate populations from adult and embryonic sources for cell transplantation and to create lineage specific cDNA libraries.

One drawback to the use of fluorescent reporters is that the fluorescent proteins used as markers take some time to mature, leaving the initial onset of gene expression devoid of fluorescent feedback. Although this is usually inconsequential, it can sometimes impede experiments requiring observation or isolation of cell types soon after the transgene is expressed. Therefore, when developing a strategy for the creation of a fluorescent transgenic, keep in mind that eGFP will mature in 1.5 to 4 h, whereas dsRED will mature in 12 to 15 h. Fortunately, new fluorescent proteins have been developed, promising improvements to existing fluorescent markers including the monomeric AcGFP, which is as bright as eGFP though it folds at the same rate, and FarRed and dsRED-Express, which fold faster than dsRED while maintaining the same fluorescence intensity (Clontech).

Upon injection into the embryo, DNA is first amplified and then integrated into the chromosomes as large concatamers. The rapid cell division of the early embryo and the delay in integration leads to incorporation of introduced DNA in only a small fraction of cells within the embryo, thus the efficiency of germ-line transmission is very low. Expression of transgenes is highly mosaic and there is an invariable decline in the number of cells expressing DNA a few days postinjection. However, in the cells that maintain expression, DNA is detectable for weeks after injection and can also be used to drive even transient tissue-specific expression.

For the creation of transgenics, it is critical to inject the embryo early in development, prior to or at the beginning of the one-cell stage. The embryo membrane is particularly tender at this time, facilitating rapid injections. More importantly, there is a higher frequency of integration when DNA is introduced early and in close proximity to the nucleus ***(30)***. Embryos are raised to adulthood to test for germ line transmission of the transgene in their progeny. Transgenic founders may be as rare as 1 to 5% of all injected fish assayed, but can be as high as 25%. The level of transgene expression varies between lines, most likely because of differences in integration location and copy number, and it is therefore worthwhile to screen through several independently derived lines for each construct.

To generate a transgenic line that reproducibly recapitulates expression of the endogenous gene, we recommend that at least 100 fish are raised to adulthood for every construct, which equates into the injection of approx 1000 embryos. Some researchers prefer to screen for transient endogenous expression at the embryonic stage, which is time consuming and in our experience does not ultimately translate into a higher percentage of founders.

Screening through hundreds of fish for transgenic founders is a laborious process, but can be facilitated by a mass mating approach, followed by smaller mating combinations, and eventually crossing candidates to a wild-type line (i.e., AB, Tü, WIK). The type of transgenic fish generated will direct the screening criteria, yet in concept, both direct and PCR-based approaches are identical; candidate founders are mated either in mass mating cages or individually, and the resulting progeny are screened for transgenic expression. For transgenics expressing a fluorescent marker, it is more efficient to directly screen embryos for reporter gene expression using fluorescence microscopy. If screening by reporter expression, we advise dechorionating the embryos to optimize visualization of the signal. For transgenics lacking reporter gene expression, founders can be identified by performing PCR for the transgene on genomic DNA isolated from their progeny. Some researchers prefer screening by PCR because it provides a more sensitive assay than screening by reporter gene expression. This tedious procedure can be expedited by pooling progeny from multiple crosses for the initial screening.

3.8.1. Preparation of DNA

1. Linearize the DNA with appropriate restriction enzymes. DNA insert should be cut from vector sequence and then purified (*see* **Note 26**).
2. Dilute the DNA between 50 and 300 ng/μL in 200 m*M* KCL. Store the prepared solution at 4°C for up to 2 wk or indefinitely at –20°C (*see* **Note 27**).

3.8.2. Screening Embryos for Transgene Expression by PCR

Embryos and solutions should be kept on ice unless otherwise noted.

1. Mate potential founder fish to each other or to a wild-type stock line. Collect and dechorionate (**Subheading 3.2.1.**) embryos from at least 100 to 200 candidates. Embryos can be stored in methanol at –20°C. Methanol should be completely removed prior to extracting DNA; this can be achieved by incubating the embryos uncovered at 65°C for 10 to 15 min.
2. Transfer 100 embryos to a microfuge tube containing 1 mL of extraction buffer, incubate at 98°C for 10 min to lyse cells, quench on ice.
3. Add 100 μL of proteinase K (10 mg/mL stock) to digest proteins, incubate at 55°C for at least 2 h. This incubation can also go overnight; longer incubations tend to yield cleaner DNA.
4. Incubate at 98°C for 10 min to inactivate proteinase K, quench on ice. For older embryos aspiration with a pipet may be necessary to homogenize the tissue.
5 Centrifuge at 18,000*g* for 10 min at room temperature to pellet embryo debris. Pool 10 samples by combining 10 μL of each sample into a new microfuge tube. Save the remaining extract at –20°C for future use. Precipitate the DNA in the pooled samples by adding 300 μL of 100% ethanol, wash with 70% ethanol, dry, resuspend in 100 μL of sterile water.
6. Perform standard PCR on the isolated genomic DNA to identify pools that contain the transgene of interest. Include an internal control that detects an endogenous zebrafish gene, i.e., ef1α. For a positive control use DNA isolated from a pool of one positive transgenic animal in a total of 500 embryos, ensuring that the primer set and conditions are sensitive enough to detect the transgene at a low frequency. A negative control should be included to rule out contamination.
7. Once a positive pool is identified, perform PCR on the individuals constituting the pool to identify the founder fish. Confirm these results by evaluating progeny from the candidate by other methods (Southern blotting or observation of transgene expression; *see* **Note 28**).
8. Transgenic founder (F_0) fish can be bred to generate homozygous populations that maintain transgene integration. F_0 fish are crossed to wild-type fish and their progeny (F_1) are grown to adulthood. The transgene can be detected visually by reporter gene expression, or by PCR on genomic DNA isolated from caudal fin clips (*see* **Note 29**).
9. Mate positively identified F_1 siblings, which should yield among their progeny (F_2), 25% transgenic homozygous, 50% heterozygotes, and 25% homozygous wild type. Raise only the F_2 fish carrying the transgene (heterozygous and transgenic homozygous) to maturity and mate individual F_2 fish to wild-type fish. The resulting F_3 fish should be screened for the transgene by direct observation of reporter expression or by PCR. A homozygous F_2 fish will pass the transgene to 100% of its progeny when mated to a wild-type fish whereas a heterozygous F_2 fish will pass the transgene to 50% of its progeny. The identified homozygous F_2 fish can be mated together to create a large population of homozygous transgenics.

3.9. Flow Cytometry of Zebrafish Hematopoietic Cells

3.9.1. Lineage Separation of Adult Kidney Tissue

The analysis of hematopoietic cells in the adult zebrafish has thus far been restricted by a paucity of reagents for lineage purification. This limitation has recently been circumvented by taking advantage of zebrafish hematopoietic tissue characteristics

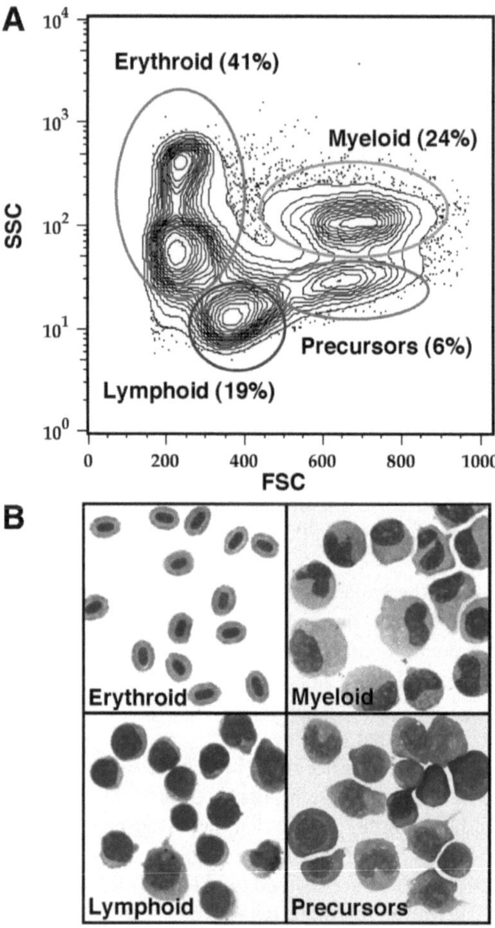

Fig. 4. **(A)** Lineage separation of adult kidney by forward scatter (FSC) and side scatter (SSC). **(B)** Blood lineages isolated by flow cytometry in **(A)** were stained with May/Grünwald-Giemsa.

that enable separation into discrete populations on the basis of light scatter characteristics (R. A. Wingert and L. I. Zon, submitted). Analysis of kidney tissue by flow cytometry reveals populations of the major blood lineages, enabling their isolation: mature erythrocytes are found within a forward scatter $(FSC)^{low}$ population, myelomonocytic cells within a FSC^{high} side scatter $(SS)^{high}$ population, lymphoid cells within a FSC^{int} SS^{low} population, and immature precursors within a FSC^{high} SS^{int} population (**Fig. 4**). This recent advance, coupled with increasingly available transgenic lines expressing fluorescent blood reporters, creates a powerful tool for the identification and quantification of adult hematopoietic tissue in wild-type, mutant, and genetically altered zebrafish.

3.9.2. Preparation of Adult Kidneys for Flow Cytometry

Keep solutions and tissues on ice as much as possible throughout the procedure.

1. Lethally anesthetize adult zebrafish in 0.2% Tricaine prior to kidney collection.
2. The kidney is a thin membrane that extends nearly the full length of the abdominal cavity and is pigmented by melanocytes, making it dark and glistening. To remove the kidney, make a ventral midline incision from the anus to the level of the gills. Using forceps, carefully remove the internal organs, being careful not to rupture the intestines, exposing the kidney immediately beneath the swim bladder. The kidney can be removed by gentle teasing, starting at the head kidney (anterior), which is more concentrated with hematopoietic tissue, and working towards the posterior. The dorsal aorta is intimately associated with the kidney and will inevitably be removed as well.
3. Transfer the dissected kidneys into a 1.5-mL microfuge tube containing 0.9X PBS/FCS.
4. Homogenize the tissue by aspirating with a pipet fitted with a P1000 tip.
5. Gently tease apart the tissue using a plunger from a 1-cc syringe atop a 40-μm nylon mesh filter over a 50-mL conical tube.
6. Add 25–50 mL of 0.9X PBS/FCS, pellet cells by spinning at 200 to 300*g* for 5 min at 4°C and remove the supernatant except for approx 750 μL. Wash cells three times with a large volume of 0.9X PBS/FCS; cells should be gently but thoroughly resuspended with each wash (*see* **Note 30**).
7. After the last wash, resuspend to a concentration of approx 5–10 × 10^6 cells/mL, add PI to 1 μg/mL to exclude dead cells (*see* **Note 31**).

3.9.3. Flow Cytometry of Cells Expressing Fluorescent Reporters

As discussed previously (**Subheading 3.8.**), the isolation of cell populations from transgenic adults and embryos on the basis of fluorescent markers has numerous applications, including purification for cell transplantation, preparation of cDNA libraries, and quantification of cell types in mutant or morpholino knockdown embryos. Kidneys from adult transgenics should be prepared as in **Subheading 3.9.2.**

3.9.4. Preparation of Embryos for Flow Cytometry

1. Transfer embryos (dechorionation is optional) to a 1.5-mL microfuge tube, wash three times with 0.9X PBS/FCS. Do not add more than 500 μL of embryos to the tube.
2. Homogenize embryos using a pellet pestle
3. Filter and wash as described in **Subheading 3.9.2., steps 5–7**. Resuspend 250 to 500 μL of embryos in 1 mL of 0.9X PBS/FCS/PI for flow cytometry.

3.9.5. Flow Cytometry

For sorting, ensure that the UV laser is blocked since we have observed toxicity to erythrocytes, and have collection tubes containing 200 μL of 0.9X PBS/FCS to help protect the cells from lysing. For lineage separation, FACS analysis should be performed on the basis of PI exclusion, forward scatter, and side scatter. To isolate based on reporter gene expression, FACS analysis should be performed on the bases of PI exclusion and GFP or RFP fluorescence (*see* **Note 32**).

4. Notes

1. Make 50X E3 stock, dilute to 1X for working concentration, can be stored for 2 wk at room temperature as a 1X dilution. Methylene blue should be added to 1X E3 as a fungicide.

2. Dissolve PFA in PBS at 65°C; if it does not dissolve readily add one to two drops of 1 *M* NaOH solution to pH 7.5. PFA should be used fresh or stored frozen in aliquots at –20°C.
3. Levamisole inhibits acidic phosphatases, which can, depending on the stage of the fixed material, lead to staining in tissues expressing phosphatases, such as the retina and intestinal tissues. Dissolve levamisole in staining buffer at 1 m*M*. If using Fast Red tablets, levamisole is already included.
4. The indoxyl-nitroblue tetrazolium (BCIP–NBT) reaction is very slow and intermediates (indoxyls) diffuse away from the source, causing a reduction of signal and making it difficult to localize the site of hybridization. The addition of polyvinyl alcohol (PVA) of high molecular weight (40–100 kDa) enhances the BCIP–NBT reaction and prevents diffusion of intermediates, resulting in a twenty fold increase in sensitivity without increasing background ***(31)***. Add PVA to the staining buffer at 10% w/v, boil to dissolve, allow solution to cool before use, and then add Tween-20 (0.1%), forming a viscous buffer. The addition of PVA is highly recommended if using Fast Red as a chromogenic substrate.
5. An alternate chromogenic marker is the BM Purple substrate from Roche. Mix well before removing from the bottle and use straight or dilute 1:1 with staining buffer, warm to room temperature before adding to samples.
6. DEPC-treated water should is not recommended for injection purposes. Sterile Milli-Q water is sufficiently RNase free for RNA overexpression analysis. The Ambion web site (www.ambion.com) has extensive information on preventing RNase contamination.
7. Use large volumes of solution for washing unhybridized probe and unbound antibody and for equilibrating embryos. For other steps (including proteinase K, re-fixation with PFA, hybridization, block, and antibody addition) conserve solutions by adding enough to cover the embryos. For example, if using 5.5-mL glass vials, 500 μL is a sufficient volume.
8. Embryos less than 18 somites are easily damaged by pronase treatment and so we recommend manual dechorionation. If the embryos are older than 20 somites, it is best to dechorionate the embryos with pronase prior to fixation to ensure that the embryos are not fixed in a curved position. The fixation step is critical and we advise using freshly prepared or freshly thawed PFA to maintain embryo integrity and to prevent high background.
9. The addition of concentrated pronase requires diligent attention to ensure the preservation of embryo integrity. Alternatively, add 10 μL of pronase to a dish of embryos, swirl to mix, leave the embryos in pronase overnight, and rinse in the morning. It may be necessary to forcefully pipet the embryos with a plastic transfer pipet to completely remove the chorions.
10. If necessary, embryos can be left in fixative longer than overnight as this does not usually affect experimental results; long-term storage in PFA will color the yolk dark yellow.
11. For bleached embryos, try cutting the suggested time in half to keep tissue intact. Usually the yolk disintegrates first, leaving the embryo proper. While unaesthetic, these embryos can still be evaluated for gene expression by *in situ* hybridization and if less than 18 somites can be flat-mounted prior to taking a photograph (**Subheading 3.5.**).
12. Total probe concentration should not exceed 1 μg/mL. If background is a problem, increase temperature and formamide concentration, or decrease the salt concentration in the hybridization buffer to increase stringency of probe binding.
13. The antibodies can be preabsorbed against zebrafish powder or whole zebrafish embryos, though some would contend that the low titer of antibody used (1:5000) does not necessitate preabsorption. For absorbing against whole embryos, pre-absorb the antibody 1:1000 in blocking solution with different stages of fixed, dechorionated, dehydrated, re-hydrated

embryos, keep at room temperature for an hour, swirling occasionally, and then transfer to ice. When ready to use, remove the pre-absorbed antibody and dilute to 1:5000 with blocking solution.

14. PBST, which is easier to make, can be used as a replacement for MABT at this step.
15. Fluorescein-labeled probes are less stable at acidic pH and the HYB^+ should be adjusted to pH 6.5.
16. Removal of unincorporated nucleotides will prevent high background as they are very sticky. Linearized template can be purified by a phenol/chloroform and chloroform extraction, followed by precipitation with 3 *M* NaOAc and ethanol.
17. Template removal is optional as the amount of transcribed probe far exceeds the residual template.
18. Approximately 5 to 10 μg of labeled probe are transcribed from 1 μg of linearized template; larger amounts can be obtained by scaling up the reaction components. The amount of synthesized labeled RNA depends on the amount, size, and purity of the template DNA; longer incubations will not increase the yield.
19. If there is high background, incubate the embryos in methanol at –20°C for a minimum of 30 min, clear the embryos with a 2:1 benzyl benzoate:benzyl alcohol solution, rinse with methanol, and store at –20°C in methanol.
20. A widely used and well-established alternative to this technique makes use of a series of grooves that are angled on one side to allow the needle access to the embryo and a perpendicular wall against which the embryos are pressed ***(21,22)***. This technique is easier to learn and is relatively faster at first, though the depth of agarose utilized restricts visibility and is therefore not recommended for the creation of transgenics.
21. We recommend using a razor blade to gently scrape the bottom of the Petri dish to remove any residual agarose as this will impede the insertion of embryos under the ledge. Rinse the dish several times after use to prolong the lifespan of the injection mold.
22. It is also possible to use a standard pipet tip by expelling a drop on the butt end of the needle and waiting for the solution to descend to the tip.
23. Try to avoid injecting into the cytoplasm through the yolk; while this is functionally sound, the yolk is sticky and is more likely to block the needle. Phenol Red can be obtained from Sigma and is used at 0.5%.
24. $V = {}^4/_3\pi R^3$; V: volume, R: diameter.
25. Some lots of morpholino oligos contain residual acid from the synthesis reaction, causing a high mortality rate when injected. It is possible to identify contaminated morpholinos by using Phenol Red, which, in addition to being an injection tracer, will also turn yellow if the morpholino solution is acidic.
26. Run the digested DNA on a gel containing 0.5 μg ethidium bromide, excise the DNA fragment with a clean razor blade, and purify using a gel purification kit (i.e., GENECLEAN II or Qiagen Gel Purification). Dialyze the DNA against 2 L of 0.5X TE overnight on a floating dialysis membrane. Spin-down the DNA solution and transfer supernatant to a fresh Microfuge tube, taking care not to disturb the precipitate. Check the DNA on a gel for purity.
27. 50 to 100 ng/μL will yield good results, though higher concentrations can be injected as long as the DNA is very pure. Higher concentrations can increase gene expression levels, but often result in increased lethality and non-specific DNA toxicity, often presented as a dorsalized phenotype with a reduction of the tail and trunk. However, abnormal embryos often have the highest expression levels, so it is critical to find a balance between the expression level and the survival rate.

28. Of the cells that will ultimately give rise to the germ line, only a small fraction will incorporate the transgene, leading to mosaicism within the germ line. As a result, founders will give rise to transgenic offspring at a frequency lower than the expected Mendelian frequency (50%), and in some founders the transgene will be present in only 1% of the embryos. Therefore, candidates that lack transgene expression in their progeny should be screened several times before concluding that the candidate is not a founder. Positive founders should be reconfirmed by outcrossing to a wild-type line.
29. Extraction of DNA from individual embryos or adult caudal tail fin clips should be performed in individual tubes, which can be facilitated by using a 96-well PCR plate. The extraction protocol used for individual embryos can be used for tail clips (**Subheading 2.9.2.**), though the fish should be sub-lethally anesthetized with Tricaine prior to fin clipping. Adjust the volume of extraction buffer (50–100 μL) and proteinase K (5 μL); all other steps are identical.
30. In the event that red blood cells are not desired, lyse red blood cells with the following red cell lysis buffer, also known as buffered ammonium chloride, or AKT: 155 m*M* NH_4Cl, 10 m*M* $KHCO_3$, 0.1 m*M* etheylene diamine tetraacetic acide, adjust pH to 7.4. Incubate on ice for 5 min, pellet at 200 to 300*g* for 5 min at 4°C, remove supernatant, resuspend pellet and rinse twice with large volumes of 0.9X PBS/FCS to stop the lysis reaction.
31. Each kidney contains on average 1.3×10^6 hematopoietic cells (D. Traver and L. I. Zon, submitted).
32. If the cell suspension is too concentrated or not filtered properly the flow cytometer will become clogged. Filter, pellet the suspension, resuspend, wash with a large volume, and re-suspend in 0.9X PBS/FCS/PI to an appropriate concentration.

Acknowledgments

We thank Alan Davidson for providing Fig. 1 and David Traver for Fig. 4. We would also like to thank Alan Davidson for providing expertise in various techniques including *in situ* hybridization, microinjection, and embryo flat-mounting, Hao Zhu for advice on creating transgenics, and David Traver for providing expertise in flow cytometry. We thank David Traver and Hao Zhu for careful review of this manuscript and Alan Davidson, Rebecca Wingert, and Kimberly Dooley for helpful discussions.

References

1. Amatruda, J. F. and Zon, L. I. (1999) Dissecting hematopoiesis and disease using the zebrafish. *Dev. Biol.* **216,** 1–15.
2. Dooley, K. and Zon, L. I. (2000) Zebrafish: a model system for the study of human disease. *Curr. Opin. Genet. Dev.* **10,** 252–256.
3. Driever, W., Solnica-Krezel, L., Schier, A. F., Neuhauss, S. C., Malicki, J., Stemple, D. L., et al. (1996) A genetic screen for mutations affecting embryogenesis in zebrafish. *Development* **123,** 37–46.
4. Ward, A. C. and Lieschke, G. J. (2002) The zebrafish as a model system for human disease. *Front. Biosci.* **7,** d827–d833.
5. Haffter, P. and Nusslein-Volhard, C. (1996) Large scale genetics in a small vertebrate, the zebrafish. *Int. J. Dev. Biol.* **40,** 221–227.
6. Ransom, D. G., Haffter, P., Odenthal, J., Brownlie, A., Vogelsang, E., Kelsh, R. N., et al. (1996) Characterization of zebrafish mutants with defects in embryonic hematopoiesis. *Development* **123,** 311–319.

7. Weinstein, B. M., Schier, A. F., Abdelilah, S., Malicki, J., Solnica-Krezel, L., Stemple, D. L., et al. (1996) Hematopoietic mutations in the zebrafish. *Development* **123,** 303–309.
8. Ekker, S. C. and Larson, J. D. (2001) Morphant technology in model developmental systems. *Genesis* **30,** 89–93.
9. Nasevicius, A. and Ekker, S. C. (2000) Effective targeted gene knockdown in zebrafish. *Nat. Genet.* **26,** 216–220.
10. Al-Adhami, M. A. and Kunz, Y. W. (1977) Ontogenesis of haematopoietic sites in *brachydanio rerio. Dev. Growth. Differ.* **19,** 171–179.
11. Detrich, H. W., 3rd, Kieran, M. W., Chan, F. Y., Barone, L. M., Yee, K., Rundstadler, J. A., et al. (1995) Intraembryonic hematopoietic cell migration during vertebrate development. *Proc. Natl. Acad. Sci. USA* **92,** 10,713–10,717.
12. Willett, C. E., Cortes, A., Zuasti, A., and Zapata, A. G. (1999) Early hematopoiesis and developing lymphoid organs in the zebrafish. *Dev. Dyn.* **214,** 323–336.
13. Bennett, C. M., Kanki, J. P., Rhodes, J., Liu, T. X., Paw, B. H., Kieran, M. W., et al. (2001) Myelopoiesis in the zebrafish, Danio rerio. *Blood* **98,** 643–651.
14. Lieschke, G. J., Oates, A. C., Crowhurst, M. O., Ward, A. C., and Layton, J. E. (2001) Morphologic and functional characterization of granulocytes and macrophages in embryonic and adult zebrafish. *Blood* **98,** 3087–3096.
15. Brownlie, A., Hersey, C., Oates, A. C., Paw, B. H., Falick, A. M., Witkowska, H. E., et al. (2003) Characterization of embryonic globin genes of the zebrafish. *Dev. Biol.* **255,** 48–61.
16. Catton, W. T. (1951) Blood cell formation in certain teleost fishes. *Blood.* **6,** 39–60.
17. Rowley, A. F., Hunt, T. C., and Page, M. (1988) *Vertebrate Blood Cells*, Cambridge University Press, Cambridge, NY, pp. 19–128.
18. Jagadeeswaran, P., Sheehan, J. P., Craig, F. E., and Troyer, D. (1999) Identification and characterization of zebrafish thrombocytes. *Br. J. Haematol.* **107,** 731–738.
19. Jowett, T. and Lettice, L. (1994) Whole-mount *in situ* hybridizations on zebrafish embryos using a mixture of digoxigenin- and fluorescein-labelled probes. *Trends Genet.* **10,** 73–74.
20. Sprague, J., Doerry, E., Douglas, S., and Westerfield, M. (2001) The Zebrafish Information Network (ZFIN): a resource for genetic, genomic and developmental research. *Nucleic Acids Res.* **29,** 87–90.
21. Westerfield, M. (ed.) (1994) *The Zebrafish Book: A Guide for the Laboratory Use of Zebrafish (Brachydanio rerio)*, University of Oregon Press, Eugene, OR.
22. Nüsslein-Volhard, C. and Dahm, R. (eds.) (2002) *Zebrafish*, Oxford University Press, New York, NY.
23. Trede, N. S. and Zon, L. I. (1998) Development of T-cells during fish embryogenesis. *Dev. Comp. Immunol.* **22,** 253–263.
24. Schorpp, M., Wiest, W., Egger, C., Hammerschmidt, M., Schlake, T., and Boehm, T. (2000) Genetic dissection of thymus development. *Curr. Top. Microbiol. Immunol.* **251,** 119–124.
25. Lieschke, G. J., Oates, A. C., Paw, B. H., Thompson, M. A., Hall, N. E., Ward, A. C., et al. (2002) Zebrafish SPI-1 (PU.1) marks a site of myeloid development independent of primitive erythropoiesis: implications for axial patterning. *Dev. Biol.* **246,** 274–295.
26. Jowett, T. (2001) Double in situ hybridization techniques in zebrafish. *Methods* **23,** 345–358.
27. Hudziak, R. M., Barofsky, E., Barofsky, D. F., Weller, D. L., Huang, S. B., and Weller, D. D. (1996) Resistance of morpholino phosphorodiamidate oligomers to enzymatic degradation. *Anti. Nuc. Acid Drug Dev.* **6,** 267–272.
28. Long, Q., Meng, A., Wang, H., Jessen, J. R., Farrell, M. J., and Lin, S. (1997) GATA-1 expression pattern can be recapitulated in living transgenic zebrafish using GFP reporter gene. *Development* **124,** 4105–4111.

29. Jessen, J. R., Jessen, T. N., Vogel, S. S., and Lin, S. (2001) Concurrent expression of recombination activating genes 1 and 2 in zebrafish olfactory sensory neurons. *Genesis* **29,** 156–162.
30. Higashijima, S., Okamoto, H., Ueno, N., Hotta, Y., and Eguchi, G. (1997) High-frequency generation of transgenic zebrafish which reliably express GFP in whole muscles or the whole body by using promoters of zebrafish origin. *Dev. Biol.* **192,** 289–299.
31. DeBlock, M. and Debrouwer, D. (1993) RNA-RNA *in situ* hybridization using digoxigenin-labeled probes: the use of high molecular weight polyvinyl alcohol in the alkaline phosphatase indoxly-nitroblue tetrazolium. *Anal. Biochem.* **216,** 88–89.

13

Imaging Early Macrophage Differentiation, Migration, and Behaviors in Live Zebrafish Embryos

Philippe Herbomel and Jean-Pierre Levraud

Summary

Because zebrafish embryos are transparent, cell behaviors and interactions can be directly imaged noninvasely in live embryos using differential interference contrast-Nomarski light microscopy. We found that the imaging quality can be much improved by coupling differential interference contrast-Nomarski to true (analogical) color video so as to visualize the image in real time on a high-resolution colour video monitor. We explain here how to apply this approach to the in vivo imaging of embryonic macrophages, which constitute a distinct early macrophage lineage, that originates from the rostral-most lateral mesoderm -adjacent to the cardiac field, differentiate in the yolk sac, and rapidly spread in embryonic tissues, although still retaining proliferative capacity.

Key Words: Zebrafish; macrophages; DIC microscopy; Nomarski; video microscopy; embryo; hematopoiesis.

1. Introduction

The zebrafish has recently become one of the major model species in vertebrate developmental biology. Fertilized eggs can be obtained virtually at will, in high numbers, on a daily basis. The embryos grow in water at room temperature and are optically transparent from fertilization to beyond hatching. Thus, using differential interference contrast (DIC) or "Nomarski" microscopy *(1,2)*, one can explore non invasively the detailed histology and cell behaviors throughout the live zebrafish embryos. Although DIC microscopy is routinely used in zebrafish labs worldwide, we found that its investigative power for zebrafish embryos can be dramatically enhanced by coupling it properly to video. The method that we describe here for the dynamic imaging of primitive macrophages can therefore be applied to the high-resolution study of any cell behaviors or tissue structure in live zebrafish embryos *(3–5)*. Even intracellular organelles such as mitochondria and lysosomes can be visualized in live embryos with this method.

From: *Methods in Molecular Medicine, Vol. 105: Developmental Hematopoiesis: Methods and Protocols.*
Edited by: M. H. Baron © Humana Press Inc., Totowa, NJ

2. Materials

1. A small zebrafish facility (≥ two tanks).
2. Embryo medium: Hank's buffered saline 0.1X, supplimented with 1 m*M* $CaCl_2$, 1 m*M* $MgCl_2$ (store at 4°C).
3. Methylene blue (1000x): 1g/L in H_2O; store at room temperature).
4. 1-Phenyl-2-thiourea (PTU), also known as phenylthiocarbamide (Sigma P7629). Make a 50X stock solution (1.5 g/L) in water and keep at 4°C. PTU is not very soluble; therefore, overnight stirring and mild heating is recommended for dissolution.
5. Tricaine (MS-222; amino benzoic acid ethyl ester; Sigma A5040). Make a 25X solution by diluting 400 mg of powder in 98 of mL water, adjust pH to approx 7.0 by addition of about 2 mL of 1 *M* Tris, pH 9.0. Prepare 5-mL aliquots and keep at –20°C. Once thawed, an aliquot kept at 4°C can be used for several wk.
6. Thermoregulated (28.5°C) incubator.
7. Dissecting microscope, preferably with transillumination.
8. A pair of very fine forceps (Dumont no. 5).
9. A very small paintbrush or another very fine, soft tool.
10. Wide-bore Pasteur pipets (smoothened glass or plastic).
11. Thin depression slides (26 × 76 × 1.5 mm) from different suppliers, providing different depression depths.
12. 20 × 20 mm No. 1 glass cover slips.
13. Upright microscope equipped with Nomarski optics.
14. Analogical Tri-CCD color video camera.
15. High-resolution color video monitor.
16. Time-lapse S-VHS video tape recorder.
17. DV (digital video) tape recorder.
18. Portable DV tape recorder (such as a mini DV camcorder).
19. Computer with DV image capture software (e.g., BTV Pro Carbon).

3. Methods

3.1. Preparing and Mounting Zebrafish Embryos

Methods for raising zebrafish will not be described here. Such methods, together with all main methods in zebrafish research, are described in the Zebrafish Book, available online at the central website of the zebrafish research community (http://zfin.org). Raising and breeding zebrafish is easy and cheap; a minimum of two 10-gallon tanks—one for raising, one for breeding—is sufficient for the purposes described here.

1. Collect fertilized eggs in the morning, transfer them to Petri dishes filled with "embryo medium" supplemented with 1 mg/L Methylene blue, and keep them at 28.5°C. The developmental times that we will mention here always refer to growth at 28.5°C, the standard growth temperature for zebrafish embryos, used to name developmental stages in terms of developmental time (http://zfin.org and **ref. *6***); for example, at 23 h post-fertilization (hpf), the embryo has 28 somites, and so on. However, because mating and egg-laying usually occur at about 9 to 10 AM (induced by onset of light), observing embryos from 20 hpf onwards, as suggested below (*see* **Subheading 3.3.2.1.**), would mean 5 AM! Therefore, we take advantage of the fact that zebrafish embryos actually develop normally at any temperature between 20°C and 33°C and accelerate or slow down their development by changing the growth temperature. The correspondence between growth temperature and growth rate is indicated in the staging series (http://zfin.org and **ref. *6***), but to give an idea: development at 25°C is 25% slower than at 28.5°C.

2. At the end of the d, just before leaving the lab, add PTU at 0.003%. PTU, a tyrosinase inhibitor, prevents the synthesis of melanin in the nascent melanophores and pigmented retinal epithelium, that would otherwise obscure some parts of the embryo from d 2 onwards. Divide the embryos in two dishes: one is kept at the standard temperature of 28.5°C, and the other is left at room temperature (typically 22–24°C), to slow down development and thus have earlier developmental stages also available the next d.
3. The next morning, remove the chorion from a dozen embryos manually under the dissecting scope, tearing it away with no. 5 fine forceps. Examine the embryos if possible under oblique transillumination, moving and rolling them carefully with a soft and fine tool (no. 10 brush, pulled yellow cone, hairloop) to check their developmental stage (*see* the staging series in **ref. *6***, which also is available on the zebrafish community website http://zfin.org).
4. Using a wide-bore pasteur pipet, transfer a few of these dechorionated embryos to a 2-cm petri dish containing 3 mL of embryo medium supplemented with 150 μL of tricaine. Tricaine, also called MS-222, is a commonly used anesthetic for fish and amphibians.
5. Transfer one embryo in a drop of medium and tricaine onto a glass depression slide (26 × 76 mm, choose slides of minimal thickness, typically 1.5 mm. The depression has a diameter of about 15 mm, and a depth at its center of about 0.2 mm. (0.5 mm depression slides from different suppliers have slightly different depression depths, which happen to be best adapted to embryos of different stages). The drop of medium must be big enough to overfill the depression; this will prevent the formation of bubbles in the next step. One can set up to four embryos per slide.
6. Put a 20 × 20 mm no. 1 glass cover slip on the slide, aside from the depression, then slide it slowly over the depression, while keeping control of the embryos with the fine tool. Just before the cover slip closes the depression, maintain the embryo in the desired orientation with the fine tool and slightly jam it in this position between the depression bottom and the cover slip.
7. Blot excess water carefully from the sides of the cover slip with Kleenex; this will seal the cover slip. The cover slip should slightly compress the embryo so that its position remains stable, yet not too tightly, which would block the blood flow. Embryos set up in this fashion will be happy for several hours (*see* **Subheading 3.3.3.**).
8. When the observation is over, the embryos can be easily recovered, left to develop under standard conditions, and be observed again at later times. To recover the observed embryos, water is added at the borders of the cover slip to unseal it, then the cover slip is delicately slid aside from the depression, the embryos are sucked in a wide-bore pasteur pipet and put back into PTU-supplemented embryo medium.

3.2. Video-DIC Imaging

3.2.1. DIC-Nomarski Microscopy

1. Use a microscope with true DIC optics, not ersatz. Keep in mind that DIC uses polarized light, therefore use only glass slides and cover slips, never plastic (which alters the polarization of light). As in any bright-field microscopy, the condenser should be centered and focused to achieve Köhler illumination. However, with objectives of 40X and higher, the depression slide is too thick to bring the condenser close enough to the sample to be correctly focused; therefore just center it properly, then raise it until it gently touches the slide. Open the field diaphragm as for Köhler illumination or less, and the aperture diaphragm to about 80%. Then, most important, tune the Nomarski prism properly. First find the position of maximum extinction, then move slightly away from it until you reach the best image. Note that moving the prism to the left or to the right of the position of maximal extinction provides contrasts—and resulting relief effects—of opposite signs.

One of the two makes much more sense to our brain than the other, for it can be more easily related to our perception of objects from shadowcast in real life: wherever individual cells stand out over the background, as in the blood, the cells should look convex to the observer (i.e., as bumps, not depressions). In dense tissues where the cells do not stand out individually over a background, the same rule actually applies: structures that are less aqueous (more refringent) than their environment, for example, nuclear membrane, mitochondria, nucleoli, should appear as bumps and worms, not as depressions or ravines, whereas vacuoles should appear as depressions (for discussion of interpretation of Nomarski/DIC images, *see* the primary **refs. *1*** and ***2***).

2. Once the Nomarski prism has been tuned, don't hesitate to re-tune the field diaphragm until you obtain the most satisfactory image. Each move to a new part of the embryo may benefit from some minute tuning of the Nomarski prism and field diaphragm.
3. DIC at highest magnification (100×) requires much light but is less sensitive to diaphragm conditions, therefore to provide more light, you may open the aperture diaphragm at 100%, and move the Nomarski prism slightly more away from extinction, without affecting image quality significantly.
4. We have used 40× and 100× oil objectives, plus an optional 0.80× lens built in the microscope; several manufacturers now offer long-working-distance water objectives, which are also quite satisfactory for DIC imaging of zebrafish embryos, and can give access to deeper tissues.

3.2.2. Contrast Enhancement and Further Magnification Through Video

Use an analogical tri-CCD color video camera that delivers a Y/C (luminance/chrominance) signal (through a four-pin Y/C cable) to a high-resolution 21-cm color video monitor (*see* **Note 1**; *see also* **Fig. 1**). We have used a Hitachi HV-C20 and its higher-performance, recently released sister, the HV-D25, with much satisfaction. Within the camera settings menu, set off all functions that alter the original signal from the CCD sensor, for example, "contrast," "gamma," "automatic gain control," for all these functions reduce the image contrast. Only one function should be set on, if present: the sharpening filter (called 'DTL filter' on Hitachi cameras, for which the maximum value, called 'high,' is best). The resulting image on the video screen has two advantages relative to that seen by the observer through the microscope eyepieces. First, it is further magnified. The final magnification depends on 1) the length of the microscope derivation that sends part of the light to the camera; 2) the size of the CCD sensor of the camera, (which can be one-third, one-half, or two-thirds of an inch; the smaller the sensor, the higher the magnification; ours is half an inch); and 3) the size of the video monitor. For instance, on our set-up, a tissue viewed through the 100× objective is enlarged 4000× on the screen of the 21-cm video monitor vs 1000× through the eyepieces (*see* **Note 2**). Second, the contrast is higher. This holds especially when using high-magnification objectives, such as 63× or 100×. With zebrafish embryos for instance, in the absence of video, the 100× objective is essentially useless because of insufficient contrast, whereas on the video screen, nicely contrasted images are obtained (**Figs. 2C**; **3D–F**; **4C,E,F**).

3.2.3. Recording and Processing Video Images

3.2.3.1. Recording Video Sequences

We record our video explorations on a S-VHS video tape recorder with a time-lapse option, and only later digitize selected images from the S-VHS video tapes. We

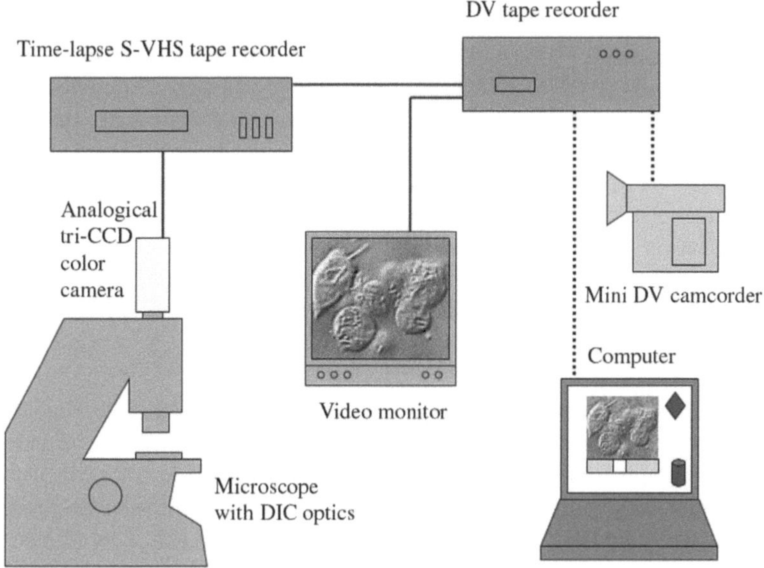

Fig. 1. Nomarski-DIC video-microscopy setup. Continuous lines represent connections through a four-pin Y/C cable, dotted lines represent digital "Firewire" (IEEC 1394) connections.

have used a Panasonic AG6730 (but also check Hitachi products). The tape recorder receives the Y/C video signal from the camera through a standard four-pin Y/C cable (**Fig. 1**).

3.2.3.2. Editing and Preparing Video Sequences for Presentations

We first select the most interesting sequences from the S-VHS tapes and copy them onto DV tapes, using a DV tape recorder (Sony DHR-1000) linked to the S-VHS tape recorder through a four-pin Y/C cable (**Fig. 1**). Because the images are encoded digitally on the DV tape, there is no detectable quality loss in the copying process and once on DV tape, the video sequences can be copied over and over from one DV tape to another with no quality loss. From this material we derive two kinds of products: 1) videos to be shown in seminars and conferences, and 2) still images and digitized movies.

To copy from one DV tape to another (for instance, to edit a precisely adjusted series of videos to be shown in seminars and conferences), a second DV player is needed. We use a mini DV camcorder to read the DV tapes and send the DV signal to the Sony DHR-1000 (through the dedicated Firewire cable), with which the precise editing is performed on a new tape. Once the final edited movie is achieved, the mini-camcorder can play it in conferences: it will send an analogical Y/C video signal to the videoprojector, again through a standard four-pin Y/C cable, and be played by the 'S-video' channel of the videoprojector (*see* **Note 3**). Thus, between the initial video capture from the microscope and the public projection of the final edited movie, there has been no perceptible loss in image quality.

3.2.3.3. Digitizing Single Images From the Videos for Publication

To prepare figures for papers, we digitize single images from the DV tapes on a PC or Mac using the Sony DVK-2000 capture board. Unfortunately, Sony no longer markets this quite convenient hard/software. However, several sharewares that do the job are available from individual programmers through the internet. For Mac users, we recommend BTVPro, which also includes time-lapse capture, image averaging, and an excellent manual explaining everything you always wanted to know about image formats, digitization of videos and existing compression protocols (http://www.bensoft ware.com; *see* **Note 4**). Once digitized, DIC images can be fruitfully processed with Adobe Photoshop to increase contrast and sharpness.

3.2.3.4. Digitizing Videos Into QuickTime Movies for Publication

Videos need to be digitized to be made available on the internet as supplementary material to a published article. A major problem is that 1 min of full-size video, once digitized (uncompressed), becomes a 800 megabyte (Mb) file (200 Mb if digitized from a DV tape, which already includes a fourfold compression), whereas presentation through the internet presently requires file sizes of only a few Mb. Therefore, to reduce the final file size, digitization softwares include various compression algorithms, which will reduce file size by 4- to 10-fold. It is thus necessary to further reduce file size through a heartbreaking process of impoverishing your video sequence, for example, by taking only one frame out of five, etc. We chose to digitize our movies through the Media Recorder software of a Silicon Graphics workstation, for in addition to the usual ways of reducing file size common to various softwares, Media Recorder allows you to reframe your video sequence so as to keep only the part of the image where the biologically relevant phenomenon is occurring. In many instances, this can save significant file size, reducing the need to impoverish the video sequence by undersampling it (*see* **Note 5**). However, some impoverishment is unavoidable. The overall scheme of our Nomarski/DIC videomicroscopy facility is shown in **Fig. 1**. If necessary, the cost of the facility can be reduced by omitting the DV tape recorder and choosing a mini DV camcorder that can also function as a tape recorder (many do).

3.3. Application to the Imaging of Early Macrophages in Zebrafish Embryos

3.3.1. Background

In all vertebrate species examined so far, the first leukocytes to arise in the embryo are macrophages, which first appear in the yolk sac, then spread through the embryo's mesenchyme, mainly of the head, and from there actively invade the forming organs before these have become vascularized *(4,5,7–18)*. These 'early' or 'primitive' or 'fetal' macrophages express the macrophage colony-stimulating factor (M-CSF) receptor yet do not seem to arise through the classical differentiation pathway involving monocytes. Indeed, monocytes are not found yet at such early stages. Also, once in the tissues, these early macrophages are often seen undergoing mitosis, whereas monocyte-derived macrophages are considered postmitotic. Based on this proliferation potential and on following the later kinetics of appearance of antibody-marked leukocytes in various tissues, Sorokin and Hoyt, using the rat, and Naito and Takahashi, using the mouse, provided data suggesting that these early macrophages may actually give rise to various self-renewed tissue macrophage and dendritic cell populations in the neonatal rodent (dermal and alveolar macrophages, Kupffer cells, Langerhans cells, and microglial cells; **refs.** ***9–11,19,20***; *see also* **refs.** ***18***). However, their actual fate in the adult remains to be directly investigated.

In mammals and birds, the origin of early macrophage precursors before they differentiate in the yolk sac is not known. In the zebrafish, we could trace their embryologic origin back to gastrulation. The surprising finding was that unlike all other hemopoietic lineages in amniotes—and probably also in zebrafish—their precursors did not originate from the caudal lateral plate mesoderm, but from the rostral-most lateral plate mesoderm, just next to the cardiac field ***(4)***. This rostral origin of early macrophages is not some exotic feature of the zebrafish. *Xenopus* early macrophages were recently found to arise from the very same region, that is, next to the atrial end of the cardiac field ***(15)***. In the zebrafish, we also found that this small region of rostral-most lateral mesoderm from which the early macrophages originate also gives rise to endothelial cells, that will notably make up the carotids ***(4)***. It thus conforms to the rule that emerged from mammalian and avian studies that hematopoietic lateral plate mesoderm is always also vasculogenic ***(21)***.

As these rostralmost lateral mesoderm cells complete their convergence to the embryo's midline, beneath the paraxial mesoderm and neural tube, the early macrophage precursors among them already segregate from the endothelial precursors, both in terms of markers and cell behaviour ***(4)***. These cells, already expressing hemopoietic markers (PU.1, draculin, CBP-β), but still with mesodermal morphology, then emigrate as single cells to the neighboring anterior aspect of the yolk sac, where they evolve into a homogeneous cell type with hemopoietic blast morphology, that we named the 'premacrophages' (**Fig. 2B**): round cells, 12 μm in diameter, with little cytoplasm and with obvious dot-like nucleoli, that divide frequently and reveal a steady 'miniblebbing' behavior on time-lapse video recordings. These cells then acquire more cytoplasm and become wandering young macrophages (**Fig. 2C**). Our 'pre' and 'young' macrophages are likely homologous to the 'primitive' and 'fetal' macrophages described by Naito and Takahashi in the mouse yolk sac ***(8)***. Then the young macrophages progressively become competent for phagocytosis—both of apoptotic bodies and of microbes—in the next few hours (typically by the onset of blood circulation, at 25 hpf). At about the same time, increasing numbers migrate to the embryonic head mesenchyme, a process that is M-CSF receptor-dependent, unlike all other aspects of their differentiation and fate that we could check ***(5,7)***.

3.3.2. Where and When (a Guide to Your Photo Safari in the Zebrafish Embryo)

3.3.2.1. The Yolk Sac

The best place to image these macrophages and the one to start with is the yolk sac, not only because they differentiate there, but also because the yolk sac has a very simple histological structure. Most of it is a big yolk mass, enveloped/surrounded by a thin syncitial cortex called the yolk syncitial layer (YSL), which distributes the yolk products to the embryo. Above this giant syncitial yolk cell, there is nothing but the body wall, which at this stage still consists in a thin ectodermal monolayer, termed

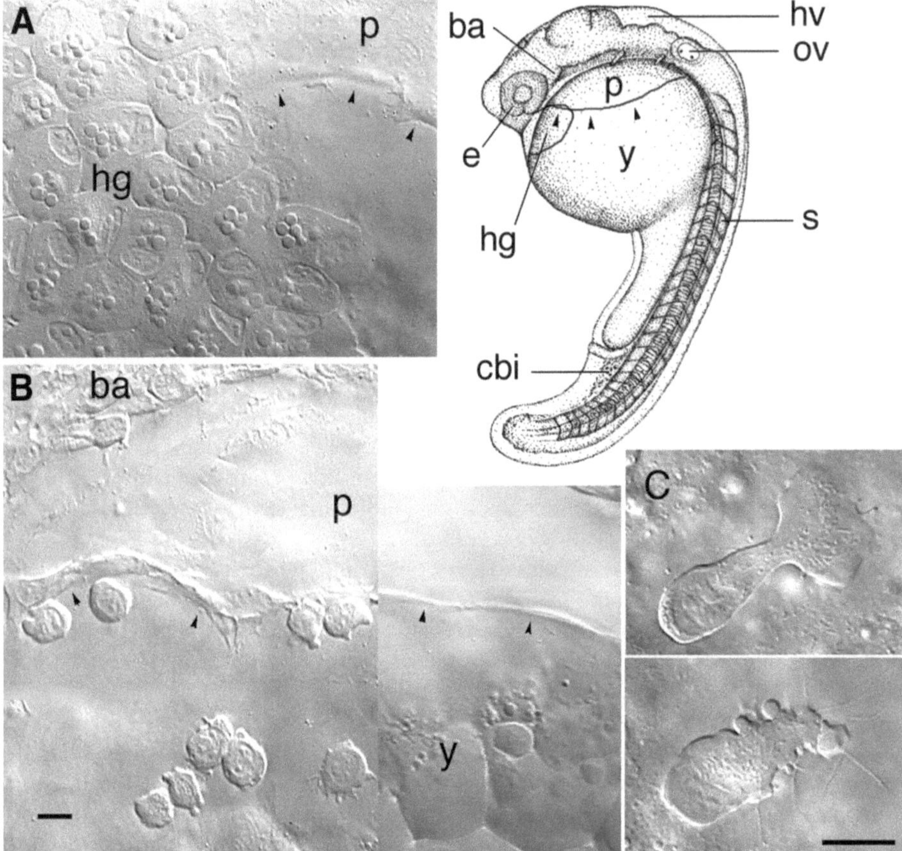

Fig. 2. Locating the differentiating early macrophages in the yolk sac of a live zebrafish embryo by DIC microscopy. The drawing on the top right ([from **refs.** ***1*** and ***2***] © Wiley-Liss, 1995; reprinted with permission of Wiley Liss, Inc., a subsidiary of John Wiley & Sons, Inc.) depicts the relevant landmarks in a zebrafish embryo at the stage (22 h after fertilization) and in the orientation (lateral) used to make the DIC pictures of a live embryo in **A–C**. The yolk ball is about 0.5 mm in diameter; the borders of the pericardial envelope (arrowheads) and hatching gland, both lying above the yolk ball, are delineated. **(A)** On the anterior quarter of the yolk sac, at this focal plane, the big hatching gland cells, with their large secretory granules and obvious eccentric nucleus, cover most of the pericardial hinge, thus only visible here to the right of the hatching gland cells (arrowheads). **(B)** At a slightly deeper focus, the same frame now reveals (beneath the hatching glands cells) the rest of the pericardial hinge (arrowheads), above which some cells and nuclei of the pericardial epithelium can be seen. The round, loose cells, some hanging onto the pericardial hinge, others a little away from it, beneath the hatching gland cells, are 'pre-macrophages.' Note their scant cytoplasm, clear dot-like nucleoli, and mini-blebs. Yolk platelets that make up the yolk ball are visible at the bottom right. **(C)** Still in the yolk sac but 1 h later (23 hpf): two successive views, 3 min apart, of a young macrophage wandering on the basal side of the overlying epidermis, about 50 μm away from the hatching gland. hg, Hatching gland; p, pericardium; ba, branchial arches; e, eye; y, yolk; hv, hindbrain ventricle; ov, otic vesicle; s, somites; cbi, caudal blood island. Scale bars, 10 μm.

epidermis, overlaid by an equally thin, protective squamous epithelium, the periderm (**Fig. 3A,B**). The early macrophages differentiate and then wander in the free space between the YSL and the epidermis, most of the time attached to and creeping on the basal side of the epidermis. This provides optimal DIC imaging conditions, for they are separated from the cover slip only by the very thin (about 4 μm) body wall. Moreover, since the yolk sac is spherical, the orientation of the embryo is not crucial in this case, for there is always some part of the yolk sac surface that lies tangential to the cover slip.

The differentiation of the wandering early macrophages from the blast-like 'premacrophages' can be easily imaged since about 21 hpf. Because this occurs on the anterior aspect of the yolk sac, we need to introduce two other tissues present there: the pericardial envelope and the hatching gland. The large pericardial envelope, which contains the heart, lies on the yolk cell dorsoanteriorly, beneath the eyes. Unlike the pericardial cells, which are exceedingly thin, the lateral border of the pericardium is very easy to find, for it is lined by an obvious line of fibroblast-like cells, which we call the pericardial hinge (**Fig. 2**, arrowheads). Many pre-macrophages are hanging onto the pericardial envelope at or close to the hinge, or stand a little away from it, under the adjacent hatching gland (**Fig. 2A,B**). Hatching gland is a somewhat misleading term, for this is merely a crescent-shaped monolayer of large, thick cells that are easily recognizable by their accumulation of large secretion granules, which locally interrupts the thin epidermal layer, just beneath the periderm (**Fig. 3B**). Each of these cells will pierce a short distance in between the periderm cells, to secrete out of the body its granules full of proteases that will locally degrade the chorion by 50 hpf, allowing the embryo to hatch. Thus, to find the premacrophages, take embryos at 20 to 23 hpf, first locate the hatching gland on the anterior-lateral aspect of the yolk sac, then focus a little deeper, and/or find the adjacent, also obvious pericardial hinge, as shown in **Fig. 2**.

At 24 hpf, cells of another hemopoietic lineage enter the yolk sac: the embryonic proerythroblasts. Unlike in mammals or birds or some other fish species, these cells in the zebrafish are not born in the yolk sac, but in the ventral side of the tail, at about the same site where later on the definitive hemopoietic precursors arise (**Fig. 2**). Quite intriguingly, 2 h before the onset of blood circulation, the proerythroblasts migrate from the tail to the yolk sac *(23)*, where they meet the young macrophages, in the space between the yolk cell and body wall. Upon their arrival there, they lose their motility, becoming strictly round pro-erythroblasts with no protrusions, that will divide frequently (**Fig. 4C**). A few of them die, and these are the first apoptotic cells that the early macrophages phagocytose (**Fig. 3E,F**).

At 25 hpf, the blood circulation slowly starts. Here the zebrafish displays a unique and experimentally very convenient feature among other teleosts: just downstream of the point where the veins carrying the blood from the head and the trunk merge into what would be the ducts of Cuvier, there is no blood vessel: the blood flows freely into the yolk sac, in between the YSL and body wall, only channelled by a depression on the YSL surface that we call the 'yolk sac circulation valley' (one valley on either side of the yolk sac; **Fig. 3A–C**). This blood flow takes most erythroblasts and some of the macrophages from the yolk sac away, first into the heart, and from the heart into the whole vasculature. But many of those macrophages that have remained in the yolk sac (instead of migrating to the head tissues through the mesenchyme) are now standing in the blood flow, mostly attached to the overlying epidermis **(Fig. 3B)**. When circulating

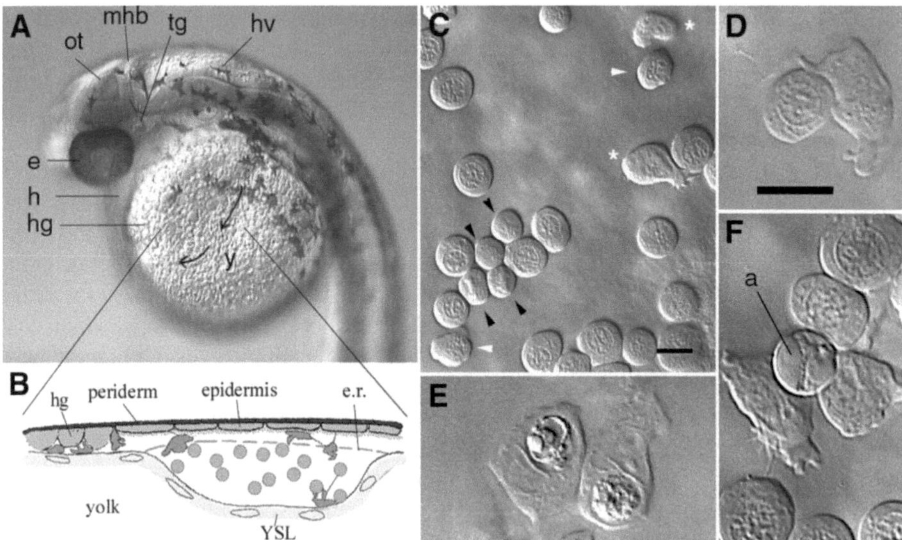

Fig. 3. The yolk sac circulation valley: an ideal window to image blood cell interactions. (**A**), and (**C–F**) are all DIC images of live embryos. (**A**) zebrafish embryo at 28 hpf (grown without PTU, hence the pigmented eye and scattered star-shaped neural crest-derived melanophores), that is, 3 h after the onset of blood circulation. Arrows show the path of the blood flow on the yolk ball, in the 'circulation valley' a mere depression on the yolk ball surface, as illustrated by the drawing in (**B**), which depicts a cross section through the valley; the YSL, with its oval nuclei, makes up the cortex of the yolk ball. In the valley, circles represent erythroblasts, and irregular shapes macrophages. Even though no vessel encloses the blood flow there, an endothelial sheet does slowly grow from 24 to 48 hpf from the trunk/cephalic veins over the yolk sac valley, progressively making up an 'endothelial roof' (depicted by a dotted line) covering the valley, though not on the ventral-most aspect, where the two valleys (from either side of the yolk sac) merge (our unpublished data). (**C**) 26 hpf, in the valley: erythroblasts divide frequently (black arrowheads, showing two pairs of freshly separated sister cells); a few erythroblasts still retain some irregular shape (white arrowheads) a remnant of their motile phase 2 h earlier, just before circulation onset (*see* text). (**D**) Early macrophages commonly adhere to the erythroblasts, seemingly exploring their surface. (**E**) Two macrophages that both phagocytosed an apoptotic body (from erythroblasts). (**F**) Another common situation at this developmental stage: an erythroblast has undergone apoptosis (a), two macrophages are in contact with it, yet will not phagocytose it for at least 1 to 2 h. y, Yolk; hg, hatching gland; h, heart; e, eye; ot, midbrain optic tectum; mhb, midbrain/hindbrain boundary; tg, trigeminal ganglion; hv, hindbrain ventricle. Scale bars, 10 μm.

erythroblasts touch them, these macrophages often stop them, explore them (**Fig. 3D**), and release them after a while to the circulation. When microbes are injected intravenously, they become quickly phagocytosed by the early macrophages. Again, the yolk sac circulation valley provides excellent conditions for imaging these macrophage/microbe interactions *(4,7)*.

3.3.2.2. Blood Vessels: The Caudal Vein

Some macrophages are continuously taken by the blood circulation. The most accessible vessel to image them is the caudal vein (*see* **Note 6**). In fact, as long as they flow in the caudal artery, they flow just like erythroblasts, but as soon as they enter the caudal vein, their behavior changes radically: they now roll on the vessel walls, just as mammalian leukocytes do in veinules—but here, the rolling can be imaged much more easily than in mice.

3.3.2.3. Embryonic Tissues

Outside the yolk sac and circulatory system (i.e., in the cephalic tissues, where they mostly emigrate, by 24–35 hpf), it is less easy to recognize the macrophages just by DIC, because of the more complex histological structure. As a visual help, the live embryos can be incubated for 5 to 8 h in 2.5 µg/mL of neutral red (in embryo medium), then rinsed for 30 min to 1 h in normal embryo medium. The neutral red readily penetrates the embryonic tissues and accumulates in the lysosomes of the most actively endocytic cells: above all, in the macrophages *(5)*. Although about two-thirds of these just show dark red dot-like, moving lysosomes, one third accumulate neutral red as one big spot, making them easily visible in any tissue (**Fig. 4C,D**). Comparison of the distribution of these heavily stained macrophages with the *in situ* hybridization data shows that they represent an evenly distributed sampling of the total population. Therefore, the vital staining with neutral red is a convenient tool to visualize their common habitats in the tissues. It is not appropriate for video-recording their motility, for heavily stained macrophages have clearly reduced motility.

Without vital staining, the macrophages in the cephalic mesenchyme can be clearly identified when they phagocytose apoptotic bodies, which happens for instance among neurons of the trigeminal ganglion around 24 to 30 hpf (**Fig. 4A**). Other sites where they can be readily identified are the body cavities: the pericardial cavity, the heart, and later (from 36 hpf) the hindbrain ventricle, which usually contains two to four resident macrophages, usually at its posterior end (**Fig. 4B**).

Among the epithelial tissues that become colonized from about 28 hpf onwards (brain, retina, epidermis; **ref. 5**), it is virtually impossible to recognize the macrophages within the dense brain or retinal neuroepithelium using only DIC (only their movement can be seen a posteriori, on rare time-lapse movies in which a macrophage happened to keep moving in the focal plane *[5]*). In contrast, they can be readily identified and followed up in the epidermis *(5)*, which at this stage is essentially a two-dimensional tissue: a thin cell monolayer, only containing 1) bulk, large and flat, epidermal cells; 2) ovoid mucous cells, and 3) less numerous macrophages. The trick is not to confuse mucous cells, which at a certain stage of their maturation have some motility, and macrophages (**Fig. 4E**).

From 40 hpf onwards, many mesenchymal and epidermal macrophages acquire refringent, highly motile granules, which facilitate their identification (**Fig. 4F**). The collective movement of these granules in the cytoplasm always anticipates the direction of the cell's movement.

At 55 hpf, all macrophages in the brain and retina simultaneously undergo the same phenotypic transformation, regardless of how long they have already resided in these tissues. Their gene expression pattern changes and they become much more avidly endocytic: upon vital staining with neutral red, they incorporate so much of the dye that they can be seen individually under a dissecting scope *(5)*. Since the transformation is brain and retina-specific, we have called the resulting cells 'early microglial cells'. From that stage onwards (55 hpf), any new macrophage that will enter the brain or retinal tissue will immediately adopt the early microglial phenotype. Such is the case of the numerous macrophages that colonize the optic tectum of the midbrain between 60 and 84 hpf *(5)*. Again, eventhough they can be very easily visualized by vital staining with neutal red, their heavy load of dye then hinders their motility, precluding a dynamic study.

These limitations on the embryonic tissues in which the macrophages can be recognized and imaged in vivo will vanish when a transgenic zebrafish line bearing specifically fluorescent (e.g., green fluorescent protein [GFP]-expressing) macrophages becomes available.

3.3.3. Time-Lapse Video Recording

Once the macrophages have been located, a time-lapse movie to document their behaviour can be made by using the 'time-lapse' option of the tape recorder. In this mode, instead of recording 25 frames/s, the standard video rate in thc PAL system (or 30 frames/s in the North American NTSC system), it will record them less frequently, by a factor that can be chosen from 4- to 80- or 240-fold, depending on the recorder. This will become the acceleration factor when the recorder plays back the sequence at the standard video rate. To perform a time-lapse sequence, the microscope stage must be perfectly stable (no drift in the *z*-axis; we sometimes stabilize it with scotch tape). Yet the embryo itself may drift a little, if only because it is developing; therefore, it is good practice to check the focus every 15 min or so.

Embryos up to 48 hpf can be kept in the depression slide mount previously described for several hours of observation, then be recovered and develop normally. Whenever their heartbeat decreases, during a long observation, just add some water with a Pasteur pipet at the edges of the cover slip (still under the objective). Very soon the heartbeat will come back to normal and you can continue the observation—you will just need to refocus the objective, because of the expansion caused by the added water.

3.3.4. DIC Microscopic Analysis of Fixed Embryos Subjected to Whole-Mount In Situ *Hybridization (WISH)*

WISH is a widely used, quite efficient method for visualizing the patterns of gene expression in zebrafish development. Although fixed embryos are less transparent

---

Fig. 4. *(opposite page)* DIC imaging of early macrophages in various embryonic tissues. Asterisks label the macrophage nuclei wherever visible. **(A)** 30 hpf; a phagocytic macrophage among neurons of the trigeminal ganglion (with their large nuclei containing one central nucleolus), in the cephalic mesenchyme. **(B)** 36 hpf; two macrophages in the hindbrain ventricle, one adherent to the hindbrain neuroepithelium, the other to the ventricle roof. **(C)** Neutral red staining (black) in the yolk sac circulation valley. Two macrophages display one large spot of neutral red, the other two only dot-like stained lysosomes; erythroblasts are unstained. **(D)** Two neutral red stained macrophages in the cephalic mesenchyme, close to the hindbrain basal lamina.

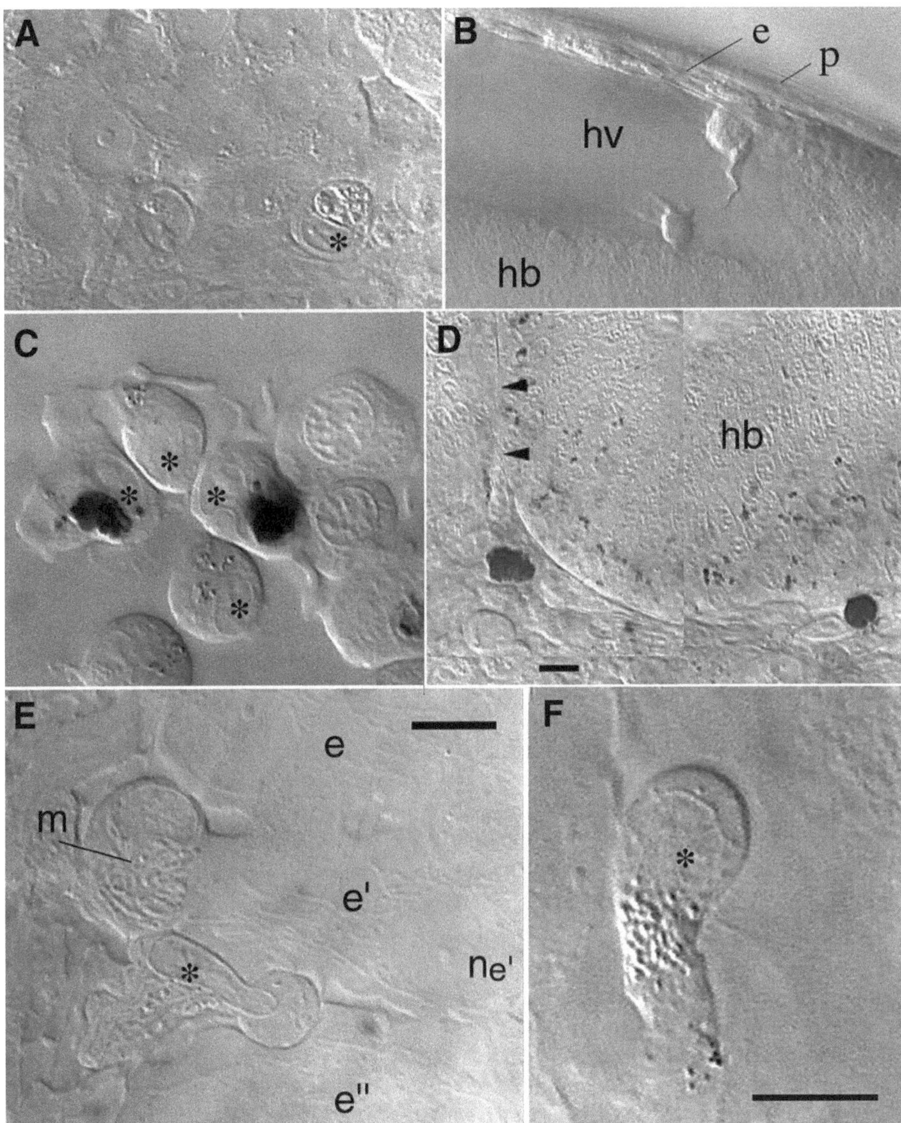

Fig. 4. *(continued)* Newly differentiated neurons in the ventral (bottom) part of the hindbrain also incorporate neutral red, thus demonstrating higher endocytic activity than the neuroepithelium. Arrowheads point at the midbrain-hindbrain boundary (*see* 'mhb' in **Fig. 2A**). **(E)** Yolk sac epidermis at 30 hpf. The three cell types are present here: three bulky, large and flat epidermal cells (e, e', e'') with clear worm-like mitochondria and nucleus (ne'), a mucus cell (m), and a macrophage. Two nuclei apparently bridging epidermal cells e and e' actually belong to the overlying periderm. **(F)** From 40 hpf onwards, many epidermal and mesenchymal macrophages now harbor refractile, highly mobile granules. hb, Hindbrain; hv, hindbrain ventricle; e, epidermis; p, periderm. Scale bars, 10 μm.

than live ones, DIC video microscopy can still be performed on them; the variety of histological details that are still recognizable despite the harshness of the WISH treatment is rather striking. Thus, using complementary ribonucleic acid probes such as L-plastin or fms that light up the early macrophages and exploring the resulting WISH-treated embryos with DIC video-microscopy, the precise relationship of the macrophages to anatomical microstructures can be visualized readily *(5)*. This is much faster and gives an easier three-dimensional rendering than going through the painstaking process of resin embedding and serial sectioning. Also, unlike with sectioned material, if the initial angle of analysis is not appropriate to understand the precise position of certain macrophages in the tissues—and it cannot be so for all of them—it can be changed at will.

3.4. Perspectives

Future developments in the in vivo imaging of zebrafish early macrophages should occur in two directions. First, when a transgenic zebrafish line harboring fluorescent (e.g., GFP or DsRed positive) macrophages becomes available, it will make it possible to follow the dynamics of the entire macrophage population in the embryo in real-time, using conventional confocal fluorescence microscopy, or the more recent spinning-disk confocal or two-photon microscopy. Such a transgenic line will also make it possible to identify every macrophage in the tissues and then to perform DIC Nomarski microscopy to reveal its cytological details. A combined fluorescence and DIC-Nomarski approach will be especially useful for following up the interactions of macrophages with microbes and apoptotic cells (*see* **Note 7**). Second, finer inter-cellular details of these interactions may become accessible by implementing in the basic DIC video microscopy set-up that we have described here: the real-time image processing techniques that made video-enhanced DIC microscopy so powerful in cell biology (namely, background substraction and image averaging, typically over 10–30 successive frames), making it possible to visualize microtubule dynamics and vesicle trafficking in intact cultured cells *(22)* many years before the advent of GFP-tagged proteins.

4. Notes

1. Here we mean real, analogical video, as opposed to the digital set-up used nowadays in most laboratories, in which a CCD camera sends digital signals to a computer. Such digital cameras are primarily designed for capturing fluorescence. They provide higher nominal resolution than analogical cameras such as the one we use (typically 1200 × 1200 pixels vs 768 × 576) but less contrast. In DIC microscopy, the limiting factor for image quality is not resolution, but contrast. Hence the use of analogical video. In addition, in our experience, DIC optics create false colors, which contribute to the contrast (aesthetic effects at low magnification may also be striking), and thus far, analogical video set-ups provide much better colour rendering than digital set-ups.
2. Although this magnification bonus does not change the resolution of the image, which only depends on the numerical aperture of the objective and condenser, it clearly improves our perception and understanding of details.
3. Alternatively, the DV camcorder can also deliver a 'normal' (composite) video signal to the 'video' channel of the videoprojector, through a standard RCA connector. Although the normal video signal is in principle of lower quality than S-video, at this final stage

this does not affect detectably the quality of the image projected on the screen.

4. When you select an image from the video on the screen of the video monitor and send it to the computer, which digitizes it, the resulting image on the computer screen most often does not look as good as the original. Don't conclude that the digitizing software has impoverished your image; this is only because of the lower performance of computer screens as compared with high-resolution video monitors.
5. Video sequences can be readily digitized from DV tapes at no cost, on any recent Mac computer, by entering the DV signal through the Firewire port and using the free iMovie2 software. This convenient but limited software is not sufficient to optimize the conversion of the videos into the small QuickTime movie files required for the Internet, but it is appropriate for making larger movie files that can be used in PowerPoint presentations.
6. Because the caudal part of the embryo is much thinner than the rest of the body, it tends to lie on the bottom of the slide's depression, far from the cover slip. Hence it is more often accessible using a long working distance water objective. We use these just as oil objectives, putting a drop of water instead of oil on the cover slip surface.
7. However, combining analogical DIC-Nomarski imaging with digital fluorescence imaging is not trivial, and will require dedicated automation.

References

1. Allen, R. D., David, G. B., and Nomarski, G. (1969) The Zeiss-Nomarski differential interference equipment for transmitted-light microscopy. Z. Wiss. Mikroskopie. u. *Mikroskopische Technik* **69,** 193–221.
2. Padawer, J. (1967) The Nomarski interference-contrast microscope. An experimental basis for image interpretation. *J. Royal Microsc. Soc.* **88,** 305–349.
3. Herbomel, P. (1999) Spinning nuclei in the brain of the zebrafish embryo. *Curr. Biol.* **9,** R627–R628.
4. Herbomel, P., Thisse, B., and Thisse, C. (1999) Ontogeny and behaviour of early macrophages in the zebrafish embryo. *Development* **126,** 3735–3745.
5. Herbomel, P., Thisse, B., and Thisse, C. (2001) Zebrafish early macrophages colonize cephalic mesenchyme and developing brain, retina and epidermis through a M-CSF receptor-dependent invasive process. *Dev. Biol.* **238,** 274–288.
6. Kimmel, C. B., Ballard, W. W., Kimmel, S. R., Ullmann B., and Schilling T. F. (1995) Stages of embryonic development of the zebrafish. *Dev. Dyn.* **203,** 253–310.
7. Davis, J. M., Clay, H., Lewis, J. L., Ghori, N., Herbomel, P., and Ramakrishnan, L. (2002) Real-time visualization of Mycobacterium-macrophage interactions leading to initiation of granuloma formation in zebrafish embryos. *Immunity* **17,** 693–702.
8. Takahashi, K., Yamamura, F., and Naito, M. (1989) Differentiation, maturation, and proliferation of macrophages in the mouse yolk sac. *J. Leuk. Biol.* **45,** 87–96.
9. Takahashi, K., Naito M., and Takeya, M. (1996) Development and heterogeneity of macrophages and their related cells through their differentiation pathways. *Pathol. Int.* **46,** 473–485.
10. Sorokin, S. P., Hoyt, R. F., and McNelly, N. A. (1992) Macrophage development: II. Early ontogeny of macrophage populations in brain, liver, and lungs of rat embryos as revealed by a lectin marker. *Anat. Rec.* **232,** 527–550.
11. Sorokin, S. P., McNelly, N. A., and Hoyt, R. F. (1992) CFU-rAM, the origin of lung macrophages, and the macrophage lineage. *Am. J. Physiol.* **263,** L299–L307.
12. Cuadros, M. A, Coltey, P., Nieto, M. C., and Martin, C. (1992) Demonstration of a phago-

cytic cell system belonging to the hemopoietic lineage and originating from the yolksac in the early avian embryo. *Development* **115,** 157–168.

13. Cuadros, M. A., Martin, C., Coltey, P., Almendros, A., and Navascues, J. (1993) First appearance, distribution, and origin of macrophages in the early development of the avian central nervous system. *J. Compar. Neurol.* **330,** 113–129.
14. Ohinata, H., Tochinai, S., and Katagiri, C. (1990) Occurence of non-lymphoid leukocytes that are not derived from blood islands in *Xenopus laevis* larvae. *Dev. Biol.* **141,** 123–129.
15. Smith, S. J., Kotecha, S., Towers, N., Latinkic, B. V., and Mohun, T. J. (2002). XPOX2-peroxidase expression and the XLURP-1 promoter reveal the site of embryonic myeloid cell development in *Xenopus*. *Mech. Dev.* **117,** 173–186.
16. Kurz, H. and Christ, B. (1998) Embryonic CNS macrophages and microglia do not stem from circulating, but from extravascular precursors. *Glia* **22,** 98–102.
17. Lichanska, A. M., Browne, C. M., Henkel, G. W., Murphy, K. M., Ostrowski, M. C., McKercher, S. R., et al. (1999) Differentiation of the mononuclear phagocyte system during mouse embryogenesis: the role of transcription factor PU.1. *Blood* **94,** 127–138.
18. Alliot, F., Godin, I., and Pessac, B. (1999) Microglia derive from progenitors originating from the yolksac and which proliferate in the brain. *Dev. Brain Res.* **117,** 145–152.
19. Mizoguchi, S., Takahashi, K., Takeya, M., Naito, M., and Morioka, T. (1992) Development, differentiation, and proliferation of epidermal Langerhans cells in rat ontogeny studied by a novel monoclonal antibody against epidermal Langerhans cells, RED-1. *J. Leuk. Biol.* **52,** 52–61.
20. Naito, M., Hasegawa, G., and Takahashi, K. (1997) Development, differentiation, and maturation of Kupffer cells. *Microsc. Res. Technol.* **39,** 350–364.
21. Pardanaud, L., Luton, D., Prigent, M., Bourcheix, L-M, Catala, M, and Dieterlen-Lièvre, F. (1996) Two distinct endothelial lineages in ontogeny, one of them related to hemopoiesis. *Development* **122,** 1363–1371.
22. Allen, R. D. (1985) New observations on cell architecture and dynamics by video-enhanced contrast optical microscopy. *Ann. Rev. Biophys. Chem.* **14,** 265–290.
23. Detrich, H. W. III, Kieran, M. W., Chan, F. Y., Barone, L. M., Yee, K., Rundstadler, J. A., et al. (1995) Intraembryonic haematopoietic cell migration during vertebrate development. *Proc. Natl. Acad. Sci. USA* **92,** 10,713–10,717.

14

In Vivo Methods to Analyze Cell Origins, Migrations, Homing, and Interactions in the Blood, Vascular, and Immune Systems of the Avian and Mammalian Embryo

Françoise Dieterlen-Lièvre, Sophie Creuzet, and Josselyne Salaün

Summary

In vivo experimental approaches that have been designed to study the ontogeny of the hematopoietic system in higher vertebrates are described in the present chapter. The avian embryo is directly available to manipulations *in ovo* during gastrulation and organogenesis. This permissiveness has led to the design of various approaches that provided crucial insights into the ontogeny of the hematopoietic system, particularly regarding traffic of progenitors between different compartments. In contrast, experimental manipulation of the developing mouse *in utero* is possible only during the second half of gestation, that is, the fetal period. This approach has been very useful in understanding how the immune system learns to distinguish self from nonself.

Key Words: Avian embryo; mouse embryo and fetus; embryogenesis; hematopoietic stem cells; *in ovo* microsurgery; grafts; *in utero* manipulation.

1. Introduction

Embryogenesis is characterized by extensive migrations of cell sheets or of individual cells. Concerning the hematopoietic system, which retains these migratory properties into adulthood, blood stem cell traffic is a particularly important feature in the embryo or fetus. A distinctive aspect of the blood forming system is that hematopoietic stem cells form in central locations and then radiate to various microenvironments, where they multiply and differentiate. These migrations may cover long distances and are not constrained in their directions. Consequently, although the mechanisms of cell movements, attraction, recognition, and interactions may be studied in vitro, the actual origins and trajectories of cells as well as the distinct fates resulting from different origins and influences encountered during migration and at the site of arrest must be unraveled in the embryo proper, thus requiring in vivo manipulations. These consist in replacing rudiments from one embryo with that of another (orthotopic grafts) or grafting extra rudiments in ectopic sites.

From: *Methods in Molecular Medicine, Vol. 105: Developmental Hematopoiesis: Methods and Protocols.*
Edited by: M. H. Baron © Humana Press Inc., Totowa, NJ

Regarding higher vertebrates, the model that lends itself most readily to such approaches at the stages of gastrulation, morphogenesis, and organogenesis is the avian model, whose embryo is easily accessible during development and is comparatively large. Recombinations between cells from two species, chicken and quail, serve as a basis for cell recognition ***(1,2)***. The two species are neighbors in the phylogenetic scale and have similar—although not exactly identical—rhythms of development. The yet-undifferentiated immune system does not interfere with the development of the grafts until after hatching. In contrast, the highly sophisticated approaches devised in the mouse model are genetic. These involve manipulations at the segmentation period, but refined surgery at the period of organogenesis is impossible. In vivo ectopic grafting techniques did, however, bring about significant advances in the understanding of immune development ***(3,4)***. These methods are reviewed in the present chapter. Previous papers have reviewed the methods that are applicable to the study of different developing systems in the avian embryo ***(5,6)***.

2. Materials

1. Incubator with temperature, ventilation and humidity regulators (*see* **Note 1**).
2. Stereomicroscope equipped with optic fibers (*see* **Note 2**).
3. Eggs: chicken (*Gallus gallus*) (*see* **Note 3**) and quail (*Coturnix coturnix japonica*).
4. Tables of development: for the chicken *(7)* and for the quail *(8)*.
5. Egg holders fitted with a series of round holes or with one hole.
6. Microsurgery instruments: (available from Société Moria, 11 rue George Besse, 92160 Antony, France; or Biotek, 34 rue des Chardonnerets, 92160 Antony, France; **Fig. 1**): 1) scissors; 2) Pascheff-Wolff iridectomy scissors; 3) black glass needle to manipulate grafts; 4) Barraquer surgical needle holder used for mouse *in utero* operations; 5) microscalpel (honed steel sewing needle) in a holder; 6) transplantation spoon; 7) ladle to manipulate whole embryos or large explants; 8) no. 5 Dumont forceps; 9) rhodorsil-based dissecting dish; and 10) micropipets made from microcapillaries.
7. Phosphate buffered saline.
8. Rhodorsil resin (Milian instruments SA, 35 route du Vélodrome CH 1228 Plan-les-Ouates, Genève – Ref. PU80NP).
9. India ink.
10. Carbon black.
11. Scotch tape.
12. Feulgen-Rossenbeck technique for deoxyribonucleic acid (DNA) staining.
13. QH1 antibody (Developmental Studies Hybridoma Bank, Dept. of Biological Sciences, University of Iowa, 007 BBE Iowa City, IA 52242-1324).
14. Nembutal, Avertin, or ketamine (Imalgène, Iffa-Merieux).
15. Surgical thread (Ethibond-Ethnor Paris).
16. LacZ or GFP transgenic mice.

3. Methods

3.1. Avian Embryo Manipulations

3.1.1. Opening the Egg

Freshly laid eggs from the vigorous strains of a chicken (*see* **Note 3**) obtained from a breeder should be stored at 15°C for at most 1 wk. Only if really necessary should

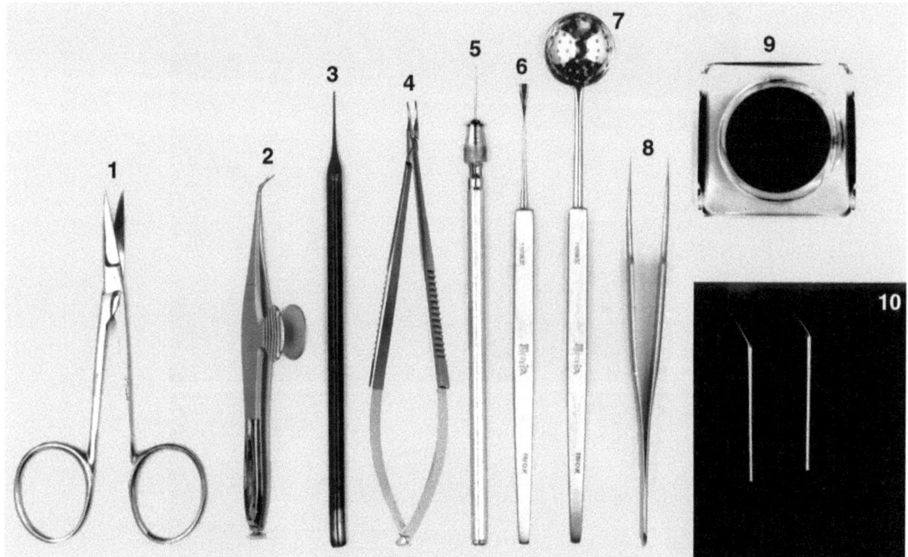

Fig. 1. Microsurgery instruments: **1**, scissors; **2**, Pascheff-Wolff iridectomy scissors; **3**, black glass needle to manipulate grafts; **4**, Barraquer surgical needle holder used for mouse *in utero* operations; **5**, microscalpel (honed steel sewing needle) in a holder; **6**, transplantation spoon; **7**, ladle to manipulate whole embryos or large explants; **8**, no. 5 Dumont forceps; **9**, rhodorsil-based dissecting dish; **10**, micropipets made from microcapillaries.

the eggs be cleaned and only then very rapidly and lightly with a humidified tissue (*see* **Note 4**). The eggs are incubated at 38 ± 0.5°C.

Eggs placed on holders can be incubated either with their long axis horizontal or vertical. The yolk rotates depending on the egg orientation, so that the blastodisk settles in the highest position. When the egg is horizontal, the embryo is more accessible, whereas the vertical position is more favorable for long-term survival and, if wanted, hatching. The blastodisk must be located exactly beneath the window made in the shell. The eggs should be incubated in the desired position for at least 24 h before manipulation. In both positions a round or oval window is cut out in the shell with small scissors above the blastodisk. Before opening, the egg is rapidly swabbed with 70% alcohol (*see* **Note 5**). As the blastodisk develops against the shell membrane, when the egg is incubated horizontally, it is necessary to draw out 2 to 3 mL of albumin through a small hole made in the pointed end of the egg to lower the blastodisk and avoid injuring it when opening the window. The hole is sealed with a drop of paraffin or a piece of tape. If the egg is incubated standing, the window is made at the level of the air chamber, where the shell membrane is split in two layers and there is no danger of injuring the blastodisk. Gently tearing away the lower layer of the shell membrane provides access to the blastodisk (**Fig. 2**).

After surgery, the window made in the shell is carefully closed with a piece of scotch tape (*see* **Note 6**).

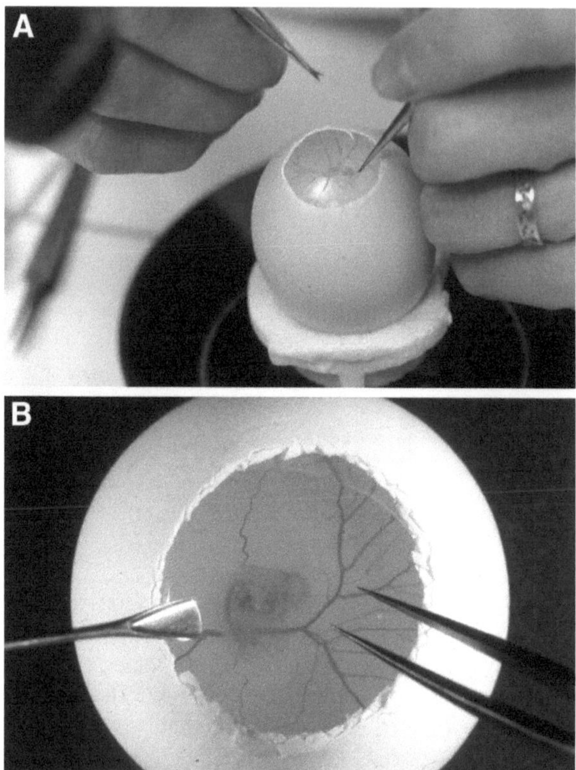

Fig. 2. Opening and accessing the chicken embryo. The egg has been positioned with its long axis vertical (**A**). The higher magnification (**B**) allows a full view of a 4-d-old embryo, with the yolk sac vascular network and the dorsal aorta.

3.1.2. Manipulation of the Embryos

Manipulations are performed under a dissecting microscope equipped with continuous magnification from 6× to 50×. Optic fibers are used to illuminate the embryo sideways. At early stages (E1, E2) it is useful to visualize the embryo against the background of the yolk, with a few drops of diluted India ink injected under the blastodisk (**Fig. 3**; **ref.** *3*). A curved glass micropipet containing the ink is inserted in the extra-embryonic area from a lateral position and pushed under the blastodisk. The particles of India ink fall to the bottom of the vitellus within a few hours and are not detrimental to development.

Microscalpels (**Fig. 1**) are prepared from stainless-steel sewing needles by honing and stropping on an Arkansas oil stone into the shape preferred by the user. Rhodorsil-bottomed dishes are prepared by mixing the two components of the resin, which are polymerized under ultraviolet light according to manufacturer's instructions. Before polymerization, carbon black is added to the resin. The advantage of rhodorsil is its resiliency, which ensures that needles do not leave a mark.

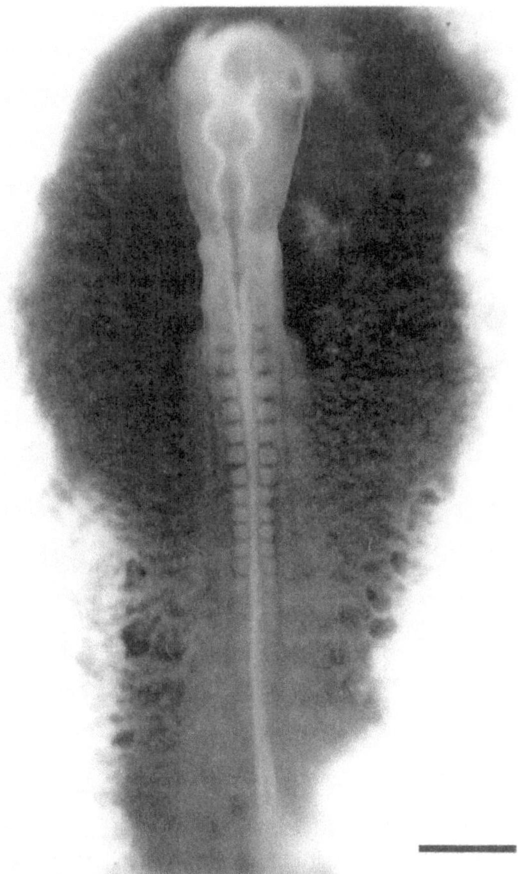

Fig. 3. Chick embryo with 15 pairs of somites prepared for in ovo surgery against a black background. A few drops of diluted India ink (1 vol/L vol phosphate-buffered saline) have been injected beneath the blastoderm using a curved glass micropipet inserted through the extraembryonic area. Scale bar: 200 μm.

3.1.3. Cell Markers

3.1.3.1. Sex Chromosomes *(9)*

In birds, the heterogametic sex is the female; the sex chromosomes are designated Z and W, the male being ZZ and the female ZW. The ZZ chromosomes of the male constitute the fifth largest pair of chromosomes. All the other pairs are minichromosomes. ZZ chromosomes may be identified by medially located centromeres. The female W chromosome, smaller than the Z, is similar in size to the seventh pair of autosomes but possesses a more medially located centromere. To obtain enough dividing cells to examine a number of metaphases, Colcemid is administered to the embryo 24 h before sacrifice.

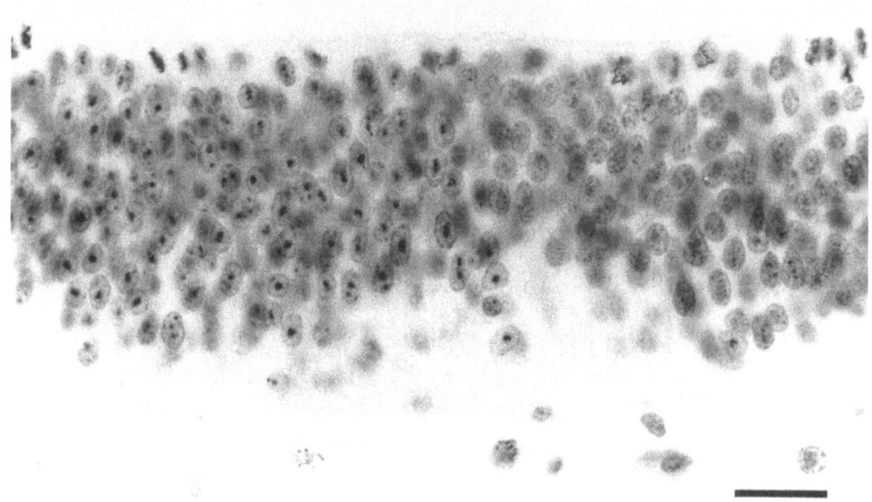

Fig. 4. Chimeric neuroepithelium at 4 d of incubation. A quail hemimesencephalon was grafted orthotopically for 2 d in a 2-d-old chick embryo. Quail cell nuclei (to the left) show the typical quail nucleolus with a large heterochromatin clump, whereas chick cells (to the right) display dispersed heterochromatin. Note the perfect merging of graft and host tissues, without any cell mixing in this type of graft. The section is 5-μm thick; Feulgen-Rossenbeck staining without counterstain. Scale bar: 20 μm.

However, this treatment is very toxic, and a high proportion of embryos die soon after receiving it. To avoid this problem, Le Douarin et al. ***(10)*** performed the Colcemid treatment in vitro (on thymocyte suspensions from male-female quail parabionts).

3.1.3.2. Quail Chick Combinations (*See* **Note 7**)

A prominent heterochromatin component in quail cell nuclei serves as a label for the progeny of quail cells grafted in chicken hosts. Chicken and quail nuclei are particularly clearly discriminated after DNA staining according to the Feulgen-Rossenbeck technique because a large mass of heterochromatin is associated with the nucleolus (or nucleoli depending on cell types) in all quail cell nuclei (**Fig. 4**). In contrast, chicken cells display small DNA dots dispersed in the whole nucleus. A number of monoclonal antibodies have been obtained that recognize cells of one species and not the other, providing excellent resolution both on tissue sections and in cell sorting. The QH1 antibody ***(11,12)*** recognizes the endothelial and hematopoietic lineages in the quail only (**Fig. 5**).

3.1.4. Heterotopic Grafts

Hematopoietic stem cells of extrinsic origin colonize the stroma of organ rudiments. This developmental dissociation in origin was discovered by means of experiments involving the transplantation of organ rudiments to heterotopic locations.

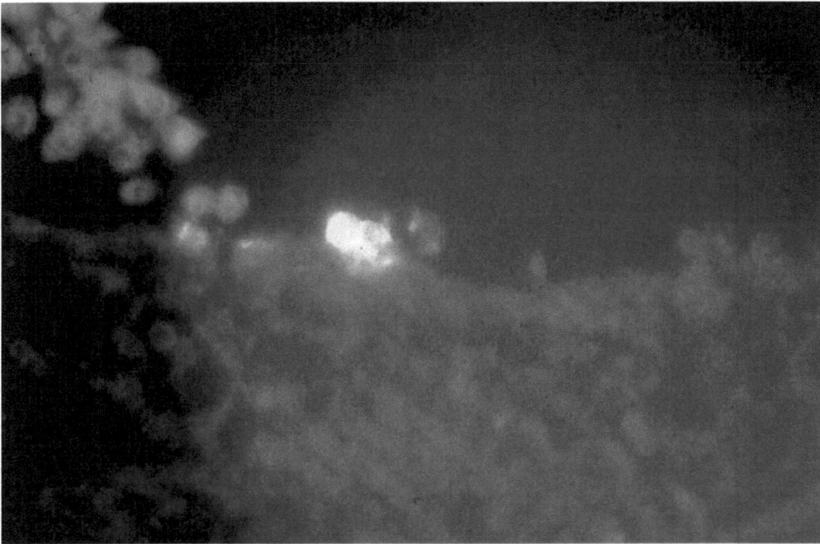

Fig. 5. Chimeric aorta in E3 chicken embryo. Twenty-four hours earlier, splanchnopleural mesoderm from a quail embryo was grafted on top of the host homologous germ layer. Quail cells, which have integrated in the host endothelium and are giving rise to hematopoietic cell clusters, are stained by means of the QH1 antibody (immunofluorescence). Reprinted with permission from *Development* 1996; **122,** 1363–1371.

3.1.4.1. Chorioallantoic Grafts and Injections Into Chorioallantoic Veins

The chorioallantoic membrane (CAM) is a good culture support for animal cells and tissues, providing necessary nutrients (*see* **Note 8**). The shell is opened at 6 to 10 d of incubation, at the level of the air chamber, where the shell membrane is split into two layers. The upper layer comes away with the shell. The lower layer is torn open carefully, avoiding hemorrhages, and the tissue or rudiment is deposited on the CAM in a region with no large vessels. The graft soon embeds into the CAM and becomes densely vascularized.

It is also possible to inject cells into a CAM vein. The egg, incubated for at least 12 d, is candled and a site of vascular branching is marked on the shell. Using a circular saw, a triangle is cut in the shell around this branching, taking care not to injure the shell membrane. This membrane is made transparent by the application of an oil droplet; the vessels become visible and remain adherent to the shell membrane, so that a glass needle may be inserted tangentially, without the vessel rolling away in depth.

3.1.4.2. Grafts Into the Somatopleura, Coelom, and Dorsal Mesentery

These operations are performed in embryos that have reached the approximate stage of 30 somites (52 h of incubation). The transplants are introduced through a slit made in the body wall, after the vitelline membrane and the amnion have been split away. In somatopleural grafts, the transplant is inserted in the opening **(Fig. 6)**,

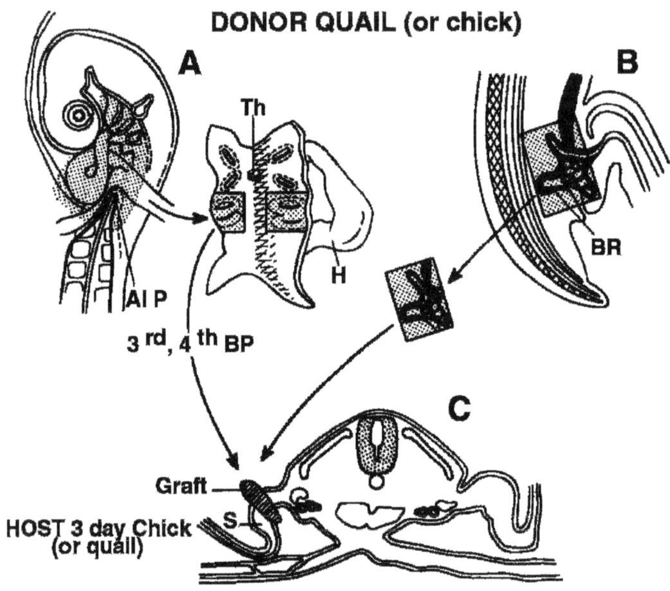

Fig. 6. Somatopleural grafting in the case of the thymus or bursa of Fabricius. (**A**) A 3-d donor for the floor of the pharynx; (**B**) a 6-d donor for the bursa rudiment (BR); and (**C**) a transverse section in the trunk of a 2-d recipient showing the position of the graft. AIP, anterior intestinal portal; BP, branchial pouch; H, heart; S, somatopleura; Th, thyroid.

whereas in coelomic grafts the transplant is pushed into the body cavity. For grafts into the dorsal mesentery, the transplant is pushed deeply in the tissues just ventral to the dorsal aorta. It is critical to avoid injury to a large blood vessel. Usually a few grains of carbon black are deposited on the transplant, facilitating its retrieval at the end of the experiment.

3.1.5. Orthotopic Grafts

These grafts ensure optimal growth of the transplants and permit more or less complete replacement of the host homologous organ. Thus, it is possible to evaluate the fate of the transplant, cell seeding to the developing embryo, and the role of the rudiment in development.

In situ thymic grafts involve in a first step the removal of the chicken host thymic primordia ***(13)***. After opening the egg at E5 (HH stage 25–26) ***(7)*** and laying bare the embryo, the tegument of the neck is incised above the vagus nerve, visible through the skin. The thymic primordia on each side, which appear as white masses between aortic arches III–IV and IV–V, are dissected and sucked out with a micropipet (0.1-mm tip internal diameter). The operation is repeated on the left side after rotating the embryo inside the amniotic cavity. Injury to the aortic arches and jugular veins must be avoided. Quail thymuses obtained from E5 (precolonization) or E6–8 (postcolonization) are inserted in the spaces created by ablation of the host primordia.

Like thymectomy, bursectomy ***(14)*** is a delicate operation because it is performed on E5 chicken embryos, which are highly vascularized. A window is made in the chorion and amnion above the posterior part of the embryo and the right limb is deflected by means of a humid cotton strand, whose ends are placed so that they adhere to the eggshell. The tail is extended with curved tweezers. The bursal rudiment is removed by a transverse cut in the anal plate, close to the ureters, and two lateral cuts. The E5 quail bursal primordium, separated from surrounding mesenchyme, is inserted in the space created by removal of the host bursa, in proper anteroposterior and dorsoventral orientations.

In situ somite transplantation has been implemented to determine the relative contributions of somites and lateral plate to the building of the vascular network and hematopoietic system. The somites selected for replacement are always the last formed (in avian embryos, the most caudal ones). Thus, no cells have begun emigrating out. One, two, or three somites or a longer string of them are dissected out from the donor and treated briefly with trypsin or pancreatin in order to remove contaminating tissue, that is, ectoderm on top and aortic roof below. Corresponding somites are mechanically dissected out from the host *in ovo*. The somites prepared for grafting are placed in the groove created by the removal of host somites and the ectoderm soon heals. This type of graft showed that the dorsal aorta has a double origin: roof and sides from the somites, hematopoietic cell-producing floor from splanchnopleural lateral plate mesoderm ***(15)***.

3.1.6. Yolk Sac Chimeras ***(16)***

This manipulation is conducted before the extraembryonic coelom has formed and consists in grafting the presumptive body of the quail embryo onto the extraembryonic area of the chicken, the latter splitting soon after into the yolk sac and amnion. Chicken and quail blastodisks, respectively incubated 36 and 30 h, are matched for stage according to their number of somites. The quail donor blastoderm is explanted onto a rhodorsil-covered Petri dish in phosphate buffered saline and trimmed to leave only a small margin around the embryonic body. The quail presumptive body is then carried onto the chick blastodisk and positioned belly down in the same cephalocaudal orientation as the chicken embryonic body. The vitelline membrane of the host is then torn away and the embryo excised. The quail embryo should be a little larger than the cavity created by the excision. It is gently transferred over the cavity and the two overlapping margins are resected simultaneously with Pascheff's scissors around the whole circumference (**Fig. 7**). The adhesive properties of embryonic tissues ensure that host and recipient tissues remain seamed together. The egg is sealed.

In a variant approach, only part of the embryonic body of the chicken is replaced by the homologous zone of the quail ***(17)***.

3.1.7. Parabiosis

In the classical technique, small holes are bored into the shells of two unincubated chicken eggs. The holes are placed facing each other and the eggs sealed together with a paraffin ring surrounding the holes ***(9)***. In the course of incubation, the chorioallantoic membranes of both embryos grow toward each other and blood vessels anastomose. In a similar technique, Le Douarin et al. ***(10)*** parabiosed two quail embryos.

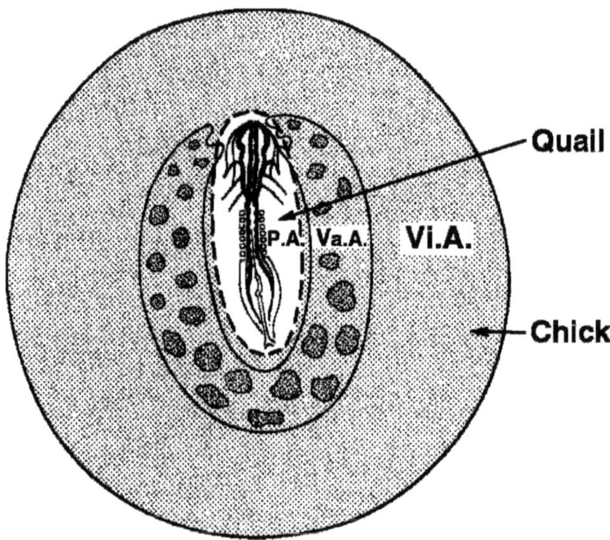

Fig. 7. Construction of a yolk sac chimera. The stippled line indicates the suture between the two components. P.A., pellucid area; Va.A., vascular area; Vi.A., vitelline area.

The shell of a chicken egg was used as a culture vessel into which the contents of two unincubated quail eggs were poured (before incubation, when the vitelline membranes have not yet ruptured). A sex-linked albino mutation was used to identify male/female pairs. Cell exchanges were detected by means of sex chromosome analysis at the end of the experiment.

3.1.8. Electroporation

Electroporation aims at transferring nucleic acid sequences into living cells. The principle is based upon a transient permeabilization of the cell membrane triggered by an electrical impulse, which enables an exogenous nucleic acid sequence to enter the targeted cells and become trapped in the cytoplasm as the cell membrane recovers its integrity. First devised in vitro, this technique has been successfully adapted to in vivo transfection in the mid nineties. It turns a unique pulse of high voltage—with an exponential decay—into a series of square low voltage iterative pulses applied to the two electrodes, anode and cathode. When placed in a polarized electric field, nucleic acids (globally negative molecules) are displaced towards the cathode. According to the above principle, the interposition of an epithelium between the nucleic acid solution and the cathode results in the directional transfer of the foreign nucleic sequence into the epithelial cells. Because of the instantaneousness and highly efficient penetration of the vector into the cells ***(18)***, this technique has rapidly conquered the field of avian embryology, in which no efficient means of transgenesis had been achieved before. This technique has allowed the study of gene function in avian developmental processes with the added feature that, in this class of vertebrates, classical embryonic tissue manipulations can be combined with molecular approaches.

Two kinds of constructs can be used to achieve either ectopic gene expression or overexpression, plasmids or retroviral vectors (*see* **Note 9**). The main drawback of plasmids resides in the non-permanent integration in the transfected-derived cells, thus leading to progressive loss of the vector and finally turning off the foreign gene expression whose Prinetics tightly defend on the preliferative rate of the recipient tissue. In contrast, the use of retroviruses that randomly integrate into the host genome by means of their long terminal repeat sequences ensures a stable transfection of the exogenous DNA. Exploiting the species-restricted infectious ability of virus into either a permissive or repellent environment provides an elegant approach to limit or promote the spread of retroviral contamination in a tissue-specific manner *(21)*.

However, one should be aware that at present this technique, very successful for epithelial cell transfection, has not been mastered for endothelial cell transfection. The latter cells are very thin and delicate and rupture when the electric impulse is applied (T. Jaffredo, personal communication). However, the whole endothelial network may be labeled by means of low-density lipoproteins *(22)* or retroviral vectors *(23)* injected into the heart of E2 to E4 chicken embryos (*see* **Note 10**). The labeling solution is inoculated by means of a borosilicated glass needle drawn into a tip approx 30 μm in diameter, in order not to damage the heart wall. The liquid is gently flushed into the circulation and distributes to the whole vascular tree.

3.2. Mouse Embryos or Fetuses

3.2.1. Anesthesia

Anesthesia is performed by intraperitoneal injections. The choice of an anaesthesic is crucial for the success of experiments. Rather than Nembutal or Avertin, used during early stages of gestation, ketamine (0.5–0.7 mL) is usually preferred between E12 and E17 for its lower abortion-inducing risk.

3.2.2. Exposing and Preparing the Uterus

A vertical incision is performed on one side of the abdominal wall in the anesthetized pregnant mouse (*see* **Note 11**). The uterus is exteriorized and the mouse is laid down on a sterile gauze cushion under a Zeiss stereomicroscope equipped with optic fibers.

3.2.3. Intraplacental Injections

In this technique, used by Fleischman and Mintz *(24)* to restore genetically anemic mice with fetal liver cells from normal fetuses, the uterine horns of pregnant mice were exposed on d 11 of gestation. The tip of a micropipet containing the cell suspension was inserted through the uterine wall into each placenta, located approx one-fourth the distance from the uterine mesometrial attachment to the antimesometrial point; $1–2 \times 10^5$ cells were injected in each placenta.

3.2.4. Intrafetal Grafting

Intrafetal grafts can been performed at later stages of gestation *(25)*. Days 14 to 17 pregnant females are anesthetized with ketamine. The abortion is lowest when only one fetus in each horn is engrafted. However, it may be necessary to engraft several or all fetuses. In this case, it is advisable to operate on fetuses in one uterine horn only.

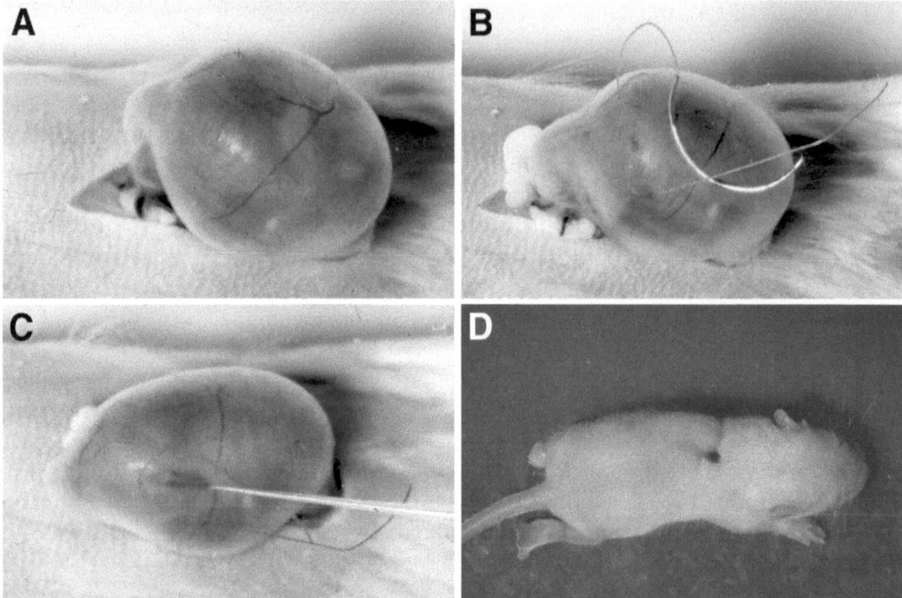

Fig. 8. (**A**) Exposure of one uterine swelling containing an E16 fetus. (**B**) A thread is passed in the uterine wall, prepared for closure of the opening after the operation. (**C**) Subcutaneous transplantation of an explant by means of a micropipet, after incision of uterus and fetal skin. (**D**) BALB/c young mouse (white strain), engrafted before birth (E16) with age-matched skin from a C57BL/6 donor (black strain).

The uterine segment containing one conceptus is exteriorized (**Fig. 8A**). A thin surgical thread (Ethibond-Ethnor Paris) is stitched around a small area of the uterine wall just above the fetus (**Fig. 8B**). Small slits are made through the uterine wall inside this area and then through the fetal thoracic cage between two ribs. The transplant is inserted in this slit using a micropipet (**Fig. 8C**). Grafts can be inserted into the coelomic cavity of the host or subcutaneously. In the latter case, the explant is placed under the skin of the back.

True skin grafts can also be performed, usually between two strains with different coat colors (**Fig. 8D**; **ref.** ***26***). A small piece of skin is removed from the host with Pascheff scissors and replaced by skin by the donor. Extra-thin surgical thread (Ethicon, BV 100, Effner framed) is used to sew up the donor skin all around. Finally, injections into the liver of fetuses on the 15 to 17 d of gestation through the fetal body wall are feasible, as the large and deeply red liver is readily visible at these stages through the uterine wall.

After each of these operations, the slit in the uterine wall is closed by tightening the Ethibond thread that was inserted previously. The uterus is then pushed back into the peritoneal cavity. The mother's abdominal wall and skin are then stitched one after the other. The operated mouse is place in a warm cage until it wakes (*see* **Note 12**).

3.2.5. Markers

Several markers are available to trace the progeny of injected cells, such as MHC antigens, Y antigen, lacZ, and green fluorescent protein. Intrafetal grafts often are marked with a few grains of carbon black so that they can be easily found at sacrifice. Carbon black can also be used to mark the injected fetuses among non-injected ones: a few grains of the powder introduced under the skin of the back make the operated animals immediately identifiable at birth.

3.2.6. Insights Obtained Using These Techniques

The existence of hematopoietic stem cells was demonstrated in the adult by the irradiation/reconstitution experiments of Till and McCulloch ***(27)*** as well as the occurrence of traffic of these cells between different organs. The approaches described here extended these findings to embryonic and fetal development in the chicken and mouse ***(9,10)***. Such manipulations in the embryo led to insights such as the extrinsic origin of hematopoietic stem cells in relation to hematopoietic organ rudiments and their sequential commitment in the yolk sac ***(9)*** and in the aorta ***(2,22,23)***. Mouse *in utero* manipulations have revealed the crucial role of the thymic epithelium in the establishment of tolerance ***(28)***.

4. Notes

1. Large incubators for industrial breeding rock the eggs at regular intervals. Automatic rocking, which best ensures proper development of the CAM and embryo, is needed when long term incubation and hatching are desired. It should be stopped when the embryos have been operated on, lest the CAM vessels become injured on the edge of the operating "windows" opened in the shell. For most experimental uses, small incubators with nonmobile trays are appropriate. Many models are available.
2. Optic fibers do not radiate heat, which is detrimental to the embryo.
3. The White Leghorn strain is the most widely used. Other strains may be useful for specific purposes.
4. The eggshell is naturally covered with a protective film and is highly permeable to small molecules.
5. The yolk is rich in lysozyme and also contains maternal immunoglobulins. The embryo is thus very resistant to contamination.
6. It is important to apply the scotch tape tightly, without creases, to avoid desiccation.
7. Usually, grafts are performed from a quail donor into a chicken host. It is advisable to verify the results in this combination with results in the reverse, when the type of operation permits.
8. Vascularization in this site is very dense, so that development of the graft may be different from that in more "normal" sites.
9. Plasmids with a combination of highly efficient regulatory sequences that link, for instance, the β-actin promoter and the cytomegalovirus enhancer (e.g., pCAGGS) ***(19)*** or duplicated β-actin promoters linked with an IRES (Internal Ribosome Entry Site) sequence (e.g., pMIW) ***(20)*** yield the highest exogenous DNA expression.
10. Younger embryos are visualized by India ink injection in the subgerminal cavity.
11. The mouse belly is first swabbed with 70% alcohol and the area to be incised is depilated.
12. Because operated newborns are frequently eaten by their mother, they are usually recovered by cesarean section and transferred to an adoptive mother with newborns of her own, from a gentle, more maternal strain (129Sv).

Acknowledgments

We are indebted to Marie-Françoise Meunier for manuscript preparation, and to Francis Beaujean and Michel Fromaget for preparing the iconography.

References

1. Le Douarin, N. (1973) A biological cell labelling technique and its use in experimental Embryology. *Dev. Biol.* **30,** 217–222.
2. Dieterlen-Lièvre, F., Pardanaud, L., Caprioli, A., and Jaffredo T. (2001) Non-yolk sac hematopoietic stem cells: the avian paradigm, in *Hematopoiesis: A Developmental Approach* (Zon, L., ed.), Oxford University Press, New York, NY, pp. 201–208.
3. Le Douarin, N. M., Corbel, C., Martin, C., Coltey, M., and Salaün, J. (1989) Induction of tolerance by embryonic thymic epithelial grafts in birds and mammals in *Cold Spring Harbor Symposia on Quantitative Biology*, vol. 65, Cold Spring Harbor Laboratory Press, Cold Spring Harbor, NY, pp. 777–787.
4. Le Douarin, N. M., Corbel, C., Bandeira, A., Thomas-Vaslin, V., Modigliani, Y., Coutinho, A., et al. (1996) Evidence for a thymus dependent form of tolerance that is not based on elimination or reactive T cells. *Immunol. Rev.* **149,** 35–53.
5. Le Douarin, N. M., Dieterlen-Lièvre, F., and Teillet, M-A. (1996) Quail-chick transplantations. *Methods Cell Biol.* **51,** 23–61.
6. Le Douarin, N. M., Dieterlen-Lièvre, F., Teillet, M-A., and Ziller, C. (2000) Interspecific chimeras in avian embryos. *Methods Mol. Biol.* **135,** 373–386.
7. Hamburger, V. and Hamilton, H. L. (1951) A series of normal stages in the development of the chick embryo. *J. Morphol.* **88,** 49–92.
8. Zacchei, A. M. (1961) Lo sviluppo embrionale della quaglia giapponese (Coturnix cotunix japonica). *Arch. Ital. Anat. Embriol.* **66,** 36–62.
9. Metcalf, D. and Moore, M. A. S. (1971) Embryonic aspects of haemopoiesis, in *Haemopoietic Cells* (Neuberger, G., and Tatum, E. L., eds.), North Holland Publications, Amderdam, The Netherlands, pp. 127.
10. Le Douarin, N. M., Dieterlen-Lièvre, F., and Oliver, P. (1984) Ontogeny of primary lymphoid organs and lymphoid stem cells. *Am. J. Anat.* **170,** 261–299.
11. Pardanaud, L., Altmann, C., Kitos, P., Dieterlen-Lièvre, F., and Buck, C. A. (1987) Vasculogenesis in the early quail blastodisc as studied with a monoclonal antibody recognizing endothelial cells. *Development* **100,** 339–349.
12. Pardanaud, L., Yassine, F., and Dieterlen-Lièvre, F. (1989) Relationship between vasculogenesis, angiogenesis and haemopoiesis during avian ontogeny. *Development* **105,** 473–485.
13. Martin, C. S. (1983) Total thymectomy in the early chick embryo. *Arch. Anat. Micr.* **72,** 107–110.
14. Belo, M., Martin, C., Corbel, C., and Le Douarin, N. M. (1985) A novel method to bursectomize avian embryos and obtain quail/chick bursal chimeras I. Immunocytochemical analysis of such chimeras by using species-specific monoclonal antibodies. *J. Immunol.* **135,** 3785–3794.
15. Dieterlen-Lièvre, F., Pardanaud, L., Bollérot, K., and Jaffredo, T. (2001) Hemangioblasts and hemopoietic stem cells during ontogeny. *C. R. Acad. Sci.* **325,** 1013–1020.
16. Martin, C. (1972) Technique d'explantation *in ovo* de blastodermes d'embryons d'oiseaux. C. R. *Séances Soc. Biol. ses Fil.* **116,** 283–285.
17. Martin, C., Beaupain, D., and Dieterlen-Lièvre, F. (1980) A study of the development of the hemopoietic system using quail-chick chimeras obtained by blastoderm recombination. *Dev. Biol.* **75,** 303–314.

18. Muramatsu, T., Mizutani, Y., Ohmori, Y., and Okumura, I. (1997) Comparison of three non-viral transfection methods for foreign gene expression in early chicken embryos *in ovo*. *Biochem. Biophys. Res. Commun.* **230,** 376–380.
19. Momose, T., Tonegawa, A., Takeuchi, J., Ogawa, H., Umesono, K., and Yasuda, K. (1999) Efficient targeting of gene expression in chick embryos by microelectroporation. *Dev. Growth Differ.* **41,** 335–344.
20. Mikawa, T., Fischman, D. A., Dougherty, J. P., and Brown, A. M. C. (1991). In vivo analysis of a new lacZ retrovirus vector suitable for cell lineage marking in avian and other species. *Exp. Cell Res.* **195,** 516–523.
21. Grammatopoulos, G. A., Bell, E., Toole, L., Lumsden, A., and Tucker, A. S. (2000) Homeotic transformation of branchial arch identity after Hoxa2 overexpression. *Development* **127,** 5355–5565.
22. Jaffredo, T., Gautier, R., Eichmann, A., and Dieterlen-Lièvre, F. (1998) Intraaortic hemopoietic cells are derived from endothelial cells during ontogeny. *Development* **125,** 4575–4583.
23. Jaffredo, T., Gautier, R., Brajeul, V., and Dieterlen-Lièvre, F. (2000) Tracing the progeny of the aortic hemangioblast in the avian embryo. *Dev. Biol.* **224,** 204–214.
24. Fleischman, R. A. and Mintz, B. (1979) Prevention of genetic anemias in mice by microinjection of normal hematopoietic stem cells into the fetal placenta. *Proc. Natl. Acad. Sci. USA* **76,** 5736–5740.
25. Salaün, J., Calman, F., Coltey, M., and Le Douarin, N. M. (1986) Construction of chimeric thymuses in the mouse fetus by *in utero* surgery. *Eur. J. Immunol.* **16,** 523–530.
26. Coutinho, A., Salaün, J., Corbel, C., Bandeira, A., and Le Douarin, N. M. (1993) The role of thymic epithelium in the establishment of transplantation tolerance. *Immunol. Rev.* **133,** 225–240.
27. Till, J. E. and McCulloch, E. A. (1961) A direct measurement of the radiation sensitivity of normal mouse bone marrow cells. *Radiat. Res.* **104,** 213–222.
28. Salaün, J., Bandeira, A., Khazaal, I., Calman, F., Coltey, M., Coutinho, A., et al. (1990) Thymic epithelium tolerizes for histocompatibility antigens. *Science* **247,** 1471–1474.

15

Mouse Embryonic Explant Culture System for Analysis of Hematopoietic and Vascular Development

Margaret H. Baron and Deanna Mohn

Summary

In vertebrates, the earliest differentiated cell types (hematopoietic and endothelial) arise from mesoderm induced during the process of gastrulation. These cells become organized into the blood islands of the extraembryonic yolk sac and are morphologically apparent by around d 7.5 in the mouse. Additional waves of hematopoietic and vasculogenic/angiogenic activity later result in the development of definitive hematopoietic lineages and in the formation of the allantois and cardiovascular system of the embryo proper. In part because of the limited accessibility of the mammalian embryo to experimental manipulation in vivo, regulation of these events is still not well understood. Both in the yolk sac and within the embryo proper, prospective hematovascular mesoderm differentiates in the vicinity of endodermal tissues. Here we describe an embryonic explant culture system that permits the dissection of mesodermal and endodermal contributions to hematopoietic and endothelial cell formation during gastrulation. This system can be used to assay for soluble or endodermal cell-associated molecules involved in mediating critical interactions between mesoderm and endoderm in the formation of the hematopoietic and endothelial lineages during embryonic development.

Key Words: Embryo culture; mouse embryo; explant; visceral endoderm; epiblast; transgenic mouse; lacZ; GFP; hematopoiesis; vasculogenesis.

1. Introduction

Embryonic blood and endothelial cells form within the yolk sac blood islands by around 7.5 d of development in the mouse and arise from extraembryonic mesoderm *(1)*. The close apposition of primitive (visceral) endoderm (VE) and the posterior epiblast (embryo proper) and between VE and extraembryonic mesoderm in the yolk sac raised the possibility that interactions between these two tissue layers might be required for the formation of blood islands. Classical transplantation studies performed almost 40 y ago in the chick embryo had implicated interactions between primitive endoderm and extraembryonic mesoderm in formation of blood and vascular tissues *(2,3)*.

From: *Methods in Molecular Medicine, Vol. 105: Developmental Hematopoiesis: Methods and Protocols.*
Edited by: M. H. Baron © Humana Press Inc., Totowa, NJ

To assess the role of VE signaling in specifying posterior mesodermal (hematopoietic and angioblastic) cell fates in the mouse, we devised an explant culture system in which pre- or early-primitive streak epiblasts (ectoderm) carrying an ε-globin/lacZ reporter transgene are recombined with non-transgenic VE ("induction assay," **Fig. 1A**; **ref. *4***). The transgenic epiblasts serve as a potential source of marked primitive erythroid cells. Epiblasts stripped of VE are unable to form blood or endothelial cells or to activate endogenous markers of these lineages in explant cultures. Recombination of epiblasts with VE results in the activation of hematopoietic and endothelial development, demonstrating that the primitive endoderm is necessary for these processes around the onset of gastrulation. Primitive endoderm signaling is required only during a narrow window of time. Early gastrulation stage VE can respecify anterior ectoderm (fated to form neurectoderm) to develop into posterior (hematopoietic and angioblastic) cell lineages ("reprogramming assay," **Fig. 1B**). The VE signals that mediate both the induction and reprogramming activities are soluble ***(4,5)***. One of the signals is Indian hedgehog (Ihh; e.g., *see* **Fig. 1C**) and may function, in part, through upregulation of Bone Morphogenetic Protein-4 (Bmp4) ***(5)***.

In this chapter, we describe both assays as well as several protocols for their analysis. It is worth noting that, in combination with various genetically engineered mouse lines, the assays are potentially quite versatile. For example, an array of lacZ or GFP transgenic or knockin mice could be used as a source of epiblasts to assess activation of markers of stem/progenitor (e.g., Flk1-lacZ or Runx1-lacZ, **ref. *5***) or of more differentiated cell types (e.g., ε-globin-lacZ or -GFP) ***(4,5)***. In principle, VE from knockout mouse lines could be used in recombination experiments. Recombinant forms of various extracellular signaling molecules can be assayed directly in culture or more indirectly in coculture studies, for example, using appropriate transfected cell lines. Finally, inhibitory substances (blocking antibodies or small molecule inhibitors) can be added to the culture to assess their effects on specific signaling pathways.

2. Materials

2.1. Equipment and Tools

Dissecting tools and other equipment should be set up near dissecting microscope.

1. Inotech instrument sterilizer Steri 350 (**Fig. 2**).
2. Nunc four-well tissue culture dishes; Nunc cat. no. 17640 (**Fig. 3**).
3. Mouth pipet: 0.2-μm filter placed between mouthpiece and tubing (**Figs. 3,4**).
4. Dissecting scissors, large (Roboz RS-6702) and for finer work, Fine Science Tools (FST) 14060-09 or Roboz RS-5882 (**Fig. 3**).
5. Vannas (spring) scissors, dvd. 0.3 mm, 3 in. Roboz RS-5601 or mini-Vannas curved spring scissors from FST (15000-10) with a 3-mm cutting edge and 1-mm blade width (**Fig. 3**; *see* **Note 1**).

Fig. 1. *(opposite page)* Explant culture assays for analysis of tissue interactions in activation of hematopoiesis and vasculogenesis in the mouse embryo. **(A)** Induction assay. **(B)** Reprogramming assay. **(C)** RT-PCR analysis of ε-globin gene expression in IHH-treated and control explant cultures. No template controls, -NT (Lane 8 on top and Lane 9 on bottom); whole embryo controls, C (Lane 9 on top and Lane 10 on bottom). (Reproduced with permission from **ref. *15***.)

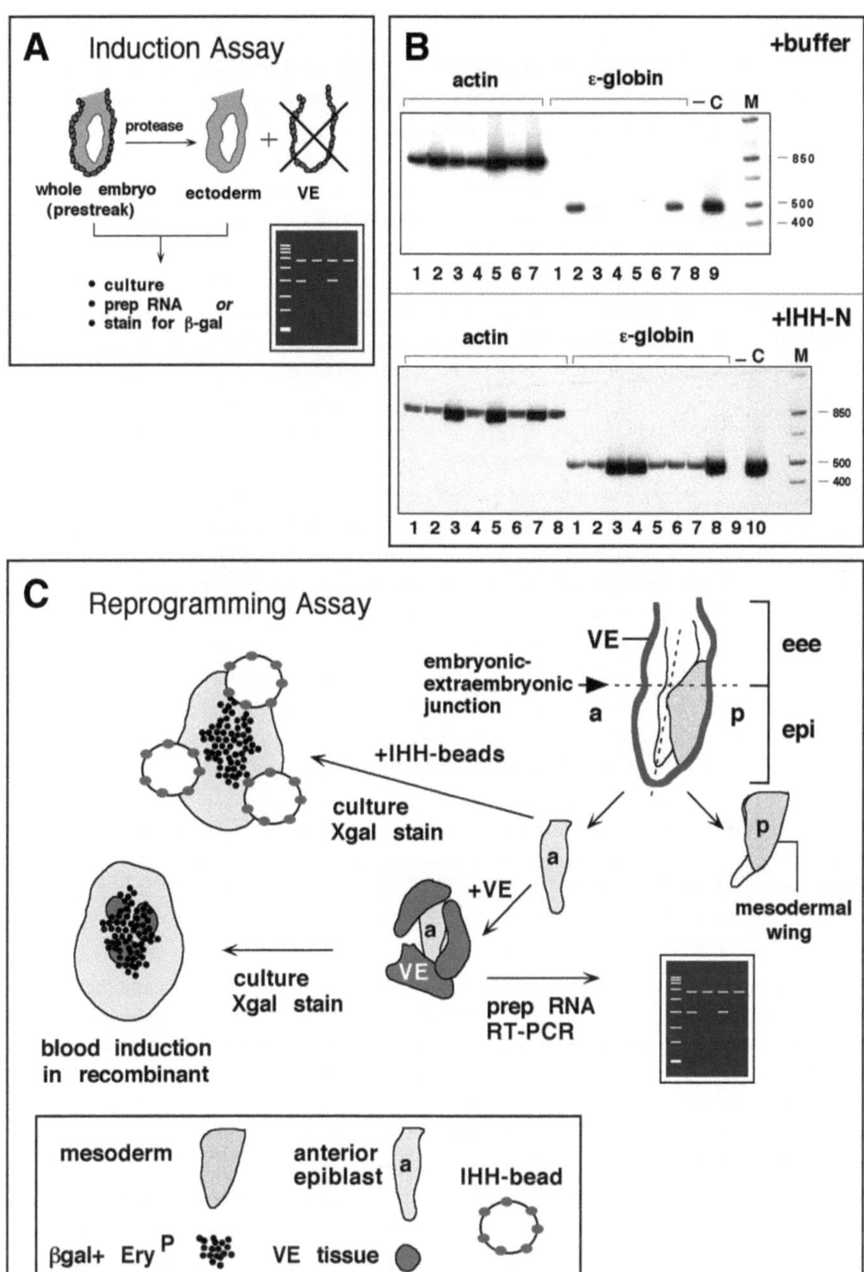

Fig. 1. *(continued)* VE, visceral endoderm; eee, extraembryonic ectoderm; epi, epiblast; a, anterior; p, posterior; IHH-bead, heparin-acrylic beads incubated with recombinant human Indian hedgehog amino-terminal fragment; βgal+ EryP, β-gal-expressing primitive erythroblasts.

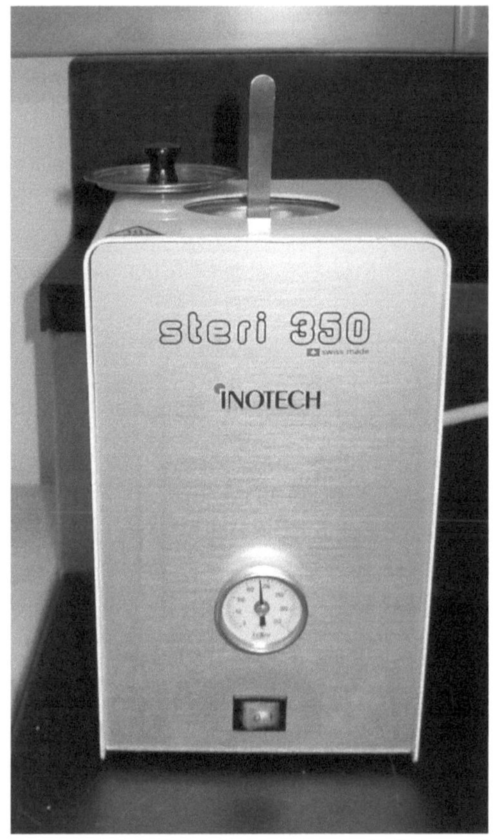

Fig. 2. Inotech instrument sterilizer Steri 350 used for sterilizing dissecting tools.

6. Watchmaker's forceps, Dumont no. 5, 55 (available from FST, Roboz and others; **Fig. 3**; *see* **Note 1**).
7. Sterile plastic transfer pipets, individually wrapped, Denville P7212S (**Fig. 3**).
8. Tungsten needles: A-M Systems; cat. no. 7190, 0.004 × 3 in., sharpened as described subsequently.
9. Glass capillaries (used as holders for tungsten needles, *see* **Fig. 3**): Fisherbrand micropipets, 10 μL, cat. no. 21-164-2C). Alternatively, use insect pin holder (e.g., FST 26015-11, **Fig. 3**, or FST 26016-12), according to personal preference.
10. Small propane torch (14.1 oz) for sharpening tungsten needle or electrolytic device as described in **ref. *6***.
11. Glass capillaries for dissection, pulled out to fine tip manually, using microburner (*see* **Subheading 2.2.4.**): FHC Inc., 1.2 mm OD × 0.9 mm ID borosil capillary tubing, cat. no. 30-31-0.
12. Sharpening stone for dissecting instruments (e.g., FST 29008-01; **Fig. 3**).
13. Becton-Dickinson 3.5-cm Petri dishes, cat no. 35-1008 or Fisher 6-cm Petri dishes, cat no. 08-757-13A.

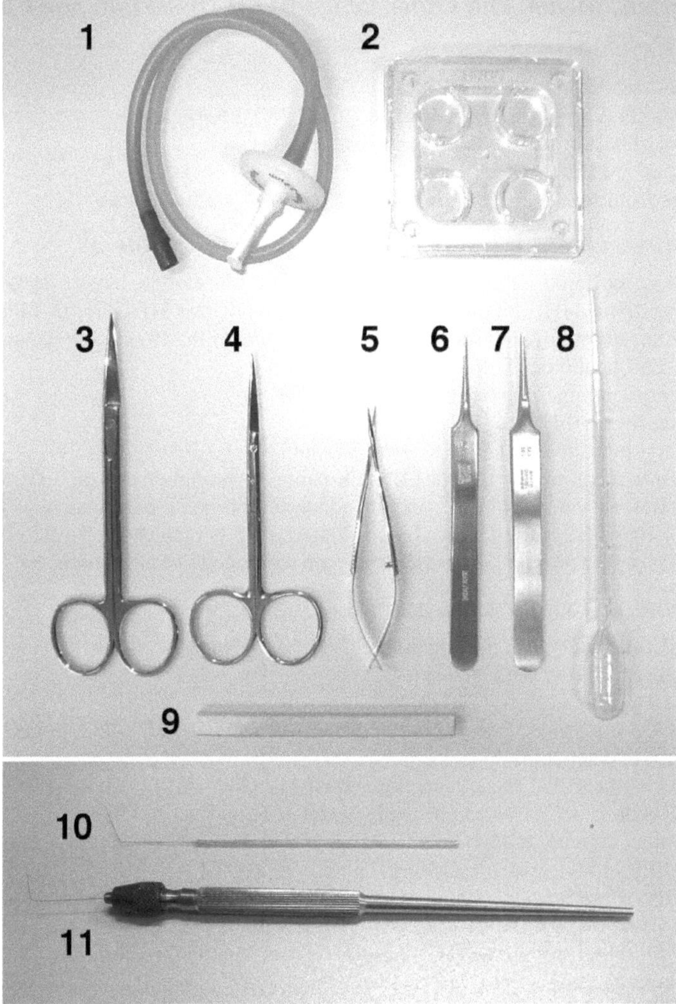

Fig. 3. Tools used in embryo dissections: **1**, mouth pipetting device for capillaries; **2**, Nunc four-well tissue culture dish; **3**, large dissecting scissors; **4**, fine dissecting scissors; **5**, Vannas (spring) scissors; **6**, Dumont watchmaker's forceps, no. 5; **7**, Dumont watchmaker's forceps, no. 5; **8**, plastic transfer pipet; **9**, sharpening stone; **10**, tungsten needle in glass capillary holder; **11**, tungsten needle in insect pin holder (brass handle).

14. Cover slips, Corning no.1.5, 18 × 18 mm square, cat. no. 2865 or Fisher cover glass no.1, cat. no. 12-545-80, 12-mm circles.
15. Water bath set at 37°C.
16. Tissue culture incubator, 37°C, 5% CO_2.
17. Leica MZ12 stereomicroscope outfitted with 1.0X Planapo objective lens (*see* **Note 2**).
18. Cigarette lighter.

2.2. Materials, Media, and Other Reagents for Dissection and Culture

2.2.1. Miscellaneous

1. Ethanol, 70%, for sterilizing tools.
2. Solution for acid washing cover slips: HCl (10%), EtOH (70%).
3. Ethanol, 95%, for rinsing acid-washed cover slips.
4. Whatman 3MM paper.
5. Figures from **ref. 7** for identification of morphological landmarks.

2.2.2. Embryo Dissection Media and Reagents (see **Note 3**)

1. Phosphate-buffered saline (PBS), Ca^{2+}/Mg^{2+}-free, 1X, Cellgro cat no. 21-040-CV.
2. Heat inactivated (HI) fetal bovine serum (FBS), HyClone SH30071.03. Filter.
3. Penicillin–streptomycin (100X; 10,000 U/mL penicillin, 10,000 µg/mL streptomycin), Gibco-BRL; cat. no. 15140-122.
4. Pancreatin, porcine; Sigma P3292.
5. Trypsin, Sigma T4799.
6. Polyvinyl pyrrolidone (PVP), Sigma PVP-360.
7. Dissection medium (37°C): 1X PBS, 1X penicillin–streptomycin, and HI-FBS (10% or 30%). Before removal of the visceral endoderm in trypsin–pancreatin (*see* **Subheading 3.1.2.**), 10% FBS is used. After trypsinization, FBS is included at 30% to inactivate the enzymes and subsequent dissection steps are continued in this medium (*see* **Note 4**).

2.2.3. Embryo Culture Media and Reagents

1. Rat tail collagen type I, Sigma cat. no. C7661 (*see* **Note 5**).
2. Acetic acid, HOAc, 0.02 *N*.
3. 1*N* NaOH, Sigma cat. no. S2770.
4. PBS, 10X, Ca^{2+}/Mg^{2+}-free, pH 7.2, Gibco-BRL; cat. no. 70013-032. For dilution of collagen for explant culture.
5. Dulbecco's modified Eagle's medium (DMEM), Gibco-BRL; cat. no. 11960-044.
6. FBS, HyClone SH30071.03 (*see* **Note 6**). HI at 55°C for 1 h. Filter.
7. Glutamine, 200 m*M*, Gibco-BRL; cat. no. 25030-081.
8. 1 *M* HEPES buffer, pH 7.4, Cellgro; cat. no. 25-060-Cl.
9. Penicillin–streptomycin (100X; 10,000 U/mL penicillin, 10,000 µg/mL streptomycin), Gibco-BRL; cat. no. 15140-122.
10. α-Methyl thioglycerol (α-MTG), Sigma; cat. no. M6145 (*see* **Note 7**).
11. Explant culture medium: DMEM, FBS (30%), 2 m*M* glutamine, 20 m*M* HEPES pH 7.4, 200 U/mL penicillin, 200 µg/mL streptomycin, and 0.7 m*M* α-MTG.
12. Heparin-acrylic beads (Sigma; cat. no. H5263), 125–250 µm in diameter.

2.2.4. Preparation of Capillaries for Use in Dissection

Use a microburner (*see* **ref. 6**) to briefly warm the center of a capillary pipet (**Subheading 2.1., step 11**). Pull the capillary from both ends until the center portion is very thin but the bore is still open. Remove capillary from flame and snap into two halves. The fine tips are used to transfer embryos and remove the visceral endoderm. It is important to prepare pipets that contain openings of different widths to accommodate variation in embryo size.

2.2.5. Preparation of Tungsten Needles for Use in Dissection

Cut tungsten needle into two halves and insert one into the end of a capillary pipet (**Subheading 2.1., step 9**). Melt the end of the capillary around the needle or use melted paraffin wax to secure it in place. Bend the tungsten needle at the far end to a right angle. Sharpen to a fine tip using a propane torch or electrolytic device *(6)*. The needle will be used to cut the epiblasts into anterior and posterior pieces, as described in **Subheading 3.1.3.**

2.2.6. Sterilization of Dissecting Tools

1. Sterilize capillaries and tungsten needles by UV treatment (15–20 min) in tissue culture hood. During dissection, to maintain sterility, submerge the tips of the capillaries in a dish of 70% ethanol. Be sure to rinse ethanol out of capillaries before using them (this is conveniently done by rinsing in medium in a part of the dish where there are no embryos). A butane cigarette lighter can be used during dissections to flame the end of the tungsten needle to remove adherent tissue and to sterilize.
2. For sterilization of metal instruments during dissection, an Inotech Steri 350 is used. Place the tip of the dissecting instrument into the container of heated glass beads in the Steri 350 for about 20 s (*see* **Note 8**).

2.2.7. Acid Washing of Cover Slips (see **Note 9**)

1. Acid wash the contents of one box of cover slips for 2 min in a large beaker containing HCl/EtOH solution (*see* **Subheading 2.2.1.**).
2. Decant HCl/EtOH. Rinse twice with H_2O.
3. Rinse twice with 95% EtOH.
4. Air dry cover slips on layers of Whatman 3MM paper. Arrange cover slips between layers of Kim wipes or 3MM paper in a large glass Petri dish and autoclave.

2.2.8. Preparation of Trypsin–Pancreatin

Trypsin-pancreatin solution is 0.5% trypsin, 2.5% pancreatin, and 0.5% PVP in PBS.

1. Dissolve the PVP in PBS.
2. Add trypsin and stir gently.
3. Add pancreatin and stir at 4°C for 30 min.
4. Spin in centrifuge for 30 min at approx 15,000*g*. Filter supernatant and store in 5-mL aliquots at –20°C.

2.2.9. Preparation of Collagen

1. Resuspend rat tail collagen type I at 5 mg/mL in filtered 0.02 *N* acetic acid. Keep on ice during preparation; collagen forms a gel at 37°C. Aliquot and store at 4°C.
2. For explant cultures, prepare 100-μL diluted collagen (here, 70%, but *see* **Note 5**) as follows: 10X PBS (10 μL); 0.1 *M* HEPES, pH 7.4 (7 μL); 0.1 *N* NaOH (13 μL); collagen (5 mg/mL; 70 μL);
3. Using pH paper, check that pH is 7.2 to 7.5. This is critical. Use 5-μL collagen per explant.

2.3. Analysis of Cultured Explants

2.3.1. X-Gal Staining of LacZ Transgenic Explants

1. Glutaraldehyde (25%), Sigma; cat. no. G5882. Store at –20°C.
2. X-gal (5-bromo-4-chloro-3-indolyl β-D-galactopyranoside), Denville Scientific cat. no. CX3000-3. Dilute 1 g in *N,N*-dimethylformamide at 100 mg/mL (100X stock). Store in the dark at –20°C. If necessary to dissolve crystallized material, warm briefly to 37°C after thawing.
3. PBS.

4. Sodium phosphate ($NaPO_4$) buffer, pH 7.3, 1 *M*: NaH_2PO_4 (23 mL of 1 *M* stock), Na_2HPO_4 (77 mL of 1 *M* stock).
5. Potassium hexacyanoferrate (III) ($K_3Fe(CN)_6$, Sigma P8131) and potassium hexacyanoferrate (II) trihydrate ($K_4Fe(CN)_6$, Sigma P9387), 100 m*M* stocks. Store at room temperature in aluminum foil-covered bottle. Prepare fresh every 3 mo.
6. Solution A: 0.1 *M* $NaPO_4$, pH 7.3; 2 m*M* $MgCl_2$, 5 m*M* ethylenebis(oxyethylenenitrilo)-tetraacetic acid.
7. Solution B: 0.1 *M* $NaPO_4$, pH 7.3; 2 m*M* $MgCl_2$, 0.01% (w/v) Na-deoxycholate (Sigma D-6750), 0.02% (v/v) NP-40 (Sigma I-8896; *see* **Note 10**).
8. Staining (developing) solution (prepared in PBS): 0.1 *M* $NaPO_4$, pH 7.3; 2 m*M* $MgCl_2$, 0.01% (w/v) Na–deoxycholate, 0.02% (v/v) NP-40, 5 m*M* $K_3Fe(CN)_6$, 5 m*M* $K_4Fe(CN)_6$, 1 mg/mL X-gal. Prepare just before use. Add X-gal to warm developing solution to avoid formation of precipitate.

2.3.2. Preparation of Ribonucleic Acid (RNA) From Cultured Explants (see **Note 11**)

1. Guanidinium isothiocyanate (GuSCN, Fluka; cat. no. 50990).
2. *N*-Lauroyl sarcosine (sarcosyl, Sigma; cat. no. L5125).
3. Sodium citrate, EM Science SX0445-3.
4. Glycogen, 20 mg/mL (Roche; cat. no. 901-393). Aliquot and store at –20°C.
5. DNase I (10 U/μL, Roche; cat. no.776-785). Store at –20°C.
6. Diethylpyrocarbonate (DEPC), Sigma D5758. Store with desiccant at 4°C.
7. DEPC-treated H_2O: TE buffer pH 7.5: 10 m*M* Tris-HCl, pH 7.5, 1 m*M* ethylenediamine tetraacetic acid (EDTA).
8. GuSCN solution: 4 *M* GuSCN, 25 m*M* Na citrate, pH 7.0, and 0.5% sarcosyl. Heat to 65°C to dissolve. Filter using 0.45-μm Nalgene filter and store in 5-mL aliquots at –20°C.
9. Solution D: GuSCN solution containing 0.1 *M* β-Mercaptoethanol (2-ME, Amersham Pharmacia Biotech; cat. no. 17-1317-01). Add 36 μL of β-ME per 5 mL of GuSCN stock solution. Best prepared fresh, but can be used for 1 to 2 wk. Store in brown glass or foil-covered bottle.
10. Sodium acetate (NaOAc), 3 *M*, pH 5.5. Prepare using DEPC-treated H_2O. Titrate pH using HOAc.
11. H_2O-saturated (acidic) phenol: American Bioanalytical; cat. no. AB01600. Saturate with Milli-Q H_2O. Store in the dark at 4°C.
12. Neutral phenol: American Bioanalytical; cat. no. AB01616.
13. Chloroform ($CHCl_3$).
14. Isoamyl alcohol (IAA).
15. Isopropanol (iPrOH).
16. Ethanol (EtOH), 100% and 75%, preferably chilled at –20°C.
17. DNase I buffer (10X): 0.25 *M* Tris-HCl, pH 7.5, 0.1 *M* $MgCl_2$, 1 m*M* EDTA in DEPC-treated H_2O. Store in aliquots at –20°C.
18. Phenol (neutral)/$CHCl_3$-IAA: 50:49:1. Store in the dark at 4°C.
19. Siliconized (silanized) Eppendorf tubes, Fisher; cat. no. 02-681-320.
20. Siliconized (silanized) pipet tips: P200, Fisher cat. no. 21-381-8A; P1000, Fisher cat. no. 21-381-8B.

2.3.3. Synthesis of Complimentary Deoxyribonucleic Acid From Cultured Explants

1. Oligo-$d(T)_{12\text{-}18}$ (Amersham; cat. no. 277858-02). Dilute to 0.25 mg/mL in DEPC-treated H_2O.

2. Reverse transcriptase (RT) buffer (10X): 0.5 *M* Tris-HCl, pH 8.3; 100 m*M* $MgCl_2$; 300 m*M* KCl. Store in aliquots at –20° or –70°C.
3. Bovine serum albumin (molecular biology grade; New England Biolabs, cat. no. B9001S). Store in aliquots at –20° or –70°C.
4. RNasin Ribonuclease inhibitor (Promega; cat. no. N251A). Store at –20°C.
5. Dithiothreitol, Sigma D9779, molecular biology grade. Prepare 0.2 *M* stock in DEPC-treated H_2O. Store in aliquots at –70°C.
6. Deoxynucleotide solution set (100 m*M* each, New England Biolabs cat. no. N0446S). Combine equal volumes of each nucleotide for a 25 m*M* final stock mix. Store in aliquots at –70°C.
7. AMV RT (Life Sciences; cat. no. AMV007). Store at –70°C.

2.3.4. Semi-Quantitative Polymerase Chain Reaction (PCR)

1. Triton X-100, Sigma T-9284.
2. Molecular biology grade $MgCl_2$: Sigma M1028.
3. Deoxynucleotide solution set, 100 m*M* each, New England Biolabs cat. no. N0446S. Combine equal volumes of each nucleotide for a 25 m*M* final stock mix and store at –70°C.
2. Oligonucleotide primers (10–20 pmol each per reaction): *see* **Table 1**.
3. PCR buffer (10X): 0.5 *M* KCl, 100 m*M* Tris-HCl, pH 9.0; 1% Triton X-100; $MgCl_2$ must be titrated for each primer set.
4. EasyTides, [α-^{32}P]-deoxyadenosine (dATP) or deoxycytidine 5' triphosphate (dCTP), 3000 Ci/mmol, 10 mCi/mL; Perkin Elmer cat. no. NEG512H or cat. no. NEG513H.
5. *Taq* polymerase (*see* **Note 12**).
6. Tris–borate–EDTA (TBE) buffer (10X): 432 g TRIS base, 220 g boric acid, 37.2 g EDTA, dilute to 4 L with Milli-Q H_2O.
7. Polyacrylamide stock: 30% polyacrylamide:bis-acrylamide (29:1).
8. Ammonium persulfate, 10% (w/v).
9. *N,N,N',N'*-tetramethyl-ethylenediamine (TEMED).
10. 1 kb Plus DNA ladder, GibcoBRL cat. no. 10787-026.
11. Gel loading buffer (5X) "Stop & Sink:" 25% glycerol (v/v), 0.05% Bromphenol blue, 0.05% xylene cyanol FF (XC), 0.5% sodium dodecyl sulfate, 10 m*M* EDTA.

2.3.5. Cryosectioning of Explants

1. Sucrose, 25% (w/v) in PBS.
2. OCT compound, Tissue-Tek 4583.
3. Cryomolds, for example, Peel-a-way S22 polyethylene squares, 22 × 22 × 20 mm, Polysciences; or, for smaller samples, Tissue Tek Cryomolds 4565 (volume 0.5 mL).
4. Cryotome.
5. Counterstain such as Nuclear Fast Red (Kernechtrot, Vector Labs H-3403) or Eosin Y, 0.5% alcoholic solution (Polysciences; cat. no. 09859).
6. Permount, Fisher Sci. SP15-100.
7. Superfrost Plus® slides (VWR) and cover slips.

2.3.6. Hematopoietic Progenitor Analysis in Secondary Cultures

2.3.6.1. Dissociation of Explants to Single-Cell Suspension

1. Collagenase, Sigma C0130.
2. Trypsin (0.25%), Mediatech #25-053-CI.
3. Collagenase solution: dissolve collagenase at 0.25% (w/v; 1 g in 400 mL) into PBS containing 20% FBS. Filter sterilize and freeze in single use (e.g., 5 mL) aliquots. Two rounds of filtration may be required. Alternatively, dissolve in PBS, filter, then add FBS and filter again. Thaw once and do not refreeze.

Table 1
Oligonucleotide Primers Used for Semi-Quantitative RT-PCR

Gener	cDNA length (bp)	Temp (°C)	Forward primer (5' to 3')	Reverse primer (5' to 3')
β-actin	929	55–60	GAGGCCCAGAGCAAGAG	CCGGACTCATCGTACTC
ε^{Y}-globin	487	55	GGAAAAAACCCTCATCAATG	ATTCATGTGCAGAGAGGAGGCATA
β_{maj}-globin	442	55	GGTGCACCTGACTGATG	AGTGGTACTTGTGAGCC
Gata-1	473	58	ACGAGGAACCGCAAGGCA	CGGGAGGTAGAGGCAGGA
CD-34	612	55	GTTACCTCTGGGATCCCTTC	GAGGTGACCAATGCAATAAG
Flk1	508	55	CCATACCGCCTCTGTGACTT	ACACGATGCCATGCTGGTCA
Pecam-1	384	55	TGCGATGGTGTATAACGTCA	GCTTGGCAGCGAAACACTAA
Vezf1	804	55	CCATGTGAGGTCTCATGAAGG	TCATTGCTATATTGAGA
vWF	209	62	GCGGACGGATCATGACCC	CAGGCTCCTCACATGTGTC
Tie2	301	60	ACCCAATACCAGTGGATGT	ATCGTGTGCTAGCATTGAGG
Fgf4	542	55	GGCAAGCTCTTCGGTGTG	CAGGCAGGCCTTTCCAGT
Brachyury	545	55	GTCTTCTGGTTCTCCGATGT	CTACTCTAAGGCAACAAGGG
Bmp4	566	55	TGTGAGGAGTTTCCATCACG	TTATTCTTCTTCCTGGACCG
AFP	402	55–60	GCTCCGGCCTCTGTCCCACC	GATGTGAGCCACATCCAGGGCC

2.3.6.2. Primitive Erythroid (EryP) Colony Assays

1. Methylcellulose powder, Fluka cat. no. 64630 (*see* **Note 13**).
2. Recombinant human erythropoietin (Epogen), 2000 U/mL, Amgen cat. no. 3107402.
3. Iscove's modified Dulbecco medium (IMDM) powder, Gibco-BRL cat. no. 12200-036.
4. Penicillin-streptomycin, 100X (5000 U/mL penicillin, 5000 μg/mL streptomycin), Gibco-BRL cat. no. 15070-063.
5. Fetal bovine platelet poor plasma-derived serum, Animal Technologies (Tyler, TX, www.animaltechnologies.com), cat. no. FBP-186.
6. Protein-free hybridoma media (PFHM-II), Gibco cat. no. 12040-077.
7. Ascorbic acid, Sigma A4544. Prepare solution at 5 mg/mL.
8. L-glutamine, 200 m*M*, Gibco cat. no. 25030-081.
9. α-Momothioglyceral (α-MTG), Sigma M6145. Store in aliquots at –20°C. Optimal concentration should be determined empirically, as for explant cultures (*see* **Note 7**).
10. 16-gage blunt-end needles, Stem Cells Technologies cat. no. HCC-8110.
11. Petri dishes, 3.5 cm, Becton Dickinson Falcon cat. no. 35-1008.
12. Corning tubes, 15 mL, cat. no. 430791.
13. Tissue culture plates, 15 cm, Becton-Dickinson Falcon cat. no. 351013.
14. IMDM/Pen-Strep/α-MTG (2X): prepare one packet of IMDM according to instructions from Gibco-BRL, except that final volume will be 500 mL. Before diluting to 500 mL, add 10 mL of Pen-Strep (100X stock) and a-MTG to 0.3 mM. Sterile filter.
15. Preparation of methylcellulose/IMDM (MC/IMDM) mix: prepared in a 1-L volume in a 2-L Erlenmeyer flask. In a preweighed 2-L Erlenmeyer flask, boil 450 mL Milli-Q water. When the water has started to boil, remove the flask from heat and add 20 g methylcellulose powder. Swirl to disperse powder. Reheat and return to a boil, with repeated swirling (this is absolutely essential, to avoid overflowing). Continue until a homogeneous slurry is obtained. This process is required both to dissolve and to sterilize the methylcellulose. Cool to room temperature (no longer than 45 min). Add 500 mL of sterile 2X IMDM/Pen-Strep/α-MTG and swirl to mix. Adding sterile H_2O, adjust final mass of the methylcellulose/IMDM mixture to 1000 g (weigh flask containing methylcellulose/IMDM mixture; final mass of the mix minus the mass of the flask should be 1000 g). Allow to cool overnight at 4°C; methylcellulose will thicken during this time. Swirl the mixture several times during the first hour of this cooling period to prevent separation of the methylcellulose and medium. Store in 100 mL aliquots at –20°C. Once thawed, the aliquot of methylcellulose/IMDM can be kept at 4°C until ready for use in EryP culture.
16. EryP medium (similar to protocol for EryP assay for cells from embryoid bodies, **ref.** ***8***): for each 10 mL, use the following recipe:

Ingredient	Volume added	Concentration
MC/IMDM mix	5.5 mL	1.1% MC
Plasma-derived serum	1.0 mL	10%
PFHM-II	500 μL	5%
Glutamine (200 m*M*)	100 μL	2 m*M*
Ascorbic acid (5 mg/mL)	50 μL	25 μg/mL
α-MTG (26 μL/2 mL IMDM)	30–40 μL	0.45-0.6 m*M*
Epogen (2000 U/mL)	20 μL	4 U/mL
1X IMDM/Pen-strep	to 10 mL total	1X

The concentration of α-MTG indicated above does not include that contributed by the MC/IMDM mix (an additional 1.5 m*M*); thus, the actual final concentration of α-MTG in the EryP medium will be 0.6–0.75 m*M* (*see* **Note 7**). Methylcellulose is extremely viscous; therefore, prepare more EryP medium than needed for the samples to be plated.

2.3.6.3. Definitive Hematopoietic Colony Assays

1. Methocult®, Stem Cells Technologies cat. no. M3434. Contains Epo and other cytokines.
2. 16-gage blunt-end needles, Stem Cells Technologies cat. no. HCC-8110.
3. Petri dishes, 3.5 cm, Becton Dickinson Falcon cat. no. 35-1008.
4. Tissue culture plates, 15 cm, Becton-Dickinson Falcon cat. no. 351013.
5. Preparation of Methocult®: per Stem Cell Technologies procedure manual, thaw bottle and shake well. Allow bubbles to disperse and aliquot 3 mL per 15-mL Corning tube, using 16-gage blunt-end needle. Store at –20°C. Thaw tube once and do not refreeze.

2.3.6.4. Materials for May-Grünwald Giemsa Staining

1. Methanol, MeOH.
2. May-Grünwald (Sigma MG-500).
3. 20–70 m*M* Tris, pH 7.2.
4. Giemsa (Sigma GS-500).
5. Superfrost Plus® slides (VWR) and cover slips.
6. ImmEdge pen, Vector Labs H-4000.
7. Hair dryer.
8. Permount, Fisher Sci. SP15-100.

3. Methods

3.1. Dissection of Embryos (Fig. 4)

3.1.1. Harvesting of Embryos

1. Sacrifice pregnant females on d 6.25 to 6.75 pc (depending on the assay to be used; *see* **Subheading 3.2.**) according to the institutional IACUC regulations (we use compressed CO_2). *See* **Note 14**.
2. Wet the abdomen with 70% EtOH (for convenience, use a spray bottle). Open the abdomen with large dissecting scissors, as described ***(9)***. Use the finer scissors to open the peritoneum, taking care not to damage any internal organs.
3. Using the fine dissecting scissors, gently push away the intestines and attached omentum so that the uterus comes into view. The uterus should contain pea-size swellings of implanted embryos.
4. Cut one horn of the uterus below the oviduct, grasping the tip of the horn with no. 5 forceps. Pulling gently on the uterine horn, trim away the mesometrium using the fine scissors. Cut across the cervix and, continuing to pull, trim the mesometrium from the contralateral uterin horn. Free the entire uterus by cutting across the second utero-tubal junction. Transfer the intact uterus to a dish of warm dissection medium.
5. Grasp one end of the uterine horn with the no. 5 forceps and insert the tip of the Vannas spring scissors into the opening. Gently push the scissors forward along the antimesometrial wall of the uterus, sliding them along so that the decidua can be visualized. Cut along the wall, taking care not to damage the decidua (**Fig. 4A**). The decidua can be shelled out individually as shown or, with some practice, in one movement, as follows. Grasp one end of the opened uterus, using the no. 5 forceps. Open and place a second pair of forceps in front of (away from you) and perpendicular to the first pair so that the uterine tissue is in between the blades of the forceps. Close the forceps and push gently away from the first pair, sliding the top blade of the forceps below the decidua so that the individual decidua are shelled out, one after the other (*see* **Note 15**). Transfer decidua to dish of clean dissecting medium.

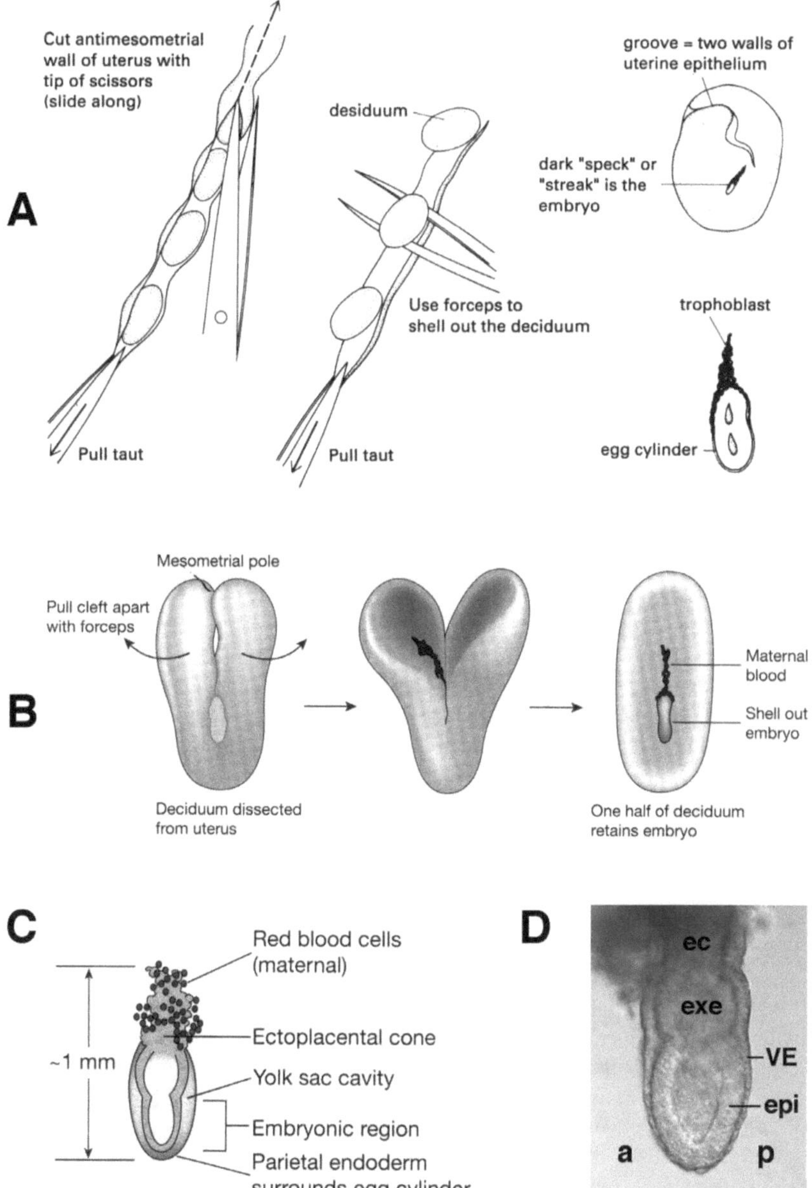

Fig. 4. Methods for dissection of early-to-mid-streak embryos. (**A**) Removal of decidua (approx 6.5 d post coitus) from uterine horns. (**B**) Dissection of early-to-mid-streak embryos from decidual tissue. (**C**) Illustration of dissected embryo. (**D**) Photograph of early-streak embryo. (A–C reproduced with permission from **ref. *6***.) a, Anterior; p, posterior; ec, ectoplacental cone; exe, extraembryonic ectoderm; VE, visceral endoderm; epi, epiblast.

6. Adjust the mirror and transmitted light on the dissecting microscope so that the decidua are transilluminated. Adjust the fiberoptic light so that the groove in the walls of the uterine epithelium (**Fig. 4A**) are easily seen.
7. Pull apart the halves of the deciduum. It may be necessary to gently cut through using fine forceps. Inside, against one half of the uterine epithelium, there is a small groove containing the embryo (**Fig 4B**). The tiny ectoplacental cone and its associated maternal blood cells are most easily spotted (**Fig. 4C**); the embryo itself is transparent.
8. Using the tips of the forceps, gently scoop out the embryo. It may be necessary to grasp the ectoplacental cone with the forceps and pull. Transfer the embryo to a dish of clean, warmed dissection medium, using a mouth pipet with capillary (**Fig. 5**; *see* **Note 16**).
9. Remove Reichert's membrane using the no. 55 forceps (**Fig. 6A,B**). Use one forceps to pin down the embryo and the second to tear away the membrane. This step, which is nicely described in **ref.** ***9***, may take some practice. Effective transillumination is essential, and it is worthwhile taking the time to adjust the mirror below the microscope stage so that membrane layers are easily distinguished. Removal of Reichert's membrane is easier if the overhead fiberoptic lights are not used.
10. Cut off the ectoplacental cone (if it has not already detached during earlier steps) by pinching with the no. 55 forceps or by cutting with a tungsten needle (**Fig. 6C**). Do not cut away the extraembryonic region of the embryo.

3.1.2. Enzymatic Separation of VE and Embryo (see **Note 17**)

1. Using the photographs in **ref.** ***7*** as a guide, select embryos at the desired stages for the induction assay (pre- or early streak) or for the "reprogramming assay" (mid-streak) as described in **refs.** ***4,5***; *see* **Note 18**. It is a good idea to photograph the embryos and make notes about their appearance and which ones will be used for the planned assay.
2. Rinse serum from embryos by transferring them (mouth pipet with capillary, **Fig. 5**) to warmed, serum-free PBS or DMEM. Contaminating serum may interfere with enzymatic digestion.
3. Transfer embryos with minimal amount of PBS (or DMEM) possible to sterile, ice-cold trypsin–pancreatin (in four-well or 35-mm dish). Swirl gently to dilute out any transferred PBS and set timer or follow second hand on watch. Timing of enzymatic treatment must be titrated for different lots of enzyme, but in general, 15–20 s is sufficient. Do not over digest. Keep dish on ice during this step.
4. Transfer the embryos to a 6-cm dish containing pre-warmed dissecting medium (30% FBS). The high FBS is used to quench the enzymes used in the previous step.
5. Allow the embryos to "recover" for a couple of minutes. During this time, select glass capillaries with appropriate bore sizes. Briefly fire polish the tips. Capillaries can be reused many times as long as they are carefully washed and re-sterilized.
6. Remove the visceral endoderm layer by gently sucking the embryo (from whichever end is narrower, usually the distal tip, **Fig. 6D**) into a drawn-out glass capillary (*see* **Note 16**). The bore of the capillary should be slightly smaller than the diameter of the embryo. Aspirate the embryo in and out of the capillary once; it may be necessary to repeat this process to remove the VE completely. The endoderm should detach from the ectoderm as a slipper or sleeve-like structure (may not always be intact). If the extraembryonic portion of the VE does not come off, do not use the rest of the VE (separated from the embryo) for recombination experiments. (*see* **Note 19**).
7. Transfer separated VEs to ice-cold dissecting medium. Keep the embryos well separated, as they become quite sticky after the enzymatic treatment.

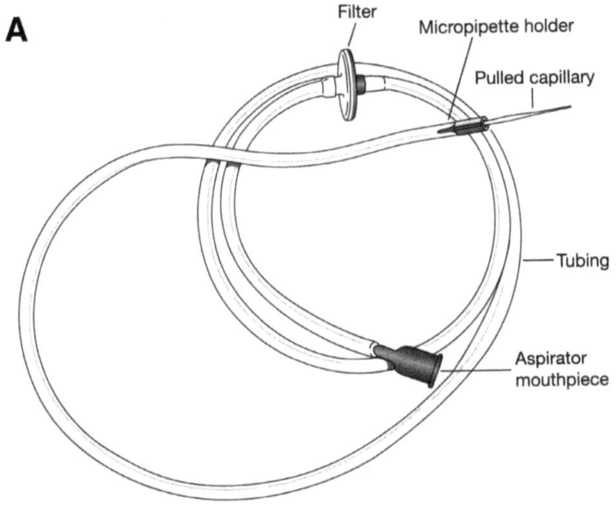

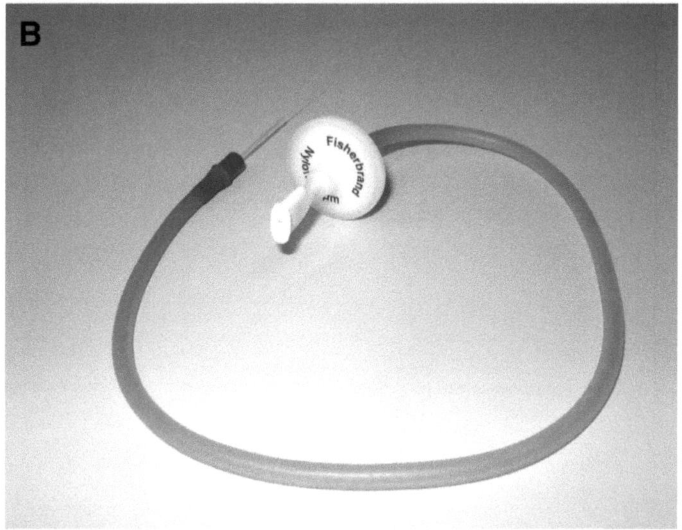

Fig. 5. **(A)** Mouth pipet used for embryo manipulation. (Illustration adapted with permission from **ref. *9*.**) **(B)** Photograph of mouth pipetting device used in authors' lab. A drawn-out Pasteur pipet may be inserted into the rubber tubing in place of a capillary.

8. For the "induction assay" in which whole pre- or early streak-stage embryos are used, the extraembryonic ectoderm can be removed using a tungsten needle. We have not observed any inhibitory effect of the extraembryonic ectoderm on activation of hematopoiesis or vascular development in this assay *(4)*.
9. For the reprogramming assay, proceed to **Subheading 3.1.3.** For the induction assay, proceed to **Subheading 3.2.**

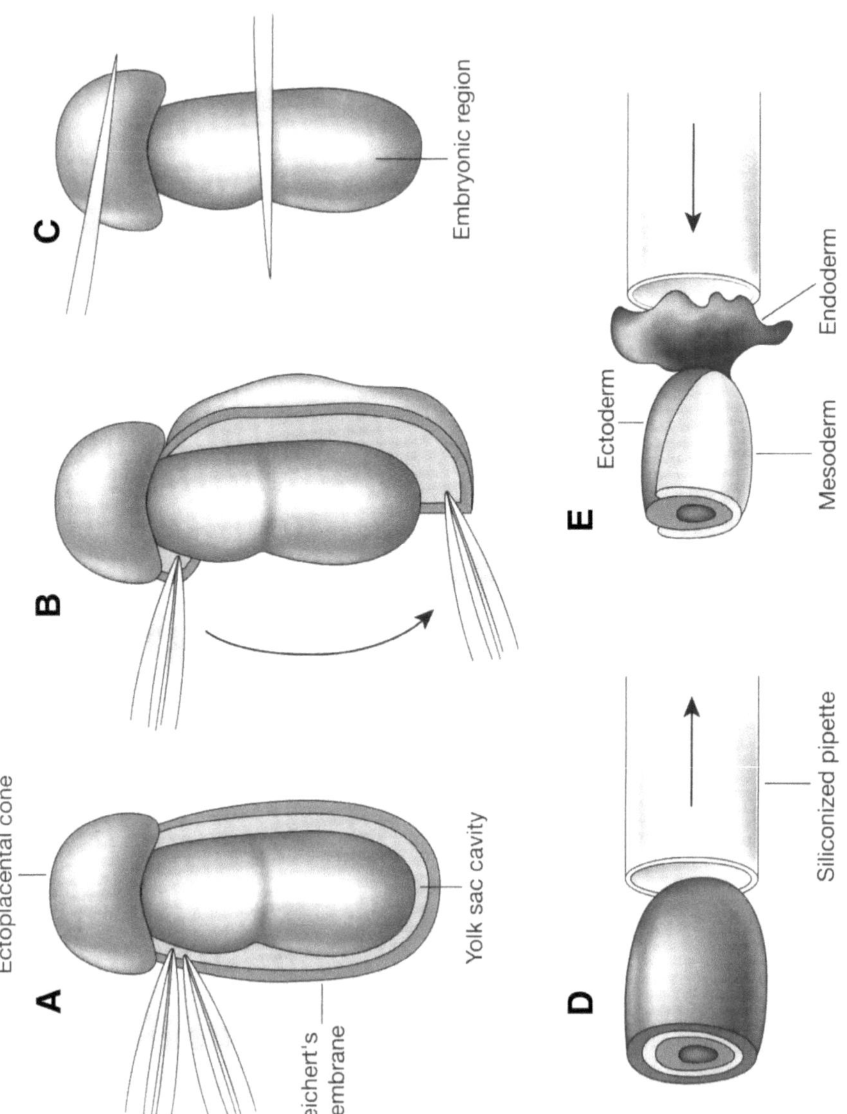

Fig. 6. Separation of VE and epiblast tissues. (Reproduced with permission from **ref. *9***.)

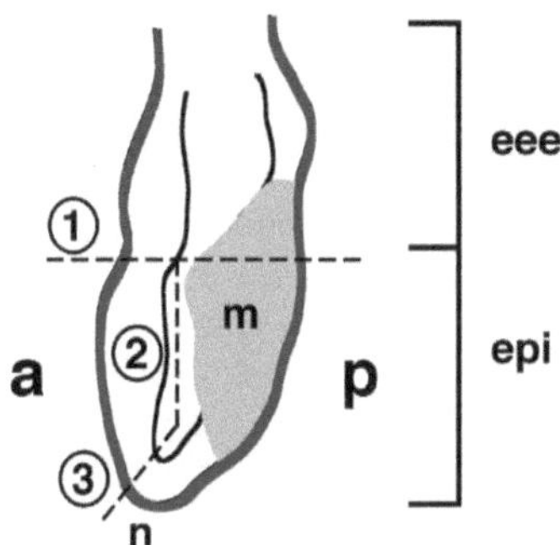

Fig. 7. Illustration indicating cuts to be made in dissecting anterior epiblasts from mid-streak embryos. The order of cuts no. 2 and 3 is interchangeable.

3.1.3. Transection of Epiblasts Into Anterior and Posterior Portions

1. Using a tungsten needle, cut the embryo at the embryonic/extraembryonic junction (**Fig. 7**, cut no. 1). Discard the extraembryonic ectoderm.
2. Orient the embryo such that anterior is to the left, posterior to the right, using morphological landmarks *(7)*. It may be easier to differentiate anterior from posterior before cutting the embryo into its embryonic and extraembryonic halves. You should be able to see the outline of the mesodermal wing (**Fig. 7**).
3. Make a longitudinal cut (no. 2, **Fig. 7**), taking care to avoid mesodermal contamination.
4. Make a third cut (no. 3, **Fig. 7**) just anterior to the node (n), freeing the piece of anterior epiblast. The posterior piece (with its associated mesodermal wings) is kept as a control for tissue viability *(5)*. Transfer both pieces to a single well of a 4- or 24-well dish (containing warm culture medium) until ready for the next step of the assay. Use a different well for the anterior and posterior pieces of each individual epiblast. The anterior and posterior pieces are easily distinguished by size.
5. Continue dissecting anterior epiblasts, placing the pieces from one embryo into a separate, numbered well.

3.2. Explant Culture (Fig. 1)

3.2.1. Setting Up Recombinants in Collagen Droplets

1. Prepare 100-mL collagen as described earlier. Dispense 5 mL of collagen into one well of a four-well dish. For convenience, this is done at the microscope.
2. Assemble the recombinant (*see* **Note 20**):
   a. Using a drawn-out glass capillary in a mouth pipet, place three VEs into the collagen and push them to the bottom of the droplet using forceps or tungsten needle.
   b. On top of the VEs, place a single pre- or early-streak epiblast or a dissected mid-streak anterior epiblast (*see* discussion of dose effects in **ref. *4***). Note that, once the VE has been removed from the epiblast, anterior and posterior aspects of the tissue can no longer be distinguished.
   c. If necessary, push tissues closer together using forceps or tungsten needle.
   d. Repeat for two more wells of the four-well dish. The fourth well contains sterile water for humidification.

e. Allow collagen to set for minimum time (preferably 5 min or less) at 37°C.
f. Gently pipet explant culture medium (300 μL) into each well of the dish (*see* **Note 9**).
g. Culture in 37°C, 5% CO_2 tissue culture incubator for up to 4 d. Change medium after 48 h.
h. For the reprogramming assay: place each posterior epiblast into a separate collagen droplet. Keep track of the origin of each anterior and posterior epiblast cultured.
i. Continue plating additional anterior epiblasts and VEs in collagen droplets (*see* **Note 21**).

3.2.2. Explant Co-Culture on Cell Monolayer

This assay can be performed using a particular cell type (as, for example, with the use of the VE-like cell line END-2, **ref. 5**) or using COS, Chinese hamster ovary, or other cells engineered to express recombinant molecules of interest.

1. Prepare monolayer of cells on which explants are to be cultured, in individual wells of 4- or 24-well dishes. This can be done on the previous day or on the morning before dissection of embryos. The density of cells in the monolayer should be adjusted according to the proliferation rate of the cells, so that during the culture period, the medium does not become acidic.
2. Place dissected explants into each well. Explants should be cultured one to a well if keeping track of the embryo origin of the explant is desired (e.g., so that an anterior epiblast can be compared with its posterior partner).
3. Change medium at least after 48 h. Examine each well to determine whether the explant has adhered to the monolayer or is still in suspension. If the explant has not adhered, replace only about half of the medium, to avoid loss of the explant. Culture for up to 4 d.

3.2.3. Explant Culture With Recombinant Protein, Blocking Antibodies, or Small Molecules

1. Set up anterior explants in collagen droplets as described in **Subheading 3.2.1.** (*see* **Note 22**).
2. Add desired recombinant protein or other molecules (blocking antibodies, small molecule agonists, etc.) directly to the explant culture medium. If recombinant protein is added in another form (e.g., as protein-soaked heparin-acrylic beads), incubate beads and protein for 1 h on ice, then transfer beads to liquid collagen droplet containing explant. Allow collagen droplet to set.
3. Change medium at least after 48 h or, as required by the particular experiment, more frequently. Culture for up to 4 d.

3.3. Analysis of Cultured Explants

3.3.1. General Considerations

1. Careful notes should be kept on the apparent developmental stage of the embryos based on morphological landmarks *(7)* and only embryos which have developed to the desired stage should be used. It is important to include as many untreated control samples as possible so that a false-positive response (e.g., owing to contaminating mesoderm) can be excluded.
2. For the "induction assay" untreated epiblasts should appear healthy and show evidence of some cell proliferation. Selection of embryos at the correct developmental stage is critical. If mesodermal wings are observed, the embryo has developed too far to be useful for

the analysis (hematopoietic and endothelial induction will occur in the absence of VE or added inducer such as recombinant hedgehog). For the "reprogramming assay" lacZ transgenic explants are scored according to the following criteria: 1) for each anterior epiblast, the matching posterior ectoderm should show evidence of significant cell proliferation and should stain heavily for β-galactosidase activity; and 2) both treated and control anterior epiblast explants should appear healthy and also show evidence of cell proliferation. Anterior epiblasts that do not fulfill both criteria are excluded from further analysis ***(5)***.

3. For secondary clonogenic culture in methylcellulose, to identify hematopoietic progenitors, the explants should be harvested at earlier times (1–3 d after initiation of culture). The numbers of progenitors decrease as differentiation occurs.
4. Vascular development can be investigated using secondary culture on Matrigel®.

3.3.2. X-Gal Staining for β-Galactosidase Activity

It may be necessary to perform the following steps under a dissecting microscope to avoid loss of samples during fixation, washing or staining. All steps are at room temperature unless otherwise indicated. Fixed explants can also be counterstained (e.g., with eosin) and can be cryosectioned ***(4)***.

1. Fix explants in 0.5% glutaraldehyde/PBS for 5 to 10 min. Do not over fix.
2. Wash 2X (approx 2 min each) with PBS.
3. Incubate in Solution A for 30 min.
4. Wash 2X with PBS.
5. Incubate in Solution B for 5 min.
6. Wash 2X with PBS.
7. Incubate in freshly prepared Staining (Developer) Solution containing X-gal (1 mg/mL) for 1 to 2 h at 37°C in the dark.
5. Wash once with PBS.
6. Photograph explants (dark field or bright light, as appropriate).

3.2.3. RT-PCR Analysis of Explants

3.2.3.1. Preparation of RNA

1. Gently aspirate medium from the well containing the explant.
2. Add 400 μL of freshly prepared Solution D. Carefully transfer contents of well to siliconized Eppendorf tube (make sure you have the explant). Vortex hard. Continue for each sample. At this point, samples can be frozen at –20°C, if necessary.
3. To each sample, add 20 μg of glycogen carrier and 27 μL of 3 *M* NaOAc, pH 5.5. Vortex.
4. Add 400 μL of H_2O saturated (acidic) phenol. Vortex.
5. Add 85 μL of $CHCl_3$. Vortex. Leave tubes on ice for ≥15 min.
6. Spin tubes in microfuge for 20 min at 4°C.
7. Transfer aqueous layer to clean, labeled siliconized Eppendorf tube.
8. To the aqueous phase, add an additional 20 μg of glycogen.
9. Add 400 μL of iPrOH. Vortex well.
10. Chill at –20°C for 3 h to O/N.
11. Spin in microfuge for 20 min at 4°C.
12. Carefully remove all supernatant and discard. Pellet should have translucent appearance.
13. Resuspend each pellet in 300 μL of Solution D (this essentially constitutes a wash of the RNA).

14. Add 300 µL of iPrOH. Vortex well. Chill at –20°C for 3 h to O/N.
15. Spin in microfuge for 20 min at 4°C.
16. Carefully remove supernatant and discard.
17. Add 1 mL of 75% EtOH and vortex.
18. Spin in microfuge for 5 to 10 min at 4°C.
19. Carefully remove supernatant and discard. Pellet will now be opaque and will be smaller than before. If any of the pellets appear to contain residual salt (large white pellet), rewash with 75% EtOH (**steps 17** and **18**). Air dry briefly, on bench.
20. Resuspend pellets in 50 µL of DEPC-treated H_2O using a plugged pipet tip. Incubate for 10 min at 55 to 60°C to resuspend thoroughly.
21. Add 5.6 µL of 10X DNaseI buffer and 1 µL of RNase-free DNaseI. Vortex, quick spin, and incubate at 37°C for 30 min.
22. Add 200 µL of DEPC-treated TE buffer, pH 7.5, and 20 µg of glycogen. Mix.
23. Add equal volume phenol (neutral)/$CHCl_3$-IAA. Vortex hard.
24. Spin in microfuge for 5 to 10 min at 4°C.
25. Transfer aqueous layer to clean, labeled siliconized Eppendorf tube.
26. Add 200 µL of $CHCl_3$. Vortex.
27. Spin in microfuge for 5 to 10 min at 4°C.
28. Transfer aqueous layer to clean, labeled siliconized Eppendorf tube.
29. Add 0.1 volume 3 *M* NaOAc pH 5.5, 20 µg of glycogen, and three volumes of 100% EtOH. Mix well.
30. Chill at –20°C for 3 h to O/N, to precipitate RNA.
31. Spin in microfuge for 20 min at 4°C.
32. Carefully remove supernatant and discard.
33. Wash pellet with 1 mL of 75% EtOH (**steps 17** and **18**) and air dry briefly. Do not allow pellet to dry completely or it may be difficult to resuspend (next step).
34. Resuspend pellet in 10 µL of DEPC-treated H_2O or TE buffer, pH 7.5. Use 5 µL for cDNA synthesis.

3.2.3.2. cDNA Synthesis

1. Prepare RT mix: 1X RT buffer, 50 µg/mL bovine serum albumin, 1 m*M* dithiothreitol, 20 U RNasin, 500 µ*M* dNTPs, and 4 U AMV reverse transcriptase.
2. Aliquot RNAs into labeled tubes, on ice. For explants, use 5 µL per reaction. For mRNAs of known concentration, for which quantity is not limiting, use 0.5 to 1 µg per reaction.
3. Add 1 µL of 0.25 µg/µL oligo-$dT_{(12–18)}$ to each tube.
4. Heat in a water bath at 65°C for 4 min to denature secondary structure in mRNA. Place tubes on ice.
5. Quick spin the samples, place back on ice, and add 14 µL of RT mix.
6. Incubate at 48°C for 30 min (*see* **Note 23**).
7. Proceed to PCR or store cDNAs at –20°C until ready for use.

3.2.3.3. PCR Analysis of Explant mRNA

All samples are first normalized for expression of β-actin, which serves as an internal control ***(4,5,10)***. Normalized samples are then analyzed for expression of other genes using appropriate primer pairs. Although it is desirable to perform multiplex PCR in which two or more primer pairs are included in the same reaction (e.g., *see* **refs. *4,10***), we have sometimes found that the presence of additional primers can influence amplification of the other product. If RNA samples have not been treated with RNase-free DNase, control reactions minus reverse transcriptase are critical, particularly if primer pairs have not been chosen to flank an intron. We also include a "no-template" control in all experiments. Finally, the cycle number and amounts of primer and template cDNA that yield nonsaturating amplification should be determined empirically in each case ***(10)***.

1. Dilute cDNA 1:5 with dH_2O. Use 5 µL per reaction.
2. Prepare PCR mix (20 µL per reaction): 1X PCR buffer, 1.5 m*M* $MgCl_2$, 200 µ*M* dNTPs, 1 to 20 pmol for each primer, 0.25 µCi [α-^{32}P]-dATP or dCTP, and 0.25 to 0.5U Taq polymerase (the amount will depend on the type of polymerase used; *see* **Note 12**).
3. Add 20 µL of PCR mix to each cDNA sample.
4. Insert tubes into block of programmed thermal cycler and run PCR.
5. Add "Stop & Sink" dye to 1X. Resolve a portion of each sample on a 5 to 6% nondenaturing polyacrylamide gel (1X TBE). Run a gel 20 × 20 cm, using 0.4 mm or 1.5- to 2-mm spacers (for the latter, dry the gel after electrophoresis is complete). Gel components and conditions for electrophoresis (6% gel) are as follows:

	0.4-mm spacers	2-mm spacers
Milli-Q H_2O	21.0 mL	42.0 mL
10X TBE	3.0 mL	6.0 mL
30% Acrylamide (29:1)	6.0 mL	12.0 mL
10% Ammonium persulfate	0.45 mL	0.9 mL
*N,N,N',N'*tetramethyl-ethylenediamine	22.5 µL	45.0 µL
Constant current	20–25 mA	70 mA

Run the gel until the Bromphenol blue dye has just run off the end.

6. For markers, end-label the 1 kb Plus DNA ladder using T4 DNA polymerase (according to the manufacturer's instructions) and [α-^{32}P]-dCTP or -dATP.
7. Subject gel to autoradiography with or without an intensifying screen, as appropriate.

*3.2.4. Cryosectioning of Explants **(4,5)***

Cryosections can be prepared from X-gal-stained explants and then counterstained or they can be used for immunostaining.

1. For lacZ transgenic samples stained with X-gal: wash 3X for 5 min in PBS after staining and post-fix in 4% paraformaldehyde in PBS for 2 h at room temperature. Wash 3X in PBS as before. (For nontransgenic samples, wash, fix in paraformaldehyde/PBS, and wash again.)
2. Detach collagen drops containing the explants from the underlying plastic or cover slip and transfer to tubes containing 25% sucrose/PBS. Infuse with sucrose at 4°C for 2 h.
3. Embed samples in OCT compound. Store at –20°C.
4. Cut 10- to 20-µm cryosections using standard methods (e.g., **ref.** ***11***).
5. Counterstain using Nuclear Fast Red (Kernechtrot) or Eosin Y according to the manufacturer's instructions.

3.2.5. Clonogenic Assays for Hematopoietic Progenitor Cells

The following assays described have been used for pooled explants and have not been optimized for single explants.

3.2.5.1. Preparation of Single-Cell Suspensions (*see* **Note 24**)

1. Transfer explants to a single 15-mL Corning tube using a mouth pipet fitted with glass capillary or a 3-mL plastic transfer pipet. Examine the culture dish under a dissecting microscope to ensure that all embryos have been transferred. A separate Corning tube should be used for each explant treatment.
2. Remove as much medium as possible from pooled explants using a mouth pipet fitted with glass capillary or a 3-mL plastic transfer pipet fitted with a sterile, P200 tip.
3. Wash explants twice with 10 mL of PBS. Allow explants to settle between washes. Remove excess PBS using a mouth pipet fitted with glass capillary or a 3-mL plastic transfer pipet fitted with a sterile, P200 tip.
4. Add 1 mL of collagenase. Transfer explants/collagenase to single well of a 12-well tissue culture dish. Make sure that all explants have been transferred by washing the bottom of the Corning tube with small amount of collagenase. Pool with explants in collagenase.
5. Incubate at 37°C for 10 min, with rocking. Gently agitate suspension using a 1-mL transfer pipet. Examine explants using an inverted tissue culture microscope to ensure dissociation of explants. Explants and dissociated cells should appear healthy (single cells should be round and refractile).
6. Incubate at 37°C for another 10 min, with rocking. Gently agitate suspension of explants/collagenase using a 1-mL transfer pipet. Check progress of explant dissociation using a microscope, as in **step 5**.
7. If necessary, incubate at 37°C for an additional 10 min, with rocking.
8. Gently aspirate the explants 3 to 5X using a 3-mL syringe fitted with 22-gage needle. Check explants under microscope.
9. If large clumps of cells remain, add 1 mL of trypsin and incubate another 5 min at room temperature.
10. Aspirate 3 to 5X using a 3-mL syringe fitted with a 22-gage needle. If a good single cell suspension has been obtained, add ice cold FBS to 30% to quench trypsin (*see* **step 11**). If large clumps remain, incubate another 5 min at room temperature. Disperse 3 to 5X using a 3-mL syringe fitted with a 22-gage needle.
11. Add FBS (30% in PBS) to inhibit trypsin. Transfer contents of well to a 15-mL Corning tube. Rinse the well with FBS (30% in PBS) and pool with suspension in Corning tube.
12. Repeat rinsing step for the tissue culture well for a total of three washes until all cells have been transferred. Dilute to a final volume of 14 mL using ice cold FBS (30% in PBS). Invert tube to mix.
13. Spin in Beckman GP tabletop centrifuge or equivalent at approx 300*g* for 7 to 8 min.
14. Gently aspirate medium from pellet using first a 10-mL pipet and then a transfer pipet fitted with a P200 tip.
15. Tap pellet to loosen and resuspend in 100 to 300 μL of IMDM containing 2% FBS.
16. Count viable cells using Trypan blue exclusion.

3.2.5.2. EryP Progenitor Assay

1. Aliquot cells into separate 15-mL Corning tubes as desired for experiment.
2. Adjust volume of cells in Corning tube to 10 mL with 1X IMDM/10% FBS.
3. Spin in Beckman G3 table top centrifuge (or equivalent) at approx 300*g* for 7 to 8 min.
4. Aspirate supernatant using a transfer pipet. Tap pellet to loosen. Add 1 mL of methylcellulose/IMDM mix to 10 to 15,000 cells.
5. Vortex. Allow tube to sit for 5 min (bubbles will settle out).
6. Plate onto 3.5-cm Petri dishes using a 3-mL syringe fitted with 16-gage blunt-end needle.

7. Place up to seven 3.5-cm Petri dishes into one 15-cm Petri dish along with one 3.5-cm dish filled with water (for humidification).
8. Culture in a tissue culture incubator (37°C, 5% CO_2).
9. Count EryP colonies between d 4 and 5 of culture.

3.2.5.3. Assay for Definitive Hematopoietic Progenitors (*see* **Note 25**)

1. Aliquot cells as appropriate. Add up to 0.1 mL cells to 1 mL of Methocult® in a 15-mL Corning tube to a final concentration of 15,000 cells/mL.
2. Vortex. Allow tube to sit for 5 min (bubbles will settle out).
3. Plate 1 mL onto each 3.5-cm Petri dish using a 3-mL syringe fitted with 16-gage blunt-end needle.
4. Place up to seven 3.5-cm dishes into one 15-cm Petri dish along with one 3.5-cm dish filled with water (for humidification).
5. Culture in a tissue culture incubator (37°C, 5% CO_2).
6. Count definitive hematopoietic colonies starting on d 5 of culture.

3.2.5.4. Cytospin Preparations From Dissociated Explants

Deposit dispersed cells from explant or colonies from secondary methylcellulose cultures onto Superfrost Plus® slides (VWR) by cytocentrifugation (Shandon Cytospin 3) at 114*g* for 4 min. Slides are then stained with X-gal, May-Grünwald-Giemsa, etc., as appropriate (e.g., *see* **ref. 5**).

3.2.5.5. May–Grünwald Giemsa Staining

1. Cytospin cells, dry. Alternatively, pick a colony using a mouth pipet, smear it around in 5 μL of PBS on a slide, then blow slowly to smear and dry the cells. These slides can be stored for a day or two. Use ImmEdge pen to mark location of cells on slide.
2. Fix for 2 min in MeOH.
3. Stain in May–Grünwald for 5 min.
4. Rinse in 20 to 70 m*M* Tris, pH 7.2, for 1 to 5 min.
5. Dilute Giemsa (Sigma GS-500) 1:20 to 1:30 with deionized H_2O.
6. Place slides in Geimsa for 15 to 20 min.
7. Wash 3 to 5X in deionized H_2O.
8. Dry with hair dryer.
9. Mount cover slips with Permount (Fisher SP15-100).

4. Notes

1. It is important to rinse off blood and bits of tissue from dissecting tools during work. First rinse in beaker of water and then submerge the tips of the forceps and scissors in a 10-cm Petri dish of water. Avoid standing the watchmaker's forceps vertically in a beaker, as the tips bend very easily.
2. The superior optics afforded by a high-quality objective lens is critical for clear visualization of morphological landmarks in embryos at this early stage.
3. All reagents are prepared under sterile conditions, in a tissue culture hood.
4. Serum, which is high in proteins, is included in the dissection medium to prevent the embryos from sticking to tools and dishes. Explant viability also is improved when serum is used during dissections.
5. Each new lot of collagen should be tested at different concentrations to minimize both setting time and collagen concentration. Collagen droplets (5 μL) should set within about

5 min. Longer times can result in drying out of the sample and poor explant growth in culture. If you find that the time required for the collagen to set has become more extended, prepare a fresh lot of collagen. The goal is to add medium to the sample as quickly as possible, to avoid drying. The collagen concentration should be no higher than required for rapid setting. Note that for collagen dilutions other than the one suggested here (70%), the amount of NaOH will need to be adjusted to maintain pH within the range 7.2 to 7.5.

6. New lots of FBS must be tested to optimize explant viability in culture. Heat inactivate serum for 30 min at 55°C, filter (0.45 μm) then store frozen in aliquots at –20°C.
7. Store at –70°C in small, single-use aliquots. Each new lot should be titrated to determine optimal concentration of α-MTG for explant viability (for this purpose, whole epiblasts can be tested). The concentration of α-MTG is critical. This reagent should be diluted into medium just prior to use; do not reuse thawed aliquots.
8. Do not lean the metal dissecting instrument against the wall of the Steri 350 during sterilization, or it will become too hot to touch and may cause severe burns.
9. In general, we have found that the collagen droplets (5 μL) used for the explant cultures adhere adequately to the plastic surface of tissue culture plates. However, some lots of collagen adhere less well and wash off upon addition of medium to the plate or well. In these cases, we have found that acid washed cover slips placed into the dish or well serves as an effective substrate for adherence of the collagen droplet.
10. NP-40 is no longer commercially available. We are currently using Igepal CA-630, (octylphenoxy)polyethoxyethanol (Sigma I-8896), which is chemically indistinguishable from NP-40.
11. The protocol described here is essentially that of Chomczynski and Sacchi ***(12)***, with minor modifications, and is the one we have used for many years. More recently, we have used a commercially available kit (Trizol, Invitrogen Life Technologies; cat. no. 15596-026), with a few modifications (e.g., precipitation of RNA in the presence of glycogen carrier, addition of a DNase step). Either approach permits isolation of high-quality mRNA.
12. We generally use purified recombinant *Taq* polymerase prepared in our laboratory (M. Baron, unpublished) but in our hands, several other commercially available enzymes give comparable results.
13. Each lot of methylcellulose powder should be tested at several concentrations to be sure it is viscous enough for colony assays. To obtain the correct consistency, the methylcellulose stock must be frozen prior to use; an aliquot can be thawed and used the following day.
14. CD1 (ICR) Mice are preferred because of their large litter size and the strongly maternal behavior of the females. The morning of discovery of the plug is taken as d 0.5 pc. In practice, we set up large numbers of cages each containing one male and three or four females. In a large facility, females can be housed with males based on their estrus cycle ***(6)***. If personnel are a limiting factor, then it is easier to set up large numbers of cages and plan on multiple experiments during the week when embryos are at the correct developmental stage. We have attempted to manipulate time of conception and litter size using hormone injections but found litter size too difficult to control (very large litters generally contain smaller embryos, some of which may not have developed to the desired developmental stages).
15. Alternatively, open the uterus and shell out the dedidua while one end of the uterus is still attached at the utero-tubal junction, as described ***(9)***. Transfer the decidua immediately to warm dissecting medium.
16. We have not found siliconizing the capillaries to be necessary. However, if embryo sticking becomes a problem, the capillaries can be siliconized as described ***(9)***. Keep around a few pipets with different diameters, because there may be substantial variability in

embryo size within a litter. It may be helpful to examine a group of capillaries under the dissecting microscope before beginning to work with the embryos. Capillaries may be reused until they break. It may be necessary to gently flame the edge of the capillary if edge is jagged.

17. Although dissections are not done in a hood, every effort is taken to maintain sterile conditions by using sterile medium and re-sterilizing instruments as needed in 70% or using the Steri 350. Bottles of media are opened in a sterile hood and the medium dispensed using sterile pipets (**do not pour**), in the hood.
18. We recommend that you scan the original figures from this very valuable reference, print them out on high quality paper, and keep them available for reference at the dissection bench.
19. It is possible to remove VE without use of enzymes. This approach reportedly results in VE with much higher viability than that of trypsinized tissue ***(13,14)***. For either approach, you can confirm the fidelity of tissue separation (absence of cross-contamination) using an RT-PCR assay with primers specific for VE (AFP, *see* **Table 1**) and for the epiblast (e.g., Fgf4) as described ***(10)***.
20. Alternatively, place anterior explant into the collagen and then place the three VEs around it, pushing them close together using a tungsten needle.
21. We advise against dissecting more than four mice in one session to avoid having explants sit around for too long. In practice, for an experienced investigator, dissection of three mice for harvesting of VEs and one mouse for anterior epiblasts works well.
22. For these assays, explants can in principle be cultured in suspension rather than in collagen droplets. However, the collagen droplet method has the important advantage of minimizing the chances of losing the explant during changes of medium and facilitates identification of the tissue (which is very tiny) at the end of the culture period.
23. We have found 48°C to give superior results compared with the usual 42°C RT reaction, when the product is then used in the PCR described in this chapter. A water bath gives more uniform heat distribution than heat block.
24. More recently, we have been experimenting with Liberase3 Blendzyme (Roche; cat. no. 1-814-184), with satisfactory results.
25. This is just one example of how hematopoietic progenitors might be assayed. Any standard assay can be adapted for this purpose (e.g., *see* Chapter 18 by Palis and Koniski, this volume).

Acknowledgments

The authors thank M. Belaoussoff, S. Farrington, and M. Dyer for their roles in developing these assays. This work has been supported by NIH grants RO1 DK52191 and HL62248 to M.H.B.

References

1. Haar, J. and Ackerman, G. A. (1971) A phase and electron microscopic study of vasculogenesis and erythropoiesis in the yolk sac of the mouse. *Anat. Rec.* **170,** 199–224.
2. Miura, Y. and Wilt, F. H. (1969) Tissue interaction and the formation of the first erythroblasts of the chick embryo. *Dev. Biol.* **19,** 201–211.
3. Wilt, F. H. (1965) Erythropoiesis in the chick embryo: the role of the endoderm. Science **147,** 1588–1590.
4. Belaoussoff, M., Farrington, S. M., and Baron, M. H. (1998) Hematopoietic induction and respecification of A-P identity by visceral endoderm signaling in the mouse embryo. *Development* **125,** 5009–5018.

5. Dyer, M. A., Farrington, S. M., Mohn, D., Munday, J. R., and Baron, M. H. (2001) Indian hedgehog activates hematopoiesis and vasculogenesis and can respecify prospective neurectodermal cell fate in the mouse embryo. *Development* **128,** 1717–1730.
6. Hogan, B., Beddington, R., Costantini, F., and Lacy, E. (1994) *Manipulating the Mouse Embryo: A Laboratory Manual*, 2nd Ed., Cold Spring Harbor Laboratory Press, Cold Spring Harbor, NY.
7. Downs, K. M. and Davies, T. (1993) Staging of gastrulating mouse embryos by morphological landmarks in the dissecting microscope. *Development* **118,** 1255–1266.
8. Keller, G. A., Webb, S., and Kennedy, M. (2001) Hematopoietic development of ES cells in culture, in *Hematopoietic Stem Cell Protocols* (Klug, C. A. and Jordan, C. T., eds.), Humana Press, Totowa, NJ.
9. Nagy, A., Gertsenstein, M., Vintersten, K., and Behringer, R. (2003) *Manipulating the Mouse Embryo: A Laboratory Manual*, 3d Ed., Cold Spring Harbor Laboratory Press, Cold Spring Harbor, NY.
10. Farrington, S. M., Belaoussoff, M., and Baron, M. H. (1997) *Winged-Helix, Hedgehog* and *Bmp* genes are differentially expressed in distinct cell layers of the murine yolk sac. *Mech. Dev.* **62,** 197–211.
11. Ausubel, F. M., Brent, R., Kingston, R. E., Moore, D. D., Seidman, J. G., Smith, J. A., et al. (1997) *Current Protocols in Molecular Biology*, John Wiley & Sons, New York, NY.
12. Chomczynski, P. and Sacchi, N. (1987) Single-step method of RNA isolation by acid guanidinium thiocyanate-phenol-chloroform extraction. *Anal. Biochem.* **162,** 156–159.
13. Wells, J. M. and Melton, D. A. (1999) Vertebrate Endoderm Development. *Annu. Rev. Cell Dev. Biol.* **15,** 393–410.
14. Wells, J. M. and Melton, D. A. (2000) Early mouse endoderm is patterned by soluble factors from adjacent germ layers. *Development* **127,** 1563–1572.
15. Baron, M. H. (2001) Induction of embryonic hematopoietic and endothelial stem/progenitor cells by hedgehog-mediated signals. *Differentiation* **69,** 175–185.

16

Hematopoietic Stem Cell Enrichment From the AGM Region of the Mouse Embryo

Catherine Robin and Elaine Dzierzak

Summary

Hematopoietic stem cells (HSCs) constitute a pool of very rare cells able to self-renew, proliferate, and/or differentiate to all the blood cell lineages during the life span. The first murine adult transplantable HSCs appear in the intraembryonic aorta–gonad–mesonephros region at embryonic day (E) 10.5. After E11, these HSCs are thought to seed the liver and then the bone marrow just before birth. So far, many questions concerning the origin, properties, and functionality of these HSCs have not been answered. To address these issues, it is necessary to isolate and purify them. One of the major problems concerning embryonic HSCs, as compared with their adult counterpart, is that they share many markers with endothelial cells at this early stage of development, making their purification very difficult. This review presents the best methods (sorting based on specific antibody staining, transgenic markers, cell cycle) for the purification and isolation of HSCs from the mouse embryo.

Key Words: Hematopoietic stem cells; aorta–gonad–mesonephros (AGM) region; embryo; aorta; transgenic mice; cell surface markers; cell cycle; FACS.

1. Introduction

All blood cells are derived from a small cohort of hematopoietic stem cells (HSCs) localized in the bone marrow (BM) of the adult. HSCs are characterized by 1) their ability to balance self-renewal against differentiation, 2) their hematopoietic lineage multipotency, and 3) their extensive proliferative capacity *(1,2)*. HSCs have a profound clinical importance in blood-related genetic deficiencies and leukemia. Fundamental research, particularly during early developmental stages, has provided important insight into the origin, properties, and functionality of HSCs.

The organization of the hematopoietic system during the development is complex. At least two independent anatomical sites are responsible for hematopoietic fate determination, with the appearance of terminally differentiated hematopoietic cells and progenitors in the extraembryonic yolk sac (YS) *(3)* preceding the appearance of first adult transplantable HSCs in the intraembryonic aorta–gonad–mesonephros (AGM) region *(4,5)*. The first adult-type HSCs emerge only beginning at mouse embryonic

From: *Methods in Molecular Medicine, Vol. 105: Developmental Hematopoiesis: Methods and Protocols.*
Edited by: M. H. Baron © Humana Press Inc., Totowa, NJ

day E10.5 in cell clusters on the floor of the dorsal aorta and the vitelline and umbilical arteries ***(6–9)***. After E11, these HSCs are thought to seed the liver and possibly the YS through the circulation. Later, HSCs are thought to migrate to the BM, where they constitute a pool of rare cells, with an estimated frequency of $1/10^5$ murine BM cells ***(10,11)***; for review, *see* **refs. *12,13***.

At all stages of development, it is impossible to directly recognize HSCs on the basis of morphology or to completely purify them because of the absence of uniquely HSC-specific antigenic surface markers. Moreover, in contrast to mature hematopoietic cells, HSCs can only be retrospectively identified by their functional properties to reconstitute an irradiated recipient after in vivo transplantation ***(1,14)***. Several markers commonly used to purify BM HSCs vary in their expression on HSCs as a function of the development stage ***(15,16)***, localization, and also vary between strains and species (i.e., Thy-1, CD38, AA4.1, CD34; *see* **refs. *17,18***). Furthermore, hematopoietic and endothelial markers that normally characterize these two lineages of cells in the adult are coexpressed by HSCs in the embryo (for review, *see* **ref. *19***). This close phenotypic relationship between hematopoietic and endothelial cells during development is not surprising based on the hypothesis of a common precursor in the YS blood islands for both lineages called the hemangioblast ***(20,21)***. Within the AGM region functional HSCs also express hematopoietic and endothelial markers, and clusters of HSCs are specifically localized, in close relation with the endothelium, in the ventral part of the dorsal aorta ***(9,22)***. Recent reports have suggested two candidates for the precursor cells to HSCs: 1) endothelial cells beneath the aortic hematopoietic clusters or 2) hemangioblasts or less-differentiated mesodermal cells underlying the aortic endothelium (for review, *see* **ref. *23***). The endothelial/hematopoietic relationship during the development poses special problems in the isolation of AGM HSCs compared with adult HSCs. Nonetheless, surface markers and transgenic markers of the earliest adult transplantable HSCs have been used for their enrichment for functional as well as gene expression investigations. In this review, we present the most recent methods for the purification and isolation of HSCs from the embryo.

2. Materials

2.1. Dissection of Embryonic Tissues

1. Dissection needles: sharpened tungsten wire of 0.375-mm diameter (Agar Scientific) attached to metal holders typically used for bacterial culture inoculation or microfine needles on syringes used for insulin injection.
2. Dumont fine forceps no. 5.
3. Dissection microscope: with magnification range from X7–40 with a black background stage and cold light source.
4. Culture plates: 60 × 15-mm plastic tissue culture dishes.
5. Medium: phosphate-buffered saline (PBS) with 10% heat-inactivated fetal calf serum (FCS), penicillin (P, 100 U/mL), and streptomycin (S, 100 μg/mL; PBS/FSC/PS; *see* **Note 1**).

2.2. Preparation of a Single-Cell Suspension From Dissected Embryonic Tissues

Collagenase type I (Sigma): make a 2.5% stock solution in PBS and freeze aliquots at –20°C. For use, make a 1:20 dilution of stock collagenase in PBS/FCS/PS. One milliliter of 0.12% collagenase will disperse approx 10 embryonic tissues when incubated at 37°C for 1 h.

2.3. Staining of Single-Cell Suspension

1. Buffers: PBS supplemented with 10% FCS for basic staining; PBS with Ca^{2+} and Mg^{2+} supplemented with 10% FCS for Annexin-V staining; DMEM supplemented with 10% FCS and MilliQ water for FDG staining; and L15 medium supplemented with 2% FCS and 10 m*M* HEPES buffer (L15+) for Hoechst staining.
2. Monoclonal antibodies: They are used for flow cytometric sorting and analysis or for immunohistochemical staining (i.e., from Pharmingen, Caltag or Becton Dickinson). They are either directly conjugated with fluorochromes (fluorescein-5-isothiocyanate (FITC), phycoerythrin (PE) or cy5) or with biotin or are unconjugated. Cells are secondarily labeled with fluorochrome-conjugated streptavidin or fluorochrome-conjugated goat anti-rat IgG, respectively, when required.
3. Fixation and permeabilization of cells: Cytofix/Cytoperm solution (BD Pharmingen).
4. Viability dye: Trypan blue is used to exclude dead cells during cell counting; Propidium iodide (PI, Sigma) and 7-aminoactinomycin D (7AAD, Molecular Probes) are used for FACS analysis; and Hoechst 33258 is used for sorting procedure.
5. Cell cycle:
   a. Hoechst 33342 (Molecular Probes, 10 mg/mL). Make 1 mg/mL stock in milliQ water.
   b. Pyronin Y (Molecular Probes). Follow manufacturers directions.
   c. 5-bromo-2'-deoxyuridine (BrdU) Flow Kit (BD Pharmingen). Follow manufacturers directions.
   d. FITC-conjugated mouse anti-human Ki67 monoclonal antibody set (BD Pharmingen).
6. LacZ β-D-galactosidase activity:
   a. 10X fluorescein-di-galactoside (FDG) solution preparation (Molecular Probes): make a 1:1 mixture of ethanol and dimethyl sulfoxide (20°C); add 76 µL of this mixture to 5 mg of FDG (one vial stored at –20°C); mix gently; add 305 µL of sterile MilliQ (37°C) and mix gently; aliquot 50 µL in Eppendorf tubes; and store at –20°C.
   b. Stockage: FDG is stocked in a 10X concentrated solution at –20°C and diluted in prewarmed milliQ water just before use (final concentration 2 m*M* or 1.31 mg/mL) to avoid precipitation.

3. Methods

3.1. Embryonal Tissue and Cell Preparation

3.1.1. Tissue Isolation and Dissection

1. Mouse embryos are obtained from timed pregnancies. Adult males and females of the desired mouse strain (wild type or transgenic) are mated in the late afternoon and the d of vaginal plug observation is considered embryonic d 0 (E0).
2. Pregnant females are sacrificed on the chosen d of gestation (usually from E8 to E12; *see* **Note 2**) and embryos removed from the uterus and placed into a tissue-culture dish in PBS/FCS/PS.
3. Dissections are performed under a dissection microscope (about 8× magnification). Reichert's membrane, the thin tissue layer surrounding the YS, and the placenta are removed from the conceptus using fine forceps. The YS is then carefully separated from the vitelline and umbilical arteries with the forceps. The embryo body, removed from the amnion, is now clearly visible and somite counts are performed to identify the gestational

stage of each individual embryo (*see* **Note 2**). Subsequently, different organs are dissected. Before E10, the para-aortic splancnopleura (P-Sp) is isolated. From E10 to E12, whole AGM (structure derived from the P-Sp) is dissected or subsequently subdissected into the aorta with its surrounding mesenchyme and the urogenital regions. Vitelline and umbilical arteries are removed with a special care from the YS and the embryo body. Various organs can also be collected (e.g., fetal liver, gut, etc.).

3.1.2. Preparing a Single Cell Suspension

1. Tissues are placed in a 5-mL snap cap tube (or in 1.5-mL Eppendorf) and treated in a 0.12% collagenase in PBS/FCS/PS. For one to five tissues, collagenase treatment is performed in 0.5 mL and for six or more in 1 mL. Tubes are incubated at 37°C for 1 h and the tube frequently tapped to disperse the tissues.
2. After incubation, the tissues are placed on ice and disrupted by pipetting 1 to 5 mL of PBS/FCS/PS back and forth up to 20 times with the blunt end of the pipet held against the bottom of the tube.
3. Wash cells twice.
4. Viable cell counts are performed using Trypan blue dye exclusion. Cell viability after collagenase treatment is expected to be 50 to 75% of the embryonic cells (*see* **Note 1**).

3.2. Detection and Sorting of HSCs by Specific Antibody Staining and Other Fluorochrome Markers

The expression of cell surface or intracytoplasmic molecules (growth factor receptors, adhesion and cell matrix molecules, cytokines, signaling molecules) or nuclear transcription factors can be used to identify and isolate cells in different stages of the hematopoietic lineage differentiation hierarchy. Some such molecules are classified with a CD number (clusters of differentiation) and many monoclonal antibodies specific for these molecules are commercially available. These antibodies when associated with different fluorochromes (directly or after a second staining step) can be used for cell sorting by flow cytometry or for immunostaining on tissue sections to visualize the precise localization of specific cells *in situ*. Some antibodies (i.e., against Thy1 or Sca1 in mouse) are polymorphic markers and therefore it is important to know the strain and background of mice with which you are working.

The best strategy to purify HSCs is to deplete, in a first step, the cells expressing mature lineage markers. Indeed, adult BM HSCs do not express many of the surface antigens that are characteristic of terminally differentiating hematopoietic cells. These lineage markers are well known, that is, CD45R/B220 for B lineage, Thy-1/CD3/CD4/CD8 for T lineage, NK1-1 for NK lineage, CD11b/Mac-1 or Gr-1 for myeloid lineage, and TER-119 for erythroid lineage in mouse (and for humans, the markers are CD19 for B lineage, CD3/CD4/CD8 for T lineage, CD56 for NK lineage, CD15 or CD11b for myeloid lineage, and GPA for erythroid lineage). Thus, the removal of such lineage-positive cells leaves a suspension of predominantly lineage negative immature cells (Lin$^-$). The Lin$^-$ cells can then be stained by antibodies characterizing immature progenitors and HSCs and sorted for these positive markers.

Mouse adult BM Lin$^-$ HSCs are phenotypically well defined and express the two glycophosphatidyl inositol-linked immunoglobulin superfamily molecules, Sca-1 (stem cell antigen 1, Ly6A/E) and Thy-1 (at low level; **ref. *18***). They also highly express the c-Kit receptor tyrosine kinase *(24)*. Hence, the c-Kit$^+$Thy-1^{low}Sca1$^+$Lin$^-$ population contains all multipotent progenitors and can be further subdivided based on the expression of other markers. For example, the CD34$^{-/low}$ fraction is enriched in self-renewing long-term repopulating HSCs, the Mac-1^{low} fraction is enriched in short-term repopulating HSCs, and the CD34^{low}Mac-1^{low} fraction is enriched in clonogenic multipotent progenitors *(25)*. Only 50% of HSCs in the E11 AGM express Sca1 and Mac1 *(17,26,27)*, whereas 100% are c-Kit$^+$ and AA4-1$^+$. In the human, HSCs are in the c-Kit^{low}CD34$^+$Thy-1$^+$CD38$^-$Lin$^-$ fraction *(28)*. They also express other markers like the vascular endothelial growth factor receptor 2 (VEGF-R2, Flk-1 in the mouse and KDR in the human) *(29,30)* or CD133 (glycosylated protein recognized by the AC133 monoclonal antibody) *(31)* that is selectively expressed on CD34^{bright} hematopoietic stem and progenitor cells derived from FL, BM, and blood.

The expression pattern of CD34 (cell surface sialomucin), considered for a long time to be the most critical marker for HSCs, is particularly interesting in light of the fact that some HSCs have been found to be CD34$^-$Lin$^-$ *(32)*. CD34 is age dependent in its expression. Indeed, in mice, all HSCs in the embryo and from perinatal to 5 wk of age express CD34. However, beginning at 7 wk of age (until 20 wk), the majority of HSCs are CD34$^-$ (only approx 15–20% of adult HSCs express CD34; **ref.** ***33,34***). CD34 expression also is influenced by the activation-state of stem cells (i.e., in vivo by 5-FU or in vitro by cytokines stimulation; **ref.** ***35***). Moreover, when G-CSF-mobilized murine stem cells expressing CD34 migrate into the BM after injection, they become CD34$^-$ as steady state is achieved *(36)*; for review, *see* **refs.** ***37,38***. Thus, the expression of cell surface markers on mouse and human cells is somewhat heterogeneous and is dependent upon the hematopoietic compartment and/or ontogenic stage.

3.2.1. Antibodies Detecting HSC Surface Markers on Embryo-Derived Cells

Unlike the adult BM, embryonic HSCs are more difficult to purify. The embryo contains fewer HSCs than the adult, and they are dispersed in several anatomically distinct sites. Depletions with mature hematopoietic lineage specific antibodies do not aid in the enrichment procedures, because few mature hematopoietic cells are present, particularly in the AGM region. Moreover, expression of some of the molecules commonly used as markers for adult BM HSCs are not hematopoietic specific in the embryo.

During development, there is a close relation between the hematopoietic and endothelial lineages. Many surface markers (i.e., flk1, tie-2, CD31, CD34, c-kit, AA4.1, Sca1, Flt-3 ligand, VEGFR1 and 2, VCAM-1, and VE-cadherin) and transcriptional factors (SCL, GATA-2, LMO-2) are, thus, commonly expressed by both hematopoietic and endothelial cells; for review, *see* **refs.** ***19,39–42***. In the human embryo (*see* **refs.** ***43,44***), CD45 appears to exclusively mark hematopoietic cells. Thus, the differential expression of CD34/CD31 and CD45 allows the discrimination of intra-aortic hematopoietic cell clusters from adjacent endothelial cells *(19,45–47)*. CD34$^+$ cells in the clusters express some transcriptional factors (SCL/Tal1, GATA2 and 3, c-myb; **refs.** ***29,46,48***) and also many molecules involved in homing and adhesion (CD44/HCAM, WASP, CD106/V-CAM1, VE-cadherin, CD31/PECAM; (**ref.** ***19***).

A candidate marker for the hemangioblast is the receptor tyrosine kinase VEGF-R2 (Flk1 in mouse and KDR in human). VEGF-R2 is expressed by endothelial cells and is essential for vessel formation. KDR is expressed in 0.1 to 0.5% of the CD34$^+$ blood cells postnatally. It is expressed both on endothelial cells lining the wall of the dorsal aorta and on hematopoietic cells within the associated intra-aortic clusters in the 5-wk human embryonic AGM ***(29,46)***. The expression of KDR marks very early human hematopoietic progenitor cells (only 5 to 10 KDR$^+$ cells, CD34$^+$CD38$^-$KDR$^+$) are necessary for restoring full hematopoiesis in lethally irradiated mice) ***(30)***.

All HSCs in the embryo are c-kit$^+$. Most are CD45$^+$ and about 50% are Mac1$^+$ ***(17)***. In contrast to adult stem cells, all/majority of HSCs in the AGM, YS, and liver are CD34$^+$ ***(17)***. Endothelial cells also are CD34$^+$ (E8-10). After E10, clusters in the aorta and in the major arteries express CD34 and CD31, with CD31 expression often restricted to the cells closest to the lumen. The majority of cells in the clusters are van Willebrand factor (vWf)$^-$, whereas the area underlying the hematopoietic clusters is vWf$^+$. The majority of cells are lectin BSLB4$^-$. In the liver the discrimination between endothelial and HSCs is easier, because CD34 expression is restricted to hematopoietic cells and CD31 to endothelial cells. It is important to remark that the expression of some endothelial markers is variable during the development and depends also on the localization and the size of vessels. For example, all endothelial cells are CD34$^+$ and CD31$^+$, but vWf and FGF-R expression are restricted to the large vessels and BSLB4 to the capillaries (for review, *see* **ref. *19***). Several markers (CD31, vWf, or BSLB4) are present from the onset of blood vessel development ***(49)***. In E11 AGM, around 3% of cells are Sca-1$^+$ ***(26)***. **Table 1** summarizes the information concerning the molecules, expression patterns and antibodies used for the phenotypic characterization of HSCs in mouse embryo.

3.2.2. Antibody Staining and Sorting Procedure

3.2.2.1. Antibody Staining

1. After collagenase treatment and washing (as described in **Subheading 3.1.**), cells are suspended in PBS/FCS/PS.
2. Single-cell suspensions are incubated with specific monoclonal antibodies of interest for 20 to 30 min at 4°C in PBS/FCS/PS.
3. Cells are then washed twice and subsequently incubated with fluorochrome-conjugated streptavidin or goat anti-rat IgG (when using biotin conjugated or unconjugated first antibodies, respectively).
4. To determine background level fluorescence, some cells are left unstained and some others are stained with appropriate immunoglobulin isotype controls.
5. After washing, PI (0.5 μg/mL) or 7AAD (2 μg/mL) are added for dead cell identification (*see* **Note 3**).
6. Cells are then ready for flow cytometric analysis or sorting (*see* **Subheading 3.2.2.2.**).

3.2.2.2. Sorting Procedure

1. After antibody staining (*see* **Subheading 3.2.2.1., steps 1–4**), cells are washed twice and filtered through a 0.45-μm nylon mesh screen (Falcon) to remove cell clumps prior the sorting.

Table 1
Summary of the Molecules Expressed on Mouse HSCs and/or Endothelium and the Specific Antibodies Available for Flow Cytometric Analysis

		Expression pattern		
Molecules	Full/alternative name	Intra-aortic hematopoietic clusters	Endothelium lining the dorsal aorta	Antibody clone
CD31	Platelet endothelial cell adhesion molecule (PECAM-1)	+	+/–	MEC 13.3
CD34	—	+	+	RAM34
CD45	Leukocyte common antigen (LCA), Ly-5	+	–	30-F11
c-kit	Stem cell factor receptor (SCF R), CD117	+	+ or –	2B8
Sca-1	Stem cell antigen 1, Ly6A/E	+/–	+/–	E13-161.7
Flk-1	Fetal liver kinase 1, Vascular endothelial growth factor receptor 2 (VEGF-R2), kinase insert domain receptor (KDR), Ly-73	+ or –	+	Avas 12a1
AA4.1	—	+	+	
vWF	Van Willebrand factor	–	+	
Endomucin	—	+	+	
BMP4	Bone morphogenetic protein 4	+/–	–	
Tie-1	Tyrosine kinase with Ig and EGF homology domains 1	+	+	
Tie-2	Tyrosine kinase with Ig and EGF homology domains 2, angiopoietin 1 receptor, TEK	+	+	
LMO2	—	+	+/–	
SMA	Smooth-muscle actin, tenascin C	–	–	
GATA2	—	+	+	
AML-1	Acute myeloid leukaemia 1, Cbfa2, Runx1, PEBP2	+	+	

Note: All antibodies mentioned below are available from commercial sources such Pharmingen.

2. In all cases, Hoechst 33258 (1 μg/mL) is added for subsequent dead cell identification and exclusion.
3. Cells are sorted using a FACS Vantage SE (Becton Dickinson) or other flow cytometric sorter.
4. Collection gates for marker-positive cells are set by comparison to cells stained with fluorochrome-conjugated immunoglobulin isotype controls. Viable fluorescent positive cells are collected in pure FCS and reanalyzed for purity and counted using Trypan blue dye exclusion (*see* **Note 3**).
5. Embryo-derived cells must be sorted slowly (less than 1000 events/s) owing to high-pressure sensitivity resulting from collagenase treatment. In this case, the cell viability is improved and the purity of the sorted cells ranges from 80 to 98%.

3.2.3. Transgenic Markers of HSCs in the Mouse Embryo

In addition to the use of antibodies in the purification of HSCs from the mouse embryo, transgenic mice specifically expressing an enzymatic marker (LacZ) or a fluorescent marker (GFP) have proven to be advantageous. Antibody mediated detection of HSCs is limited by the number of molecules expressed on the cell surface and by expression of the molecule on other cell lineages. In contrast, the transgenic approach offers the use of HSC specific expression vectors and the possibility of high-level expression caused by multiple copy transgene integration. GFP transgenic mice, for example, have been generated using the gene regulatory elements for Sca-1 (Ly-6A gene), which is the most widely used HSC marker. As expected with the Sca-1 antibody, flow cytometry analysis and in vivo transplantation data demonstrate Ly-6A GFP transgene expression in all adult BM HSCs. More interestingly in the AGM region, long-term transplantation experiments showed that HSCs are equally distributed in both Sca-1^+ and Sca-1^- fractions of AGM cells and not only in the Sca-1^+ fraction as expected. Unlike the Sca-1 molecule, the Ly-6A GFP transgene expression marks all HSCs in the AGM region and more precisely in the aorta-mesenchyme region. This difference is most likely owing to the limiting nature of Sca-1 protein on the surface of these HSCs as they are emerging in the aorta, compared to a more intense fluorescence signal produced by GFP. Indeed, the transgenic mice contain eight copies of the transgene as compared to the normal diploid copy of the endogenous Ly-6A/E gene encoding Sca-1. Furthermore, GFP is a cytoplasmic protein that does not require the processing steps necessary to get the Sca-1 protein properly displayed on the cell surface. Hence, the Ly-6A GFP transgene appears to be an optimally expressed reporter in AGM HSCs and is an excellent marker for HSC isolation from the embryo (*see* **Note 4**).

In the absence of specific knowledge concerning transcriptional regulatory elements of interesting genes, it is possible by homologous recombination to insert a lacZ or GFP gene into the specific gene locus and follow the expression pattern of desired gene. This is particularly important for analysis of transcription factor expression in HSCs in the embryo. For example, studies on the expression of the Runx1 transcription factor, which is required for the generation of HSCs in the AGM region ***(50–52)*** have been facilitated through the use of a Runx1 lacZ knockin allele ***(8,27)***. Cells from the AGM region were permeabilized and FDG, a fluorescent substrate for lacZ, allows for flow cytometric sorting. When such lacZ$^+$ and lacZ$^-$ sorted cells were transplanted into irradiated adult recipients it was found that all AGM HSCs are Runx lacZ$^+$. Further experiments used this FDG staining in combination with antibodies that discriminate between hematopoietic, endothelial and mesenchymal cells. These results demonstrate that HSCs are found in all three lineages expressing the Runx1 transcription factor (at a haploid dose) ***(27)***.

3.2.3.1. FACS-FDG Staining Procedure for LacZ β-D-Galactosidase

The classical FDG procedure is appropriate for embryonic cell staining. Nevertheless, it is recommended to stain the cells with some precautions (*see* **Note 5**).

1. Prewarm MilliQ water to 37°C.
2. Cells obtained after collagenase-treatment of embryonic tissues (as described in **Subheading 3.1.**) are suspended in DMEM/FCS at the maximal concentration of 2 × 10^6 cells per 50 µL of medium in 4-mL FACS tube with lid and kept on ice.
3. Place the cells 1 min before use in a 37°C water bath.
4. Dilute 1 min before use 50 µL of 10X FDG stock with 450 µL of warmed MilliQ water and make sure that the solution is without any precipitate.
5. Add 50 µL of 1X FDG to 50 µL of cells. Mix rapidly and thoroughly, and leave at 37°C for exactly 1 min.
6. Stop FDG loading at end of the 1 min by adding 1 mL of ice cold DMEM/FCS and place the tube deep in ice.
7. Leave for at least 30 min on ice before regular staining with fluorescent antibodies directed against various markers of interest. It is recommended to stain the cells first with FDG and subsequently with fluorescent antibodies directed against the markers of interest.
8. Add PI for live/dead cell discrimination and keep cells on ice until FACS analysis. LacZ staining is read in the FITC channel.

3.2.4. Live Apoptotic/Dead Cell Discrimination

Discrimination between live and dead cells is very important with the use of embryonic material because of the particular fragility of the cells. The dissection of tissues and cell preparation must be done as fast as possible to favor a good cell viability (around 70%). As with all careful flow cytometric analysis or sorting, the inclusion of fluorescent dyes able to discriminate live from dead cells (particularly because of the non-specific staining of apoptotic/dead cells) improves the final result.

3.2.4.1. Propidium Iodide/7AAD and Annexin-V

Propidium iodide (PI) and 7-amino-actinomycin D (7AAD) are two fluorescent nuclear dyes currently used to discriminate live from dead cells. 7-AAD and PI are fluorescent intercalators of DNA and are detected in the far-red range of the spectrum (650-nm long pass filter) and in the orange range of the spectrum (562- to 588-nm band pass filter), respectively. Viable or early apoptotic cells that maintain membrane integrity are not stained by dyes that cannot cross the plasma membrane. In contrast, late apoptotic/dead cells that have lost the membrane integrity become permeable to the dyes and thus, are positively stained.

The use of Annexin-V (a 35- to 36-kDa Ca^{2+}-dependent phospholipid binding protein with a high affinity for the membrane phospholipid phosphatidylserine [PS]) allows a more precise discrimination of cells at the different steps of the apoptotic process. Indeed cells that enter in the earliest apoptotic process have a translocation of the PS from the inner to the outer leaflet of the plasma membrane. Extracellular binding sites on PS become then available for Annexin-V. Fluorochrome conjugated Annexin-V, used in combination with 7AAD or PI, allows the discrimination of cells that are in earlier stages of apoptosis (Annexin-V^+7AAD/PI^-) from those that are in later stages of apoptosis or already dead (Annexin-V^+7AAD/PI^+).

1. Live/dead cell staining: after antibody staining (as described in **Subheading 3.2.2.1.**), PI (0.5 μg/mL) or 7AAD (2 μg/mL) is added to cells just before FACS analysis or sorting.
2. Annexin-V staining: cells obtained after collagenase treatment of tissues (as described in **Subheading 3.1.**) are incubated with Annexin-V-FITC for 20 to 30 min at 4°C in PBS with Ca^{2+} and Mg^{2+}/FCS/PS. To analyze the degree of apoptosis inside a particular population, cells can be labeled simultaneously with another antibody (PE or Cy-5).
3. Cells are then washed twice and subsequently incubated with 7AAD at 0.5 μg/mL or with PI at 1 μg/mL.

3.2.4.2. Hoechst 33258

Hoechst 33258 is a cell-permeable bis-benzamide dye that specifically binds to the minor groove of double-stranded DNA. Hoechst can be excited with ultraviolet light (350 nm; *see* **Note 6**).

1. After staining with the appropriated antibodies (as described in **Subheading 3.2.2.1.**), labeled cells are washed twice and resuspended in PBS/FCS/PS containing 1 mg/mL Hoechst 33258 (Molecular probes).
2. Viable cells are defined by exclusion of Hoechst 33258-positive cells on a FACS Vantage cell sorter (Becton Dickinson).

3.3. Cell Cycle Analysis of Embryonal Hematopoietic Cells

HSCs can be discriminated according to their position in the cell cycle. They are normally quiescent (G_0/G_1) and are not high in metabolic activity. It is possible to quiescent discriminate cells by using different dyes. For example, Hoechst 33342 dye allows the separation of cells in G_0/G_1 from the cells in S/G_2-M. When a cell suspension stained with this dye is examined under two distinct wave lengths, a side population (SP), characterized by weak fluorescence, can be identified and sorted ***(53,54)***. The dye efflux property of these cells is caused by the activity of the *mdr* (multidrug resistance) gene, which encodes a protein responsible for the building of a canal, which serves to extrude toxins from the cells. Moreover, Pyronin Y (a nucleic acid dye that has affinity for RNA), in association with Hoechst 33342, allows the separation between cells in G_0 ($Pyronin^-$) and cells in G_1 ($Pyronin^+$; **ref. *55***). Staining with antibodies against BrdU or Ki67 allows also the discrimination between cells at different phases of the cell cycle ***(56,57)***.

3.3.1. Hoechst Staining Procedure

The nucleic acid stain most frequently used for cell-cycle analysis is the Hoechst 33342 (which more rapidly permeates cells than Hoechst 33258). The ability to discriminate Hoechst SP cells is based on the differential efflux of Hoechst 33342 by a multidrug resistance-like transporter. Optimal resolution of the profile is obtained after great attention is paid to the staining conditions. Indeed, the Hoechst concentration, staining time, and staining temperature are all critical. The classical technique used to discriminate BM SP-cells does not allow a precise separation of SP cells from AGM, YS, or FL, so it is recommended to stain the cells with some precautions (*see* **Note 7**).

Pyronin Y (final concentration 1 mg/mL or 3.3 μ*M*) stains the RNA content of cells already stained with Hoechst 33342. Pyronin Y staining allows the discrimination between cells with low RNA content (cells in G_0) from cells expressing higher levels of RNA as they progress through G_1. Hoechst/Pyronin Y staining allows the separation of cells in G_0 from cells in G_1 or in S/G_2+M phases.

1. Prewarm L15+ medium at precisely 37°C.
2. Single-cell suspensions from embryonic tissues are prepared in L15+ and count.
3. Spin cells down 10 min at 1300 rpm at 4°C. Remove supernatant.
4. Resuspend at 10^6 cells/mL or less in prewarmed L15+ and mix well.
5. Add Hoechst to a final concentration of 5 μg/mL (5 μL of 1 mg/mL stock for each milliliter of cell suspension) and mix well.
6. Incubate 90 min exactly in the 37°C water bath. Make sure the staining tubes are well submerged in the bath water to ensure that the temperature of the cells is maintained at 37°C. Tubes should be mixed several times during the incubation.
7. No washing step. At this point cells must be kept on ice until the FACS analysis or can be further stained with antibodies.

3.3.2. BrdU Labeling and Staining Procedure

It is also possible to study the cell cycle status of embryonic cells by using the BrdU. BrdU incorporates into newly synthesized DNA of cells entering and progressing through the S phase of the cell cycle. BrdU can be used to stain single-cell suspensions, cells maintained in culture or cells in the intact embryonic tissue cultured as explant. The incorporated BrdU is secondarily detected in the cells with fluorescent dye-labeled anti-BrdU antibodies, and the addition of 7AAD or PI allows the discrimination of the total DNA content. The flow cytometric analysis of stained cells allows the separation between cells in G_0/G_1 (resting/active noncycling cells with diploid DNA content), in S (DNA-synthesizing cells), or G_2/M (cells with tetraploid DNA content/dividing cells) phases of the cell cycle (during the time of BrdU pulse). The staining of BrdU-pulsed cells with fluorescent antibodies directed against various markers provides further characterization of cell subsets with respect to cell cycle status. To study the cell cycle status of embryonic cells we use the BrdU flow kit from BD Pharmingen. BrdU incorporation by labeled cells is analyzed by flow cytometry by comparing with controls (*see* **Note 8**). An overview of the different steps of the BrdU staining protocol is described as follows:

1. In vitro labeling of cells with BrdU: we use BrdU to stain cells in the intact embryonic tissue cultured as explant. We found that a overnight pulse is necessary for the identification of actively cycling cell populations in explant culture (final concentration 20 μ*M* or 6.14 μg/mL).
2. Immunofluorescent staining of cell surface antigens: as described in **Subheading 3.2.2.1.**, in staining buffer.

3. Fixation and permeabilization of cells: using cytofix/cytoperm buffer.
4. Permeabilization of cells: using Cytoperm Plus buffer.
5. Re-fixation of cells: using Cytofix/Cytoperm buffer.
6. Treatment of cells with Dnase to expose BrdU epitopes.
7. Immunofluorescent staining: with FITC conjugated anti-BrdU and appropriate intracellular antigen specific.
8. Stain total DNA for cell cycle analysis using 7AAD.
9. Suspend cells in staining buffer and analyze by flow cytometry.

3.3.3. Ki67 Labeling and Staining Procedure

Ki67, a nuclear cell proliferation-associated antigen, is expressed in all active stages of the cell cycle (G_1 and S/G_2) but not during G_0. Cells expressing Ki67 are revealed by fluorescent-labeled anti-Ki67 antibodies and flow cytometric analysis.

1. Antibody staining: single-cell suspensions are incubated with specific monoclonal antibodies of interest for 20 to 30 min at 4°C in PBS/FCS/PS. Cells are then washed twice and subsequently incubated with fluorochrome-conjugated streptavidin or goat anti-rat IgG (when using biotin conjugated or unconjugated first antibodies, respectively).
2. Fix and permeabilize cells: a) wash cells twice in PBS with 1% FCS and thoroughly resuspend them; b) add 250 μL of cytofix/cytoperm solution per tube; c) incubate 20 min at 4°C; and d) wash twice in PBS with 1% FCS and thoroughly resuspend them.
3. Ki67 staining: a) add Ki67-FITC antibody (20 μL/tube) or IgG1 control (*see* **Note 8**); and b) incubate 30 to 45 min at 4°C in the dark and wash.
4. After washing, add 7AAD (2 μg/mL).
5. Cells are then ready for flow cytometric analysis.

4. Notes

1. To obtain the best cell viability, cells must be kept at 4°C at every step. Moreover, FCS and collagenase must be tested before use because of large variations between different commercially available lots. The serum must be heat-inactivated to prevent complement-mediated cell lysis.
2. Embryos to be used for experiments are staged following three major criteria (**Table 2**): a) the number of somite pairs (sp), b) the eye pigmentation, and c) the shape of the limb buds ***(58)***.
3. In contrast to human/adult cells, the discrimination of live/dead cells from embryonic tissues is essential because of the cell mortality occurring during the dissection and collagenase treatment steps. Moreover, for the best viability after sort, cells are collected in pure 0.2-μm filtered FCS.
4. Special considerations must be made in FACS compensation parameters for GFP transgene expression in combination with antibody staining, particularly if GFP expression is high.
5. We have found that the FDG staining results are dependent on cell concentration and staining medium. Therefore, we recommend staining the cells in DMEM medium with 10 % FCS and at a maximum concentration of 2×10^6 cells per 50 μL of medium. All procedures must be conducted at 4°C to avoid fluorescein leakage out of the positive cells (and to stain negative cells).
6. The detection of Hoechst stained cells, instead of PI or 7AAD stained cells, requires a UV laser (i.e., FACS Vantage). The advantage in using a different laser (UV) is: a) the absence of contamination with the other fluorescent signals read by another laser, and b) the possible use of antibodies with three different fluorochromes.

Table 2
Staging Criteria for Mouse Embryos

Embryonic stage	No. of sp	Eye and limb characteristics
E8–8.5	1–7	No eye pigmentation
E8.5–9	8–14	No limb bud
E9–9.5	13–20	No eye pigmentation
E9.5–10	21–30	No limb bud
Early E10	30–35	Progressive partial eye pigmentation ring
Mid E10	36–37	(starting at 36–37 sp)
Late E10	38–40	Progressive limb bud formation
E11	>40	Eye pigmentation ring closed
		Round limb buds with the beginning of internal digital segmentation

7. For the Hoechst 33342 staining, we find that the use of L15+ medium instead of DMEM+ medium and avoidance of washing step at the end of the procedure significantly improves the results. Also 90 min of staining are optimal to stain mouse cells. When the staining process is over, the cells must be maintained at 4°C to avoid further dye efflux.
8. Controls are particularly important to analyze correctly the cell cycle status by flow cytometry (for BrdU or Ki67 staining). Those controls must include: a) cells fixed and permeabilized only; b) cells fixed and permeabilized and stained with BrdU or Ki67-FITC; c) cells fixed and permeabilized and stained with IgG1-FITC control and an other antibody-PE of interest; d) cells fixed and permeabilized and stained with 7AAD; e) cells fixed and permeabilized and stained with IgG1-FITC control, an other antibody-PE of interest and 7AAD.

Acknowledgments

The authors thank all the members of the laboratory, particularly past members Maria-Jose Sanchez, Corne Snoys, and Marella de Bruijn for their dedicated contributions to developing sorting procedures for functional AGM HSCs. This work is supported by La Ligue Nationale Contre Le Cancer (CR), EC Marie Curie fellowship 99-1 (CR), KWF 2001-2442 (ED) and the NIH RO1 DK54077 (ED).

References

1. Lemischka, I. R. (1991) Clonal, in vivo behavior of the totipotent hematopoietic stem cell. *Semin. Immunol.* **3,** 349–355.
2. Spangrude, G. J., Smith, L., Uchida, N., Ikuta, K., Heimfeld, S., Friedman, J., and Weissman, I. L. (1991) Mouse hematopoietic stem cells. *Blood* **78,** 1395–1402.
3. Moore, M. A. and Metcalf, D. (1970) Ontogeny of the haemopoietic system: yolk sac origin of in vivo and in vitro colony forming cells in the developing mouse embryo. *Br. J. Haematol.* **18,** 279–296.
4. Medvinsky, A. and Dzierzak, E. (1996) Definitive hematopoiesis is autonomously initiated by the AGM region. *Cell* **86,** 897–906.

5. Muller, A. M., Medvinsky, A., Strouboulis, J., Grosveld, F., and Dzierzak, E. (1994) Development of hematopoietic stem cell activity in the mouse embryo. *Immunity* **1,** 291–301.
6. de Bruijn, M. F., Speck, N. A., Peeters, M. C., and Dzierzak, E. (2000) Definitive hematopoietic stem cells first develop within the major arterial regions of the mouse embryo. *EMBO J.* **19,** 2465–2474.
7. Garcia-Porrero, J. A., Godin, I. E., and Dieterlen-Lievre, F. (1995) Potential intraembryonic hemogenic sites at pre-liver stages in the mouse. *Anat. Embryol. (Berl).* **192,** 425–435.
8. North, T., Gu, T. L., Stacy, T., Wang, Q., Howard, L., Binder, M., et al. (1999) Cbfa2 is required for the formation of intra-aortic hematopoietic clusters. *Development* **126,** 2563–2575.
9. Tavian, M., Hallais, M. F., and Peault, B. (1999) Emergence of intraembryonic hematopoietic precursors in the pre-liver human embryo. *Development* **126,** 793–803.
10. Harrison, D. E., Jordan, C. T., Zhong, R. K., and Astle, C. M. (1993) Primitive hemopoietic stem cells: direct assay of most productive populations by competitive repopulation with simple binomial, correlation and covariance calculations. *Exp. Hematol.* **21,** 206–219.
11. Harrison, D. E., Stone, M., and Astle, C. M. (1990) Effects of transplantation on the primitive immunohematopoietic stem cell. *J. Exp. Med.* **172,** 431–437.
12. Cumano, A. and Godin, I. (2001) Pluripotent hematopoietic stem cell development during embryogenesis. *Curr. Opin. Immunol.* **13,** 166–171.
13. Robin, C., Ottersbach, K., de Bruijn, M., Ma, X., van der Horn, K., and Dzierzak, E. (2003) Developmental origins of hematopoietic stem cells. *Oncol. Res.* **13,** 315–321.
14. Orlic, D. and Bodine, D. M. (1994) What defines a pluripotent hematopoietic stem cell (PHSC): will the real PHSC please stand up! *Blood* **84,** 3991–3994.
15. Lansdorp, P. M., Dragowska, W., and Mayani, H. (1993) Ontogeny-related changes in proliferative potential of human hematopoietic cells. *J. Exp. Med.* **178,** 787–791.
16. Morrison, S. J., Wandycz, A. M., Akashi, K., Globerson, A., and Weissman, I. L. (1996) The aging of hematopoietic stem cells. *Nat. Med.* **2,** 1011–1016.
17. Sanchez, M. J., Holmes, A., Miles, C., and Dzierzak, E. (1996) Characterization of the first definitive hematopoietic stem cells in the AGM and liver of the mouse embryo. *Immunity* **5,** 513–525.
18. Spangrude, G. J., Heimfeld, S., and Weissman, I. L. (1988) Purification and characterization of mouse hematopoietic stem cells. *Science* **241,** 58–62.
19. Garcia-Porrero, J. A., Manaia, A., Jimeno, J., Lasky, L. L., Dieterlen-Lievre, F., and Godin, I. E. (1998) Antigenic profiles of endothelial and hemopoietic lineages in murine intraembryonic hemogenic sites. *Dev. Comp. Immunol.* **22,** 303–319.
20. Flamme, I., Frolich, T., and Risau, W. (1997) Molecular mechanisms of vasculogenesis and embryonic angiogenesis. *J. Cell Physiol.* **173,** 206–210.
21. Nishikawa, S. I., Nishikawa, S., Hirashima, M., Matsuyoshi, N., and Kodama, H. (1998) Progressive lineage analysis by cell sorting and culture identifies FLK1+VE-cadherin+ cells at a diverging point of endothelial and hemopoietic lineages. *Development* **125,** 1747–1757.
22. Wood, H. B., May, G., Healy, L., Enver, T., and Morriss-Kay, G. M. (1997) CD34 expression patterns during early mouse development are related to modes of blood vessel formation and reveal additional sites of hematopoiesis. *Blood* **90,** 2300–2311.
23. Dieterlen-Lievre, F. (1998) Hematopoiesis: progenitors and their genetic program. *Curr. Biol.* **8,** R727–R730.
24. Ikuta, K. and Weissman, I. L. (1992) Evidence that hematopoietic stem cells express mouse c-kit but do not depend on steel factor for their generation. *Proc. Natl. Acad. Sci. USA* **89,** 1502–1506.

25. Morrison, S. J. and Weissman, I. L. (1994) The long-term repopulating subset of hematopoietic stem cells is deterministic and isolatable by phenotype. *Immunity* **1,** 661–673.
26. de Bruijn, M. F., Ma, X., Robin, C., Ottersbach, K., Sanchez, M. J., and Dzierzak, E. (2002) Hematopoietic stem cells localize to the endothelial cell layer in the midgestation mouse aorta. *Immunity* **16,** 673–683.
27. North, T. E., de Bruijn, M. F., Stacy, T., Talebian, L., Lind, E., Robin, C., Binder, M., Dzierzak, E., and Speck, N. A. (2002) Runx1 expression marks long-term repopulating hematopoietic stem cells in the midgestation mouse embryo. *Immunity* **16,** 661–672.
28. Baum, C. M., Weissman, I. L., Tsukamoto, A. S., Buckle, A. M., and Peault, B. (1992) Isolation of a candidate human hematopoietic stem-cell population. *Proc. Natl. Acad. Sci. USA* **89,** 2804–2808.
29. Labastie, M. C., Cortes, F., Romeo, P. H., Dulac, C., and Peault, B. (1998) Molecular identity of hematopoietic precursor cells emerging in the human embryo. *Blood* **92,** 3624–3635.
30. Ziegler, B. L., Valtieri, M., Porada, G. A., De Maria, R., Muller, R., Masella, B., et al. (1999) KDR receptor: a key marker defining hematopoietic stem cells. *Science* **285,** 1553–1558.
31. Yin, A. H., Miraglia, S., Zanjani, E. D., Almeida-Porada, G., Ogawa, M., Leary, A. G., et al. (1997) AC**133,** a novel marker for human hematopoietic stem and progenitor cells. *Blood* **90,** 5002–5012.
32. Osawa, M., Hanada, K., Hamada, H., and Nakauchi, H. (1996) Long-term lymphohematopoietic reconstitution by a single CD34- low/negative hematopoietic stem cell. *Science* **273,** 242–245.
33. Ito, T., Tajima, F., and Ogawa, M. (2000) Developmental changes of CD34 expression by murine hematopoietic stem cells. *Exp. Hematol.* **28,** 1269–1273.
34. Szilvassy, S. J., Humphries, R. K., Lansdorp, P. M., Eaves, A. C., and Eaves, C. J. (1990) Quantitative assay for totipotent reconstituting hematopoietic stem cells by a competitive repopulation strategy. *Proc. Natl. Acad. Sci. USA* **87,** 8736–8740.
35. Sato, T., Laver, J. H., and Ogawa, M. (1999) Reversible expression of CD34 by murine hematopoietic stem cells. *Blood* **94,** 2548–2554.
36. Tajima, F., Sato, T., Laver, J. H., and Ogawa, M. (2000) CD34 expression by murine hematopoietic stem cells mobilized by granulocyte colony-stimulating factor. *Blood* **96,** 1989–1993.
37. Engelhardt, M., Lubbert, M., and Guo, Y. (2002) CD34(+) or CD34(-): which is the more primitive? *Leukemia* **16,** 1603–1608.
38. Ogawa, M. (2002) Changing phenotypes of hematopoietic stem cells. *Exp. Hematol.* **30,** 3–6.
39. Keller, G., Lacaud, G., and Robertson, S. (1999) Development of the hematopoietic system in the mouse. *Exp. Hematol.* **27,** 777–787.
40. Nishikawa, S. I. (2001) A complex linkage in the developmental pathway of endothelial and hematopoietic cells. *Curr. Opin. Cell Biol.* **13,** 673–678.
41. Shivdasani, R. A. and Orkin, S. H. (1996) The transcriptional control of hematopoiesis. *Blood* **87,** 4025–4039.
42. Zhu, J. and Emerson, S. G. (2002) Hematopoietic cytokines, transcription factors and lineage commitment. *Oncogene* **21,** 3295–2313.
43. Bonnet, D. (2002) Haematopoietic stem cells. *J. Pathol.* **197,** 430–440.
44. Marshall, C. J. and Thrasher, A. J. (2001) The embryonic origins of human haematopoiesis. *Br. J. Haematol.* **112,** 838–850.
45. Jaffredo, T., Gautier, R., Eichmann, A., and Dieterlen-Lievre, F. (1998) Intraaortic hemopoietic cells are derived from endothelial cells during ontogeny. *Development* **125,** 4575–4583.

46. Marshall, C. J., Moore, R. L., Thorogood, P., Brickell, P. M., Kinnon, C., and Thrasher, A. J. (1999) Detailed characterization of the human aorta-gonad-mesonephros region reveals morphological polarity resembling a hematopoietic stromal layer. *Dev. Dyn.* **215,** 139–147.
47. Tavian, M., Coulombel, L., Luton, D., Clemente, H. S., Dieterlen-Lievre, F., and Peault, B. (1996) Aorta-associated CD34+ hematopoietic cells in the early human embryo. *Blood* **87,** 67–72.
48. Bernex, F., De Sepulveda, P., Kress, C., Elbaz, C., Delouis, C., and Panthier, J. J. (1996) Spatial and temporal patterns of c-kit-expressing cells in WlacZ/+ and WlacZ/WlacZ mouse embryos. *Development* **122,** 3023–3033.
49. Sporn, L. A., Marder, V. J., and Wagner, D. D. (1989) Differing polarity of the constitutive and regulated secretory pathways for von Willebrand factor in endothelial cells. *J. Cell Biol.* **108,** 1283–1289.
50. Cai, Z., de Bruijn, M., Ma, X., Dortland, B., Luteijn, T., Downing, R. J., and Dzierzak, E. (2000) Haploinsufficiency of AML1 affects the temporal and spatial generation of hematopoietic stem cells in the mouse embryo. *Immunity* **13,** 423–431.
51. Okuda, T., van Deursen, J., Hiebert, S. W., Grosveld, G., and Downing, J. R. (1996) AML1, the target of multiple chromosomal translocations in human leukemia, is essential for normal fetal liver hematopoiesis. *Cell* **84,** 321–330.
52. Wang, Q., Stacy, T., Binder, M., Marin-Padilla, M., Sharpe, A. H., and Speck, N. A. (1996) Disruption of the Cbfa2 gene causes necrosis and hemorrhaging in the central nervous system and blocks definitive hematopoiesis. *Proc. Natl. Acad. Sci. USA* **93,** 3444–3449.
53. Bunting, K. D. (2002) ABC transporters as phenotypic markers and functional regulators of stem cells. *Stem Cells* **20,** 11–20.
54. Goodell, M. A., Brose, K., Paradis, G., Conner, A. S., and Mulligan, R. C. (1996) Isolation and functional properties of murine hematopoietic stem cells that are replicating in vivo. *J. Exp. Med.* **183,** 1797–1806.
55. Shapiro, H. M. (1981) Flow cytometric estimation of DNA and RNA content in intact cells stained with Hoechst 33342 and pyronin Y. *Cytometry* **2,** 143–150.
56. Gerdes, J., Lemke, H., Baisch, H., Wacker, H. H., Schwab, U., and Stein, H. (1984) Cell cycle analysis of a cell proliferation-associated human nuclear antigen defined by the monoclonal antibody Ki-67. *J. Immunol.* **133,** 1710–1715.
57. Gratzner, H. G. (1982) Monoclonal antibody to 5-bromo- and 5-iododeoxyuridine: A new reagent for detection of DNA replication. *Science* **218,** 474–475.
58. Samoylina, N. L., Gan, O. I., and Medvinsky, A. L. (1990) Development of the hematopoietic system: splenic colony forming units in mouse embryogenesis. *Sov. J. Dev. Biol.* **21,** 127–133.

17

Hematopoietic Stem Cell Development During Mouse Embryogenesis

Julien Y. Bertrand, Sebastien Giroux, Ana Cumano, and Isabelle Godin

Summary

The progress of the last few years in the understanding of hematopoietic cell development during embryogenesis resulted from a combination of experimental approaches used in hematology and developmental biology. This methodology has been particularly powerful for the analysis of the earliest steps of hematopoietic ontogeny because it allows for the first time the demonstration of the existence of two independent sites of hematopoietic cell generation. Here, we describe the methods used in our laboratories to characterize the phenotype and differentiation potential of the primordial hematopoietic precursors as well as their localization in the mouse embryo. This multidisciplinary approach is required to explore the mechanisms of hematopoietic cell generation.

Key Words: AGM; flow cytometry; FTOC; *in situ* hybridization; hematopoiesis; mouse embryo; ontogeny; organ culture; stem cells; yolk sac.

1. Introduction

Hematopoietic progenitors are first detected in the yolk sac (YS) of mouse embryos between 7 and 7.5 d post-coitus (dpc) *(1)*. These YS hematopoietic precursors can either be expanded in vitro or transplanted in vivo. Reconstitution of the hematopoietic lineage in recipient adult mice cannot be obtained under these conditions. Only erythroid cells are generated after in vitro expansion of YS hematopoietic progenitors under culture conditions that allow the differentiation of all hematopoietic lineages. Nowhere in the embryo proper can we find other hematopoietic cells at this stage of development *(2,3)*.

Later, between 8 and 8.5 dpc, before the establishment of circulation between the YS and the embryo proper, hematopoietic precursors can also be detected in the intraembryonic compartment (splanchnopleura [Sp]: *see* following paragraph), but only if an organ culture step precedes in vitro differentiation or in vivo transplantation.

From: *Methods in Molecular Medicine, Vol. 105: Developmental Hematopoiesis: Methods and Protocols.*
Edited by: M. H. Baron © Humana Press Inc., Totowa, NJ

Under these conditions, Sp precursors can generate all hematopoietic lineages when transferred to the appropriate differentiation culture systems and provide hematopoietic long-term reconstitution in natural killer-deficient mice, illustrating the presence of hematopoietic stem cells. In contrast, YS isolated from the same embryos generate only precursors with erythroid and/or myeloid potential and do not provide hematopoietic long-term reconstitution *(3)*.

The extraembryonic and intraembryonic sites capable of generating hematopoietic cells before the onset of fetal liver hematopoiesis as well as their evolution during development are schematically described in **Fig. 1**. The extraembryonic YS provides for immediate erythropoiesis from 7 dpc. The hematopoietic determination of mesodermal cells takes place in the caudal intraembryonic Sp beginning at the presomitic stage (7.5 dpc). In both hemogenic sites, mesoderm is associated with endoderm, a combination termed Splanchnopleura. After the 15-somite stage, the tissues derived from the Sp comprise the endoderm of the developing gut, the dorsal aorta, the omphalomesenteric artery, and the splanchnopleural lining of these tissues. This site is now referred to as Para-aortic Sp (P-Sp: 8.5–10 dpc; **ref.** ***4***). When fetal liver colonization by hematopoietic stem cells begins, the P-Sp develops further and comprises, besides the aorta, the developing gonads and the mesonephros (AGM region: 10–11.5 dpc; **refs.** ***5–8***).

2. Materials

2.1. Dissection of Embryo

1. 70% Ethanol.
2. Phosphate-buffered saline (PBS) with calcium and magnesium.
3. Dissecting tools. Dissecting tools are all from BioTek Microsurgery, 34 Rue Des Chardonnerets, 92160 Antony, France; Web site: biotek-online.com:
   a. Curved-serrated forceps: P-95-BC;
   b. Fine forceps: DU-110-AUF
   c. Ultra-fine forceps: DU-110-A
   d. Sieve used for embryo transfer: S-20-P

2.2. Whole-Mount and In Situ *Hybridization*

1. Labeling solution: ribonucleic acid (RNA) labeling with digoxigenin-UTP by in vitro transcription with appropriate RNA polymerases (Boehringer), DIG RNA labeling. Mix (1X final), transcription buffer (1X final), RNA polymerase (40 µL), RNAsine (10–20 µ*M*/µL) and complemented with RNA free H_2O to a 20 µL of final volume.
2. TE: 10 m*M* Tris-HCl, 1 m*M* ethylenediamine tetraacetic acid (EDTA; pH 8.0), make up with RNAse-free water and autoclave
3. WISH-FIX: Whole-mount embryo *in situ* hybridization fixative solution (for 50 mL), 5 mL 37% formaldehyde, 200 µL of 0.5 *M* EDTA (pH 8.8) and 150 µL of 1 *M* NaOH in PBS without Ca^{2+}/Mg^{2+}.
4. WISH buffer: Whole-mount embryo *in situ* hybridization buffer (for 200 mL), 100 mL of formamide, 13 mL of 20X SSC (pH 5.0), 2 mL 0.5 *M* EDTA (pH 8.0), Torula (50 µg/mL), 400 µL of Tween-20, 1 g of CHAPS and heparin (100 µg/mL) in H_2O.
5. ISH-Fix buffer: *in situ* hybridization fixative buffer (for 200 mL): 8 g of sucrose, 24 µL of 1 *M* $CaCl_2$, 77 mL of 0.2 *M* $NaHPO_4$, and 23 mL of 0.2 *M* NaH_2PO_4 in H_2O.

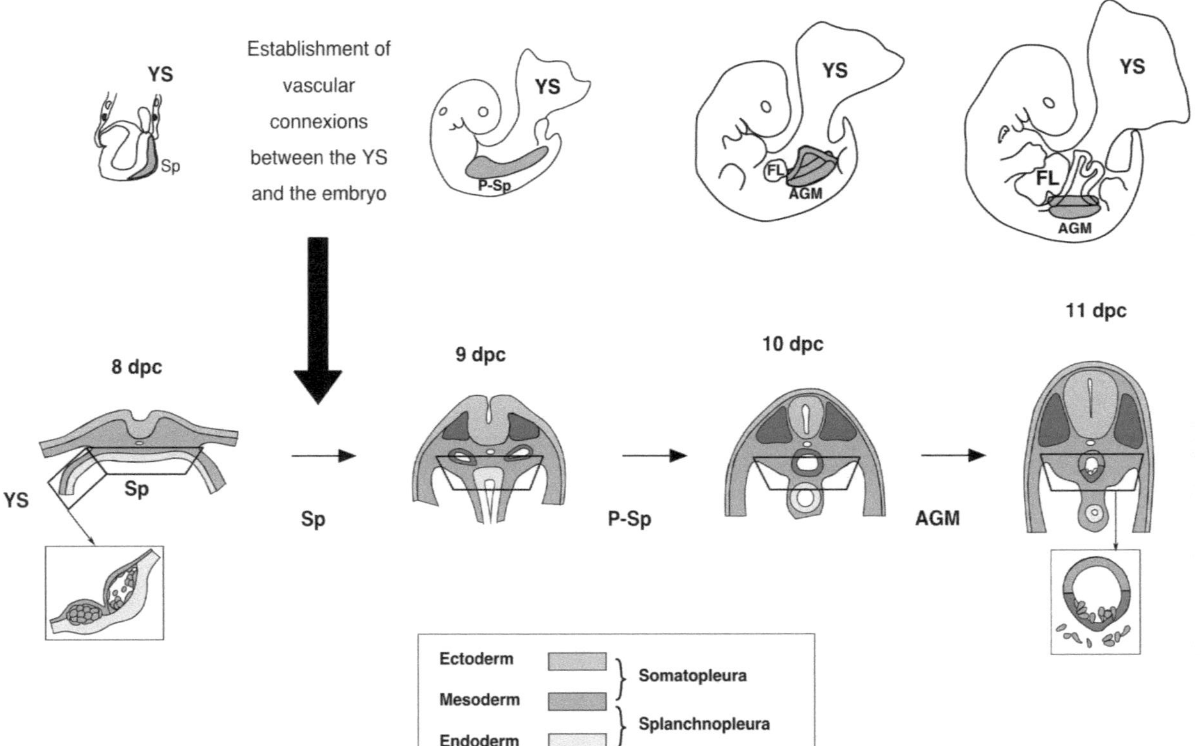

Fig. 1. Localization of embryonic sites capable of hematopoietic cell generation. Top drawings display the location of extra- and intraembryonic hemogenic sites in whole embryos. Bottom line: the extra- and intraembryonic regions involved in generation of hematopoietic precursors are shown in boxes.

6. ISH-FIX: *in situ* hybridization fixative solution (for 200 mL, add 8 g of paraformaldehyde in prewarmed ISH buffer.
7. ISH buffer: *in situ* hybridization (for 10 mL), 1 mL of 10X salt, 5 mL of formamide, 2 mL of 50% dextran sulfate, 200 µL of 50X Denhardt's and Torula Yeast (1 mg/mL) in H_2O.
8. PBT: PBS containing 0.1% Tween-20.
9. MABT (for 1 L; pH 7.5), 11.6 g of maleic acid, 807 g of NaCl, and 10 mL of Tween-20 in H_2O.
10. Anti-digoxigenin-AP: Fab fragment from an anti-digoxigenin antibody from sheep, conjugated with alkaline phosphatase.
11. NTMT (for 100 mL): 2 mL of 5 *M* NaCl, 5 mL of 2 *M* Tris-HCl (pH 9.5), 1 mL of Tween-20 and 2.5 mL of 2 *M* $MgCl_2$ in H_2O.
12. Washing solution: 1X standard saline citrate (SSC), 50% formamide, 0.1% Tween-20.
13. Staining solution: 100 mL of NTMT + 450 µL of NBT + 350 µL of BCIP.

2.3. *Organ Culture* In Toto *and Analysis of Hematopoietic Potential*

1. 24-Well plate (TPP).
2. OptiMEM (Invitrogen).
3. Fetal calf serum (ICN).
4. Penicillin–streptomycin (Invitrogen).
5. β-mercapto-ethanol (Invitrogen).
6. OP9 stromal cells (T. Nakano, S.-I. Nishikawa, Kyoto, Japan).
7. Trypsin–EDTA (Invitrogen).
8. 96-Well plate (TPP).
9. Hanks balanced salt solution (HBSS; Invitrogen).
10. Trypan blue (Invitrogen).
11. Irradiator (X-ray or cesium source).
12. IL-7 supernatant. We use the supernatant of J558 cells transfected with the cDNA encoding IL-7, a kind gift from F. Melchers (Basel, Switzerland). Cells are grown to confluency, and the supernatant is collected. Titration is done in 2E8 cells, a kind gift from P. Kincade (Oklahoma City, OK), dependent on IL-7 for growth. The supernatant is serially diluted on the 2E8 cells and growth is scored 3 d later, either by counting the cells or by thymidine incorporation. The highest dilution that gives maximum proliferation is chosen.
13. Flt3-Ligand (Flt3-L) supernatant. We use the supernatant of Sp2.0 myeloma cells transfected with the cDNA encoding Flt3-L and Baf3 cells transfected with the cDNA encoding Flt3, kind gifts from R. Rottapel (Toronto, Canada). Supernatant collection and titration is performed as described in **step 12**.
14. c-Kit-Ligand (c-Kit-L) supernatant. We use the supernatant of CHO cells transfected with the cDNA encoding c-Kit-L, a kind gift from Genetics Institute (Boston, MA). Titration is performed on freshly prepared bone marrow mast cells cultured for 1 wk in c-Kit-L, essentially as described in **step 12**.
15. Terasaki plates (Nunc).
16. Millipore filters. ATTP 0.8 µm (Millipore).
17. Hemostatic sponge (Helistat Colla-Tec, Plainsboro, NJ).

2.4. *Flow Cytometry Analyses*

2.4.1. Monoclonal Antibodies From Pharmingen (Becton Dickinson)

1. CD19-FITC (clone 1D3).
2. Ter119-PE.

3. Mac-1- APC (clone M1/70).
4. CD4-PE.
5. CD8-APC.
6. Ly5.1- FITC.

2.4.2. Other Products

1. PBS, 1X.
2. Fetal calf serum (ICN).
3. Round bottom 96-well plate (CML).
4. Propidium iodide (Sigma).

3. Methods

3. 1. Dissection of Embryonic Sites Involved in Hematopoietic Development

3.1.1. Mating and Embryo Recovery

1. Place females and one male in cage either overnight or for 4 consecutive days (*see* **Note 1**). Mating is ascertained by the presence of a copulation plug the following morning, which is then considered d 0.5 of gestation.
2. Pregnant mice at the appropriate stage are sacrificed by cervical dislocation (or by appropriate method required by the investigator's institution) and placed on their back. Uterine horns are dissected as shown in **Fig. 2A**.
3. Cleanse abdomen with 70% ethanol.
4. A skip-incision is made perpendicular to the axis.
5. Reflect the skin towards the head and tail and make a similar incision in the muscle layer. Displace the intestines to expose the uterine horns.
6. The cervical segment of the uterine horn is grabbed with a pair of blunt ended forceps and sectioned below the ovary. The horns are then lifted from the peritoneal cavity and the mesometrium and fat are trimmed away to produce a string of concepti.
7. The concepti, surrounded by the muscular layers, are individually sectioned and placed in a Petri dish containing PBS with calcium and magnesium.
8. Under a dissecting microscope, open the uterine muscle layers by splitting along the antimesometrial side with thin forceps. Reflect the muscle layer towards the mesometrial side. Compression of the deciduoma during this procedure would damage the embryo and should be avoided.
9. The embryos surrounded by the deciduoma are located at the anti-mesometrial side. Embryos should be removed from the deciduoma by cutting the top third of the egg-shaped structure opposite from the mesometrial side and by pulling the embryo and surrounding YS away from the deciduoma. Transfer embryos (up to 9.0 dpc) to a clean Petri dish containing PBS with calcium and magnesium using a Pasteur pipet. For later stage embryos, use a sieve designed for embryo transfer (Biotek; *see* **Note 2**).

3.1.2. Embryo Staging

During presomite stages, embryos are staged according to the criteria of Downs and Davies *(9)*. The developmental stages of P-Sp and AGM explants are ascertained by somite counting.

3.1.3. YS and Sp Dissection: 7.5–8 dpc, Up to 4S (Fig. 2B)

YS is explanted by cutting with ultra-fine forceps, all along its connection with the embryo body (**Fig. 2B,3**). The amnion is cut medially, up to the trunk (**Fig. 2B,4**) and

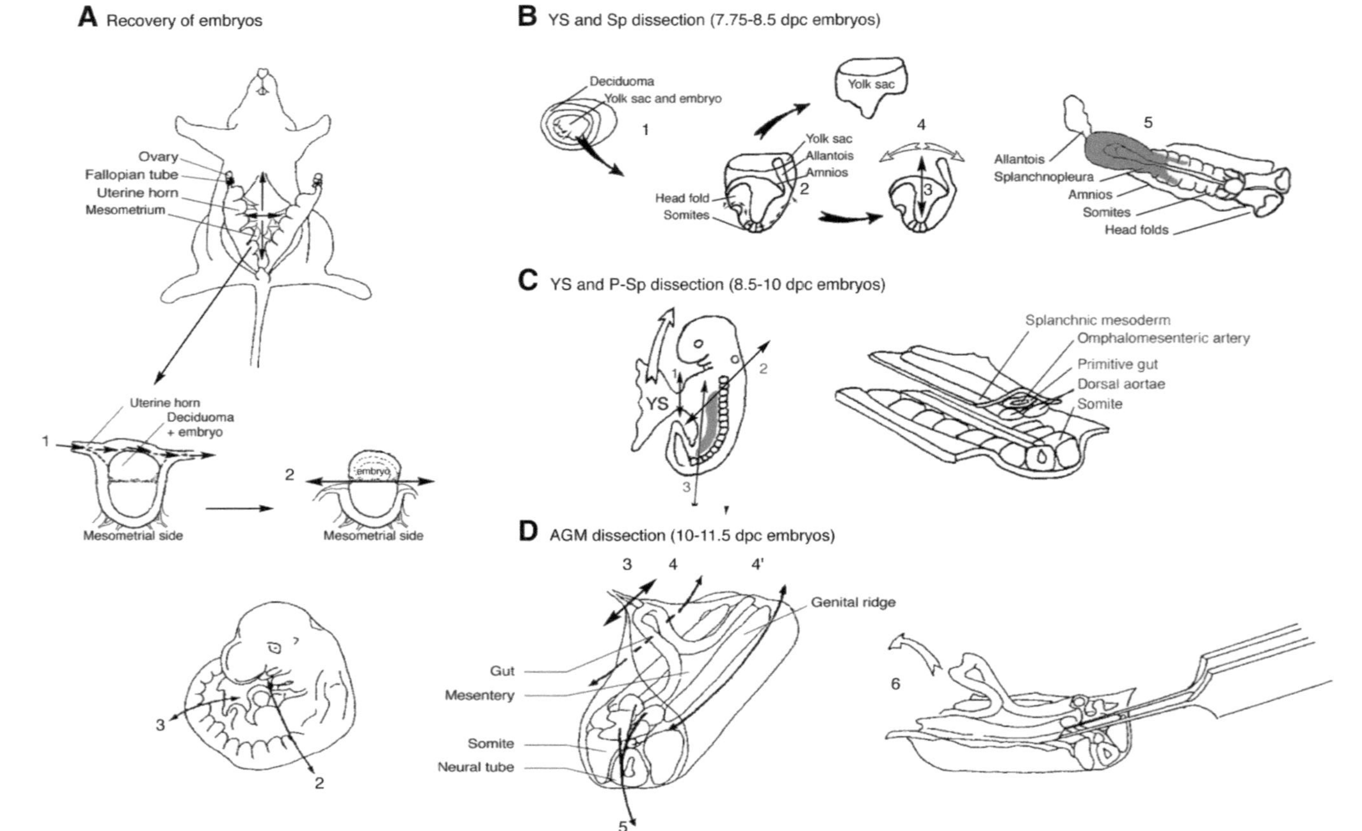

Fig. 2. Dissection of embryonic sites involved in hematopoietic development. **(A)** Embryo recovery from pregnant mice. **(B)** YS and Sp dissection: 7.5–8 dpc, up to 4S; **(C)** YS and P-Sp dissection: 8.5–10 dpc; 5-30S. **(D)** YS and AGM dissection: 10–11.5 dpc; 30–45S.

the embryo flattened by pulling the amnion towards the head and tail (**Fig. 2B,5**). Sp (in grey) is removed by grabbing it at the base of the allantois and pulling it towards the heart region.

3.1.4. YS and P-Sp: 8.5–10 dpc; 5-30S (Fig. 2C)

1. Explant the YS by sectioning it close to the body wall and by tearing it apart.
2. To reveal the P-Sp and free it from anatomical connections that would prevent its removal, dissect the trunk region as shown in **Fig. 2C**. Remove the P-Sp (in grey) by grabbing it anteriorly, below the somite, and pulling it towards the caudal region.

3.1.5. YS and AGM: 10–11.5 dpc; 30–45S (Fig. 2D)

1. Explant the YS by tearing it apart and sectioning it close to the body wall.
2. AGM is freed from anatomical connections to the body wall by three cuts, as shown in **Fig. 2D**. Carefully remove the fetal liver and lung buds. Grab the AGM anteriorly, at the edges of the genital ridges. Lift up and pull towards the caudal region of the embryo. Care should be taken at this stage to remove all the fetal liver.

3.2. In Situ *Hybridization With Cryostat Sections and Whole Mouse Embryos*

3.2.1. Riboprobe Synthesis and Purification

1. Mix linearized template deoxyribonucleic acid (DNA) equivalent to 1 μg with probe in labeling solution.
2. Incubate mixture at 37°C for 2–3 h for in vitro transcription.
3. Add 2 μL of DNAse I and 1 μL of RNAsin to the reaction tube, place on ice, and then spin down, to terminate the reaction.
4. Digest away plasmid DNA by incubation at 37°C for 30 min.
5. Terminate DNase reaction by addition of 200 μL of TE.
6. Precipitate RNA by addition of 20 mL of 4 *M* LiCl and 600 μL of ethanol. Incubate for 30 min at –80°C or overnight at –20°C.
7. Collect RNA pellet by centrifugation for 30 min at 15,500*g*. Remove the supernatant.
8. Add 1 mL of 70% ethanol, mix and centrifuge for 15 min at 15,500*g*.
9. Remove the supernatant and air dry the pellet.
10. Dissolve the RNA probe in 100 μL of 10 m*M* EDTA. The probe may be checked on an agarose minigel (1X TBE) and the concentration determined (1.0 A_{260} OD corresponds to single stranded RNA at 40 μgmL).

3.2.2. Fixation, Storage, and Processing

1. For whole-mount embryo *in situ* hybridization (WISH), embryos are soaked in whole-mount *in situ* hybridization fixative solution (WISH-FIX) overnight at 4°C and washed in PBT. The embryos may be treated at this stage or dehydrated through a MeOH/PBT series (25:75%, 50:50%, 75:25%) finishing with MeOH (100%) and stored up to 1 mo at –20°C.
2. For *in situ* hybridization (ISH), embryos are soaked in ISH fixative solution (ISH-FIX) and washed first in ISH buffer, then in phosphate 0.12 *M*, 15% sucrose buffer. All steps are performed overnight at 4°C. The embryos are first placed in 0.12 *M* phosphate, 15% sucrose, 7.5% gelatin buffer (predissolved at 37°C) for at least 1 h at 37°C, then placed in the appropriate orientation in the same mixture in small plastic dishes and allowed to cool at room temperature. After trimming, the embedded embryos are placed in isopentane (frozen at –80°C in liquid nitrogen) for 1 min and stored at –80°C. The embedded embryos are cryosectioned at 10–15 μm and transferred to Superfrost slides. These can be stored at –20°C for up to 1 yr.

Table 1
Duration of PK Treatment Depending on Developmental Stage of Embryos

Stage	Presomitic stage	0-10 s	10-20 s	20-30 s	30-35 s	35-40 s	40-50 s
Duration	2–3 min	5 min	10 min	15 min	20 min	25 min	30 min

3.2.3. Prehybridization Washes and Hybridization

1. WISH: embryos stored in MeOH must be rehydrated in MeOH/PBT (5 min in each: 75%:25%, 50%:50%, 25%:75%, finishing with PBT). Then, they are treated with proteinase K (PK: 10 μg/mL in PBT) to allow easy access of probes and antibodies. The duration of the PK treatment depends on the developmental stage of the embryos (**Table 1**). The reaction is performed at room temperature and stopped by a 5-min wash in PBT. Embryos may then be re-fixed in 4% formaldehyde, 0.1% glutaraldehyde in PBT for 20 min at room temperature to better maintain its structure. Then, the embryos are rinsed twice in PBT, once in PBT/WISH-buffer (1:1). Embryos can be stored at –20°C up to 1 mo, after a final wash in WISH buffer. The embryos in WISH buffer are placed at 70°C for at least 1 h. Then, they are incubated in preheated hybridization mix containing the labelled probe overnight at 70°C. Total probe concentration should not exceed 1 μg/mL.
2. ISH: Sections are defrosted at room temperature for at least half an hour while prewarming ISH buffer (65°C) and lining a Perspex box with Whatman paper wetted with 1X salt and 50% formamide buffer. The probe is diluted in prewarmed ISH buffer (0.1–1 μg/mL) and denatured for 5 to 10 min at 70°C. One hundred microliters of probe is added to each slide, which is then covered with a cover slip. It does not matter if the probe does not cover completely all the sections at this stage, as it spreads during hybridization. Hybridization is carried out overnight at 70°C in sealed Perspex box.

3.2.4. Blocking and Antibody Staining

1. WISH: unbound probe is rinsed twice and washed 2 × 30 min in hybridization buffer, then 2 × 20 min in mixture of hybridization buffer/MABT (1:1) at 70°C on a shaker. Embryos are rinsed twice and washed twice for at least 1 h in MABT at room temperature on a shaker.
2. ISH: slides are transferred into a rack and washed 15 min at 65°C in washing solution to allow cover slips to fall off, then washed 2 × 30 min in the same solution. After, they are washed 2 × 30 min in MABT at room temperature.
3. Nonspecific binding sites are blocked before antibody treatment by placing the embryos or sections in blocking solution (MABT containing 2% blocking reagent and 20% heat inactivated goat serum) and incubating at room temperature on a shaker for at least 1h.
4. Embryos for WISH are incubated on a shaker in blocking solution containing a 1/2000 dilution (0.375 U/mL) of Fab fragments from an anti-digoxigenin antibody coupled to alkaline phosphatase overnight at room temperature. The embryos are rinsed and washed three times for 1 h in MABT then twice for 10 min in NTMT (prepared just before use) at room temperature.
5. For ISH, each slide is covered with 100 μL of blocking solution with antidigoxigenin antibody (as in **step 4**) and covered with a cover slip, placed in a PBS or water humidified chamber and incubated overnight at room temperature. After allowing cover slips to fall off during the MABT wash, sections are further washed four to five times in MABT for 20 min at room temperature.

3.2.5. Staining Reaction

Incubation with staining solution is performed in the dark at 37°C. Staining may appear rapidly in the embryonic regions in which the mRNA is strongly expressed. Because development of staining is usually slower for cells expressing low levels of the mRNA, several hours to a few days may be required to obtain full expression (*see* **Note 3**). When color has developed to the desired extent, wash embryos or sections 3 times in PBT (**Fig. 3**).

3.3. Organ Cultures of YS and Sp Explants From 7.5 to 8 dpc Mouse Embryos

1. Explant YS and Sp at 7.5 to 8 dpc as shown in **Fig. 2B**.
2. Using a siliconized Pasteur pipet, deposit individual explants into single wells of 24-well plates containing 2 mL of Complete Medium per well.
3. Incubate plates at 37°C, 5% CO_2 for 2 to 4 d.
4. At the end of the organ culture, YS and Sp explants have developed. **Figure 4** shows YS and Sp explants after a 4-d organ culture. The explants can now be enzymatically dissociated and the cells obtained tested for the presence of hematopoietic progenitors in in vitro and in vivo experiments, in bulk or after cell sorting *(2)*.

3.3.1. Dissociation Protocol

1. Remove two-thirds of the culture medium. Dissociate explant by gently passing through 26-gage needle attached to 1-mL syringe (from BD Plastipak, 300015) 10 times.
2. Allow debris to sediment by gravity.
3. Collect the suspension above the debris (*see* **Note 4** for a procedure to increase cell recovery).

3.4. Hematopoietic Potential Analysis in Suspension Cultures

3.4.1. Culture Conditions

3.4.1.1. Feeder Cells

Hematopoietic progenitors cannot develop in suspension without the presence of feeder cells. We use the OP9 stromal cell line, derived from bone marrow of the *op/op* mouse, as feeders *(10)*. OP9 cells can be amplified and maintained in OptiMEM 10% fetal calf serum (FCS), 1% antibiotics and 5×10^{-5} *M* β-mercaptoethanol at 37°C, 5% CO_2. Plates seeded with OP9 feeder cells should be prepared 1 d before the start of culture. We have also successfully used S17 stromal cells in this protocol.

3.4.1.2. Preparation of Culture Plates Coated With OP9 Stromal Cells

1. Add 4 mL of trypsin–EDTA to OP9 cell monolayer in culture flask (75-cm^2 flask). Incubate for 10 min at room temperature.
2. Collect cells and wash once in HBSS containing 5% of FCS.
3. Centrifuge cells and resuspend pellet in 1 mL of Complete Medium (OptiMEM 10% FCS 1% antibiotics).
4. Count OP9 after dilution in Trypan blue.
5. Plate cells at a concentration of 5×10^4 living cells per milliliter of Complete Medium.
6. Dispense 50 µL of stromal cell suspension per well of a flat bottomed 96-well plate or 500 µL per well of a 24-well plate.
7. Incubate OP9 cells overnight in an incubator.
8. Irradiate OP9 cells at 400 rads to stop their proliferation.

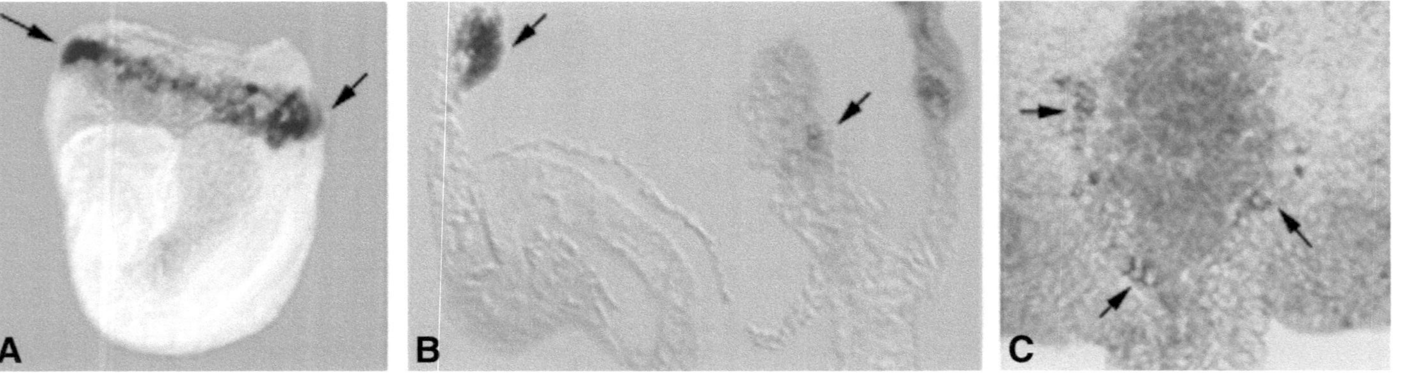

Fig. 3. ISH. **(A)** WISH on 8 dpc mouse embryo: erythroid cells that express the embryonic globin gene bH1 can be detected in the YS (arrows). **(B)** Section of an 8 dpc embryo previously WISH-hybridized with a probe against the Lmo-2 transcription factor to detect expression in YS hematopoietic precursors. **(C)** GATA-3 detection by ISH on section of 10.5 dpc embryo. Expression of this transcription factor is seen in the AGM (arrows).

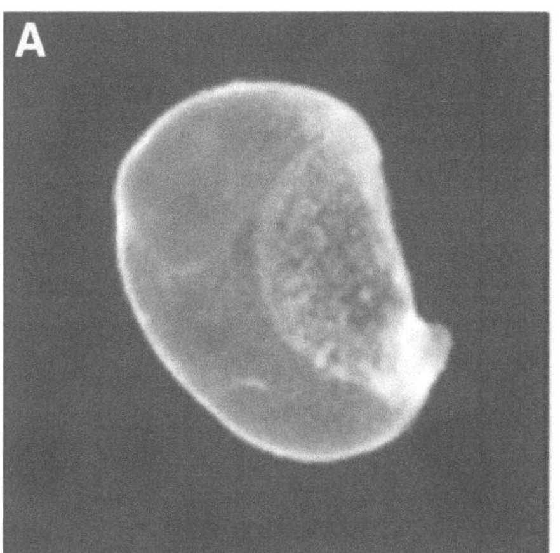

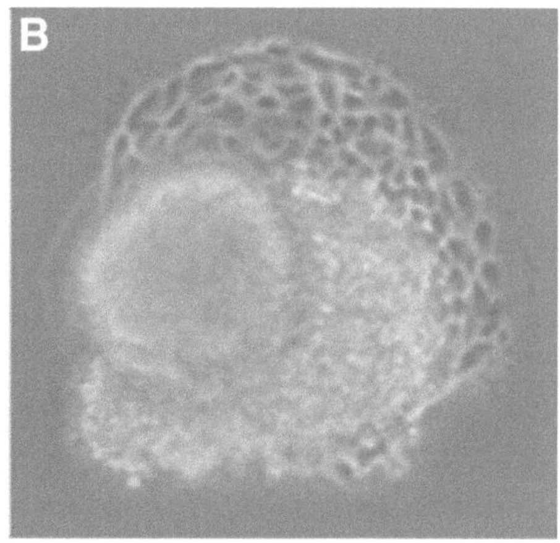

Fig. 4. (**A**) 8 dpc YS after 3 d in organ culture. (**B**) 8 dpc Sp after 3 d in organ culture.

3.4.1.3. Hematopoietic Cultures

1. Suspend putative hematopoietic precursors in Complete Medium.
2. Deposit 50 μL of this suspension into each well containing an OP9 stromal cell layer. Each well now contains 100 μL (OP9 + progenitors; *see* **Note 5**).
3. OP9 cells cannot produce M-CSF and FLT3-L, but express c-kit-L and IL-7, though in limited amounts. For this reason, we add cytokines to the medium to provide an appropriate environment for proliferation and differentiation. Complete Medium supplemented with c-Kit-L, IL-7, and FLT3-L (each of those twice concentrated) is then prepared and 100 μL added to each well. Under these conditions, multipotent hematopoietic precursors can differentiate towards lymphoid, myeloid and erythroid lineages. (If differentiation of the erythroid lineage is to be studied, erythropoietin should be added to the cytokine cocktail at a concentration of 8 U/mL).
4. Culture for 12 to 14 d at 37°C, 5% $C0_2$.
5. On d 6 of culture, remove half of the medium from each well. (Carefully remove the medium with a multi-channel pipet, preferably at the surface, to avoid removing developing cells). Replace with 100–150 μL of fresh medium supplemented with FLT3-L and IL-7 only. Excess of c-Kit-L in the culture favors the development of mast cells that can overgrow.
6. At the end of the culture period, analyze the well contents by flow cytometry.

3.4.2. Fetal Thymic Organ Cultures (FTOCs)

1. Suspension cultures do not allow the differentiation of T lymphocytes. When T-cell potential is to be analyzed, FTOCs must be performed ***(11)***.
2. Isolate 14 to 15 dpc embryos. Recover individual thymic lobes using a fine forceps. Place in HBSS.
3. Irradiate thymic lobes at 3000 rads to deplete proliferating endogenous hematopoietic precursors.
4. FTOCs are done in a two-step process:
   a. Colonization of thymic rudiment is achieved by a hanging drop culture. Wells of Terasaki plates are seeded with 30 μL of cell suspension. Individual lobes are then

placed in each well and the plate is turned upside down. Terasaki plates are incubated (37°C, 5% CO_2) in an inverted position for 1 to 2 d.

b. The second step consists of a 14-d culture on a filter. To this end, 35mm culture dishes are filled with 3.5 to 4 mL of complete medium. A filter is then gently placed floating on the medium. The Terasaki plate is placed in upright position and the lobes are transferred onto the floating filter with a fine forceps (*see* **Note 6**). After the 14-d culture, lobes are dissociated and single cell suspension is analyzed by flow cytometry. To be sure that the developing lymphocytes are of donor origin, we use a congenic combination of thymic lobes expressing the Ly5.2xLy5.1 isoform of CD45 and colonizing cells from Ly5.2 embryos.

3.5. Phenotypic Analysis of the Hematopoietic Progeny

3.5.1. Flow Cytometry Analysis

1. After a 2-wk culture, cells from each well are analyzed by flow-cytometry for the presence of lineage-specific surface markers: CD19 for lymphoid B cells, CD4 and CD8 for T-cells, Mac-1 for myeloid cells, and Ter119 for erythrocytes (**Fig. 5**). Other antibodies can be used for a more precise analysis.
2. Transfer cells from each culture well into wells of a round-bottomed 96-well plate. Spin down the plate for 2 to 3 min at 4 to 500*g*, 4°C. Excess medium in the wells is flicked off by inverting the plate vigorously on a paper towel.
3. Prepare staining mix in PBS containing 3% FCS and 10 m*M* sodium azide (Facs Medium). We use CD19-FITC, Ter119-PE, and Mac-1-APC, for the suspension culture. For FTOC, we use CD4-PE, CD8-APC, and Ly5.1-FITC (exclusion of recipient cells) at previously determined dilutions. Resuspend each cell pellet in 25 µL of the staining mix. Incubate 15 to 20 min at 4°C in the dark.
4. At the end of the incubation period, wash the cells in Facs medium. Add 200 µL per well, then spin 2 to 3 min at 4 to 500*g*, 4°C.
5. During the spin, prepare Facs medium with propidium iodide (PI, 0.5 µg/mL). PI is a DNA intercalator, passively entering the nucleus of dead cells. PI gives equal fluorescence in the flow cytometer for filters detecting phycoerythrin and Cy5–phycoerythrin conjugates. It also permits exclusion of dead cells that appear on the diagonal of the plot of both parameters.
6. Wash stained cells. Resuspend the pellets in Facs medium-PI and analyze by flow cytometry. Use the SSC parameter in linear mode so that you can easily distinguish between mononuclear cells (low SSC) and granulocytes (high SSC).

4. Notes

1. Breeding schedule: for occasional experiments, it is better to set up a large number of cages (e.g., 18), each containing two females and one male, overnight. To obtain a regular supply of embryos or to obtain embryos at various developmental stages for the same experiment, it is advantageous to mate four females with a single male for four consecutive days. In this case, the number of breeding males is about eight. To optimize breeding efficiency, record the number of plugs obtained for each male. For the breeding colony, keep only those males that mate efficiently.
2. Explant transfer: embryonic explants are small and fragile and tend to collapse at the liquid/medium interface during transfer or to stick to the Pasteur pipet. We overcome this difficulty by: a) filling the culture dishes up to the top; b) using siliconized Pasteur pipets; and c) monitoring the transfer under a binocular microscope

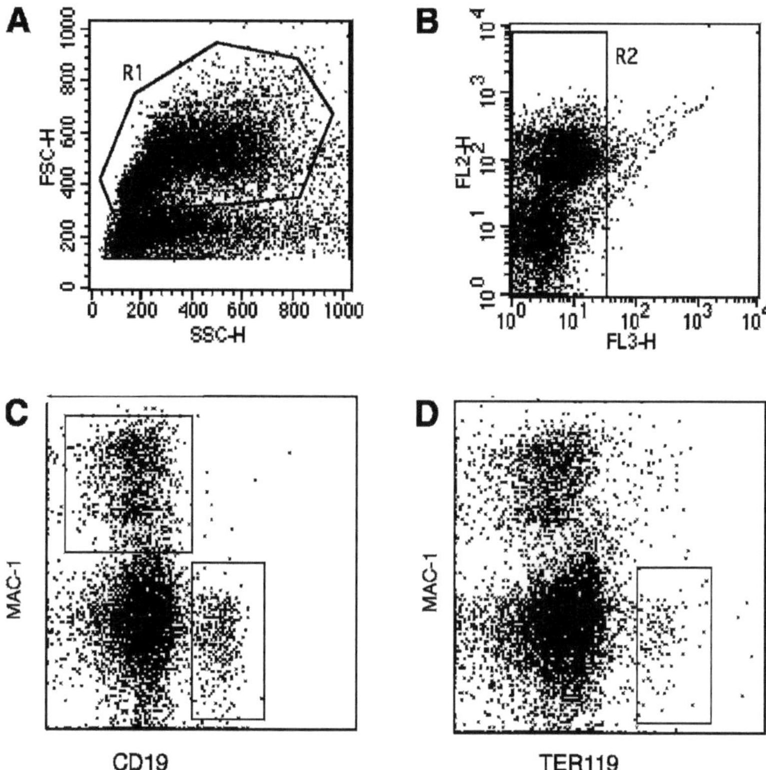

Fig. 5. FACS analysis of suspension culture well. The progeny of a single AGM progenitor was analyzed after 12-d suspension culture, as described. Cells were scored for the presence of erythroid (Ter119), myeloid (Mac-1), and lymphoid (CD19) markers. FSC/SSC plot **(A)** shows gate R1 excluding debris. **(B)** FL2/FL3 plot, gated on R1 cells, shows gate R2 excluding dead cells (the fluorescence on the diagonal is the result of PI incorporation). Plots **(C,D)** gated on R1 and R2 cells, show the repartition of cultured cells in the main lineages: erythroid, myeloid and lymphoid. Knowing that a single cell gave rise to these progeny, multipotentiality could be ascribed to this cell.

3. Visualization of ISH staining: to optimize the hybridization signal, staining speed may be controlled by incubation at room temperature or 4°C. The reaction can even be stopped for up to 2 d by a wash in MABT, followed by incubation in a new staining solution, when necessary. To ensure that the full expression pattern has been obtained, it is useful to terminate the staining reaction at different times for groups of embryos, until over-expression is observed.
4. Optimization of cell recovery: although YS grow in organ culture in a three-dimensional manner and are therefore easy to recover from the plate, Sp explants grow tightly attached to the dish (*see* **Fig. 4**). To maximize Sp cell recovery, medium is flushed laterally to the explant with a 1-mL syringe fitted with a 26-gage needle. Lifting of the whole explant from the culture plate is ascertained by inspection under an inverted microscope.

After mechanical dissociation of the explant, debris can be further subjected to a trypsin–EDTA treatment for 5 min at room temperature. Inactivate trypsin by addition of FCS and collect cells by centrifugation.

5. Culture conditions on OP9 and S17 stromal cells: OP9 stromal cells are contact inhibited and they do not overgrow the cultures. Irradiation can, therefore, be omitted. When using other stromal cell lines such as S17 cells, irradiation (2Gy) is required. Under these conditions, all stromal cells have died after 5 d. Immature B cell precursors have a strict requirement for stromal cells. However, we have not seen improvement in the yield of hematopoietic cells if cultures are passed onto a freshly irradiated feeder layer.
6. For optimal FTOC growth, care should be taken that: a) the lobe falls in the meniscum of the drop, when the Terasaki plate is turned upside down; b) the filter is still floating on the medium after transfer of the colonized lobes; and c) the plates are shaken during the incubation period. If you have problems keeping the filters floating at the air-medium interface, you can use hemostatic sponges in the culture medium.

Acknowledgments

The work is supported by grants from the French Ministry of Research (ACI Developmental Biology) to A.C. and I.G. and grant no. 4441 from the "Association pour la Recherche sur le Cancer" to I.G. The Unité du Développement des Lymphocytes is supported by the "Ligue Nationale de la Recherche contre le Cancer" as a registered laboratory. J.Y.B. is supported by the French Ministry of Research and Education.

References

1. Palis, J., Robertson, S., Kennedy, M., Wall, C., and Keller, G. (1999) Development of erythroid and myeloid progenitors in the yolk sac and embryo proper of the mouse. *Development* **126,** 5073–5084.
2. Cumano, A., Dieterlen-Lievre, F., and Godin, I. (1996) Lymphoid potential, probed before circulation in mouse, is restricted to caudal intraembryonic splanchnopleura. *Cell* **86,** 907–916.
3. Cumano, A., Ferraz, J. C., Klaine, M., Di Santo, J. P., and Godin, I. (2001) Intraembryonic, but not yolk sac hematopoietic precursors, isolated before circulation, provide long-term multilineage reconstitution. *Immunity* **15,** 477–485.
4. Godin, I., Dieterlen-Lievre, F., and Cumano, A. (1995) Emergence of multipotent hemopoietic cells in the yolk sac and paraaortic splanchnopleura in mouse embryos, beginning at 8.5 days postcoitus. *Proc. Natl. Acad. Sci. USA.* **92,** 773–777.
5. Medvinsky, A. L., Samoylina, N. L., Muller, A. M., and Dzierzak, E. A. (1993) An early pre-liver intraembryonic source of CFU-S in the developing mouse. *Nature* **364,** 64–67.
6. Medvinsky, A. and Dzierzak, E. (1996) Definitive hematopoiesis is autonomously initiated by the AGM region. *Cell* **86,** 897–906.
7. Godin, I., Garcia-Porrero, J.A., Dieterlen-Lievre, F., and Cumano, A. (1999) Stem cell emergence and hemopoietic activity are incompatible in mouse intraembryonic sites. *J. Exp. Med.* **190,** 43–52.
8. Manaia, A., Lemarchandel, V., Klaine, M., Max-Audit, I., Romeo, P., Dieterlen-Lievre, F., et al. (2000) Lmo2 and GATA-3 associated expression in intraembryonic hemogenic sites. *Development* **127,** 643–653.
9. Downs, K. M. and Davies, T. (1993) Staging of gastrulating mouse embryos by morphological landmarks in the dissecting microscope. *Development* **118,** 1255–1266.

10. Nakano, T., Kodama, H., and Honjo, T. (1994) Generation of lymphohematopoietic cells from embryonic stem cells in culture. *Science* **265,** 1098–1101.
11. Jenkinson, E. J., Anderson, G., and Owen, J. J. (1992) Studies on T cell maturation on defined thymic stromal cell populations in vitro. *J. Exp. Med.* **176,** 845–853.

18

Analysis of Hematopoietic Progenitors in the Mouse Embryo

James Palis and Anne Koniski

Summary

All mature blood cells are derived from hematopoietic progenitors that have been defined by their ability to generate colonies of cells in semisolid media. Investigation of the cellular components of these colonies has confirmed the existence of unilineage, bilineage, and multilineage progenitors. Furthermore, it has led to a better understanding of the relationships that exist among the erythroid, myeloid, and megakaryocyte lineages that compose much of the hematopoietic hierarchy in the adult. More recently, the development of hematopoietic progenitors has been investigated in the mammalian embryo. The first progenitors arise in the yolk sac and subsequently expand in the fetal liver before settling into the postnatal bone marrow. This chapter describes the methodologies for the culture and identification of unipotential and multipotential hematopoietic progenitors in the mouse embryo.

Key Words: Hematopoiesis; embryo; yolk sac; mouse; progenitor; colony-forming cell.

1. Introduction

Hematopoietic stem cells undergo progressive restrictions in lineage fate and proliferative potential to generate multipotential and unipotential progenitor cells that in turn produce mature blood cells. The ability of progenitors to form colonies of blood cells in semisolid media has greatly contributed to our understanding of the dynamics of the hematopoietic system. Initially, soft agar was used to grow "colony-forming units in culture" (CFU-C), that gave rise to colonies of myeloid cells *(1)*. This was followed by the use of plasma clots for the growth of colonies of erythroid cells *(2,3)*. Currently, methylcellulose is the semisolid medium of choice because it supports the growth of erythroid, multiple myeloid, and megakaryocyte progenitors and easily permits the physical isolation and transfer of colonies onto microscope slides for the evaluation of their cellular components. The association of granulocytes and macrophages in the same colony led to the identification of bipotential (CFU-GM) progenitors. Colonies containing cells of three or more lineages are derived from earlier multipotential (CFU-mix) progenitors *(4)*. Another multipotential progenitor termed the high proliferative potential colony-forming cell (HPP-CFC) generates macroscopic

From: *Methods in Molecular Medicine, Vol. 105: Developmental Hematopoiesis: Methods and Protocols.*
Edited by: M. H. Baron © Humana Press Inc., Totowa, NJ

colonies with >50,000 myeloid cells and is considered the earliest hematopoietic precursor that can be cultured in stroma-free conditions *(5)*.

The yolk sac is the first site of blood cell development in the mammalian embryo. Blood islands originate from gastrulating mesoderm cells that migrate into the yolk sac after exiting the posterior primitive streak. Studies of the spatial and temporal emergence of hematopoietic progenitors in the mouse embryo indicate that commitment to hematopoietic fates occurs soon after the start of gastrulation *(6)*. In contrast to hematopoiesis in the bone marrow, embryonic hematopoiesis consists of a restricted set of lineages. There are two waves of erythroid progenitors in the yolk sac. The first wave consists of primitive erythroid progenitors (EryP-CFC) that give rise to the embryo's first red blood cells. Subsequently, there is a second wave of definitive erythroid progenitors (BFU-E and CFU-E) that are later found in the bloodstream and ultimately expand in numbers within the fetal liver. These give rise to definitive erythrocytes that enter the bloodstream beginning at E12.5. This chapter will present the materials and methods necessary to explore the development of unipotential and multipotential hematopoietic progenitors in the post-implantation mouse embryo.

2. Materials and Reagents

2.1. Mice

We primarily use outbred strains of mice because they have higher fecundity and increased litter size compared to inbred strains (*see* **Note 1**). Early postimplantation embryos derived from Swiss Webster ICR mice (Taconic, Germantown, NY) contain similar numbers and display similar kinetics of hematopoietic progenitors compared with embryos from CD-1 mice (Charles River, Wilmington, MA). Timed pregnant mice can be obtained from all major mouse suppliers. Alternatively, in-house colonies of mice can be maintained to generate timed pregnancies (*see* **Subheading 3.1.**).

2.2. Mouse Embryo Dissections

1. Dissection forceps no. 5 (Dumoxel; Fine Science Tools, Foster City, CA; cat. no. 11252-30). Forceps can be sharpened using an Arkansas oil stone and mineral oil.
2. Tungsten needles (Fine Science Tools; cat. no. 10130-10) attached to metal holders (Fine Science Tools; cat. no. 26018-17).
3. Dissection stereomicroscopes with external fiber-optic light source are available from many manufactures, including Leica, Nikon, and Olympus.
4. Embryos are dissected in PB-1 solution:

Dulbecco's phosphate-buffered saline (PBS) with calcium chloride (GibcoBRL 21300-025)	1-L packet
Calcium chloride (provided w/PBS)	1 package
Glucose (GibcoBRL 15023-021)	1.0 g
Bovine serum albumin (BSA; Sigma A9647)	3.0 g
Sodium pyruvate (Sigma P2265)	0.036 g
Tissue culture-grade water to	1 L

   Sterile filter through a 0.2-μm filter and store at 4°C.
5. Calcium/magnesium free PBS (GibcoBRL; cat. no. 70013-032). This 10X stock is diluted with tissues culture grade water to make a 1X working solution.
6. Trypsin (Worthington Biochemical Corporation, Lakewood, NJ; cat. no. LS003667). Prepare a 0.25% trypsin, 1 m*M* ethylenediamine tetraacetic acid (EDTA) solution in calcium/magnesium free PBS. Sterile filter and store at 4°C.

7. Collagenase Type 1 (Worthington Biochemical Corp.; cat. no. 4194). 100 mg/mL is dissolved in sterile tissue culture grade water. Aliquots are stored frozen at –20°C.

2.3. General Tissue Culture Reagents

1. All glassware used for reagents should be hand rinsed in deionized distilled water without the use of dishwashing detergents. All media and reagents should be made with tissue culture grade water.
2. Cytokines can be purchased from a number of different suppliers and reconstituted according to manufacturer's instructions. We use human recombinant EPO (Amgen), GM-CSF (Peprotech; cat. no. 315-03), IL-1α (Peprotech; cat. no. 211-11A), IL-3 (Peprotech; cat. no. 213-13), IL-6 (Peprotech; cat. no. 216-16), IL-11 (Peprotech; cat. no. 200-11), M-CSF (Sigma; cat. no. M9170), SCF (Peprotech; cat. no. 250-03), human recombinant thrombopoietin (TPO; Peprotech; cat. no. 300-18), and VEGF (Peprotech; cat. no. 450-32). All cytokines, except those noted, are murine recombinant.
3. Sera. Different sera are used in the various hematopoietic progenitor assays since they support different colony types. Furthermore, different lots of serum must be tested to ensure appropriate biological activity. Sera are heat inactivated by treatment at 56°C for 15 min and sterile filtered.
   a. Plasma-derived serum, platelet poor (PDS; Animal Technologies, Tyler, TX). PDS supports the growth of primitive erythroid progenitors *(7)*, as well as embryonic megakaryocyte progenitors. PDS will form a white precipitate during heat inactivation that can be removed by filtration (*see* **Note 2**).
   b. GemCell fetal bovine serum (FBS), ES cell qualified (Gemini Bio-Products, Woodland, CA; cat. no. 100-500).
4. 35 × 10-mm Petri dishes (BD Falcon, cat. no. 351008 or Corning nontreated suspension culture dishes, cat. no. 430588). Each lot of dishes must be tested to ensure that colonies do not attach to the plastic.
5. 60 × 15-mm Gridded Petri dish (Nunc, cat. no. 169558).

2.4. Agar Cultures

1. Bacto-Agar (Difco, cat. no. 0140-01) 1% and 0.66% agar are made in distilled water, autoclaved, and stored at room temperature.
2. 200 mM L-glutamine (100X stock; Gibco BRL, cat. no. 25030-081). Store aliquots of 1 to 2 mL at –20°C. Thaw aliquots at 37°C and store at 4°C less than 2 wk.
3. Sodium bicarbonate (Sigma; cat. no. S5761). Make a 5.6% solution fresh monthly.
4. Minimal Essential Medium α (αMEM) medium:

   αMEM 5X Stock:

αMEM powder (Gibco BRL 11900-024)	1-L packet
Tissue-culture grade water, make up to	200 mL

   Sterile filtered through a 0.2-μm filter. Store in 5-mL aliquots at –70°C.

   2X αMEM medium (10 mL):

αMEM 5X stock	3.2 mL
200 m*M* L-glutamine (100X stock)	0.2 mL
5.6% sodium bicarbonate	0.8 mL
FBS	4 mL
Penicillin/Streptomycin (Gibco BRL 15140-122)	0.2 mL
Tissue culture-grade water	1.6 mL

   Sterile filter through a 0.2-μm filter and store at 4°C.
   Double strength media should be made fresh from the stock weekly.

2.5. Collagen Cultures

1. Lab-Tek II two-chamber slide system (Nalge Nunc International, Naperville, IL; cat. no. 154461).
2. Filter card spacer (ThermoShandon, cat. no. 5991023)
3. Polypropylene spacers (Gelman Laboratory, cat. no. 61757). To fit the slides, cut filter in half and fit over the collagen.
4. Bovine collagen solution (Stemcell Technologies, Vancouver, Canada; cat. no. 04902)
5. 10% Detoxified bovine serum albumin (BSA; Quality Biological, Gaithersburg, MD; cat. no. 672-001-061)
6. Monothioglycerol (MTG; Sigma, cat. no. M6145). Each new batch of MTG must be tested for optimum concentration. MTG should be aliquotted and stored at –20°C. Thawed aliquots maybe used for 1 wk. A 1:10 working concentration should be made fresh before use.
7. Acetylthiocholiniodide (Sigma; cat. no. A5751). Store in –20°C in dessicator.
8. Sodium citrate buffer (Sigma; cat. no. S4641). Prepare a 0.1 *M* solution by dissolving 2.9 g in 90 mL of water, adjust to pH 6.0 with citric acid, and bring to 100 mL final volume.
9. Sodium phosphate buffer, pH 6.0 (Fisher,; cat. no. S373). Prepare a 0.1 *M* solution by dissolving 13.4 g in 490 mL of water, adjust to pH 6.0, and bring to 500 mL final volume.
10. Copper sulfate solution (Fisher; cat. no. C493). Prepare a 30 m*M* solution by dissolving 749 mg in 95 mL of water and bring to 100 mL.
11. Potassium ferricyanide solution (Sigma ACS Reagent; cat. no. P3667). Prepare a 5 m*M* solution. Protect from light.
12. 2X Iscove's modified Dulbecco's medium (2X IMDM):

IMDM powder (GibcoBRL; cat. no. 12200-036)	1-L packet
Penicillin/streptomycin	10 mL
$NaHCO_3$	3.025 g
Tissue culture-grade water, make up to	500 mL

Sterile filter through a 0.2-μm filter.

13. Preparation of Megacult media. The serum free megacult media is used for growth of Meg-CFC from postnatal bone marrow and fetal liver. The megacult substitute media supports the growth of Meg-CFC from the yolk sac.

Megacult medium (1.8X stock):

2X IMDM	8 mL
Insulin (stock 10 mg/mL, GibcoBRL; cat. no. 18125-039)	20 μL
Transferrin (stock 10 mg/mL, Sigma; cat. no. T0665)	0.4 mL
200 m*M* L-glutamine (100X stock)	0.2 mL
β-mercaptoethanol (bME, 1:100; Sigma; cat. no. 3148)	7 μL
10% Detoxified BSA	2 mL
Tissue culture-grade water	2 mL

Megacult substitute (1.8X stock):

2X IMDM	8 mL
Insulin (stock 10 mg/mL, GibcoBRL; cat. no. 18125-039)	20 μL
Transferrin (stock 10 mg/mL)	0.4 mL
200 m*M* L-glutamine (100X stock)	0.2 mL
MTG (1:10)	2.5 μL
PDS	2 mL
Tissue culture-grade water	2 mL

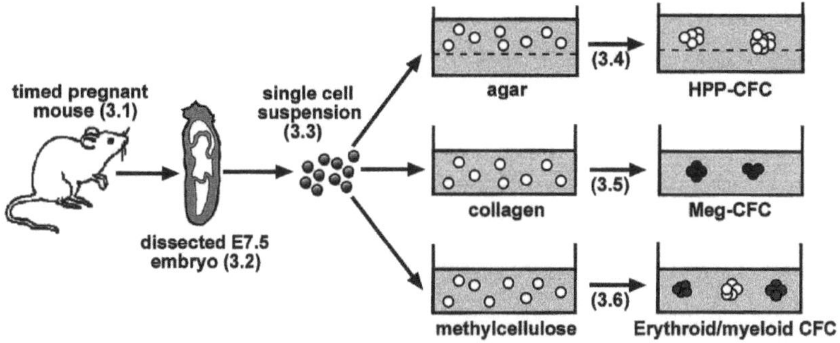

Fig. 1. Experimental approach discussed in this chapter. Embryos from timed pregnant mice are dissected and staged. Specific tissues are isolated, dissociated into single cells, and plated in semisolid media with serum and growth factors. After incubation for 2 to 16 d, colonies are examined with an inverted microscope and enumerated. Multiple methods can be used to aid in colony identification, including colony morphology, cell morphology on cytospins, and *in situ* staining with benzidine or acetylcholinesterase.

2.6. Methylcellulose Cultures

1. Methylcellulose (Methocel®; Fluka; cat. no. 64630), *see* **step 5** for preparation.
2. Protein-free hybridoma medium (GibcoBRL; cat. no. 12040-077).
3. Benzidine dihydrochloride (Sigma; cat. no. B-0386). The benzidine stock is prepared by solvating 100 mg of benzidine dihydrochloride with 50 mL of 0.5% acetic acid. This stock solution can be stored in the dark at room temperature for several months. Care must be taken when handling benzidine because it is a carcinogen.
4. Hydrogen peroxide, 50% (EM Science; cat. no. HX0630-1).
5. Preparation of methylcellulose:
    a. Autoclave a 2-L Erlenmeyer flask containing a large stir bar and 27 g of methylcellulose. Use two layers of aluminum foil over top of flask. Do not use a bottle with a screw cap.
    b. While the methylcellulose is still warm, add 500 mL of 37°C prewarmed sterile tissue culture grade water. While stirring the methylcellulose mix, carefully bring mixture to a boil. Immediately reduce the heat and stir for 4 to 6 h.
    c. Prewarm 500 mL of sterile filtered 2X IMDM to 37°C and add it to the warm methylcellulose mix. Stir at room temperature for 1 h.
    d. Transfer to the cold room and stir overnight.
    e. Aliquot the methylcellulose into 50-mL conical tubes and freeze at –20°C. Methylcellulose must be frozen and thawed before use.

3. Methods

An overview of the methodologies discussed in this section is outlined in **Fig. 1**. Staged embryos are derived from timed pregnant mice. After further dissection, specific tissues are dissociated into single cells and plated in semisolid media with serum and growth factors. Hematopoietic progenitors generate colonies of maturing blood cells that are identified and enumerated on an inverted microscope.

3.1. Timed Pregnancies

Mice are mated overnight by placing three to four females into a cage with one male. Mating is assumed to occur at the mid-point of the dark cycle. Vaginal plugs are checked the next morning, with noon of that day defined as embryonic d 0.5 (E0.5) if the dark cycle runs from 6 PM to 6 AM. At specific times, pregnant mice are euthanized by approved animal care protocols and the uteri removed from the peritoneum and washed with several changes of PB-1.

3.2. Embryo Dissection and Staging

The dissection strategy depends on the age of the embryos *(8)*. For E6.5 to 8.5 conceptuses, the uterine muscle is removed using no. 5 dissecting forceps and the decidual tissue is split into two halves starting from the mesometrial side. Subsequently, a tear is carefully made in Reichert's membrane and the embryos are freed from the decidual tissue at its attachment at the ectoplacental cone/chorion. The conceptuses are transferred with a pipetman to a fresh 35-mm Petri dish containing 2 to 3 mL of PB-1 and completely freed of Reichert's membrane. Further dissection into yolk sac and embryo proper tissue fractions is performed with dissecting forceps or tungsten needles. Because the mouse embryo develops extremely rapidly and there can be wide intra- and inter-litter variation, it is important to determine the stage of each dissected embryo (*see* **Note 3**).

3.3. Preparation of Single Cell Suspensions

Progenitor assays depend on plating single cells in semisolid media to ensure that each colony is clonal in nature. Both collagenase and trypsin provide effective cell separation of E6.5 to E11.5 embryos with equivalent high cell viabilities and hematopoietic progenitor plating efficiencies (*see* **Note 4**). Older embryos must be dissociated with collagenase. However, as the embryo ages and organogenesis proceeds, it becomes more and more difficult to obtain complete cell dissociation with good viabilities. Once tissues are completely dissociated, cell numbers and viability are determined after staining with trypan blue using standard tissue culture methods.

3.3.1. Dissociation With Trypsin

Embryo proper and yolk sac tissues are treated in 0.25% Trypsin/1X PBS/1 m*M* EDTA at 37°C for 10 to 20 min (*see* **Note 5**). The volume of Trypsin depends on the amount of tissue being dissociated. Yolk sacs (5–15) from E7.5 embryos are dissociated in 0.1 mL of Trypsin–EDTA. The tissue is triturated with a pipet to aid in digestion and checked microscopically to determine if the tissues are completely dissociated. If dissociation is not complete, the dishes are incubated at 37°C for another 2 to 5 min and again triturated. Once dissociated, one half volume of IMDM/20% PDS is added to stop the action of the trypsin. The cells are pelleted by centrifugation, resuspended and counted.

3.3.2. Dissociation With Collagenase

Tissues are incubated in 2.5 mg/mL collagenase/IMDM/20% serum at 37°C for 2 h and vortexed every 15 to 30 min. Yolk sacs (5–15) or embryos proper from E7.5 embryos can be dissociated in 1 to 2 mL of collagenase/IMDM/20% serum. The tissues are triturated by multiple passages through a 22-gage needle and examined for completeness of dissociation. If not completely dissociated, the tissues are incubated in collagenase for another hour.

3.3.3. Number of Cells Cultured

It is necessary to optimize the number of cells plated per milliliter of semisolid media. If plating density is too high, it may be difficult to distinguish one colony from another and nutrients can be depleted before the colonies are scored. The number of cells plated will vary depending on 1) the colony types to be assayed, 2) the stage of the embryo, and 3) the tissue source of the cells ***(6,9)***. Plating serial dilutions of the cells is helpful in establishing an optimum cell number per dish. A good starting range is 5×10^3 cells/mL to 5×10^5 cells/mL.

3.4. Culture of Multipotential HPP-CFC in Agar

Multipotential hematopoietic progenitors give rise to colonies that contain three or more hematopoietic lineages. HPP-CFC are multipotential hematopoietic progenitors that are thought to be close to, but not within, the stem cell compartment ***(10)***. They require the combined action of the four cytokines SCF, IL-1α, IL-3, and M-CSF to stimulate their growth. HPP-CFCs are cultured in a double agar system with the cytokines added to the underlayer and the cells added to the overlayer.

3.4.1. Agar Underlay

1. The 1% agar is boiled in the microwave and cooled to 40°C, in a water bath, and mixed with an equal volume of 2X αMEM medium prewarmed to 40°C.
2. The cytokines SCF (100 ng/dish), IL-1α (10 ng/dish), IL-3 (20 ng/dish), and M-CSF (10 ng/dish) are added to the bottom of each Petri dish. Multiple dishes can be prepared at the same time.
3. Pipet 1 mL of the prewarmed 1% agar/2X αMEM (from **step 1**) over the growth factors in the dishes. The dishes are gently swirled to spread the agar evenly over the surface of the dish bottom and are cooled at room temperature to harden the agar.

3.4.2. Agar Overlay

1. Melt the 0.66% agar by boiling in a microwave.
2. For each sample, aliquot 250 µL of 0.66% agar into a 3-mL tube and cool to 40°C in a water bath.
3. Add 250 µL of 2X αMEM medium to a second 3-mL tube and warm to 40°C.
4. Transfer the pre-warmed 2X αMEM to the 0.66% agar and quickly add a known number of cells in 25 µL of volume. Mix and pipet the 0.5 mL of agar/αMEM/cells over the hardened agar underlay. Allow the overlay to harden for a several minutes at room temperature.

3.4.3. Double Agar Incubation

The double agar cultures are incubated at 37°C in 10% CO_2, 5% O_2, 85% N for 14 d. We have found that the cultures in low O_2 produce approximately twofold more HPP-CFC when compared to cultures incubated in 5% CO_2 room air.

3.4.4. Colony Identification

At d 14, the agar dishes are examined with an inverted microscope. HPP-CFCs generate macroscopic colonies that are >0.5 mm in diameter and are densely packed with myeloid cells. Less dense colonies should be >1 mm in size to be scored as HPP-CFC (*see* **Note 6**). Colonies <0.5 mm are scored as low proliferative potential colony-forming cells.

3.5. Culture of Megakaryocyte Progenitors (Meg-CFC) in Collagen

Megakaryocyte colonies can be grown in several different semisolid media, including agar, methylcellulose, and collagen. The ability to dehydrate collagen offers the unique advantage of producing a permanent record of the experimental results. As a basis for growth of megakaryocyte progenitors we use the Megacult reagents and protocols from Stem Cell Technologies (Vancouver, BC). We have modified these reagents to support the growth of Meg-CFC from yolk sac tissues.

3.5.1 Collagen Culture

Multiple cytokines have been shown to support megakaryocyte maturation, including TPO, IL-11, IL-6, and IL-3. Serum can inhibit the in vitro growth of bone marrow-derived megakaryocyte progenitors, necessitating the use of serum free medium (e.g., Megacult medium). We have found that megakaryocyte progenitors in the early post-implantation yolk sac do not grow consistently in serum-free conditions. However, embryonic Meg-CFC can be supported by the addition of PDS in the culture medium (Megacult "substitute").

1. Prechill two-chamber Nunc slides on ice in the laminar flow hood. Label slides with pencil, as an ink label will be lost during fixation.
2. Prepare the cytokine mix by adding the four cytokines below to 150 μL IMDM per slide.

Cytokine	Final concentration	Stock	Use
TPO	50 ng/mL	10 ng/μL	8.25 μL
IL-3	10 ng/mL	10 ng/μL	1.65 μL
IL-6	20 ng/mL	10 ng/μL	3.3 μL
IL-11	50 ng/nL	5 ng/μL	16.5 μL

3. Preparation of collagen culture. For each well, add to a sterile 1.5 mL tube in order the following:
   75 μL of cytokine mix
   425 μL of megacult or megacult substitute
   300 μL of collagen; mix the first three and than add the cells.
   25 μL of cells (in IMDM/10% PDS)
4. Add the 825 μL to each of the four chambers of the Nunc slide. It is not necessary to spread the collagen to the edge of the well.
5. Place the slide in a covered Petri dish along with uncovered Petri dish of sterile water to maintain optimal humidity. Incubate undisturbed at 37°C, 5% CO_2 for 5 d.

3.5.2. Dehydration and Fixation of Collagen

1. Prechill 200 mL of ice-cold acetone in a glass or plastic container with a tight fitting lid. The container should be large enough to hold the slides horizontally without overlapping. The acetone should be discarded after 12 slides.
2. Take the slides from the incubator one at a time and remove the plastic walls and rubber seal according to manufacturer's instructions.
3. Cut the round polypropylene filter spacer in half and place the shiny side of the half filter on each section of collagen.

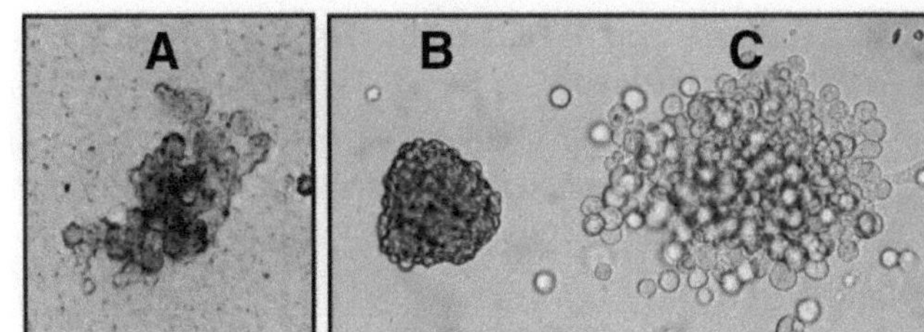

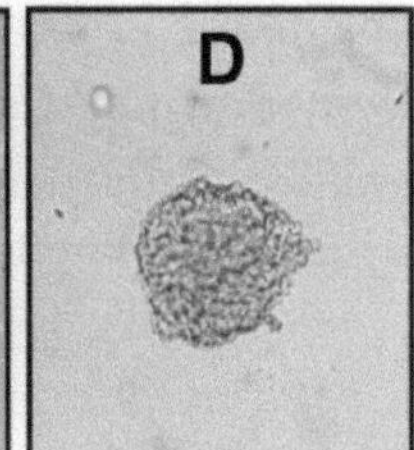

Fig. 2. Examples of murine hematopoietic colonies. (**A**) Megakaryocyte colony in collagen stained with acetylcholinesterase. (**B**) Primitive erythroid colony composed of large red cells. (**C**) Macrophage colony composed of large clear cells. (**D**) Definitive erythroid colony (derived from a BFU-E) composed of small red cells. *See* color insert following p. 80.

4. Carefully place a filter card over the spacer. The card will wet completely over 5 to 10 min Do not adjust the filter card once it is placed on the slide.
5. Remove the filter card, leaving the polypropylene spacer on the slide. Place the slides horizontally in the cold acetone and fix for 5 min on ice. The polypropylene spacer will float off in the acetone.
6. Remove the slides from the acetone and air dry. The dehydrated slides can be stained immediately or stored at 4°C or –20°C in the dark up to 1 mo.

3.5.3. Identification of Megakaryocyte Colonies by Acetylcholinesterase Stainin

Acetylcholinesterase is present in multiple hematopoietic lineages, however it is highly expressed in mature megakaryocytes. Thus, acetylcholinesterase staining provides a means of identifying megakaryocytes in collagen culture *(11)*, obviating reliance on morphology alone. We have applied acetylcholinesterase staining to methylcellulose cultures to identify megakaryocyte colonies (*see* **Subheading 3.6.3.**).

1. Dissolve 10 mg of acetylthiocholiniodide in 15 mL of 0.1 *M* sodium phosphate buffer.
2. To the acetylthiocholiniodide, add in the following order with constant stirring:

   1 mL of 0.1 *M* sodium citrate
   2 mL of 30 m*M* copper sulfate
   2 mL of 5 m*M* potassium ferricyanide solution

   The total volume of 20 mL is sufficient to stain 10 to 15 slides.
3. Allow slides to come to room temperature before staining. Pipet 0.75 to 1 mL of the stain onto the dehydrated collagen, enough to cover the dried collagen. Incubate the slides at room temperature in a humid chamber for 3.5 h to detect large mature megakaryocytes, and up to 5 h to detect immature megakaryocytes.
4. Pour off staining solution and fix the slides horizontally in 95% ethanol for 10 min.
5. Rinse slides with lukewarm tap water and air dry.
6. Megakaryocytes colonies range in size from 3 to 50 cells and stain orange-brown to brown-black depending upon the amount of acetylcholinesterase activity in the cell. A typical megakaryocyte colony derived from the E8.5 yolk sac and stained with acetylcholinesterase is shown in **Fig. 2A**.

3.6. Culture of Erythroid, Myeloid, and Megakaryocyte Colony-Forming Cells in Methylcellulose

Unilineage, bilineage, and multilineage hematopoietic progenitors can be identified by the colonies they generate when suspended in methylcellulose. Serum lots and cytokine combinations greatly influence the colony types that can be generated.

3.6.1. Preparation of Methylcellulose Cultures

Methylcellulose is very viscous, requiring a 16-gage needle for aliquotting. Each batch of methylcellulose must be tested to determine the final concentration that optimizes colony growth. We have found that the final methylcellulose concentration typically falls between 55 to 65% of the starting solution. The following growth factors, serum, and other reagents are added to the methylcellulose.

	Final concentration
Methylcellulose	55–65%
Serum (PDS or GemCell)	10%
Protein-free hybridoma medium	5%
Glutamine (100X)	1X
IL6 (5 ng/mL)	20 ng/mL
IL3 (5 ng/mL)	20 ng/mL
EPO (10,000 U/mL)	2 U/mL
SCF (100 ng/mL)	60 ng/mL
GM-CSF (5 ng/mL)	2.5 ng/mL
1X IMDM	to final volume

3.6.2. Plating Methylcellulose

1. Aliquot 1.4 mL of the methylcellulose mix per dish into a 5-mL tube and add 0.1 mL of cells at the appropriate concentration.
2. Vortex vigorously and allow the bubbles to surface for 15 to 20 min at room temperature.
3. Use a 3-mL syringe with a 16-gage needle to plate 1 mL into each 35 × 10-mm culture dish.
4. Swirl the dish to distribute the methylcellulose evenly.
5. Plate enough cells to count between 50 and 500 colonies per 35-mm dish (*see* **Note 7**).
6. Cultures are incubated at 37°C, 5% CO_2, room air for 2 to 16 d as needed to quantify colony numbers.

3.6.3. Colony Identification

The identification of colonies in semisolid media is often difficult. Colony morphology is dependent on the concentration of methylcellulose, the combination of growth factors and type of serum used, the length of time in culture, and the combination of lineages present in the colony.

1. Colony kinetics. Hematopoietic progenitors give rise to mature colonies over different periods of time, ranging from as short as 2 d for CFU-E to as long as 16 d for mast cell progenitors. The approximate times for optimal growth of the various hematopoietic progenitors are listed in **Table 1**. This wide range in colony timing necessitates examination of the dishes at multiple time-points to enumerate the various colony types.
2. Colony morphology. Each colony type has a distinct morphology and range of sizes. Myeloid and megakaryocyte colonies consist of clear cells, while erythroid colonies turn red (**Fig. 2**). Primitive erythroid colonies (e.g., EryP-CFC) are relatively small, bright cherry red colonies (**Fig. 2B**), whereas definitive erythroid (e.g. BFU-E) are larger and

Table 1
Murine Hematopoietic Progenitors That Give Rise to Distinct Colony Types

	Progenitor	Semisolid media	Timing	References
Unipotential	CFU-E	MC, PC	d 2-3	***2,15***
	BFU-E	MC, PC	d 7-10	***3***
	EryP-CFC	MC	d 5	***6***
	Meg-CFC	collagen, agar, MC	d 5	***6***
	Mac-CFC	MC, agar	d 7-10	***6,17***
	G-CFC	agar	d 7-10	***17***
	Mast-CFC	MC	d 16	***18***
Bipotential	EMeg-CFC	MC	d 5-10	
	CFU-GM	agar, MC	d 7-10	***6***
Multipotential	CFU-Mix	MC	d 14	***4,19***
	HPP-CFC	agar, MC	d 14	***5***

Several semisolid media have been used for in vitro culture including agar, methylcellulose (MC), plasma clot (PC), and collagen. Colonies mature at different rates as indicated by the optimal timing (in days). All references contain photographs of colony morphology.

more orange–red in color (**Fig. 2D**). EryP-CFCs contain large red cells whereas CFU-E and BFU-E contain much smaller erythroid cells (**Figs. 2A,B**).

The references in **Table 1** were chosen in part because they contain photographs of each of the colony types. Although the literature can serve as a starting point, colony identity should initially be confirmed by transferring the colony onto microscope slides to evaluate cell morphology. The colony is plucked out of methylcellulose, transferred into 0.2 to 0.3 mL of PBS/50% FBS, dispersed by pipetting, and then cytospun at 400 rpm for 3 to 5 min on a Shandon cytocentrifuge. After air drying, the cells on the slide are stained with May-Grüwald-Giemsa or with Wright's stain and examined to determine the different hematopoietic cell types present. A description of the morphology of the different cell types is beyond the scope of this chapter but can be found in ***(12)***.

3. *In situ* staining. a) Benzidine staining has been used to identify erythroid colonies or the erythroid component of mixed colonies in methylcellulose ***(4)***. Add 3 μL of 50% hydrogen peroxide to 1 mL of benzidine stain stock and immediately layer 0.5 mL of the benzidine/peroxide stain onto the methylcellulose dish. Dark blue–brown erythroid colonies are after evident 5 to 20 min of incubation at room temperature. b) We have adapted the acetylcholinesterase stain to identify megakaryocyte colonies in methylcellulose. The stain is prepared as described in **Subheading 3.5.3.** One milliliter of the acetylcholinesterase stain is layered onto the methylcellulose dish. Megakaryocytes stain light brown to black after a 3- to 5-h incubation at room temperature. Colonies must be scored immediately after staining is complete because methylcellulose cannot be fixed and dehydrated.

4. Notes

1. Strains of mice differ both in progenitor numbers and in progenitor kinetics. Individual variability in progenitor numbers can be mitigated by pooling tissues from several similarly staged embryos prior to plating. Because the total number of cells in the embryo increases exponentially, we have found it more useful to compare hematopoietic progenitor numbers per tissue rather than per cell number plated ***(6,9)***.

2. To heat inactivate serum under sterile conditions, serum is thawed, aliquoted into 15-mL tubes, and incubated at 56°C in a water bath. A 15-mL conical tube with 10 mL of water and a thermometer is placed in the water bath as well. The serum is incubated for 15 min after the water in the conical tube reaches 56°C. During heat inactivation PDS will form a white precipitate that can be removed by filtration. The filtration step is optional, since the precipitate in the PDS can be allowed to settle before use of the serum.
3. Although there are established times postcoitum at which specific embryonic stages tend to be present, there is significant variation in stage of embryos both within a litter and between litters. We use the criteria of Downs and Davies ***(13)*** for presomite stage embryos (E6.5–E8.25), somite counts between E8.25 and E10.5, and external morphological criteria between E10.5 and birth ***(14,15)***.
4. In our hands, mechanical dissociation with syringes and other non-enzymatic approaches, such as glycine, have led to high levels of cell death.
5. Each lot of trypsin must be tested to determine the optimum concentration yielding maximum dissociation with minimum cell death. We test serial dilutions (1:2–1:64) of the 0.25% trypsin in PBS/1 m*M* EDTA. We have also found that some lots of Trypsin can interfere with colony growth, particularly of primitive erythroid progenitors.
6. When scoring colonies with an inverted microscope, the 35 × 10-mm agar dish can be placed inside a 60 × 15-mm gridded dish. The 2-mm squares of the gridded dish are used: a) as a guide to ensure that the entire dish is counted and b) to estimate the size of the colonies. Alternatively, HPP-CFC can be assayed by plating directly in gridded dishes.
7. We have used an alternative plating strategy when cell numbers are limiting. One milliliter of the methylcellulose mix is plated into each 35 × ⁻10-mm dish and the cells, resuspended in 0.1 mL of IMDM/10% serum, are added directly to the dish. The tip of the pipet is used to mix the cells with the methylcellulose. This method leads to an uneven distribution of cells in the dishes, necessitating that the entire dish be scored. However, this plating method has the advantage of overcoming the loss of 20 to 30% of the cells because of the viscous nature of the methylcellulose.

Acknowledgments

We thank Janet Rossant, Gordon Keller, Marion Kennedy, and Merv Yoder for sharing so generously of their knowledge and expertise. We also thank our colleagues Paul Kingsley, Kathleen McGrath, and Jeff Malik. This work has been supported by funds from the National Institutes of Health and from the Strong Children's Research Center, University of Rochester, Rochester, NY.

References

1. Bradley, T. R. and Metcalf, D. (1966) The growth of mouse bone marrow cells in vitro. *Aust. J. Exp. Biol. Med. Sci.* **14,** 287–300.
2. Stephenson, J. R., Axelrad, A., McLeod, D., and Shreeve, M. (1971) Induction of colonies of hemoglobin-synthesizing cells by erythropoietin in vitro. *Proc. Natl. Acad. Sci. USA* **18,** 1542–1546.
3. Heath, D. S., Axelrod, A. A., McLeod, D. L., and Shreeve, M. M. (1976) Separation of the erythropoietin-responsive BFU-E and CFU-E in mouse bone marrow by unit gravity separation. *Blood* **17,** 777–792.
4. Hara, H. and Ogawa, M. (1978) Murine hematopoietic colonies in culture containing normoblasts, macrophages, and megakaryocytes. *Am. J. Hematol.* **1,** 23–34.
5. Bradley, T. R. and Hodgson, G. S. (1979) Detection of primitive macrophage progenitor cells in mouse bone marrow. *Blood* **14,** 1446–1450.

6. Palis, J., Robertson, S., Kennedy, M., Wall, C., and Keller, G. (1999) Development of erythroid and myeloid progenitors in the yolk sac and embryo proper of the mouse. *Development* **126,** 5073–5084.
7. Keller, G., Kennedy, M., Papayannopoulou, T., and Wiles, M. V. (1993) Hematopoietic commitment during embryonic stem cell differentiation in culture. *Mol. Cell. Biol.* **13,** 473–486.
8. Hogan, B. L. M., Beddington, R. S. P., Constantini, F., and Lacy, E. (1994) *Manipulating the Mouse Embryo: A Laboratory Manual*, 2nd Ed, Cold Spring Harbor Laboratory Press, Cold Spring Harbor, NY.
9. Palis, J., Chan, R. J., Koniski, A. D., Patel, R., Starr, M., and Yoder, M. C. (2001) Spatial and temporal emergence of high proliferative potential hematopoietic precursors during murine embryogenesis. *Proc. Natl. Acad. Sci. USA* **18,** 4528–4533.
10. Bertoncello, I. (1992) Status of high proliferative potential colony-forming cells in the hematopoietic stem cell hierarchy. *Curr. Topics Microbiol. Immunol.* **177,** 83–94.
11. Jackson, C. W. (1973) Cholinesterase as a possible marker of early cells of the megakaryocytic series. *Blood* **12,** 413–421.
12. Fredrickson, T. N. and Harris, A. W. (2000) *Atlas of Mouse Hematopathology*, Harwood Academic Publishers, Amsterdam, The Netherlands.
13. Downs, K. M. and Davies, T. (1993) Staging of gastrulating mouse embryos by morphological landmarks in the dissecting microscope. *Development* **118,** 1255–1266.
14. Kaufman, M. H. (1992) *The Atlas of Mouse Development*, Academic Press, New York, NY.
15. Cooper, M. C., Levy, J., Cantor, L. N., Marks, P. A., and Rifkind, A. R. (1974). The effect of erythropoietin on colonial growth of erythroid precursor cells in vitro. *Proc. Natl. Acad. Sci. USA* **11,** 1677–1680.
16. Burstein, S. A., Adamson, J. W., Thorning, D., and Harker, L. A. (1979) Characteristics of murine megakaryocyte colonies in vitro. *Blood* **14,** 169–179.
17. Ichikawa, Y., Pluznik, D. H., and Sachs, L. (1966) In vitro control of the development of macrophage and granulocyte colonies. *Proc. Natl. Acad. Sci. USA* **16,** 488–495.
18. Nakahata, T., Spicer, S. S., Cantey, J. R., and Ogawa, M. (1982) Clonal assay of mouse mast cell colonies in methylcellulose culture. *Blood* **10,** 352–361.
19. Pharr, P. N., Suda, T., Bergmann, K. L., Avila, L. A., and Ogawa, M. (1984) Analysis of pure and mixed murine mast cell colonies. *J. Cell. Physiol.* **120,** 1–12.

19

In Vivo and In Vitro Assays of Thymic Organogenesis

Julie Gordon, Valerie A. Wilson, Billie A. Moore-Scott, Nancy R. Manley, and C. Clare Blackburn

Summary

We describe two complementary methods for the study of early thymus organogenesis in the mouse. The first is an in vitro technique for lineage analysis, where a chosen population of cells within the mouse embryo is labeled with a fluorescent cell tracker dye. The embryos are then transferred to whole embryo culture for a defined period, after which time the location of the labeled cells is determined with respect to the developing thymus. In the second method, an in vivo assay is used to determine the ability of a specific tissue type to form a structurally and functionally normal thymus. This method uses an ectopic grafting technique where the embryonic pharyngeal endoderm containing the prospective thymus tissue is carefully isolated and transplanted under the kidney capsule of an adult mouse. Together, these techniques have allowed the cell types that make a physical contribution to the formation of the thymic epithelium to be identified.

Key Words: Thymus organogenesis; whole embryo culture; lineage analysis; kidney capsule grafting; mouse.

1. Introduction

Thymus organogenesis is a complex and dynamic process that encompasses a series of cellular interactions between several different cell types *(1)*. This chapter will focus on the early events in this process, prior to and including formation of the organ primordium. The thymus in the mouse originates from the third pharyngeal pouches, transient bilateral epithelial structures that emerge from the pharyngeal endoderm on embryonic d 9 (E9.0). The thymic lobes begin to develop at about E11 and separate from the pharynx at around E11.5. During this short time window, the developing primordia also briefly contact the surface ectoderm of the overlying third pharyngeal clefts *(2)*. This has lead to the widely accepted model of a dual origin for the development of the thymic epithelium, where both the pharyngeal endoderm and ectoderm contribute to compartments within the mature organ *(3)*. Here, we describe two techniques used to investigate the cell types that make a physical contribution to the mature thymic epithelium, and thus to differentiate between the single and dual origin

From: *Methods in Molecular Medicine, Vol. 105: Developmental Hematopoiesis: Methods and Protocols.*
Edited by: M. H. Baron © Humana Press Inc., Totowa, NJ

models briefly of thymus organogenesis. The first is a lineage trace, in which a specific population of cells within the embryo is labeled and their location with respect to the organ primordium is assessed at the end of a defined period. The second technique uses ectopic grafting to determine the ability of a single tissue type to give rise to a fully mature organ. Both permit a functional assessment of early thymus organogenesis. We have successfully used these techniques to evaluate the physical contributions of ectoderm and endoderm to thymus organogenesis ***(2)***.

2. Materials

1. Rolling bottle whole embryo culture apparatus (BTC Engineering, Cambridge, UK).
2. 95%O_2/5%CO_2 Cylinder with low flow regulator.
3. Serum-free whole embryo culture medium: Knock-Out DMEM (Gibco) containing 10% Knock-Out Serum Replacement (Gibco), 1X N2 supplement (Gibco), 2% cell culture grade albumin (Sigma), 25 U/mL penicillin, and 25 μg/mL streptomycin.
4. DMEM (Gibco) or M2 (Sigma) medium for dissection.
5. Fine dissecting forceps (no. 5, Roboz Surgical).
6. Dissecting stereomicroscope.
7. Fluorescent microscope for analysis.
8. Picopump microinjector (World Precision Instruments).
9. Fine glass needles: pull a thin-walled glass capillary tube (Clark Electromedical Instruments) using a micropipet puller (Sutter Instruments) to give a needle length of about 1 cm. Break a small piece from the tip of the needle before use.
10. CMFDA cell tracker dye (Molecular Probes).
11. Plastic transfer pipets.
12. Paraffin-embedding apparatus: graded ethanol series (70% to 100%), xylene, paraffin wax, plastic embedding molds (Polysciences), 65°C oven, microtome, glass slides, water bath, and hot plate.
13. Trypsin/pancreatin solution: 0.5 g of pancreatin, 0.1 g of trypsin, 0.1 g of polyvinylpyrrolidone in 20 mL of filter-sterilized Ca^{2+}-Mg^{2+}-free Tyrode Ringer's saline (8 g NaCl, 0.3 g KCl, 0.093 g $NaH_2PO_4 \cdot 5H_2O$, 0.025 g KH_2PO_4, 1 g $NaHCO_3$, and 2 g glucose in 1 L of sterile water, pH 7.6–7.7).
14. Eyelash tool: an eyelash held in place at the end of a fine capillary tube with parafilm.
15. 50-mm or 35-mm Petri dishes for dissection.
16. Mouth-controlled micropipet: Pasteur pipet, flame, flexible rubber tubing and mouthpiece (*see* **Subheading 3.2.3.**).
17. Avertin and Torbugesic solutions, or other small animal anesthetic.
18. Surgical instruments: scissors (Roboz Surgical, RS-5910), forceps (blunt and fine, e.g., Roboz Surgical, cat. nos. RS-5358 and RS-5045), wound clips and applier (Autoclip system, Harvard Apparatus, cat. nos. AH52-3747 and AH52-3758), suture thread and needle (Roboz Surgical, cat. no. SUT-1073-31), 1-mL syringes and 23-gage needles.

3. Methods

3.1. Ectoderm Labeling

A lineage tracing technique used to determine the physical contribution made by a specific tissue or cell population to formation of a chosen organ primordium is described in this section. A cell-tracking technique is utilized together with a novel serum-free whole embryo culture system for mid-gestation mouse embryos ***(4)***.

In this example, the surface ectoderm of the pharyngeal region is examined in relation to development of the thymic primordium.

3.1.1. Embryo Isolation

1. Dissect E10.5 embryos from the uterus in DMEM culture medium. Confirm the age of the embryos by assessing morphological criteria such as overall size, eye development, and limb bud and pharyngeal arch morphology *(5)*.
2. Completely remove the decidua, leaving the placenta intact.
3. Free each embryo from the yolk sac and amnion by making a small slit close to the placenta, taking care to maintain the integrity of the main blood supply of the yolk sac (*see* **Note 1**). After dissection, the embryo and yolk sac should remain connected to each other and to the placenta, but the embryo should be outside of the yolk sac. The embryos are now ready for manipulation and/or culture as required (*see* **Note 2**).

3.1.2. Ectoderm Labeling

1. Using a plastic transfer pipet, place an embryo in a small drop of DMEM culture medium in the lid of a 50-mm Petri dish, and orientate to expose the target pharyngeal region.
2. Using a microinjector, drop a small volume (approx 1 μL) of a 10 m*M* CMFDA solution in dimethylsulfoxide onto the surface ectoderm overlying the pharyngeal region, or other region of interest.
3. If desired, turn the embryo over to expose the opposite side and repeat the application of the cell tracker dye. Labeling of the target cells will be instantaneous.
4. Immediately transfer the embryo to culture using a plastic transfer pipet.

3.1.3. Whole Embryo Culture

1. Freshly prepare 3 mL of serum-free culture medium per embryo. Prior to use for embryo culture, equilibrate the medium for 20 min at 37°C in an atmosphere of 95%O_2/5%CO_2.
2. Using a plastic transfer pipet, transfer labeled embryos to a rolling bottle culture apparatus (BTC Engineering, Cambridge, UK) at 37°C in an atmosphere of 95%O_2/5%CO_2. One embryo is cultured in a 5-mL bottle containing 3 mL of serum-free medium for a maximum period of 30 h (*see* **Note 3**).

3.1.4. Recovery and Analysis

1. After a 30-h culture period, remove the embryos from the culture bottles, and wash in phosphate-buffered saline. Select the embryos in which development has proceeded normally as judged by morphological criteria (this is vastly dependent on individual skill, but will be about 90% in experienced hands *[4]*).
2. To determine the location of the labeled cells, assess the embryos first using a fluorescent dissecting microscope to ensure the CMFDA tracker dye has persisted in the target region. Embryos can then be sectioned for further analysis.

3.1.5. Paraffin Embedding and Sectioning

1. Fix the embryos overnight in 4% paraformaldehyde at 4°C.
2. Wash thoroughly in phosphate-buffered saline.
3. Dehydrate the embryos through a series of 15-min incubations in 50%, 70%, 80%, 90%, 90%, 100%, 100% ethanol.
4. Rinse the tissue twice, for 15 min each, in xylene.
5. Incubate in three changes of paraffin wax in 1 h at 65°C before embedding in fresh paraffin wax with plastic moulds.

6. Blocks can be stored at room temperature indefinitely.
7. Cut 8-μm sections using a microtome, expand them in a water bath at 37°C and collect them onto glass slides. Slides should be air-dried for several hours on a warm plate at 37°C before analysis, to allow the sections to adhere.
8. Dewax the sections in xylene for 10 to 15 min. The tissue is now ready for direct analysis or further histology, as required.

3.2. Kidney Capsule Grafting

The kidney capsule is well established as an ectopic site able to provide a permissive environment for thymus development (*see* **Note 4**). Described below is one application of this technique to study early thymus organogenesis. Enzyme digestion and manual dissection are used to isolate the pharyngeal endoderm from the overlying ectoderm and mesoderm of E9.0 embryos. The resulting tissue explants containing the third pharyngeal pouches are grafted under the kidney capsule of an adult mouse and the ability to form a functional organ is assessed. All steps of this procedure should be carried out under sterile conditions as far as possible.

3.2.1. Isolation of the Pharyngeal Endoderm

1. Remove E9.0 embryos (10–15 somites) from the uterus into serum-free culture medium and remove all extra-embryonic tissues. M2 medium works well as the pH does not alter when exposed to air for long periods of time.
2. Remove all structures caudal to the heart. Digest the remaining tissue in a trypsin/pancreatin enzyme mixture for 15 to 20 min on ice, then transfer to serum-containing medium and wash thoroughly (*see* **Note 5**).
3. Using an eyelash tool and a pair of fine forceps, remove the head and first pharyngeal arches. Carefully peel away the surface ectoderm, and then remove the heart and neural tube (*see* **Note 6**).
4. Carefully strip away the remaining mesenchyme using the eyelash tool, to leave a clean endodermal gut tube (*see* **Note 6**). Trim this down to include only the second and third pharyngeal pouches. Explants should be stored in M2 medium on ice until ready for grafting (*see* **Note 7**).

3.2.2. Anesthesia

1. Anesthetize mice with an intraperitoneal injection of Avertin (Tribromoethanol). For an average 40-g adult mouse, 5 to 10 mg of Avertin is required to allow approx 30 min to perform the procedure (*see* **Note 8**).
2. Administer an intraperitoneal injection of Torbugesic for pain relief. Use 0.2 mL of a 1% solution for an average 40-g adult mouse.

3.2.3. Preparation of the Tissue for Transplantation

1. Prepare a mouth-controlled micropipet: heat the shaft of a Pasteur pipet over a flame, and when molten pull into a capillary. Break the capillary about 2 cm from the shoulder of the pipet and connect the micropipet to a length of flexible rubber tubing and a mouthpiece.
2. Fill the mouth-controlled micropipet by dipping the tip into medium and allowing it to fill up by capillary action. Then draw a small column of air into the pipet to create an air bubble.
3. Pick up the tissue fragments in a small volume of fluid and position them about 5 mm from the tip of micropipet (*see* **Note 9**). Multiple tissue explants can be transplanted simultaneously (*see* **Note 10**).
4. Place the loaded micropipet on the microscope stage until required.

3.2.4. Exposure of the Kidney

1. Lay the anesthetized mouse on its side, with the head pointing either to the left or right, and sterilize the flank skin with 70% ethanol.
2. Make a 1-cm incision through the skin about 1 cm from the spine and immediately caudal to and parallel with the last rib.
3. Make a second incision of about 0.7 mm through the muscle layers to expose the kidney. Avoid blood vessels and nerves as much as possible.
4. Hold the incision open with an open pair of blunt, angled forceps and grasp the fat pad at the cranial pole of the kidney with a second pair. Pull the kidney out of the peritoneal cavity. Applying a slight pressure to the flank of body may also help ease the kidney through the incision. Use of a small incision will help prevent the kidney from sliding back into abdominal cavity.
5. Let the exposed kidney stand for about 30 s to dry the capsule slightly. This makes it easier to grasp with forceps.

3.2.5. Transplantation of the Tissue (Fig. 1A–C)

1. Pick up the kidney capsule (the thin, transparent covering of the kidney) with a pair of fine forceps and use a second pair to make a small hole in the capsule about 2 to 3 mm away from the holding forceps. Lift the holding forceps slightly to create a space between the capsule and the kidney surface.
2. Insert the micropipet containing the explants into the opening in the capsule until it is about 5 mm into the space created by the raised holding forceps (*see* **Note 9**). Blow gently into the mouthpiece to slowly expel the tissue. Use the air bubble as a guide and stop blowing just before it reaches the end of the micropipet. Carefully withdraw the pipet, maintaining a positive pressure until it is completely out of the capsule, to prevent the tissue being drawn back into the pipet. (*see* **Notes 9–11** for alternative methods.)
3. Release the holding forceps to secure the grafts between the capsule and the kidney surface.
4. Check the micropipet to ensure that the tissue has been transplanted, and examine the kidney to ascertain the position of the grafts. Depending on the size of the grafts, a microscope may be required.

3.2.6. Suture and Recovery

1. Allow the kidney to slide back into the peritoneal cavity by manipulating the wound opening.
2. Stitch the muscle layers with suture thread to seal the peritoneal cavity and close the skin with a wound clip.
3. Warm the mice slightly on a standard small animal heat pad to aide recovery from anesthesia. A slide warmer (Fisher, cat. no. 12-594) set to 37°C is also effective.

3.2.7. Graft Recovery and Analysis

After the desired period of time (*see* **Note 12**), sacrifice the mouse and remove the kidney by cutting through the skin and muscle layers at the original wound site. The grafted tissue should be evident under the kidney capsule (**Fig. 1D**). The graft can then either be freed completely, or removed together with a small piece of the underlying kidney. The grafted tissue can now be analyzed as appropriate, e.g., using standard histological or immunohistological techniques. (also *see* **Note 13**).

4. Notes

1. When dissecting embryos for whole embryo culture it is important to avoid tearing the placenta or damaging major blood vessels in the yolk sac, as this can compromise oxygen

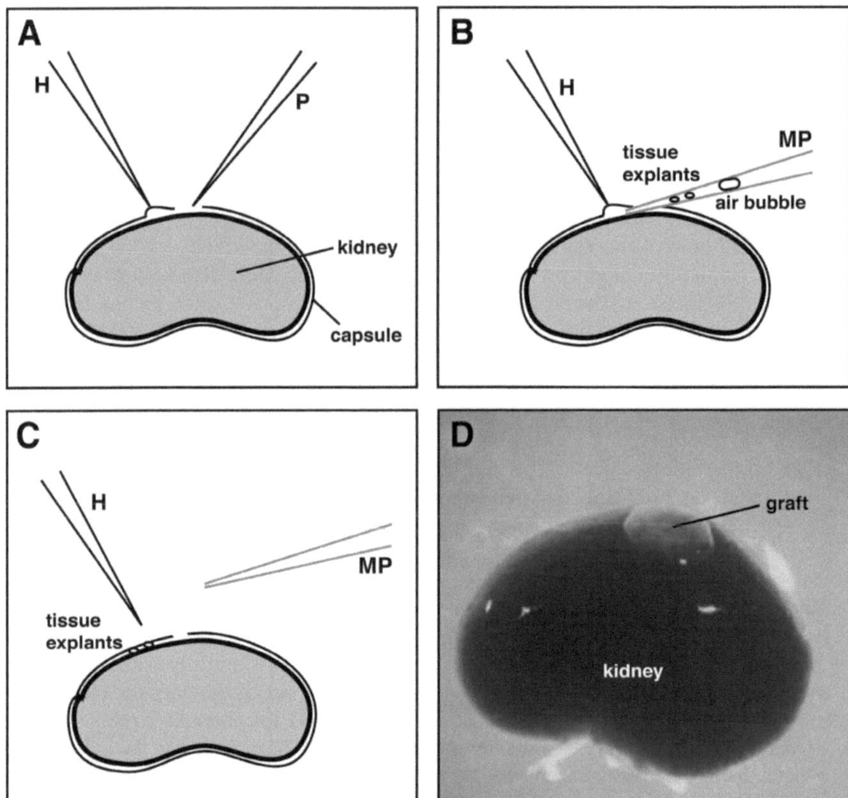

Fig. 1. Schematic representation of tissue graft transplantation under kidney capsule, following exposure of the kidney from the abdominal cavity. **(A)** Grasp the kidney capsule with a pair of fine forceps H and use a second pair P to make a small hole in the membrane. Lift the holding forceps H gently to make a space between the capsule and the surface of the kidney. **(B)** Bring in the micropipet MP containing the grafts and place into the hole created by the raised forceps H. Blow to release the grafts, stopping before the air bubble reaches the end of the pipet. **(C)** Remove the micropipet MP, maintaining a positive pressure to ensure the grafts are not taken back up into the pipet. Release the holding forceps H to secure the grafts under the capsule. **(D)** Kidney recovered 10 d after grafting. The transplanted tissue has increased substantially in size, and can be removed completely from the kidney for analysis.

and nutrient flow to the embryo. It is also important to remove tissue debris from the culture medium as this may affect embryo survival.

2. The whole embryo culture system may be utilized in many experiments. For example, it has been used successfully to allow embryonic development after injections of deoxyribonucleic acid or morpholino oligonucleotides into the third pharyngeal pouch at E10.5 (Gordon J., Manley, N. R., and Blackburn, C. C., manuscript in preparation) and in bead implant experiments (Moore-Scott, B. A., unpublished data).

3. The maximum time that an E10.5 mouse embryo will survive, grow and develop under the whole embryo culture conditions described is 30 h. This may be caused in part by poor placental development, or to the absence of an as-yet unidentified serum component *(4)*, both of which lead to a compromised nutrient supply.
4. The kidney capsule is well established as providing a permissive environment for growth and development of other organs and tissues *(6,7)*. With respect to the study of thymus development, thymi or cells from any stage may be transplanted under the kidney capsule *(8–12)*, and tissue manipulation such as cell labeling may be performed prior to the transplant. Thus, the technique could be used to extend an analysis that a whole embryo culture-based technique only permits to a limited point.
5. For the isolation of tissues for grafting, the enzyme digestion time is crucial: too long and the tissue will be destroyed, but not long enough and the layers will not separate easily. It is recommended to test an explant after 10 to 15 min and place it back into the enzyme solution if digestion was insufficient. Furthermore, it is important to wash the tissues well after this treatment, as the serum in the medium will inactivate the enzymes and therefore halt the digestion process.
6. It essential to handle the tissue delicately throughout the endoderm dissection. Alternative tools for the dissection include a very fine glass needle or tungsten needle in place of the eyelash tool. The order of dissection is not crucial and may be altered slightly to suit personal preference.
7. When grafting tissue under the kidney capsule, it is important to carry out the transplant as soon as possible after the initial dissection, as the tissue will start to disintegrate even in medium.
8. Alternative methods of anesthesia may be used to perform the grafting experiments. For example, when performing multiple grafts, a stronger dose or alternative substance may be required to allow the operating time to be increased.
9. For tissue transfer, use a minimum volume of liquid in the pipet to avoid flooding of the space under the kidney capsule and loss of the graft. It is also important to push the micropipet at least 5 mm into the space created by the raised forceps to ensure the grafts will remain in place. For grafting larger tissues, forceps may be more suitable than a mouth pipet for placing the grafts under the capsule (a wider diameter pipet will require a larger entry hole and therefore cause more damage). The procedure is more efficient if performed using a dissecting microscope to monitor placement of the tissue fragments.
10. If the tissues or cells being grafted are particularly small, it may be useful to mark the graft site with a small piece of nitrocellulose filter. This should be carefully inserted into the opening in the capsule after the tissue transfer.
11. We routinely use pouch endoderm from two embryos in a single graft. Transplanting tissue from multiple embryos together in a single graft may improve graft recovery. It is theoretically possible to perform grafts from individual embryos, although the survival rate may be reduced. This could be useful if using transgenic or knockout embryos for grafting, where the genotypes of the embryos may not be known before the transplant.
12. Grafts should be sufficiently developed after 10 d to be used for histological or immunohistochemical analysis. For analysis of T-cells in lymph nodes, grafts should be left for a minimum of 2 to 3 wk.
13. For thymus studies, an important extension of the kidney capsule grafting technique involves the use of nude mice as recipients. This allows for a functional analysis, as the host lymph nodes can be assessed for the presence of peripheral T-cells, which will be present only when a fully functional thymus has developed from the grafted tissue *(11)*.

Optimum results will be obtained using recipient mice syngeneic with the transplanted tissue, to prevent rejection of the graft, even if using nude mouse recipients.

Acknowledgments

We wish to thank the Medical Research Council (J.G. and V.A.W.), NIH grant number HD043479 and NSF grant number 0131314 (N.R.M.), and the Leukaemia Research Fund (C.C.B.) for their support. C.C.B. and N.R.M. are also supported by a Biomedical collaboration grant from the Wellcome Trust.

References

1. Manley, N. R. (2000) Thymus organogenesis and molecular mechanisms of thymic epithelial cell differentiation. *Semin. Immunol.* **12,** 421–428.
2. Gordon, J., Wilson, V. A., Blair, N. F., et al. (2004) Functional evidence for a single endodermal origin for the thymic epithelium. *Nat. Immunol.* **5,** 546–553.
3. Manley, N. R. and Blackburn, C. C. (2003) A developmental look at thymus organogenesis: where do the non-hematopoietic cells in the thymus come from? *Curr. Opin. Immunol.* **15,** 225–232.
4. Moore-Scott, B. A., Gordon, J., Blackburn, C. C., Condie, B. G., and Manley, N. R. (2003) New serum-free in vitro culture technique for midgestation mouse embryos. *Genesis* **35,** 164–168.
5. Kaufman, M. H. (1992) *The Atlas of Mouse Development.* Academic Press, London.
6. Bogden, A. E., Haskell, P. M., LePage, D. J., Cobb, W. R., and Esber, H. J. (1979) Growth of human tumor xenografts implanted under the renal capsule of normal immunocompetent mice. *Exp. Cell Biol.* **47,** 281–293.
7. Wassarman, P. M. and Depamphilis, M. L., eds. (1993) *Guide to Techniques in Mouse Development.* Academic Press, London.
8. Zinkernagel, R. M., Althage, A., Waterfield, E., Kindred, B., Welsh, R. M., Callahan, G. and Pincetl, P. (1980) Restriction specificities, alloreactivity, and allotolerance expressed by T cells from nude mice reconstituted with H-2-compatible or -incompatible thymus grafts. *J. Exp. Med.* **151,** 376–399.
9. Hoffman, M. W., Allison, J., and Miller, J. F. A. P. (1992) Tolerance induction by thymic medullary epithelium. *Proc. Natl. Acad. Sci. USA* **89,** 2526–2530.
10. Rodewald, H. R., Paul, S., Haller, C., Bluethmann, H., and Blum, C. (2001) Thymus medulla consisting of epithelial islets each derived from a single progenitor. *Nature* **414,** 763–768.
11. Bennett, A. R., Farley, A., Blair, N. F., Gordon, J., Sharp, L. and Blackburn, C. C. (2002) Identification and characterization of thymic epithelial progenitor cells. *Immunity* **16,** 803–814.
12. Gill, J., Malin, M., Hollander, G. A., and Boyd, R. (2002) Generation of a complete thymic microenvironment by MTS24$^+$ thymic epithelial cells. *Nat. Immunol.* **3,** 635–642.

20

Retroviral Transduction in Fetal Thymic Organ Culture

Bronwyn M. Owens, Robert G. Hawley, and Lisa M. Spain

Summary

T-cell development requires cytokines and intimate contact with stromal cells provided exclusively by the thymus. Consequently, an in vitro model of thymocyte differentiation, fetal thymic organ culture (FTOC), has been developed. FTOC recapitulates the normal development of T-cells derived from both mouse and human progenitor populations, providing a more rapid means to study T-cell development compared with alternative in vivo approaches. Furthermore, FTOC is easily amenable to genetic manipulation using retroviral gene transfer. In this chapter, we outline the basic FTOC technique and describe several applications, including retroviral transduction of mouse thymocyte subsets and human CD34$^+$ stem/progenitor cells.

Key Words: Thymic microenvironment; T-cell development; FTOC; gene transfer; hematopoietic stem/progenitor cell; thymocyte progenitor; retroviral transduction; CD34$^+$ cells; cord blood; human/mouse chimeras; double negative thymocyte.

1. Introduction

The differentiation of mature T-cells from hematopoietic stem and progenitor cells occurs almost exclusively in the thymus. The thymic microenvironment provides many factors important for T-cell development. Even the three-dimensional structure of the thymus itself is functionally important because thymic stromal cells do not substitute for the thymic microenvironment unless they are allowed to reaggregate into organoids (reviewed in **ref.** ***1***). However, fetal thymic organs can be very easily cultured ex vivo and will support the sequential differentiation of T-cell progenitors from CD4–CD8– double negative (DN) to CD4+CD8+double positive (DP) and finally to CD4+CD8–CD3+ and CD4–CD8+CD3+ single positive (SP) populations (reviewed in **ref.** ***2***).

Fetal thymic organ culture (FTOC) has been used to investigate the mechanisms of positive and negative selection, which tolerize the T-cell repertoire to self (reviewed in **ref.** ***3***). FTOC has also proved to be a useful method for elucidating the molecular and cellular mechanisms of T-cell development ***(1,4)***. In this latter case, gene transfer into developing T-cell precursors in FTOC provides a faster and more economical

From: *Methods in Molecular Medicine, Vol. 105: Developmental Hematopoiesis: Methods and Protocols.*
Edited by: M. H. Baron © Humana Press Inc., Totowa, NJ

method (relative to germ line transgenics or bone marrow transplantation in live animals) to explore gene function during T-cell development ***(5–10)***.

Although direct retrovirus-mediated gene transfer to thymus in FTOC has been reported ***(5,11)***, in our hands transduction of hematopoietic stem/progenitor cells followed by thymic reconstitution in vitro is more efficient and reproducible. It has been shown previously that mouse FTOC can be used for the study of the development of human thymocytes from $CD34^+$ progenitor cell populations ***(12–14)***. We extend those results and provide a detailed method here for retroviral gene transduction in human/mouse chimeric FTOCs.

2. Materials

1. Retroviral expression plasmid with fluorescent protein marker, for example MIEV ***(11,15)***.
2. 293T Cells (ATCC CRL-1573), a human embryonic kidney cell line derived from primary human embryonal kidney transformed with adenovirus E1a carrying the SV40 large T antigen.
3. Phoenix™ eco cells (Orbigen), a 293T-derived cell line with stably transduced *gag-pol* and ecotropic envelope constructs.
4. HT1080 cells (ATCC CCL-121), a human fibrocarcinoma cell line.
5. NIH3T3 cells (ATCC CRL-1658).
6. Recombinant murine interleukin-3 (IL-3; 20 ng/mL) and recombinant murine stem cell factor (SCF; 100 ng/mL; Peprotech). Transfection reagents: $CaCl_2$ solution (2.5 *M*); 2X HEPES-buffered saline (HeBS), pH 7.05. Store reagents at –20°C
7. Mouse breeder pairs (C57BL/6, BALB/cByJ, etc., Jackson or Taconic Laboratories).
8. Fetal liver and FTOC culture medium: RPMI culture medium (Invitrogen) supplemented with 10 to 15% heat-inactivated fetal bovine serum (FBS; BioWhittaker; *see* **Note 1**), 1% penicillin–streptomycin (Invitrogen), 10 m*M* HEPES, and 50 μ*M* β-mercaptoethanol.
9. 293T and HT1080 culture medium: Dulbecco's modified Eagle's medium (DMEM; Invitrogen) supplemented with 10% heat-inactivated FBS, 1% penicillin–streptomycin (Invitrogen), and 10 m*M* HEPES.
10. Human $CD34^+$ cell culture medium: X-VIVO 15 (BioWhittaker) containing 10% bovine serum albumin, insulin, and human transferrin serum substitute (BIT, StemCell Technologies), 100 μ*M* β-mercaptoethanol, 100 ng/mL each SCF and Flt-3 ligand, and 20 ng/mL each IL-3, IL-6, and thrombopoietin (Recombinant human growth factors all from Peprotech).
11. Dissecting tools (Roboz): curved forceps, Roboz cat. no. RS-5135; fine forceps, Roboz cat. no. RS-5040; rat-tooth forceps, Roboz cat. no. RS-5248; blunt-tip scissors, Roboz cat. no. S-5962; disposable scalpels, no. 11, Fisher cat. no. S17800: Microfuge tube tissue grinder; Fisher cat. no. 05-559-26.
12. Bel-Art dissecting microscope.
13. Polybrene and protamine sulfate (Sigma).
14. Terasaki dishes (Nunc).
15. Nuclepore® Polycarbonate Track Etch Membranes, pore size 8 μm (Whatman), wrapped in foil pouches and sterilized by autoclaving.
16. Gelfoam gelatin sponge (Pharmacia Upjohn).
17. Tissue culture dishes: 100 mm, six-well (Costar).
18. Fluorochrome-labeled antibodies, for example, PE, PerCP, APC, available from many sources, for example, PharMingen, Caltag.

19. Staining media: Hank's buffered saline or phosphate-buffered saline with 2 to 3% FBS and 0.01% sodium azide. Sodium azide should be omitted if flow sorting will be performed.
20. Flow cytometer capable of four-color analysis, for example, BD FACSCalibur, BD LSR.
21. Magnetic-bead-labeled anti-human CD34, anti-mouse CD4 and anti-mouse-CD8 antibodies and separation apparatus (Miltenyi Biotec).

3. Methods

In this chapter, we describe general approaches to the FTOC technique. The primary method involves the stimulation and retroviral transduction of fetal liver cells, followed by the repopulation of irradiation-depleted fetal thymic lobes. We also describe methods, based on studies by Yasuda et al. ***(16)***, for the isolation and transduction of thymocyte progenitors as an alternative to whole fetal liver. In addition to murine cells, human fetal liver and cord blood-derived $CD34^+$ cells have been used to study human T-cell differentiation and the effects of specific transgenes introduced using retroviral vectors ***(17)***. Although many previous studies have used SCID or NOD-SCID mouse thymi for repopulations, one study showed that human thymocyte differentiation can be achieved if immunocompentent thymi are first depleted using 2-deoxyguanosine ***(12)***. We show here that irradiation is also effective for depletion of thymocytes in human/mouse chimeras. Retroviral gene transfer into human $CD34^+$ cord blood cells can be achieved using amphotropic retroviral vectors or retroviral vectors pseudotyped with envelope proteins from the gibbon ape leukemia virus, the feline endogenous virus RD114 or the vesicular stomatitis virus G (VSV-G) glycoprotein ***(18)***. Here, we describe the use of VSV-G-pseudotyped retroviral vectors.

3.1. Retroviral Expression Plasmids

Efficient transduction and transgene expression in murine hematopoietic cells has been attained using retroviral vectors ***(18)***. We use here MSCV-based vectors containing an enhanced green fluorescent protein (GFP) gene as a FACS-selectable reporter ***(19–21)***. The gene of interest can be inserted into the vectors via unique restriction sites using standard molecular biology techniques.

3.2. Production of Ecotropic Retroviral Supernatants

1. Phoenix-eco cells should be kept subconfluent and passaged every 2 to 3 d to maximize transfection efficiency, (*see* Orbigen data sheet for further details).
2. Trypsinize Phoenix-eco cells and plate at 4×10^6 per 10-cm dish in DMEM + 10 % FBS the morning of the transfection. (Cells and reagents can be scaled up or down according to requirements.)
3. In the afternoon, mix the retroviral construct (10–15 μg) with sterile water to a total volume of 400 μL in a sterile tube.
4. Add 100 μL of 2.5 *M* $CaCl_2$ dropwise to the tube.
5. To a separate 15-mL tube, add 500 μL of 2X HeBS. Then add DNA/$CaCl_2$ mixture dropwise while blowing bubbles using another pipet or by vortexing the mixture.
6. Incubate at room temperature for 20 min.
7. Add 1 mL of calcium phosphate mixture to the dish of producer cells.
8. The following day, change media on producer cells (6.5 mL).
9. One day after changing the medium, collect the retroviral supernatant and pass through a 0.45-μm filter. Store at –70°C. Replace the medium on the producer cells.

10. Twenty-four h later, collect retroviral supernatants and filter as in **step 9**. Discard 293T-cells. Retroviral supernatants can be concentrated (*see* **Note 2**).
11. To titrate the virus, plate 2×10^5 NIH3T3 cells per well in six-well plates. Allow the cells to attach.
12. Make 10-fold dilutions of the viral supernatant and replace the medium on the NIH3T3 cells with 1 mL of diluted retroviral supernatants plus 6 μg/mL of polybrene.
13. Twenty-four h later, replace the viral supernatant with fresh medium.
14. After a further 24 h, trypsinize the cells and analyze on a flow cytometer for GFP expression. Retroviral infectious units per mL of the supernatants can be calculated as follows:

$$\% \text{ GFP}^+ \times \text{dilution factor} \times \text{starting cell number per well}$$

3.3. Production of VSV-G Pseudotyped Retroviral Supernatants

1. Trypsinize and plate 4×10^6 293T-cells per 10-cm dish in DMEM + 10 % FBS the morning of the transfection.
2. In the afternoon, mix retroviral construct (10–15 μg), packaging construct pEQPAM3-E (10 μg; **ref.** ***22***), and VSV-G envelope construct pMD.G (6.7 μg; **ref.** ***23***) and sterile water to a total volume of 400 μL.
3. Add 100 μL of 2.5 *M* $CaCl_2$ dropwise to the tube.
4. To a separate 15-mL tube, add 500 μL of 2X HeBS. Then add DNA/$CaCl_2$ mixture dropwise while blowing bubbles using another pipet or vortexing the mixture.
5. Proceed as described in **step 6** of **Subheading 3.2.**
6. Viral titers can be determined using the HT1080 cell line as described for titration of retroviral supernatants on NIH3T3 cells (from **step 11** of **Subheading 3.2.**).

3.4. Collections of Fetal Livers

1. Place mice together for breeding in the evening.
2. The following morning, check for vaginal plugs using a polished capillary. If females are plugged, separate from the males and date cages. Count this time point as d 0.5.
3. Dissections can be performed on the benchtop on ethanol-soaked paper towels supported by a polystyrene platform. For collection of fetal livers, sacrifice pregnant females (method determined by institutional guidelines) on d 14 of gestation (E14). Prepare the dissection site by soaking fur with 70% ethanol. Using sterile dissecting scissors and forceps, remove uterus containing fetuses and place in a 6-cm dish of complete RPMI on ice (*see* **Note 3**).
4. Remove the fetuses from the uterus and place them into a fresh dish of medium.
5. Pin down a fetus with abdomen facing upward and, using a dissection microscope, carefully slice open the abdomen with a scalpel to expose the liver. Remove the liver using curved fine tweezers and transfer to a well of a 24-well dish that contains medium. Alternatively, using fine jeweler's forceps, make a small horizontal slit in the abdomen just above the umbilicus. Holding the forceps slightly open, push down on either side of the slit: this will force the liver out, whereupon it can be pinched off with the forceps and transferred to a culture dish.
6. In a tissue culture hood, dissociate the fetal liver (FL) cells by pipetting and transfer to a 15-mL conical tube.
7. Bring the volume of the FL cells to 10 mL and allow any large tissue particles to settle to the bottom of the tube (5 min).
8. Transfer cells to a fresh tube and wash once with medium.
9. FL cells from two to three livers may be pooled and frozen in 90% FBS + 10% DMSO in liquid nitrogen for future use, or used immediately for retroviral transduction.

3.5. Collection of Fetal Thymic Lobes

1. Set up timed matings for plugged females as described in **Subheading 3.4.**
2. For fetal thymic lobes, sacrifice pregnant females according to institutional guidelines on d 15 or 16 of gestation (E15 or E16), remove fetuses and place each one in medium in a well of a 24-well plate (*see* **Note 4**).
3. Pin down the fetus at head, feet, and arms, with abdomen facing upward.
4. Using a scalpel and a dissecting microscope, carefully open the thorax to reveal the thymic lobes, which are two white organs located above the heart.
5. Using sterile fine straight forceps, tweeze out the individual lobes and place pairs of lobes into media in a well of a 24-well dish on ice. Transfer lobes to the tissue culture hood.
6. To prepare organ culture conditions, place pieces of Gelfoam sponge (0.5 × 0.5 cm) into wells of a six-well dish containing 2.5 mL of complete RPMI and completely soak the Gelfoam sponge in medium by squeezing it with a pipet tip. Place a Nuclepore® membrane shiny side up on each sponge.
7. Place up to four thymic lobes on each membrane. Thymi can be kept for up to 1 mo before use. Media should be changed weekly.

3.6. Retroviral Transduction

1. Thaw FL cells, wash and resuspend cells at 2 × 10^6 cells/mL in complete RPMI plus 20 ng/mL IL-3 and 100 ng/mL SCF for 24 to 48 h in a 37°C humidified incubator, 5 % CO_2. (Retain some GFP-negative FL cells that can be used as controls for immunophenotypic analysis as described in **Subheading 3.10.**)
2. On the day of transduction, quickly thaw retroviral supernatants in a 37°C water bath, place on ice.
3. Replate the FL cells at a concentration of 1 × 10^6 cells/mL in ecotropic retroviral supernatant plus 20 ng/mL IL-3, 100 ng/mL SCF, and 6 μg/mL polybrene in a multiwell tissue culture dish and "spinoculate" (centrifuge) cells at approx 500*g* for 1 h.
4. Place the cells in an incubator overnight. The following day, repeat spinoculation with additional ecotropic supernatant and incubate overnight.
5. After a 2-d transduction protocol, the transduced cells may be used directly in FTOC or sorted for purity based on GFP expression and then used in FTOC.

3.7. FTOC

1. Thymic lobes must be irradiated prior to incubation with transduced/sorted FL cells. Using a sterile forceps, place Gelfoam sponge with lobes into a 6-cm dish and irradiate at 2000–2500 rads in a γ irradiator (FTOC scheme is outlined in **Fig. 1**). Add 2 to 3 mL of complete RMPI to the dish until lobes are required.
2. Collect transduced FL cells, centrifuge at 500*g* for 5 min, and resuspend in 35 μL of complete RPMI medium per lobe. Typically, 2–5 × 10^5 cells are used but fewer cells are sufficient to reconstitute thymi. However, there may be a delay in reconstitution and the development of different thymocyte subsets if fewer cells are used (dose dependence of thymic reconstitution is shown in **Fig. 2**).
3. Place 35 μL of transduced cell suspension per well of a Terasaki dish. Space the drops of cells so that there is minimal risk of overflow between wells and use a separate Terasaki dish for each retroviral construct being used. Set up some untransduced cells for FTOC as negative controls.
4. Place one lobe in each aliquot of cells. Carefully invert the plate such that a hanging drop forms. Place the dishes into a humidified container, such as a Tupperware® with moist-

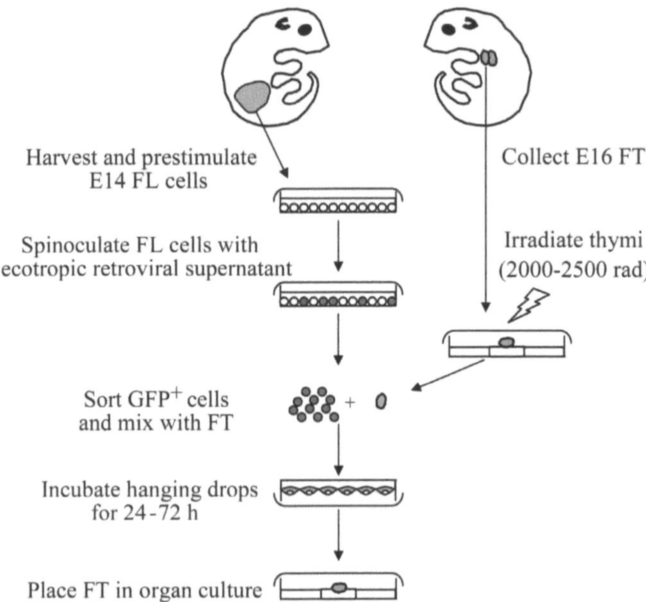

Fig. 1. Flow diagram of fetal thymic organ culture model. E14 fetal liver (FL) hematopoietic progenitor cells are incubated in cytokines IL-3 and SCF for 24 to 48 h. Retrovirally transduced cells can be sorted based on GFP expression, mixed with E16 irradiated fetal thymi (FT), and inverted in hanging drops in Terasaki dishes. After incubating for 24 to 72 h, thymi are placed in organ culture until analysis.

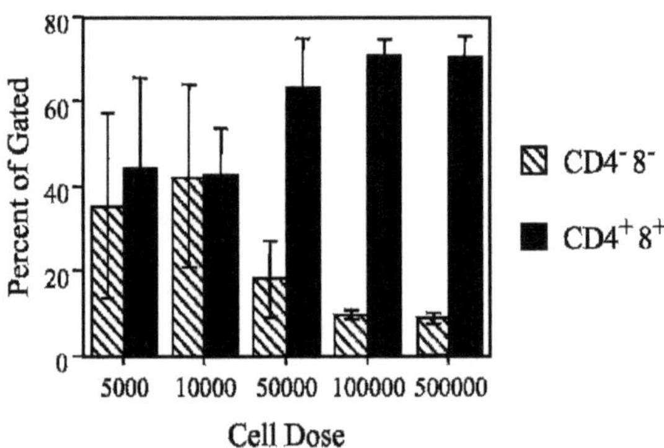

Fig. 2. Higher doses of reconstituting fetal liver cells increase the percentage of $CD4^+8^+$ thymocytes. Graded doses of fetal liver cells were delivered to irradiated fetal thymic lobes as described. The percentage of $CD4–8^-$ (hatched bars) and $CD4^+8^+$ (solid bars) thymocytes after 14 d was measured by flow cytometry. Shown are the average and standard deviation of at least three lobes per dose.

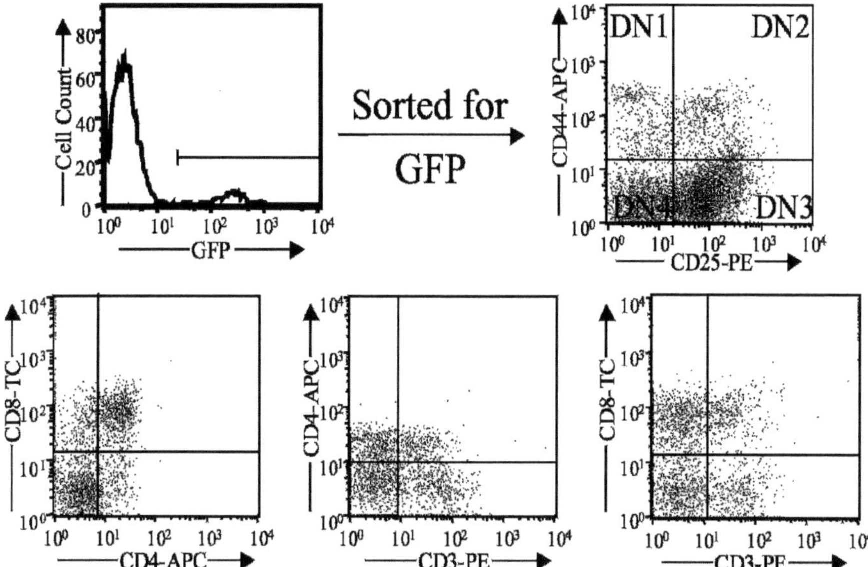

Fig. 3. DN cells reconstitute thymi. CD4/CD8 DN thymocytes selected by several rounds of negative selection using magnetic bead separation were transduced with concentrated (10X) retroviral supernatants and enriched for GFP expression (upper plots). Total DN cells (10^4 cells per lobe) were used to reconstitute irradiated E16 thymi and immunophenotyped after 15 d for differentiation into DP and SP populations.

ened paper towels that has been pre-equilibrated in the incubator. Incubate hanging drops for 24 to 72 h.

5. The following day, prepare organ culture conditions as described in **Subheading 3.5.** Change the media weekly until analysis.

3.8. Isolation and Transduction of DN Thymocytes

DN thymocytes can be isolated from fetal or young adult mice. Although the majority of cells in adult mice are CD4 and/or CD8 positive (>95%), the absolute numbers of DN cells is greater in adult than fetal mice and adults may therefore may be a preferable source of DN thymocytes.

1. Dissect thymi from 4- to 6-wk old mice and dissociate thymocytes using a sterile tissue grinder. Approximately 10^8 total cells can be isolated per mouse.
2. Label CD4 and CD8 cells with MicroBead-labeled antibodies and isolate CD4/CD8 DN cells by negative selection according to manufacturer's directions. Two rounds of negative selection may be required to ensure purified DN cells. Different DN populations can be further separated by sorting based on expression of CD25 and CD44 (**Fig. 3**).
3. Resuspend DN cells in ecotropic retroviral supernatant (neat or 10X concentrated; *see* **Note 2**) supplemented with polybrene (6 μg/mL), IL-7 (10 ng/mL), and IL-2 (10 ng/mL) and spinoculate for 1 h at 1000*g*.
4. Repeat spinoculation with additional retroviral supernatant 24 h later.

5. Twenty-four hours later, analyze GFP expression on flow cytometer and either sort GFP+ DN populations or use cells directly in place of fetal liver cells in FTOC as in **Subheading 3.7.** For reconstitution, use 104 cells/thymus.
6. Change medium on FTOC weekly until analysis. CD4/CD8 double and single positive populations develop within 2 wk.

3.9. Human/Mouse Chimeric Organ Culture

For our studies, human umbilical cord blood samples provided by the American Red Cross Cord Blood Program were obtained after informed consent, in conformity with an institutionally approved protocol. Cord blood samples are also available from several commercial sources, for example, AllCells, (Berkeley, CA) or Cambrex BioScience Walkersville, (Walkersville, MD). The thymocyte progenitor population can be transduced with retroviral constructs using VSV-G-pseudotyped retroviruses.

3.9.1. Isolation and Transduction of Human CD34+ Cells

1. Isolate mononuclear cells from anti-coagulated human cord blood using Ficoll-Paque.
2. Isolate the CD34+ cells by positive selection using anti-CD34 antibodies labeled with magnetic MicroBeads on magnetic columns, according to manufacturer's instructions (Miltenyi Biotec).
3. Evaluate the purity of the CD34+ cells by staining with a fluorochrome-conjugated anti-CD34 antibody (typically, 95% of cells should be CD34+).
4. Resuspend CD34+ cells at a concentration of 1×10^6/mL in X-VIVO 15 medium and culture cells on fibronectin-coated for 2 to 3 d in the presence of cytokines IL-3, IL-6, SCF, Flt-3, and thrombopoietin.
5. After prestimulation, resuspend cells in VSV-G pseudotyped retroviral supernatants containing cytokines and protamine sulfate (4 μg/mL) in multiwell dishes coated with recombinant fibronectin fragment (2 μg/cm^2 CH-296; Takara Shuzo, Shiga, Japan) and spinoculate at 1300*g* for 1 h. Return cells to the incubator.
6. Repeat spinoculation with fresh retroviral supernatants for 2 d longer.
7. Analyze percent transduction by fluorescence activated cell sorter (FACS) analysis. Depending on transduction efficiency, cells may need to be sorted based on GFP expression.

3.9.2. Human/Mouse Chimeric FTOC

1. Irradiate E16 fetal thymi dissected from immunocompetent or immunocompromised mice (2500 rad).
2. Centrifuge transduced human progenitors and resuspend at 10^4 cells/35 μL X-VIVO 15 medium without cytokines.
3. Place aliquots of 35 μL of cell suspension in wells of a Terasaki dish and place one lobe into each well.
4. Invert the dish and incubate in a humidified container for 48 to 72 h (*see* **Subheading 3.7., step 4**).
5. Place the thymi in organ culture as described in **Subheading 3.5.**, in complete X-VIVO 15 excluding cytokines. Replace medium weekly until analysis. If development to early (DN) stages is to be evaluated, analysis can occur within 10 d. For DP development, analysis should be performed between 10 to 16 d, and for SP development, analysis should be performed after 16 and up to 20 d.
6. Phenotype human thymocyte development using anti-human specific antibodies (**Fig. 4**).

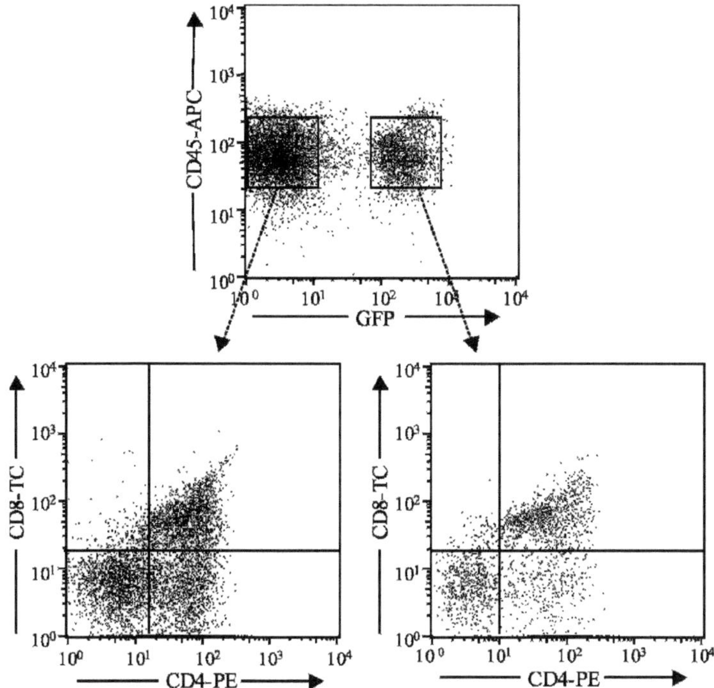

Fig. 4. Human/mouse FTOC. Cord blood-derived human $CD34^+$ cells were transduced with VSV-G pseudotyped retrovirus and enriched for GFP expression. After 25 d in organ culture, $CD45^+GFP^-$ and $CD45^+GFP^+$ cells were analyzed with human-specific antibodies for surface expression of CD4 and CD8.

3.10. Immunophenotypic Analysis

Multicolor analysis is now possible as a result of the increasing availability of a broad spectrum of fluorochrome-labeled antibodies. The procedure described next is based on four-color analysis to maximize the data that can be generated from each experiment. Since this protocol describes the use of cells transduced with GFP, it is important to have thymi reconstituted with GFP negative cells that can serve as compensation controls for FACS analysis. Four-color analysis may require the use of additional FACS software such as FlowJo (Tree Star, Inc., San Carlos, CA).

1. Place individual thymi into Eppendorf tubes with 200 μL of 2.4G2 hybridoma supernatant. This antibody pretreatment serves to block the Fc receptor and reduce Fc-mediated background staining.
2. Disrupt the thymi using a tissue grinder to release thymocytes and incubate for 15 min at 4°C in 2.4G2.
3. Aliquot the cells into one to two wells of a 96-well place. Divide the GFP-negative cells between enough wells for staining with each antibody being used. Also aliquot some GFP^+ cells for setting up compensation.

4. Using a multichannel pipet, add 200 μL of staining medium to each well and centrifuge the cells in plate holders for 5 min at 500*g*.
5. To remove the staining medium, invert the plate with a flick of the wrist. Wipe any droplets of staining medium off the surface of the plate.
6. Resuspend the cells by gently agitating the plate on a vortex mixer affixed with a plate holder. Assume that 10 μL of staining medium remains in each well, and add 2X diluted antibody cocktails (10 μL per well) to each well and individual antibodies to the cells to be used for compensation. (Titration of the antibodies will be necessary to find optimal dilution.) Incubate for 15 min at 4°C.
7. Add 150 μL of staining medium to each well and centrifuge plate.
8. Resuspend the cells in 200 μL of staining medium and transfer to 6 × 50-mm flint glass tubes and insert into FACS tubes.
9. Proceed to data acquisition.

4. Notes

1. Serum lots should be screened for efficacy in FTOC assays. Embryonic d 16 fetal thymic lobes should be placed directly into FTOC and 5-d survival, proliferation, and differentiation should be measured. Serum lots should support proliferation to 10^6 cells per lobe and DP percentages not less than 70% and CD4 percentages not less than 5%.
2. Concentration of ecotropic retrovirus can be achieved by centrifugation of viral supernatants at 10,000*g* for 16 h at 4°C ***(24)***. Viral pellet can be resuspended in 1/30 of the original volume and stored at –70°C. Concentrated supernatants should be used at 10X or 20X concentration. The transduction efficiency of refractory cells may improve with concentrated viral preparations but should be weighed against increased toxicity and inconvenience of large-scale cultures of retroviral packaging cells.
3. Dissections can be performed on the bench with minimal contamination, provided sterile dissecting tools are used and the procedures are carried out efficiently, with minimal exposure to non-sterile conditions.
4. Both fetal livers and thymic lobes can be harvested from E15 fetuses.

Acknowledgments

We thank the members of the Spain lab for continuing methodology development and Teresa Hawley of the Holland Laboratory Flow Cytometry Facility for expert assistance with cell sorting. This work was supported in part by National Institutes of Health grants A149807 and A136453 and the American Cancer Society (to L.M.S.), and HL65519 and HL66305 (to R.G.H.).

References

1. Anderson, G., Jenkinson, E. J., Moore, N. C., and Owen, J. J. (1993) MHC class II-positive epithelium and mesenchyme cells are both required for T-cell development in the thymus. *Nature* **362,** 70–73.
2. Jenkinson, E. J. and Owen, J. J. (1990) T-cell differentiation in thymus organ cultures. *Semin. Immunol.* **2,** 51–58.
3. Jameson, S. C., Hogquist, K. A., and Bevan, M. J. (1995) Positive selection of thymocytes. *Annu. Rev. Immunol.* **13,** 93–126.
4. Anderson, G., Owen, J. J., Moore, N. C., and Jenkinson, E. J. (1994) Thymic epithelial cells provide unique signals for positive selection of CD4+CD8+ thymocytes in vitro. *J. Exp. Med.* **179,** 2027–2031.

5. Crompton, T., Gilmour, K. C., and Owen, M. J. (1996) The MAP kinase pathway controls differentiation from double-negative to double-positive thymocyte. *Cell* **86,** 243–251.
6. Spain, L. M., Lau, L. L., and Takahama, Y. (2000) Retroviral infection of T-cell precursors in thymic organ culture. *Methods Mol. Biol.* **136,** 79–86.
7. Izon, D. J., Punt, J. A., Xu, L., Karnell, F. G., Allman, D., Myung, P. S., et al. (2001) Notch1 regulates maturation of CD4+ and CD8+ thymocytes by modulating TCR signal strength. *Immunity* **14,** 253–264.
8. Spain, L. M. and Liu, P. (2002) TCRbeta transmembrane tyrosines are required for pre-TCR function. *J. Immunol.* **168,** 127–133.
9. Carleton, M., Haks, M. C., Smeele, S. A., Jones, A., Belkowski, S. M., Berger, M. A., et al. (2002) Early growth response transcription factors are required for development of CD4(–)CD8(–) thymocytes to the CD4(+)CD8(+) stage. *J. Immunol.* **168,** 1649–1658.
10. Izon, D. J., Aster, J. C., He, Y., Weng, A., Karnell, F. G., Patriub, V., et al. (2002) Deltex1 redirects lymphoid progenitors to the B cell lineage by antagonizing Notch1. *Immunity* **16,** 231–243.
11. Michie, A. M., Soh, J. W., Hawley, R. G., Weinstein, I. B., and Zuniga-Pflucker, J. C. (2001) Allelic exclusion and differentiation by protein kinase C-mediated signals in immature thymocytes. *Proc. Natl. Acad. Sci. USA* **98,** 609–614.
12. Globerson, A., Kollet, O., Abel, L., Fajerman, I., Ballin, A., Nagler, A., et al. (1999) Differential effects of CD4+ and CD8+ cells on lymphocyte development from human cord blood cells in murine fetal thymus explants. *Exp. Hematol.* **27,** 282–292.
13. Plum, J., De Smedt, M., Defresne, M. P., Leclercq, G., and Vandekerckhove, B. (1994) Human CD34+ fetal liver stem cells differentiate to T cells in a mouse thymic microenvironment. *Blood* **84,** 1587–1593.
14. Robin, C., Bennaceur-Griscelli, A., Louache, F., Vainchenker, W., and Coulombel, L. (1999) Identification of human T-lymphoid progenitor cells in CD34+ CD38low and CD34+ CD38+ subsets of human cord blood and bone marrow cells using NOD-SCID fetal thymus organ cultures. *Br. J. Haematol.* **104,** 809–819.
15. Leung, B. L., Haughn, L., Veillette, A., Hawley, R. G., Rottapel, R., and Julius, M. (1999) TCR alpha beta-independent CD28 signaling and costimulation require non-CD4-associated Lck. *J. Immunol.* **163,** 1334–1341.
16. Yasuda, Y., Nishijima, I., Watanabe, S., and Arai, K. (1997) Thymocyte proliferation and differentiation in human granulocyte-macrophage colony-stimulating factor receptor transgenic mice. *J. Allergy Clin. Immunol.* **100,** S87–S96.
17. Taghon, T., Stolz, F., De Smedt, M., Cnockaert, M., Verhasselt, B., Plum, J., and Leclercq, G. (2002) HOX-A10 regulates hematopoietic lineage commitment: evidence for a monocyte-specific transcription factor. *Blood* **99,** 1197–1204.
18. Hawley, R. G. (2001) Progress toward vector design for hematopoietic stem cell gene therapy. *Curr. Gene Ther.* **1,** 1–17.
19. Cheng, L., Fu, J., Tsukamoto, A., and Hawley, R. G. (1996) Use of green fluorescent protein variants to monitor gene transfer and expression in mammalian cells. *Nat. Biotechnol.* **14,** 606–609.
20. Hawley, T. S., Telford, W. G., and Hawley, R. G. (2001) "Rainbow" reporters for multispectral marking and lineage analysis of hematopoietic stem cells. *Stem Cells* **19,** 118–124.
21. Cheng, L., Du, C., Murray, D., Tong, X., Zhang, Y. A., Chen, B. P., and Hawley, R. G. (1997) A GFP reporter system to assess gene transfer and expression in human hematopoietic progenitor cells. *Gene Ther.* **4,** 1013–1022.
22. Kelly, P. F., Vandergriff, J., Nathwani, A., Nienhuis, A. W., and Vanin, E. F. (2000) Highly efficient gene transfer into cord blood nonobese diabetic/severe combined immunodefi-

ciency repopulating cells by oncoretroviral vector particles pseudotyped with the feline endogenous retrovirus (RD114) envelope protein. *Blood* **96,** 1206–1214.

23. Naldini, L., Blomer, U., Gallay, P., Ory, D., Mulligan, R., Gage, F. H., et al. (1996) In vivo gene delivery and stable transduction of nondividing cells by a lentiviral vector. *Science* **272,** 263–267.
24. Travers, H., Anderson, G., Gentle, D., Jenkinson, E., and Girdlestone, J. (2001) Protocols for high efficiency, stage-specific retroviral transduction of murine fetal thymocytes and thymic epithelial cells. *J. Immunol. Methods* **253,** 209–222.

21

Expansion and Differentiation of Immature Mouse and Human Hematopoietic Progenitors

Helmut Dolznig, Andrea Kolbus, Cornelia Leberbauer, Uwe Schmidt, Eva-Maria Deiner, Ernst W. Müllner, and Hartmut Beug

Summary

A prerequisite for proper investigation of self-renewal and differentiation of hematopoietic cells is the possibility to obtain large quantities of homogenous primary progenitors under defined conditions, allowing meaningful biochemical and molecular analyses. These cells should show renewal and differentiation characteristics similar to the in vivo situation. The serum-free culture systems delineated in this chapter meet these requirements, employing primary hematopoietic cells derived from murine fetal liver and human umbilical cord blood, which show physiological self-renewal responses to cytokine/hormone combinations, which in vivo are involved in stress hematopoiesis. We describe the expansion and sustained proliferation of multipotent (mouse) and erythroid (mouse and human) progenitors, responding to physiological signals. Moreover, both mouse and human erythroid progenitors can be induced to undergo synchronous terminal differentiation by addition of high levels of erythropoietin. If fetal liver cells from $p53^{-/-}$ mice are used, respective multipotent and erythroid cells undergo immortalization without an obvious Hayflick crisis, but otherwise retain their primary cell characteristics. Finally, both primary and immortal mouse progenitors can be subjected to genetic manipulation via retroviral constructs with high efficiency.

Key Words: Self renewal; multipotent progenitors; primary cells; immortalized cells; serum-free culture conditions; differentiation; erythroid progenitors; erythropoiesis; mass culture; erythropoietin (Epo); stem cell factor (SCF); glucocorticoid; dexamethasone (Dex); hematopoietic development; retroviral infection; flow cytometry.

1. Introduction

Comprehensive analysis of biochemistry and molecular biology of red cell development in mammals and humans is severely hampered from the lack of suitable in vivo-like cell systems that undergo continuous proliferation in cell culture. However, available primary model systems suffer either from the heterogeneity of cell populations caused by different stages of maturation or yield only insufficient cell numbers *(1–3)*. Yet, erythroleukemic cell lines (frequently derived by transformation with the

From: *Methods in Molecular Medicine, Vol. 105: Developmental Hematopoiesis: Methods and Protocols.*
Edited by: M. H. Baron © Humana Press Inc., Totowa, NJ

Friend–virus complex or respective oncogenes, **refs. *4,5***) generally fail to execute the normal erythroid differentiation program (four to five terminal cell divisions, massive size reduction, nuclear condensation, and enucleation; **refs. *6–8***). This is even true for a recently described erythroblast system overexpressing endogenous PU-1/Spi-1 ***(9)***. These cells exhibit aberrantly timed differentiation, undergo an immediate proliferation arrest upon differentiation induction, lack proper size control, and fail to generate mature, enucleated erythrocytes. The situation is similarly problematic with respect to the expansion of multipotent progenitors because such cells can either only be expanded in a short-term fashion ***(10)*** or established as cell lines in response to introduction of exogenous genes, such as a constitutively active RARα ***(11)*** or human leukemia oncogenes (*see* **ref. *12*** and references therein).

Therefore, an obvious need exists for procedures that allow the long-term expansion of primary, immature hematopoietic cells, stimulating their ability to undergo renewal at the expense of differentiation. Recently, progress was made in this direction, starting from the observation that leukemia oncogenes such as the mutated EGF-receptor v-ErbB plus the mutated nuclear receptor v-ErbA can cause renewal in primary erythroid progenitors (for review, *see* **ref. *13***). Both physiologically and biochemically, this leukemic renewal corresponds to stress erythropoiesis, taking place in the spleen of hypoxic or anemic mice and depending on the concerted action of erythropoietin (Epo), stem cell factor (c-Kit ligand/SCF), and glucocorticoids ***(14,15)***. Although activation of the glucocorticoid receptor (GR) by dexamethasone (Dex) is functionally equivalent to v-ErbA oncogene function ***(16)***, v-ErbB activates the same signal transduction pathways (Stat5; PI3K) as the combined action of the Epo-receptor (Stat5) and c-Kit (PI3K). Exploiting these findings led to the successful long-term outgrowth of primary erythroid progenitors from murine fetal livers and human umbilical cord blood, when cultivated in serum-free media supplemented with the factors active in stress erythropoiesis (low Epo/SCF/Dex). In both cases, the cells retain an immature proerythroblast phenotype but can be induced to terminally differentiate when the renewal factors are replaced by differentiation factors (high Epo/insulin; *see* **Subheading 3.1.4.**).

The aim of this chapter is to describe a number of procedures allowing the long-term-expansion of erythroid progenitors from both murine and human sources, to provide methods allowing their synchronous terminal differentiation into erythrocytes, and to describe the use of such methods to characterize erythropoiesis in genetically modified mice ***(17–19)***. We also will describe how to expand multipotent cells in enriched cytokine/hormone mixtures, which can be shifted into erythroid progenitors by switching to erythroid renewal factors, thus allowing expansion of erythroid progenitors with erythroid renewal/proliferation defects from respective mutant mice. Furthermore, we will outline methods for efficient retroviral infection of wild type and $p53^{-/-}$ erythroid progenitors to transduce genes of interest. Finally, we will describe the somewhat different requirements of murine versus human erythroid cell systems for outgrowth and terminal differentiation.

The murine fetal liver is the major embryonic erythropoietic organ and thus harbors large numbers of erythroid progenitors. Furthermore, the fetal liver is a source of committed hematopoietic progenitors capable of differentiating towards other hematopoietic lineages (*see* **refs. *14,15,17***, and references therein). One source for human erythroid progenitors is umbilical cord blood, superior to cells from peripheral blood or bone marrow biopsies ***(21)***. Like murine fetal liver, human cord blood contains immature, nonlineage committed progenitors in CD34$^+$ fractions.

To expand immature erythroid progenitor cells, murine fetal liver cells are isolated and expanded in particular serum-free media supplemented with SCF, Epo, glucocorticoids like Dex, and insulin growth factor-1 (IGF-1; for apoptosis protection). A particular advantage of these cells in comparison to existing cell lines is that they rather faithfully recapitulate the normal erythroid differentiation program in vivo. Actively proliferating cultures contain >90–95% of proerythroblasts and very few apoptotic cells (<5%). They are thus superior to existing two- or three-step procedures for enrichment of erythroid progenitors ***(22)***, which always contain a substantial fraction of apoptotic cells and are heterogenous, containing either immature cells from other lineages or a mixture of immature, partially mature and mature erythroid cells. As already mentioned above, cultures of proliferating mouse erythroblasts can be induced to initiate terminal differentiation by replacing the self renewal factors Epo/SCF/Dex with the physiological differentiation factors Epo and insulin. Under these conditions, differentiation is highly synchronous and effectively completed within 3 d, involves three to four cell divisions, leading to an 8- to 15-fold increase in cell number during differentiation and resulting in about 70% enucleated, fully hemoglobinized cells that are morphologically similar to erythrocytes of peripheral blood ***(15,17–19)***.

The life-span of murine erythroblasts from wild type mice is sufficient to allow infection of these cells right after isolation with retroviral vectors bearing the gene of interest, co-expressing green-fluorescent-protein (GFP) via an IRES element. Fibroblasts producing high titers of infectious retrovirus are co-cultivated with the primary cells, which then can be purified by FACS. In several cases, the high efficiency (>80%) allowed immediate expansion and analysis of infected cells without further purification ***(18)***. In case of immortal erythroblasts from p53$^{-/-}$ mice, sublines stably expressing various genes of interest have been obtained and analyzed ***(15,19)***.

More immature, most likely multipotent hematopoietic cells can be expanded in a more complex cytokine/hormone mixture containing SCF, Flt3-ligand, IGF-1, IL-3, IL-6, granulocyte-macrophage–colony-stimulating factor, and Dex. If multipotent progenitors that actively proliferate in response to these factors are switched to erythroid medium (Epo/SCF/Dex/IGF-1), they continue to proliferate but acquire an erythroid set of surface markers within 5 to 6 d. Partially mature cells from other (particularly myeloid) lineages can be removed by simple step density gradients using lymphocyte separation medium and/or Percoll. The erythroid cells thus produced show a similar proliferation capacity as freshly isolated fetal liver cells, and can be normally differentiated into mature erythrocytes. By switching a mass culture of multipotent cells from mutant mice showing erythroid lineage proliferation defects into the erythroid medium, enough erythroid progenitors can be obtained to analyze their potential proliferation- and differentiation defects at the molecular level (**ref. *19***; Deiner et al., in preparation).

Long-term outgrowth of human erythroblasts requires a different type of serum-free medium, but otherwise proceeds well in the same factor combination (Epo/SCF/Dex/IGF-1). Interestingly, immature human erythroblasts can be expanded for around 40 generations, much longer than wild type mouse erythroblasts, which survive only for 12 to 15 generations. This long-term expansion of human erythroblasts required some additional medium ingredients (lipids, other steroid hormones). Likewise, the conditions for terminal differentiation of human erythroblasts differ somewhat from those used for murine cells. Furthermore, synchronous differentiation is slower (6 instead of 3 d are required for enucleated erythrocytes to form). No initial acceleration of the cell cycle and fewer differentiation divisions (two to three) are observed.

Optimal outgrowth of these primary erythroid and multipotent progenitor cells is critically dependent on the following: 1) use of pretested batches of serum-free media, including added components; 2) correct, optimized factor concentrations; 3) close maintenance of optimal cell densities; and 4) daily dilution with fresh medium plus restoration of full growth factor levels (thus requiring handling of the cells at least once daily). These safeguards are essential to prevent apoptosis and maintain the cells in an immature state by preventing spontaneous differentiation into more mature cells. Furthermore, close observation of these points is required to obtain optimal expansion levels of fetal liver/cord blood cells and prevention of genetic instability/tetraploidy/aneuploidy in the case of immortal p53 http://www.runagainstbush.org/ erythroid progenitors or multipotent cells.

2. Materials

2.1. Chemical Reagents

1. Diff Quick Red I (cat. no. 130 834) and Diff Quick Blue II (cat. no. 130 835; Dade Behring, Austria).
2. 4,6-diamidino-2-phenylindole dihydrochloride (DAPI; VWR International Merck, Darmstadt, Germany; cat. no. 24653).
3. Dimethyl sulfoxide (DMSO; Fluka, Buchs, Switzerland; cat. no. 41639).
4. Entellan (VWR International Merck; cat. no. 1.07961).
5. Erylysis-buffer (10X stock solution): 89.9 g of ammonium chloride, 10 g of $KHCO_3$, 0.37 g of ethylene diamine tetraacetic acid, H_2O, to 1000 mL (readjust pH to 7.3 immediately before use).
6. Ethanol, p.a. (high purity, VWR International Merck; cat. no. 100983).
7. Hemoglobin assay solutions (freshly prepared): 0.5 mg/mL O-phenylene-diamine dihydrochloride (Sigma, St. Louis, MO; cat. no. P1526) and 1 μL/mL of 30% H_2O_2 in 50 m*M* citric acid, 0.1 *M* Na_2HPO_4. Stop solution: 4 *M* H_2SO_4. Citric acid and stop solution can be stored for weeks at room temperature.
8. L-glutamine (100X stock solution: 200 m*M*; Invitrogen Gibco, Carlsbad, CA; cat. no. 25030-024).
9. Methanol, p.a. (high purity, VWR International Merck; cat. no. 106009).
10. *O*-dianisidine (Fast Blue; Sigma; cat. no. D 9143).
11. Phosphate-buffered saline (PBS).
12. Propidium iodide (Sigma; cat. no. P 4170).

2.2. Biological Reagents

1. Antibodies for flow cytometry:

   Mouse cells: Ter119 (cat. no. 09085B), Sca-1 (cat. nos. 01165B; 01164D), GR-1 (cat. no. 01215A), CD45R/B220 (cat. nos. 01125B; 01129A), CD135/Flk-2/FltL-3 (cat. no. 09895A), CD11b/Mac-1 (cat. no. E511019), CD117/c-Kit (cat. no. 01904D), Integrin *a*-4 (cat. no. 01735) all from PharMingen, San Diego, CA.

   Human cells: CD15 (FITC = fluorescein iso-thiocyanate labeled; Pharmingen, cat. no. 555401), CD19 (FITC; PharMingen, cat. no. 555412), CD45 (FITC; PharMingen, cat. no.

555482), GPA (glycophorin A; FITC; PharMingen, cat. no. 559943), CD33 (PE = phycoerythrin; PharMingen, cat. no. 30945X), CD38 (PE; PharMingen, cat. no. 555460), CD45RA (PE; PharMingen, cat. no. 555489), CD56 (PE; PharMingen, cat. no. 555516), CD71 (transferrin receptor; PE; PharMingen, cat. no. 555537), CD117 (c-Kit, stem cell factor receptor; PE; PharMingen, cat. no. 555714), CD3 (ECD = phycoerythrin-Texas Red; Coulter-Immunotech, Marseille, France, cat. no. IM2705), CD45 (ECD; Coulter-Immunotech, cat. no. IM2710), CD 14 (PC5 = phycoerythrin-cyanin 5.1; Coulter-Immunotech, cat. no. IM2640), CD 34 (PC5; Coulter-Immunotech, cat. no. IM2648).

2. Dexamethasone (Dex; 1000X stock: 10^{-3} *M* in ethanol, store at –20°C; Sigma, D 4902).
3. Dulbecco's modified Eagle's medium (DMEM; Invitrogen Gibco, cat. no. 31966-021).
4. Fetal calf serum (FCS; Invitrogen Gibco).
5. Highly purified bovine serum albumin (BSA; Sigma, cat. no. A0281).
6. Human recombinant insulin (Ins; 1000X stock in 0.1% BSA/PBS: 10 μg/mL = 0.4 IE/mL; Actrapid HM, Novo Nordisk, Bagsvaerd, Denmark).
7. Human recombinant insulin like growth factor-1 (IGF-1, 40 μg/mL = 1000X stock in 0.1% BSA/PBS; Promega, Mannheim, Germany, cat. no. G 5111).
8. Human recombinant erythropoietin (Epo, 10,000 U/mL; Erypo, Janssen-Cilag, Baar, Switzerland).
9. Human serum (HS, type AB, male; Sigma, cat. no. H 4522).
10. Human transferrin (17.5 mg/mL in 0.1% BSA/PBS; Sigma, cat. no. T 8158).
11. Lipids, cholesterol-rich (Sigma, cat. no. L 4646).
12. Lymphocyte separation medium (density 1078 g/mL; Eurobio, Les Ulis Cedex B; France, cat. no. CMSMSL01-01).
13. Methocel (semi solid medium basis; Invitrogen Gibco).
14. Mouse culture stock solutions of cytokines (1000X): mouse recombinant SCF (100 μg/mL), human recombinant IL-3 (2 μg/mL), mouse recombinant IL-6 (5 μg/mL), mouse recombinant Flk2/Flt3 ligand (10 μg/mL), mouse recombinant GM-CSF (3 μg/mL), (all in 0.1% BSA/PBS; all from R&D Systems, Minneapolis, MN). For suggestions to produce murine SCF (used at much higher concentration than other factors and thus quite expensive), *see* **Note 1**.
15. Penicillin/streptomycin (10,000 U/mL P, 10000 μg/mL S; Invitrogen Gibco, cat. no. 15140-122).
16. Percoll (density gradient separation medium, density 1.1 g/mL; Amersham Biosciences, Little Chalfont, UK, cat. no. 17-0891-02).
17. Polybrene transfection reagent (4 mg/mL stock solution, store at 4°C; Aldrich, Milwaukee, WI, cat. no. AL-118).
18. Polyfect transfection reagent (Qiagen, Valencia, CA, cat. no. 301105).
19. Stem-Pro-34™ serum free medium (SFM; including Nutrient supplement; Invitrogen Gibco, cat. no. 10639-011). Particular measures have to be taken to obtain medium and Nutrient supplement of sufficient quality from the purchaser and for storage of these items (*see* **Note 2**).
20. StemSpan™ SFEM (serum-free expansion medium; Stem Cell Technologies, Vancouver, BC, Canada; cat. no. 09650).
21. 3,5,3'-Triiodo-L-thyronine (T3; Sigma, cat. no. T 6397).
22. ZK112993 (ZK, 1000X stock = 3×10^{-3} *M* in ethanol, store at –20°C; not available from Schering any more, but RU486 or Mifepristone, Sigma, cat. no. M8946, can be used at similar concentrations).

2.3. Equipment

1. CASY™ cell analyzer, (Schärfe System, Reutlingen, Germany).
2. Cell strainer 70 μm (Becton Dickinson, San Jose, CA; cat. no. 352350).

3. Cytocentrifuge (Cytospin III or IV, Shandon, Pittsburgh, PA).
4. Glass slides.
5. Scissors (big: cat. no. 14001-12; small: cat. no. 14084-08, FineScienceTools, Heidelberg, Germany).
6. Tissue culture plates (mostly Nunc, Roskilde, Denmark; some types Greiner bio-one, Kremsmünster, Austria).
7. V-shaped 96-well plates, for hemoglobin assay (Greiner bio-one; cat. no. 651180).
8. Forceps (all FineScienceTools; eye dressing forceps, serrated: cat. no. 11050-10; straight forceps: cat. no. 11008-13; watchmaker: no. 7b: cat. no. 11270-20; watchmaker, curved: cat. no. 11273-20).

Some items (SCF, purified, detoxified BSA) are required in quantities that are quite cost-intensive. For some hints to lab-scale production of these items, *see* **Note 1**.

3. Methods

3.1. Expansion and Differentiation of Mouse Hematopoietic Progenitors

3.1.1. Isolation of Mouse Fetal Livers

Ideally fetal livers should be isolated at E12.5 (**Fig. 1A** and **Note 3**).

1. Sacrifice the pregnant female mouse by gassing with CO_2 or cervical dislocation.
2. Place the mouse on its back on a sterile surface and wipe the fur of the entire mouse with 70% ethanol to avoid bacterial contamination. Open the body wall by a small longitudinal cut through the skin (tear apart by grabbing with forceps on both sides of the incision). With a new pair of scissors open the peritoneum by a similar cut, without injuring the intestines, to avoid contamination. Isolate left and right uterine horns (in one piece) containing the embryos and place them in a cell culture dish containing ice-cold PBS.
3. Open the uterus with an antimesenterial cut and dissect single embryos with the deciduas. Separate the embryo and carefully remove the surrounding tissue (i.e., placenta and amniotic sac) using two tweezers. Immediately kill the isolated embryo by decapitation (the head can be used for genotyping if required).
4. On E12.5 the fetal liver is clearly visible as a red distinctive area in the center of the embryo (*see* **Fig. 1A**, top). Isolate the liver with the help of two watchmaker forceps. Use one forceps to immobilize the embryo and the second to separate the liver; remove surrounding epithelial tissue until only the red liver tissue is left over.

3.1.2. Outgrowth of Immature Hematopoietic Progenitors

The procedure for outgrowth of multipotent and erythroid progenitors is roughly the same. For the most part, the growth factor combination and optimal cell density for outgrowth are different and will be indicated separately.

3.1.2.1. Procedure for Erythroid Cells

1. Transfer the fetal liver (from above) into one well of a four-well dish (17-mm diameter, Nunc; cat. no. 176740) and resuspend it in 600 μL of twofold concentrated factor mix (2X factor medium multipotent progenitors: SCF, IL3, IL-6, GM-CSF, Flk2/Flt3 ligand, IGF-1 and Dex; erythroid progenitors: SCF, Epo, IGF-1, Dex; *see* **Note 5**) by pipetting up and down until the whole liver tissue has been homogenized (avoid bubbling). Place the dish into an appropriate cell culture incubator (set to 37°C, 5% CO_2).
2. After 24 h, carefully remove 250 μL of the supernatant, add 350 μL of fresh medium supplemented with growth factors, and mix. Transfer one half (300 μL) into a new well

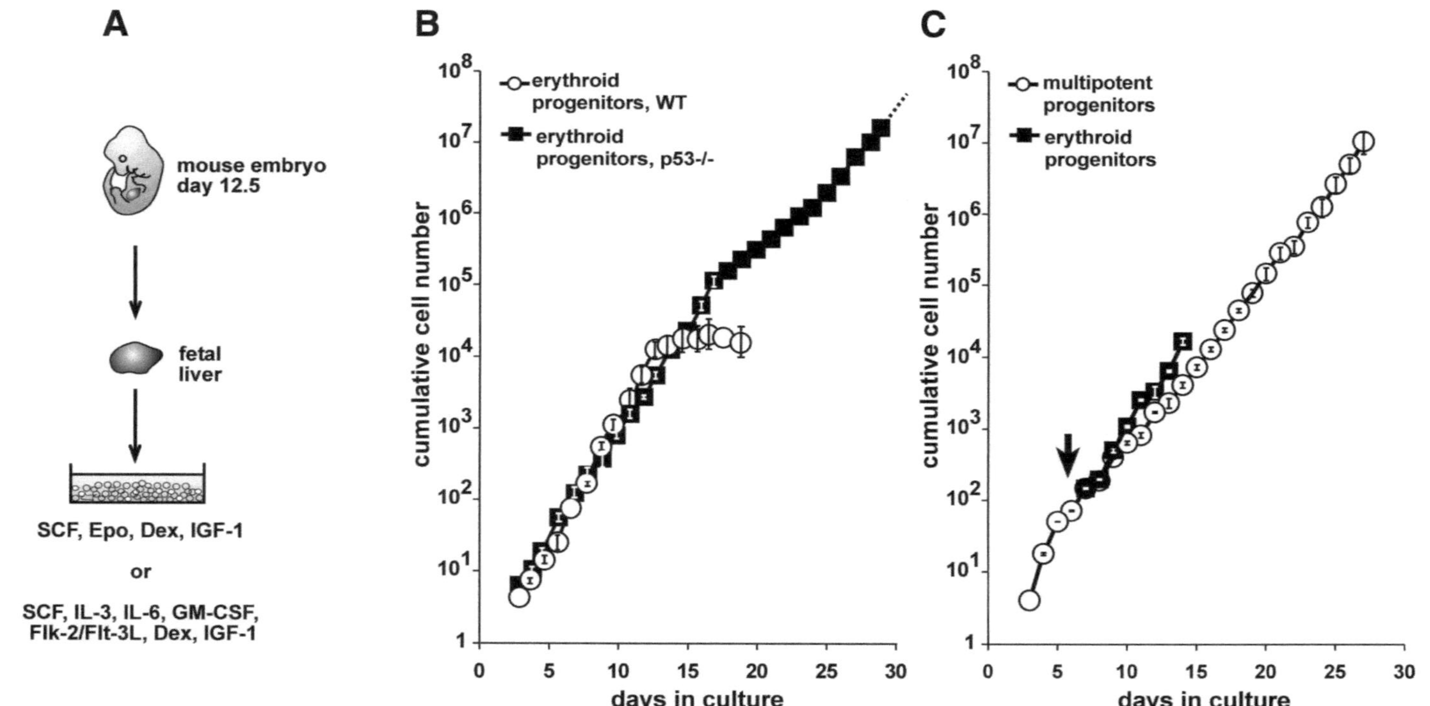

Fig. 1. **(A)** Flow chart of preparation of cultures from mouse fetal livers and factor combinations used for outgrowth of erythroid and multipotent cells. **(B)** Outgrowth of wild type (WT, open circles) and $p53^{-/-}$ (black squares) erythroid progenitors. Note that after 15 d in culture, wild type cells stop proliferating (and die), whereas erythroid cells lacking p53 keep proliferating without limit, leading to cell immortalization. Error bars depict standard deviations of at least four independent experiments. **(C)** Outgrowth of multipotent progenitors (open circles). The arrow indicates the time point of switching of a part of the culture to erythroid conditions and the outgrowth of erythroid progenitors (black squares). Error bars depict standard deviations of three independent experiments.

and add further 300 μL of fresh medium into each well (every well containing now 600 μL; *see* **Note 6**).

3. Day 2 and/or 3: big blast like cells will be visible in each well. If the blasts cover the surface of the well, pool them from both wells into a centrifuge tube and spin the cells at 250*g* for 5 min. Carefully remove the supernatant, resuspend in medium with 2X factors, and count in an electronic cell counter that also displays size distributions. If the number of blasts (size around 8–10 μm diameter) is below 1.5×10^6 cells/mL, spin the cells down again, adjust cell number to 2×10^6 cells/mL with medium containing 2X factors and transfer either into a 4-well plate (0.5–1.2 mL of medium) or to a bigger dish (>1.2 mL of medium; 3.5 cm diameter; Nunc; cat. no. 153066). If the total cell number is $>3 \times 10^6$ cells/mL, transfer into 3.5-cm dish, adjusting cell number to 2×10^6 cells/mL with fresh medium supplemented with growth factors (also *see* **Note 6**).
4. Day 4: count cells again; if $>2.5 \times 10^6$ cells /mL are obtained, transfer the whole suspension to a bigger dish (6 cm diameter; Nunc; cat. no. 150326) and add 3 mL of fresh medium with 2X factors. If the cell density is lower, let the cells sit for about 5 min in the hood (to sink to the bottom), remove 0.9 mL of the supernatant, and add 2 mL of fresh 2X factor medium (partial medium change).
5. Day 5: if the cells have again reached a density of $>2.5 \times 10^6$ cells/mL, transfer the suspension to a larger dish again (9 cm diameter; Nunc; cat. no. 150350) in a final volume of 10 mL (i.e., add 5–6 mL of 2X factor medium). If the density is lower, perform a partial medium change as described earlier, just using correspondingly higher volumes.
6. From this point onward cells are either maintained at densities between 2 and 4×10^6 cells/mL by daily partial medium changes or can be expanded to larger volumes (one or multiple 14.5-cm dishes; Greiner bio-one, cat. no. 639160 holding a total volume of 20 mL each). A typical expansion of erythroid progenitors is shown in **Fig. 1B,C**. Depending on the cell number required for different experiments, assays can be started from d 4 to 6 onwards. Alternatively, the cells can be further expanded and used for assays at later time points (e.g., proliferation or differentiation assays, FACS or biochemical analysis, histology, etc., *see* **Notes 7–9**). A typical antigen profile for renewing, immature murine erythroblasts as determined by flow cytometry is shown in **Table 1**.
7. After about d 9 in culture: The cells start to show increased spontaneous differentiation or die more easily. Dead and differentiated cells will have to be removed by density gradient purification on a regular basis (every 2 to 3 d; *see* **Note 9**). After purification, the remaining immature cells have again to be seeded at 2×10^6 cells/mL. If this results in no further increase in total cell numbers, the culture has to be considered as at the end of its life-span (*see* also **Fig. 1B**).

3.1.2.2. Procedure for Multipotent Cells

Proceed through **steps 1** and **2** as for erythroid cells. In **step 3**, the cells should be removed from adherent cells as for erythroid cells but maintained in 17-mm wells with partial medium changes using 2X factor medium until they reach a density of 4–6 × 10^6 cells/mL (counting sizes from 8 to 12 μm diameter). From **step 4** onwards, the days at which this has to be done cannot be predicted. Rather, further expansion requires maintaining the cells at a density not lower than 3 to 3.5 and not exceeding 7 × 10^6 cells/mL. It may become necessary to split the cells at ratios lower than 1:2, for example, from a 5-mL culture, remove 1.5 mL of supernatant and add 3.5 mL of fresh 2X factor medium. If cells start to grow slowly, try to keep them at higher density (>4 × 10^6) after removing dead cells by density gradient purification (*see* **Note 9**).

Table 1
Characterization of Cultured Murine Hematopoietic Cells by Flow Cytometry

Antigen	Immature erythroblast	Differentiated erythroid	Multipotent
CD117 (c-Kit)	+++	—	++
CD71 (TfR)	+++	++	+++
CD135 (Flt-3/Flk-2)	—	—	+
Sca-1	—	—	+
CD45R (B220)	—	—	+
Ter119	+	+++	+/–
CD11b (Mac1)	—	—	+
Integrin α4	+++	n.d.	n.d.

+++ > 80%
++ >41–79%
+ 11–40%
+/– 3–10%
— 0–2%
n.d., not determined.

Typical proliferation curves for multipotent and erythroid progenitors are depicted in **Fig. 1B,C**. A typical surface antigen profile of renewing, immature multipotent progenitors as determined by flow cytometry is shown in **Table 1**.

3.1.3. Development of Erythroid Progenitors From Multipotent Cultures

Depending on the cytokine cocktails used, multipotent progenitors can give rise to various myeloid lineages (e.g., monocytes, macrophages, dendritic type cells). Currently, the development of erythroblasts from multipotent cells represents the best-characterized system.

1. Expanding multipotent cells are removed from the culture, washed twice in PBS and reseeded in SCF/Epo/Dex /IGF-1 at densities between 2 to 3 × 10^6 cells/mL.
2. Proliferation of the cultures has to be monitored closely for the next 2–3 d. There may be a lag phase of 1 d but thereafter cells should resume exponential proliferation at doubling times of about 24 h.
3. If the cells have proliferated exponentially up to d 4 under erythroid proliferation conditions, subject them to a density gradient purification to remove dead and differentiated cells of other lineages. Cultivate immature cells (interphase) for 2 more days under erythroid conditions.
4. At d 6 to 7, the culture should consist of >80% pure erythroblasts. This can be ascertained by visually inspecting the homogeneity of the culture and performing flow cytometry for erythroid markers (CD71, CD117, Ter119), whereas myeloid lineage markers should be <10% (*see* **Table 1**). Like fetal liver erythroblasts, multipotent cell-derived erythroblasts can be subsequently induced to terminally differentiate into mature erythrocytes (*see* **Subheading 3.1.4.**).

3.1.4. Induction of Terminal Erythroid Differentiation

1. Immediately before the induction of terminal differentiation (**Fig. 2**), erythroblasts need to be purified by density gradient centrifugation in 1078 g/mL lymphocyte separation

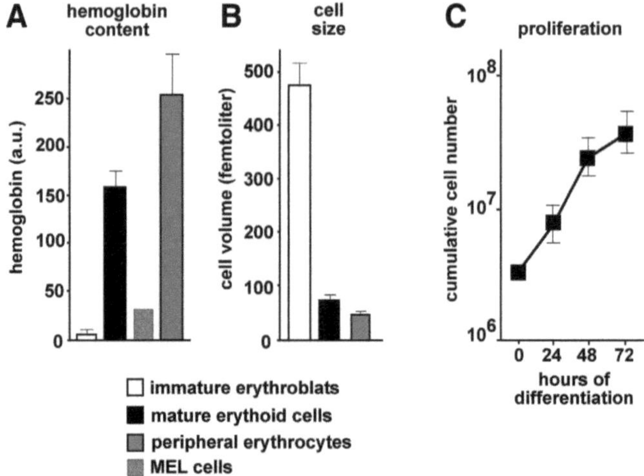

Fig. 2. **(A)** Hemoglobin content of immature erythroid progenitors. Mature erythroid cells (after 3 d of differentiation) were compared with differentiated MEL cells and mouse erythrocytes obtained form peripheral blood. **(B)** Size distribution of cells described in A. **(C)** Proliferation of erythroid cells during differentiation to mature erythrocytes.

medium to remove dead and spontaneously differentiated cells and to obtain homogeneous populations of proliferating erythroid progenitors ***(15,17)***.

2. Wash the cells twice in PBS and reseed at 2–3 × 10^6 cells/mL in Stem-Pro/Nutrient supplement differentiation medium (supplemented with 10 U/mL Epo, 4 × 10^{-4} IE Ins, 3 × 10^{-6} *M* of the GR antagonist ZK112.993 ***(23,24)***, and 1 mg/mL iron-saturated human transferrin. Differentiating erythroblasts have to be maintained at densities between 2–4 × 10^6 cells/mL. Therefore, cell number and cell size has to be monitored every 12 (first 12–40 h) to 24 h (after 48 h) and diluted or substituted with fresh differentiation medium accordingly. **Figure 2** shows the typical time course of cell proliferation (**Fig. 2C**) and cell size decrease (**Fig. 2B**) obtained with differentiating mouse erythroblasts.
3. For analysis of cell morphology and cytological staining, cyto-centrifuge the cells (50–100 μL of cell suspension; 7 min at 150*g*) onto glass slides (*see* **Note 7**). For the detection of hemoglobin, 50 or 100 μL of the cell suspension is transferred in triplicates into a 96-well plate (v-shaped) and centrifuged for 5 min at room temperature at 250*g* and washed once with 150 μL of PBS; repeat centrifugation and remove supernatant. Lyse the cells in 30 μL of water and quantitate the hemoglobin content colorimetrically with O-phenylenediamine dihydrochloride (*see* **Note 10**). A typical time course of hemoglobin accumulation in primary murine erythroblasts is depicted in **Fig. 2A**. Hemoglobin levels attained by fully differentiated Friend erythroleukemic cells and the hemoglobin content of normal peripheral murine erythroblasts are shown for comparison. Typical surface antigen profiles of terminally differentiated red cells obtained in culture are shown in **Table 1**.

3.1.5. Outgrowth of Immortal p53$^{-/-}$ Murine Erythroid Progenitors

One major drawback in using primary cultures of erythroid progenitors is the relatively short life span in vitro (15–20 d). To circumvent this problem, we have successfully established permanent cultures and clones from erythroblasts derived from p53$^{-/-}$ mice ***(15,17,18)***.

Erythroblasts from p53$^{-/-}$ fetal livers are propagated as described for wild-type cells until d 15 to 20 (*see* **Subheading 3.1.2.**), when the proliferation rate decreases and the proportion of differentiated erythrocytes increases. During this period, purify the p53$^{-/-}$ erythroblasts every 2 d for 7 to 10 d using density gradient centrifugation, and reseed them at 3 × 10^6 cells/mL. In our hands, this procedure yielded erythroblasts showing unlimited proliferation potential from 10 of 10 p53$^{-/-}$ fetal liver cultures. However, particular care has to be taken that the cells are maintained at optimum medium, factor and density conditions at all times, since these cells have an inherent genetic instability owing to the lack of p53, and thus easily become tetraploid or aneuploid. Thus if maintained at sub-optimal conditions for just a few days, the cells are not longer useful for experiments (*see* **Subheading 3.1.2.** and **Notes 2, 4,** and **5**).

3.1.6. Cloning of p53$^{-/-}$ Erythroblasts

1. After about 30 d in culture, seed 1000 and 3000 erythroid progenitors lacking p53 into 2 mL of semisolid medium (Methocel-containing StemPro medium supplemented with Nutrient supplement at a final concentration similar to liquid medium) containing mouse SCF/Epo/Dex/IGF-I, as above, into 35-mm dishes.
2. After 7 to 10 d of incubation (take care to avoid medium evaporation), large colonies are obtained with a cloning efficiency of 2 to 10%. Pick about 100 clones from dishes with well-separated colonies, and cultivate them in 96-well plates in 100 μL medium with 2X erythroid factor mix.
3. After another 4 to 6 d, inspect clones from picked colonies visually. Discard clones containing either a high proportion of mature cells, cells of irregular size/shape or exhibiting a slow proliferation rate.
4. Expand the remaining clones and subject them to quantitative analysis of proliferation kinetics, factor dependence and ability to terminally differentiate. In our experiments, about 50% of the selected clones showed optimal proliferation rates and differentiation behavior. Finally, clones should be inspected for a normal diploid deoxyribonucleic acid (DNA) content by flow cytometry after DNA staining with DAPI or propidium iodide. Clones with diploid DNA profile can be stored frozen in liquid nitrogen for further experiments.

3.1.7. Retroviral Infections

Retroviral gene transfer has turned out to be the most efficient method to deliver exogenous DNA into primary erythroid cells. Because primary erythroblasts have a limited life-span of about 15 to 20 d when taken into culture, rapid identification of infected cells is critical for the execution of subsequent experiments. Therefore, time-consuming selections with drugs are not feasible, leaving the possibility to couple the gene of interest via an IRES (internal ribosome entry site) element ***(26)*** to fluorescent proteins (mainly EGFP) or surface proteins (like signaling deficient human CD4; a gift from Meinrad Busslinger, Institute of Molecular Pathology, Vienna). Mouse stem cell virus-based vectors (pMSCV) have been shown to meet these prerequisites together with strong expression capacity of the target gene via the 5' LTR in immature erythroid and hematopoietic progenitors ***(18,19)***. To generate high titer virus, we routinely use ecotropic phoenix cells obtained from Garry P. Nolan, Stanford University (the cells should be selected for high expression of gag-pol and env proteins prior to use; *see* **Note 11**).

1. Two days before infection of primary erythroblasts (i.e., freshly prepared fetal livers or short term cultured erythroid cells), seed the phoenix cells in DMEM supplemented with 10% FCS, penicillin/streptomycin and L-glutamine in 6-well plates (3.5 cm diameter; Nunc; cat. no. 150229) at a density, which should reach 20 to 30% confluency the next day. For this purpose, plate the cells at about 10, 15, and 20% confluency into dishes of the same size.
2. The next day, decide which dishes have a density closest to 20 to 30% and take them for transfection, after partial medium change with 0.7 mL of fresh medium/well. Phoenix cells are transfected with a pMSCV-gene of interest-IRES-GFP vector using Polyfect transfection reagent. For one well of a 6-well plate, 1.5 µg of DNA is diluted to a final volume of 100 µL in Eagles basal medium/10 m*M* Hepes, pH 7.4, and mixed with 10 µL of Polyfect. After incubation for 15 min at room temperature, add the transfection mix drop-wise to the phoenix cells freshly removed from the incubator. Incubate the cells overnight.
3. Check transfection efficiency under a conventional UV microscope; 70 to 80% of green cells are expected. If the percentage of transfected cells is below that, repeat the transfection, since low transfection efficiency will result in low titer virus production. Remove the medium and add either the cell suspension equivalent of one fetal mouse liver or 1×10^6 immature progenitors resuspended in 1 mL of Stem-Pro/Nutrient supplement with 2X factors (erythroid or multipotent). Add polybrene to a final concentration of 4 µg/mL and incubate the cells overnight.
4. Carefully remove 0.7 mL of supernatant without aspirating hematopoietic cells, which are sitting on top of the phoenix producer cells at the bottom of the plate. Add 1.3 mL of fresh Stem-Pro/Nutrient supplement with 2X factor mix and polybrene (4 µg/mL) and incubate for one more day.
5. Remove the supernatant again and add 2 mL of fresh 2X factor mix medium and polybrene (4 µg/mL) and incubate until the third morning.
6. Carefully resuspend the hematopoietic cells by gently pipetting over the phoenix cells. Check under the microscope to determine whether the majority of the nonadherent cells have been removed (they tend to stick to the layer of phoenix producer cells). Be careful not to remove too many phoenix cells, (they do not adhere well to the plate at this time).
7. Count the hematopoietic cells and resuspend them at $2–3 \times 10^6$ cells/mL in fresh 1X factor medium.
8. Check GFP expression by flow cytometry. We generally obtain 10 to 85% infection efficiency, depending on the gene of interest. If the proportion of genetically modified cells is too low for the interpretation of results or biochemical analysis, they may be highly enriched by fluorescence activated cell sorting.

3.1.8. Freezing and Thawing of Cells

1. For freezing, aliquots of $1.5–2 \times 10^7$ cells are collected by centrifugation and resuspended in 0.5 mL of FCS followed by transfer to appropriate cryotubes. Subsequently, 0.5 mL of ice-cold FCS/20% DMSO is added drop-wise (final concentration of DMSO = 10%). The cells are frozen slowly to –80°C (in a styrofoam box) and transferred to liquid nitrogen storage the next day.
2. For thawing, the cryotube coming from the liquid nitrogen storage is placed into a 37°C water bath and the content transferred into a 15-mL polypropylene tube immediately after melting. Slowly, 10 mL of medium without factors are added (1 mL at a time) and the cells recollected by centrifugation to remove DMSO. Subsequently, the cells are resus-

pended at 3 × 10^6 cells/mL and incubated with full medium containing 2X factors overnight. Next morning, the culture is transferred to standard medium at 2 × 10^6 cells/mL. Cell viability is close to 100%.

3.2. Expansion and Differentiation of Human Erythroid Progenitors

Several protocols exist for expansion of human erythroid progenitors from cord blood, peripheral blood, or bone marrow. We will describe the current status of our methods to both expand and terminally differentiate human progenitors from cord blood, improving over the published procedures ***(21,22)*** with respect to both in vitro life-span of erythroid cells and their ability to undergo terminal differentiation.

3.2.1. Preparation of Mononuclear Cells From Human Umbilical Cord Blood

1. Blood is collected from the umbilical cord of full term deliveries (30–100 mL) into heparinized 50-mL polypropylene tubes and processed within 24 h (interim storage at room temperature to reduce aggregation of progenitor cells; cells should be processed as soon as possible).
2. To remove mature erythrocytes, the samples are diluted 20-fold in sterile ice-cold erylysis-buffer (50-mL tubes) and incubated with repeated agitation for 10 to 20 min at room temperature (until the liquid is observed to become transparent and cherry-red, indicating release of hemoglobin; *see* **Note 13**).
3. The cells are collected by centrifugation for 10 min at 250*g*, the supernatant is aspirated (collecting it as biohazard waste for proper disposal), and the cell pellets washed several times with ice-cold PBS (5 min 250*g*) until no red color (released hemoglobin) is visible any more, while sequentially combining the pellets into a single 50-mL tube. At this stage, the cells can be either cultivated directly or frozen as liver cells in liquid nitrogen for long-term storage.

3.2.2. Expansion of Human Erythroid Progenitors

As in the case of mouse cells, maintaining proliferation of human erythroid progenitors over extended periods critically depends on optimal culture conditions and handling, including daily partial medium changes, keeping cell density in a narrow range and using a high quality air/gas supply. Under these circumstances, committed erythroid cells can be kept proliferating routinely between 40 and 60 d with an acceptable low level of spontaneous terminal differentiation.

1. Seed the population of 5–10 × 10^7 mononuclear cells prepared from cord blood at a density of 5 × 10^6 cells/mL into StemSpan medium supplemented with Epo (2 U/mL), SCF (100 ng/mL, murine SCF can be used), Dex (10^{-6} *M*), IGF-1 (40 ng/mL), and a cholesterol-rich lipid mix (20 μg/mL). Put cultures into a humidified incubator set to 5% CO_2 (*see* **Notes 5** and **14**).
2. To remove adherent cells (mainly macrophages), the following day the culture is transferred to a fresh dish after counting (CASY cell analyzer) and the cell density readjusted to 5 × 10^6 cells/mL, accompanied by a partial medium change. For this purpose, cultures are allowed to settle for 3 to 5 min in the tissue culture hood and half of the medium (no collection by centrifugation is required, but care should be taken not to disturb the cells at the bottom of the plate) is aspirated and replaced by fresh medium with 2X factors.
3. During the next 5 to 7 d, cells are counted daily and maintained at a density between 3 to 5 × 10^6 cells/mL at all times, transferring to smaller dishes as required (because of gradual loss of mature, nonproliferating cells); as already mentioned, daily partial medium change is absolutely essential to maintain viability of emerging progenitors.

Table 2
A Differential Analysis Set-Up for the Characterization of Hematopoietic Cells

FITC	PE	PC5	ECD	Discrimination between
CD15/45	CD56	CD14	CD3	granulocytes/NK/monocytes/T-cells[a]
CD15/45	CD8	CD4	CD3	granulocytes/cytotoxic T-cells/T-helper cells/T-cells[b]
CD15	CD33	CD34	CD45	granulocytes/pluripotent/myeloidc progenitors[c]
CD19	CD45RA	CD34	CD45	B-cells/pluripotent progenitors[d]
CD15/45	CD38	CD34	CD3	granulocytes/pluripotent/lymphoide progenitors[a]
GPA	CD71	–	–	erythoid lineage[f]
CD116	CD117	–	–	monocytic/erythroid cells[g]

[a] CD15 positive signals combined with CD45 high indicates granulocytes; CD56 positive corresponds to natural killer (NK) cells; CD14 is a specific marker for monocytes and CD3 is found on all mature T-cells.

[b] CD3 versus CD4 vs CD8 allows to discriminate between subpopulations of T-cells: CD4/CD8 double positive: developing thymocyte, CD4 positive: helper T-cells, CD8: cytotoxic T-cells.

[c] CD33 is found on myeloid committed progenitors, CD34 in combination with CD45dim is a hallmark for early (potentially pluri-potent) progenitors.

[d] CD19 plus CD45 is characteristic for mature B-cells; CD45RA positive signals confirm this classification.

[e] CD38 is found on lymphoid progenitors, these cells in consequence should be CD3 negative; CD34 in combination with other markers (*see* **Notes 3** and **4**) is needed to derive mean values of CD34 positive and lineage-restricted negative populations in various compartments.

[f] To indicate erythroid commitment, GPA high can be used in conjunction with high transferrin receptor expression (CD71), since by itself its background may be too high.

[g] CD116 is found on immature monocytes; the combination with c-Kit (CD117; erythroid specific) serves no particular discrimination and just allows to measure these two cell types simultaneously.

4. Around d 8 of culture, a homogenous population of larger cells (average diameter 11 μm) becomes apparent visually and in the cell counter, consisting predominantly of committed erythroid progenitors, as analyzed by flow cytometry (*see* **Table 2** and **Subheading 3.2.4.**). From this stage on, cell density is re-adjusted daily to 2×10^6 cells/mL.
5. The cultures keep proliferating for a total of 40 to 60 d with an average expansion rate of 1.6-fold, which gradually declines towards the end. Spontaneous differentiation into mature erythrocytes necessitates density gradient purification about once a wk (*see* **Note 9**). The rates of cell death (as determined, for example, by terminal deoxynucleotidyl transferase-mediated deoxyuridine triphosphate-digoxigenin nick end labeling assay) should stay below 10% in a healthy culture at all times. As an alternative, DNA profiles can be determined after staining cellular DNA with 6 μ*M* DAPI in a flow cytometer equipped with an appropriate UV light source (e.g., Partec PAS-III, Münster, Germany), followed by computation of the percentage of cells in different cell cycle phases (particularly S phase). This also allows an estimation of the percentage of early apoptotic cells, which appear as a population with sub-G1 DNA content.
6. Freezing and thawing of cells is essentially done as described for mouse cells (*see* **Subheading 3.1.8.**) except for: a) a larger volume of freezing stock (1.8 mL for $1.5–2 \times 10^7$ cells instead of 1.0 mL) and b) an additional 1-h incubation step with 2Xfactor medium upon thawing, followed by centrifugation, aspiration of the supernatant, and resuspension before the first overnight incubation. For thawing of mixed populations of mononuclear cells frozen immediately after preparation from cord blood, *see* **Note 12**.

3.2.3. Terminal Differentiation

The changes in human erythroid progenitors undergoing terminal maturation are similar to those observed in the mouse system, with some notable exceptions. First, the whole process is protracted, taking 6 d instead of d 3 to produce fully hemoglobinized, enucleated erythrocytes. Second, there is no initial increase in proliferation rates during the early phase of differentiation induction (and thus no shortening of the G1 phase of the cell cycle).

The culture conditions to induce synchronous differentiation into mature cells are similar to those for mouse erythroblasts: the corresponding medium consists of StemSpan medium supplemented with 3% human serum, Epo (10 U/mL), insulin (4×10^{-4} IE = 10 ng/mL), T3 (10^{-6} *M*), ZK112993 (3×10^{-6} *M*), and iron saturated transferrin (1 mg/mL). In contrast to the mouse ***(17,18)***, the presence of serum is essential for successful maturation. However, either higher or lower concentrations of serum are counter-productive. Moreover, the proportion of enucleated cells is drastically increased by T3, pointing to a role for this hormone in human erythropoiesis, resembling the situation in the chicken ***(27,28)***.

Determination of hemoglobin content, cell size, morphological parameters as well as cytospin preparation/cytological staining is done as described in **Notes 7** and **10**. Mature cultivated human cells are larger (average diameter 7 μm) than mouse erythrocytes (5 μm), closely matching the sizes observed for human peripheral blood erythrocytes.

3.2.4. Characterization of Human Erythroid Progenitors by Flow Cytometry

The initial composition of mononuclear cells freshly isolated from human cord blood is similar to that observed in peripheral blood, except that in the former, depending on individual variation, the percentage of granulocytic cells may be reduced (peripheral blood: about 60%, cord blood 20–55%), resulting in a virtual "increase" of cells from other lineages.

Four-color flow cytometry (*see* **Note 8** and **Table 2** for a detailed description of suitable marker combinations) facilitates differential analysis of cord blood and cultured samples derived thereof at various time points during the gradual outgrowth of erythroid committed cells (*see* **Table 3**). In conjunction with the increase in erythroid markers, the loss of markers characteristic for mature cells of other lineages (T and B cells, monocytic and granulocytic progenitors) can be determined in parallel, to assess the effective establishment of an erythroid progenitor culture. These flow cytometry data serve to complement and corroborate the results obtained from the cell size profiles (emerging erythroid progenitors "peak" around d 8), and to demonstrate that pure but immature erythroid progenitors are indeed obtained at d 14 and thereafter. Therefore, a full-scale measurement series is not routinely performed on each culture.

4. Notes

1. Suggestions for large-scale production of murine SCF. If milligram amounts of murine SCF are required for large-scale cultures, we recommend using a c-DNA clone containing the entire coding region of murine SCF (including the leader sequence required for secretion). The c-DNA could be tagged with a 6xHis or a CD4 tag. This c-DNA should then be introduced into 293T-cells by transfecting the cells with a suitable expression

Table 3
Outgrowth of Erythroid Progenitors From Human Umbilical Cord Blood In Vitro as Analyzed by Flow Cytometry

	Day of proliferation/percentage of cells positive for				
Cell surface marker	1	6	14	20	30
CD117 (c-Kit)	0.11	20	91	73	44
CD71 (TfR)	0.33	22	98	99	98
GPA	21	21	36	56	77
CD33	8	21	47	46	15
CD38	20	11	0.42	—	—
CD34	0.43	4	0.28	—	—
CD3	7	8	0.15	—	—
CD19	2	1	—	—	—
CD14	8	2	—	—	—

— < 0.1%

vector containing a selectable marker to obtain stable transfectant clones. Cells expressing high levels of murine SCF can either be obtained by producing many subclones and testing these for secretion of SCF by proliferation assays on p53$^{-/-}$ erythroblasts (for an analogous procedure using avian erythroblasts, *see* **ref. *20***) or by sorting the highest expressor clones by flow cytometry using anti CD4 antibodies. In our hands, it is not necessary to purify the SCF from supernatants of secreting cells, but if this is desired, a procedure has been described for His-tagged avian SCF ***(20)***.

2. Recommendations for purchase and storage of Stem-Pro serum-free medium. Since the manufacturers information given on the shelf life of liquid medium (24 mo) do not at all correspond to our experience, the following recommendations are given: When ordering medium and Nutrient supplement, insist on delivery of the batch with the most recent production date. At the time of delivery, both medium and serum supplement should not be older than 3 mo. Make a reservation for large batches of both liquid medium and Nutrient supplement and obtain test samples. Test in proliferation assays against medium of proven quality, using immortalized p53$^{-/-}$ erythroblasts as control cells. Then have a large batch delivered and store liquid medium at 4°C in the dark and serum supplement at –80°C (storage at –20°C as recommended by the manufacturer leads to deterioration of the serum supplement after <6 mo). If stored in this fashion, liquid medium can be stored for 12 mo, whereas serum supplement lasts 12 to 18 mo.
3. Age of fetal livers. In general, fetal livers can be isolated from E10 until E14.5. Therefore, it is possible to use fetal livers of genetically modified mice, which die during embryonic development or at birth (e.g., Raf-1$^{-/-}$ or GR$^{-/-}$). Around E12.5, the fetal liver is clearly visible, easily accessible and contains a lot of immature hematopoietic cells. The content of any progenitor-like-cell clearly declines around E14, making the expansion of progenitor cells less efficient. Other possible sources of hematopoietic progenitors are the bone marrow (more spontaneous differentiation of erythroblasts), and spleen. The latter requires density purification with lymphocyte separation medium, density 1.077 g/mL, or treatment with erylysis-buffer to deplete mature erythrocytes before taking cells into culture.

4. Medium preparation. Thaw the tube containing Nutrient supplement (for Stem-Pro medium) in a 37°C water bath, shaking the tube occasionally. Pay attention that all of the frozen supplement is covered with warm water. The supplement should thaw rapidly and has to be absolutely clear immediately after thawing completely. "Cloudy" batches, or those which contain translucent, irregular crystal-like particles (aggregated lipid), are not to be used, because appropriate expansion of cells cannot be achieved and existing cell populations are irreversibly damaged. Similarly, liquid media aliquots (Stem-Pro as well as StemSpan) have to be completely free of even minute amounts of sediment. If this occurs, the medium is likely to be toxic (for additional information on how to avoid the formation of sediment, *see* **Note 14**). Add supplement and 5 mL each of penicillin/streptomycin and L-glutamine stock solutions to 500 mL of Stem-Pro medium. The complete medium can be stored for 4 wk at 4 to 8°C in the dark.
5. Cytokines. Stock solutions of cytokines are prepared as recommend by the manufacturer. In general, solutions are prepared in 0.1% of highly purified BSA as a 1000X stock. After preparing aliquots of desired size (multiple freezing and thawing of the aliquots should be avoided), stocks should be shock-frozen in liquid nitrogen and stored at –80°C. Twofold concentrated factor mixes. Both erythroid or multipotent factor mixtures for mouse cells can be stored in the dark at 4°C for a maximum of 4 d (for human progenitors, up to 2 d). Thus, depending on the experiment, it is recommended that media with twofold concentrated factors be prepared in volume batches of no more than 25 or 50 mL. During culture, factors in the medium are used up by the cells; in addition, they are not stable for longer than 24 h under standard incubation conditions. Final cytokine concentrations for murine multipotent expansion cultures: SCF, 100 ng/mL; IL-3, 2 ng/mL; IL-6, 5 ng/mL; Flk2/Flt3 ligand, 10 ng/mL; GM-CSF, 3 ng/mL; Dex, 10^{-6} *M*; IGF-1, 40 ng/mL. GM-CSF concentrations should be reduced to 1 ng/mL or lower if multipotent cultures tend to differentiate prematurely into monocytes (indicated by the prevalence of small, irregular shaped cells and overall slow proliferation of the cultures): Final cytokine concentrations for murine and human erythroid expansion cultures. Human Epo, 2 U/mL; SCF, 100 ng/mL; Dex, 10^{-6} *M*; IGF-1, 40 ng/mL. If cultures tend to contain many differentiated cells, reduce Epo concentration to 1 or 0.5 U/mL. This should not affect the proliferation rate of the cultures.
6. Amount of starting material. If fewer cells than expected are isolated from a fetal liver and/or cell concentrations are too low, partial medium changes may be performed instead of immediately increasing the total culture volume.
7. Cell morphology and histological staining of hematopoietic cells. For histological analyses, aliquots of hematopoietic cells at various stages of culture are cyto-centrifuged onto glass slides, dried with a hair dryer and subsequently stained with histological dyes and neutral benzidine for hemoglobin. Unprocessed cytospin slides can be kept at room temperature for several days. However, best results are obtained if the staining procedure is performed as soon as possible. Nucleated and enucleated erythrocytes (brown or yellow stained, small cells), partially mature or immature cells (larger cells with grey or blue cytoplasm) and dead cells (fragmented/condensed nuclei, disintegrated cells) can be quantified using an appropriate microscope (normally >600 cells on multiple, randomly selected fields per sample should be evaluated).

   Staining procedure:

   a. Spin cell aliquots onto slides using a cytospin centrifuge at 150*g* for 7 min.
   b. Incubate for 4 min in methanol.
   c. Incubate for 2 min in 1% benzidine solution.
   d. Incubate 1.5 min in H_2O_2 solution.
   e. Wash 0.5 min in H_2O.

f. Stain 4 min with Diff Quick Red (I).
g. Stain 20 to 40 s with Diff Quick Blue (II).
h. Rinse thoroughly in water.
i. Dry with hair dryer.
j. Add Entellan mounting media and an appropriate cover slip.

Staining materials/solutions:

a. Ethanol.
b. Methanol.
c. *O*-dianisidine.
d. Benzidine solution (1%): dissolve 2 g of *o*-dianisidine in 200 mL of methanol. Protected from light, this solution can be stored at –20°C for 4 to 6 wk. Prior to use, warm to room temperature, with stirring.
e. H_2O_2 solution: mix 75 mL of water and 75 mL of ethanol. Add 4.5 mL of 30% H_2O_2; mix again. Always prepare fresh.
f. Entellan.

8. Flow cytometry. Staining: primary cells are density purified and a total number of 1×10^6 cells incubated in 100 µL of 1% FCS/PBS for 30 min on ice in the dark with the respective antibodies directly coupled to fluorochromes. Cells are washed twice with 1% FCS/PBS, resuspended in 1% FCS/PBS plus propidium iodide (1 µg/mL). Surface marker expression is quantified using a flow cytometer (like FacsScan or LSR; Becton Dickinson, or Partec PAS-III; Paint-a-gate software of Becton Dickinson is recommended for analysis). Propidium iodide staining cannot be used with the recommended four-color analysis of human cells owing to fluorescence interference; DAPI staining and UV excitation may be used instead.
9. Density gradient purification of hematopoietic cells. Add 10 mL of a cell suspension containing a maximum of 2×10^7 cells to a 15-mL polypropylene tube. Underlay the cell suspension with 2 mL of lymphocyte separation medium using a Pasteur pipet. Be careful not to intermingle separation medium and cell suspension. Centrifuge at 600*g* for 7 min. Aspirate the interphase (containing viable and undifferentiated cells) with a Pasteur pipet and transfer to a new tube. Be sure that enough medium is aspirated together with the lymphocyte separation medium (at least half of the volume), otherwise sedimentation in the subsequent centrifugation step does not work properly. After counting and re-centrifugation (250*g* for 5 min) to remove residual lymphocyte separation solution, the cells in the pellet can be used for further experiments. Sometimes, the separation medium may not be dense enough to discriminate between immature and more mature erythroid cells. In this case, the medium can be mixed 1:1 or 2:3 with Percoll supplemented with 0.1 volume of 10X concentrated PBS and used instead of pure lymphocyte separation medium.
10. Photometric hemoglobin determination during terminal erythroid differentiation. Small aliquots (50 or 100 µL) of the cultures are removed and analyzed for hemoglobin content by colorimetry ***(25)***. For each test, prepare a fresh dye solution containing 0.5 mg/mL *o*-phenylene-diamine-dihydrochloride, 50 m*M* citric acid, 0.1 *M* Na_2HPO_4. Add 1 µL/mL of 30% H_2O_2. Sequentially add 125 µL of reagent to each well (e.g., every 2 s) and incubate for exactly 3 min at room temperature. The reaction is terminated at the appropriate time points by addition of 25 µL of 8 *M* H_2SO_4. Read the OD_{495} of samples in triplicate in a 96-well plate photometer, using a 630-nm filter as reference wavelength. Finally, hemo-globin values are normalized to cell volume and cell number (OD from colorimetric tests is divided by cell number and cell volume measured with the cell analyzer).

11. Selection of phoenix (Eco) cells for high gag, pol and env expression was performed as described excellently on the laboratory homepage of Garry P. Nolan, Department of Microbiology and Immunology at Stanford University (www.stanford.edu/group/nolan/).
12. Mononuclear cells freshly prepared from umbilical cord blood can be frozen and thawed similar to established erythroid cultures, except that:
    a. the number of cells per cryotube is increased to 5–10 × 10^7 and
    b. the first incubation step is reduced to 30 min to minimize toxic effects from dead cells remnants. Furthermore, to remove cell debris (mainly gelatinous chromatin), the use of a 70-μm cell strainer is recommended.
13. As an alternative in the preparation of mononuclear cells from cord blood, less erylysis buffer (10 volumes) can be used and the resulting cell pellet further purified by a single centrifugation through lymphocyte separation medium, collecting the cells from the interphase and discarding the red pellet at the bottom. Also, small samples of cord blood may be mixed with PBS (1 + 2 volumes) and purified directly via lymphocyte separation medium without prior lysis of erythrocytes. For large sample volumes, on the other hand, it may be advisable to generate a buffy-coat first: after centrifugation of heparinized whole blood for 10 min at 300*g* and room temperature, the whitish cell layer at the interface between plasma and erythrocytes is collected and subsequently purified further by the standard erylysis procedure. Although the yield is smaller by about 50% when buffy-coats are used, the resulting population has a reduced percentage of granulocytic cells (40% vs 70%), which may be advantageous in the further cultivation.
14. The quality of the serum-free media is the most critical point in successful cultivation of primary human erythroid progenitors. In our hands, StemSpan medium yields the most reproducible and reliable results when compared to other products. This medium is stored at –20°C and should be slowly thawed at 4°C prior to use and may be re-frozen. Aliquots of complete medium are stable about one month at 4°C. If necessary, full medium can be supplemented with antibiotics (penicillin, streptomycin–sulfate). The biological activity of proliferation promoting factors has to be tested individually for each new batch. The cells in long-term culture are also extremely sensitive to gaseous contaminants from the ventilation (disinfectants, bleach fumes, NH_3 from a nearby animal house), responding with a greatly increased rate of spontaneous differentiation and premature cell death. More information on Stem-Pro (for mouse cells) is given in **Note 13**.

Acknowledgments

Helmut Dolznig, Andrea Kolbus, Cornelia Leberbauer, and Uwe Schmidt contributed equally to the work and are therefore listed alphabetically as co-authors; Eva-Maria Deiner, Ernst W. Müllner, and Hartmut Beug should be regarded as joint senior authors.

We thank Gabi Litos for excellent technical assistance. We are grateful to Dr. Gerhard Fritsch (Childrens Cancer Research Institute, Vienna) for his valuable advice in the flow cytometry of human cells. Work in the labs of the authors was supported by the Austrian Science Foundation (FWF) and Research Training Networks of the European Union.

References

1. Udupa, K. B., Crabtree, H. M., and Lipschitz, D. A. (1986) In vitro culture of proerythroblasts: characterization of proliferative response to erythropoietin and steroids. *Br. J. Haematol.* **62,** 705–714

2. Meagher, R. C., Rothmann, S. A., Paik, I. K., and Paul, P. (1989) In vitro growth of rat bone marrow BFU-E. *Exp. Hematol.* **17,** 374–378.
3. Sitar, G., Garagna, S., Zuccotti, M., Falcinelli, C., Montanari, L., Alfei, A., et al. (1999) Fetal erythroblast isolation up to purity from cord blood and their culture in vitro. *Cytometry* **35,** 337–345.
4. Kabat, D., Sherton, C. C., Evans, L. H., Bigley, R., and Koler, R. D. (1975) Synthesis of erythrocyte-specific proteins in cultured friend leukemia cells. *Cell* **5,** 331–338.
5. Dean, A., Erard, F., Schneider, A. P., and Schechter, A. N. (1981) Induction of hemoglobin accumulation in human K562 cells by hemin is reversible. *Science* **212,** 459–461.
6. Sawada, K., Krantz, S. B., Dai, C. H., Sato, N., Ieko, M., Sakurama, S., et al. (1991) Transitional change of colony stimulating factor requirements for erythroid progenitors. *J. Cell Physiol.* **149,** 1–8.
7. Alter, B. P. (1994) Biology of erythropoiesis. *Ann. N Y Acad. Sci.* **731,** 36–47.
8. Dolznig, H., Bartunek, P., Nasmyth, K., Mullner, E. W., and Beug, H. (1995) Terminal differentiation of normal chicken erythroid progenitors: shortening of G1 correlates with loss of D-cyclin/cdk4 expression and altered cell size control. *Cell Growth Differ.* **6,** 1341–1352.
9. Tamir, A., Howard, J., Higgins, R. R., Li, Y. J., Berger, L., Zacksenhaus, E., et al. (1999) Fli-1, an Ets-related transcription factor, regulates erythropoietin-induced erythroid proliferation and differentiation: evidence for direct transcriptional repression of the Rb gene during differentiation. *Mol. Cell Biol.* **19,** 4452–4464.
10. Kusadasi, N., van Soest, P. L., Mayen, A. E., Koevoet, J. L., and Ploemacher, R. E. (2000) Successful short-term ex vivo expansion of NOD/SCID repopulating ability and CAFC week 6 from umbilical cord blood. *Leukemia* **14,** 1944–1953.
11. Tsai, S., Bartelmez, S., Sitnicka, E., and Collins, S. J. (1994) Lymphohematopoietic progenitors immortalized by a retroviral vector harboring a dominant-negative retinoic acid receptor can recapitulate lymphoid, myeloid and erythroid development. *Genes Dev.* **8,** 2831–2844.
12. Schulte, C. E., Lindern Mv, M., Steinlein, P., Beug, H., and Wiedemann, L. M. (2002) MLL-ENL cooperates with SCF to transform primary avian multipotent cells. *Embo J.* **21,** 4297–4306.
13. Bauer, A., Gandrillon, O., Samarut, J., and Beug, H. (2001) Nuclear receptors in hematopoietic development: cooperation with growth factor receptors in regulation of proliferation and differentiation, in *Hematopoiesis: a Developmental Approach* (Zon, L., ed.), Oxford University Press, Oxford, pp. 368–390.
14. Bauer, A., Tronche, F., Wessely, O., Kellendonk, C., Reichardt, H. M., Steinlein, P., et al. (1999) The glucocorticoid receptor is required for stress erythropoiesis. *Genes Dev.* **13,** 2996–3002.
15. von Lindern, M., Deiner, E. M., Dolznig, H., Parren-Van Amelsvoort, M., Hayman, M. J., Mullner, E. W., et al. (2001) Leukemic transformation of normal murine erythroid progenitors: v- and c-ErbB act through signaling pathways activated by the EpoR and c-Kit in stress erythropoiesis. *Oncogene* **20,** 3651–3664.
16. Bauer, A., Ulrich, E., Andersson, M., Beug, H., and von Lindern, M. (1997) Mechanism of transformation by v-ErbA: substitution for steroid hormone receptor function in self renewal induction. *Oncogene* **15,** 701–715.
17. Dolznig, H., Boulme, F., Stangl, K., Deiner, E. M., Mikulits, W., Beug, H., et al. (2001) Establishment of normal, terminally differentiating mouse erythroid progenitors: molecular characterization by cDNA arrays. *FASEB J.* **15,** 1442–1444.

18. Dolznig, H., Habermann, B., Stangl, K., Deiner, E. M., Moriggl, R., Beug, H., et al. (2002) Apoptosis protection by the epo target bcl-x(l) allows factor- independent differentiation of primary erythroblasts. *Curr. Biol.* **12,** 1076–1085.
19. Kolbus, A., Pilat, S., Husak, Z., Deiner, E. M., Stengl, G., Beug, H., et al. (2002) Raf-1 antagonizes erythroid differentiation by restraining caspase activation. *J. Exp. Med.* **196,** 1347–1353.
20. Beug, H., Bartunek, P., Steinlein, P., and Hayman, M. J. (1995) Avian hematopoietic cell culture: In vitro model systems to study the oncogenic transformation of hematopoietic cells, in *Oncogene Techniques* (Vogt, P. K., and Verma, I. M., eds.), Vol. 254, Academic Press Inc., New York, NY, and London, UK, pp. 41–76.
21. von Lindern, M., Zauner, W., Mellitzer, G., Steinlein, P., Fritsch, G., Huber, K., et al. (1999) The glucocorticoid receptor cooperates with the erythropoietin receptor and c-Kit to enhance and sustain proliferation of erythroid progenitors in vitro. *Blood* **94,** 550–559.
22. Migliaccio, G., Di Pietro, R., di Giacomo, V., Di Baldassarre, A., Migliaccio, A. R., Maccioni, L., et al. (2002) In vitro mass production of human erythroid cells from the blood of normal donors and of thalassemic patients. *Blood Cells Mol. Dis.* **28,** 169–180.
23. Wessely, O., von Lindern, M., Levitzki, A., Gazit, A., Ischenko, I., Mellitzer, G., et al. (1997) Distinct regulatory roles of the receptor tyrosine kinases c-ErbB and c-Kit in erythroid differentiation and proliferation. *Cell. Growth Differ.* **8,** 481–493.
24. Mikulits, W., Chen, D., and Mullner, E. W. (1995) Dexamethasone inducible gene expression optimised by glucocorticoid antagonists. *Nucleic Acids Res.* **23,** 2342–2343.
25. Kowenz, E., Leutz, A., Doderlein, G., Graf, T., and Beug, H. (1987) ts-oncogene-transformed erythroleukemic cells: a novel test system for purifying and characterizing avian erythroid growth factors, in *Modern Trends in Human Leukemia VII* (Neth, R., Gallo, R. C., Greaves, M. F., and Kabisch, H., eds.), Vol. 31. Springer Verlag, Heidelberg, Germany, pp. 199–209.
26. Holcik, M., Sonenberg, N., and Korneluk, R. G. (2000) Internal ribosome initiation of translation and the control of cell death. *Trends Genet.* **16,** 469–473.
27. Schroeder, C., Gibson, L., Zenke, M., and Beug, H. (1992) Modulation of normal erythroid differentiation by the endogenous thyroid hormone and retinoic acid receptors: a possible target for v-erbA oncogene action. *Oncogene* **7,** 217–227.
28. Bauer, A., Mikulits, W., Lagger, G., Stengl, G., Brosch, G., and Beug, H. (1998) The thyroid hormone receptor functions as a ligand-operated developmental switch between proliferation and differentiation of erythroid progenitors. *EMBO J.* **17,** 4291–4303.

22

A New Clonal Assay System for Lymphoid and Myeloid Lineages

Hiroshi Kawamoto and Yoshimoto Katsura

Summary

It has long been unclear how the pluripotent hematopoietic stem cell is restricted to the major lineage progenitors including the progenitors for myeloid, T- and B-cells. This is the result of the absence of a methodology capable of determining the developmental potential of individual progenitors to generate these major lineage cells. We have established such an assay system, termed the multilineage progenitor assay, as a modification of the fetal thymic organ culture system. By examining cells from murine fetal tissues with this assay, we have succeeded in elucidating the process of lineage restrictions in early hematopoiesis.

Key Words: Hematopoiesis; differentiation; development; lineage restriction; lineage commitment; clonal assay; single cell assay; T-cell; B-cell; myeloid cell; fetal thymus organ culture; FTOC; multilineage progenitor assay; MLP assay.

1. Introduction

All hematopoietic cells, including myelo-erythroid cells, T-cells, and B-cells, are derived from the hematopoietic stem cell (HSC). However, the development of these major lineages has long been investigated with different systems by different research groups. The most popularly used methods for studies on the differentiation of myelo-erythroid, T- and B-cell lineages have been the colony-forming unit-culture (CFU-C) assay ***(1,2)***, fetal thymus organ culture (FTOC) ***(3–5)***, and co-culture with a stromal cell line ***(6,7)***, respectively. Because these experiments are unable to determine the potential of progenitors for other lineages, it is impossible to assess the developmental relationship among lineages. Another problem is that clonal assays have not been used in most studies on T- and B-cell development (*see* **Notes 1** and **2**).

To understand the whole story of hematopoiesis, it is important to develop a system effective in determining the developmental potential of a progenitor towards all major lineages, including the myeloid, T- and B-cell lineages. The multilineage progenitor (MLP) assay that we have developed is able to determine the developmental potential of individual progenitors towards these three lineages ***(19)***. The MLP assay is based on the FTOC because T-cell development is highly dependent upon the thymic micro-

From: *Methods in Molecular Medicine, Vol. 105: Developmental Hematopoiesis: Methods and Protocols.* Edited by: M. H. Baron © Humana Press Inc., Totowa, NJ

environments. The FTOC system was modified by adding cytokines that support the growth of myeloid and B-cells, and in such an environment we cultured single progenitors. With the MLP assay, the process of hematopoiesis, especially the relationship among myeloid, T- and B-cell lineages, became much clearer ***(20–25)***. Currently we call this assay the MLP<MTB> assay, <MLP> representing the assay area, mainly myeloid (M) T- and B-call linages. Some other assay systems covering erythroid ***(26)***, natural killer ***(27)***, and dendritic cell lineages ***(28)*** have been developed so far. In this section, we will describe the detailed procedure of the MLP <MTB> assay.

2. Materials

1. 6-Well plate (Costar), 96-well V-bottom plate (Nunc), and 96-well U-bottom plate (Nunc).
2. Membrane filters (13 mm in diameter, pore size 8 μm, Nucleopore).
3. Plastic bag (25 × 38 cm, heat-sealable, with a cap; Tedlar bag, Ohmi Odo Air Service, Hikone, Japan).
4. Toothpicks.
5. 200-μL Tip with a large hole (BIO-BIK).
6. A gas cylinder containing a gas mixture of 70% O_2, 25% N_2, 5% CO_2. This high oxygen gas mixture can be replaced by injecting the air, 100% CO_2 gas, and 100% O_2 gas into a bag at an appropriate ratio.
7. 2'-Deoxyguanosine (dGuo; Nakalai Tesque, Kyoto). To make a stock solution, dGuo is dissolved at a concentration of 135 m*M* in 0.1 *N* NaOH at 50°C. 90-μL aliquots are stocked in a –20°C freezer.
8. RPMI 1640 Medium (Gibco BRL, Grand Island, NY) supplemented with 10% fetal calf serum (FCS; *see* **Note 3**), 2 m*M* L-glutamine, 1 m*M* sodium pyruvate, 2 mg/mL sodium bicarbonate, 0.1 m*M* nonessential amino acid solution (Gibco BRL), 5×10^{-5} *M* 2-mercaptoethanol (2-ME), 100 μg/mL streptomycin, and 100 U/mL penicillin.
9. Dulbecco's modified Eagle's medium (DMEM) containing 1% FCS.
10. Recombinant murine (rm) SCF, rm interleukin (IL)-3, rm IL-7 (Genzyme-Techne, Cambridge, MA).
11. C57BL/6 (B6) mice and B6Ly5.1 mice (*see* **Note 4**). Embryos at various stages of gestation were obtained from time-mated pregnant B6 and B6Ly5.1. The day of appearance of a vaginal plug was designated as d 0 postcoitum (dpc).
12. Antibodies: Anti-Ly5.1 (A20), anti-Ly5.2 (104), anti-c-kit (2B8), anti-Sca-1 (E13-161.7), TER119 ***(29)***, anti-Mac-1 (M1/70), anti-Gr-1 (RB6-8C5), anti-B220 (RA3-6B2), anti-Thy1.2 (53-2.1), anti-CD19 (1D3; BD PharMingen, San Jose, CA). A mixture of TER119, anti-Gr-1, anti-B220, anti-CD19 and anti-Thy-1.2 was used as the anti-lineage markers (anti-Lin).

3. Methods

3.1. dGuo Treatment of Fetal Thymus (FT) Lobes (Fig. 1)

3.1.1. Preparation of dGuo Solution

1. Thaw 90 μL of the dGuo solution at room temperature. If precipitation occurs, use a hair dryer to warm the solution.
2. Add 90 μL of dGuo solution to 9 mL of RPMI medium (final dGuo concentration is 1.35 m*M*).
3. Add 3 mL per well of a six-well plate.
4. Float two membrane filters per well.

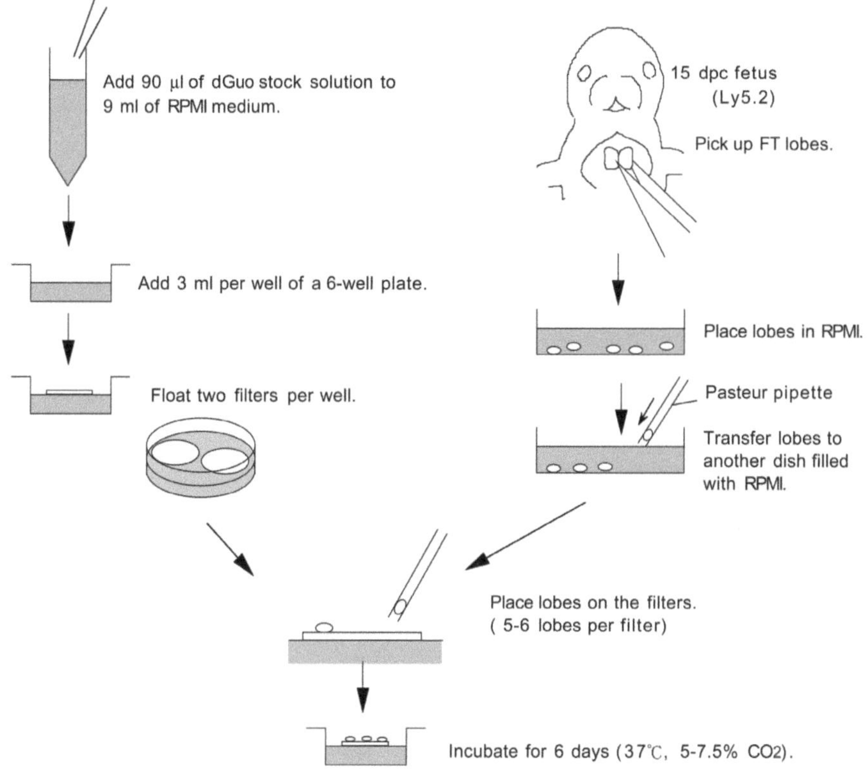

Fig. 1. dGuo treatment of FT lobes.

3.1.2. Preparation of FT Lobes

1. Remove the thymic lobes from fetuses of 15 dpc using fine forceps. Use Ly5.2 mice as a source of thymic lobes when progenitors to be examined are Ly5.1.
2. Place the lobes in RPMI medium.
3. Transfer the lobes to another dish containing RPMI medium by using a Pasteur pipet.

3.1.3. dGuo Treatment

1. Pick up the FT lobes from the RPMI medium by using a Pasteur pipet, and place them on the floating filter. Place five to six lobes per filter.
2. Incubate for 6 d (37°C, 5 to 7.5% CO_2).

***3.2. Washing of dGuo-Treated Lobes* (Fig. 2)**

1. Remove all dGuo-containing RPMI medium carefully.
2. Slowly add 3 mL of RPMI medium.
3. Incubate for 2 h in 37°C CO_2 incubator.
4. Take out the filter with FT lobes from the well by using forceps. Detach the lobes from the filter by gently brushing with forceps and place them in a new dish filled with RPMI.

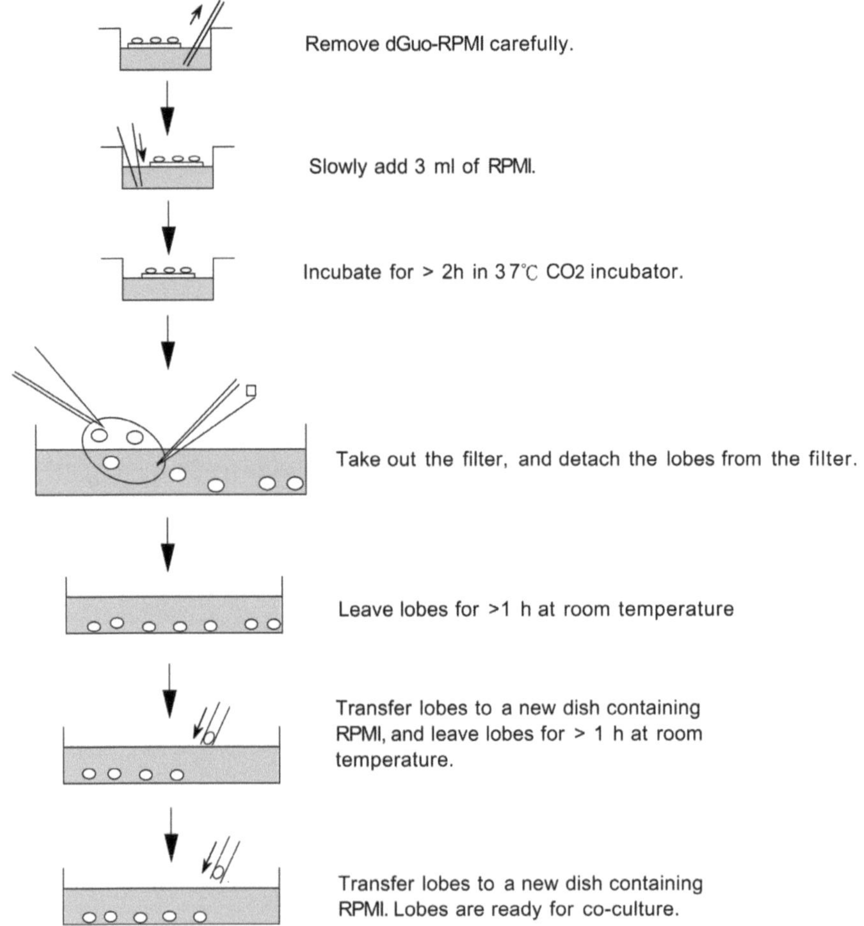

Fig. 2. Washing dGuo-treated FT lobes.

5. Leave the lobes for 1 h at room temperature.
6. Transfer the lobes to a new dish containing RPMI medium.
7. Leave the lobes for at least 1 h at room temperature. Lobes are then ready for coculture.

3.3. Seeding of a Single Cell (Fig. 3)

3.3.1. Preparation of Wells With a dGuo Lobe

1. Place 200 μL of RPMI medium into each well of 96-well V-bottom plate. The medium is supplemented with SCF (10 ng/mL), IL-7 (5 ng/mL), and IL-3 (3 ng/mL). GM-CSF (1 ng/mL) can be used instead of IL-3 (**ref.** ***22***; *see* **Notes 4** and **5**).
2. Place one dGuo-treated FT lobe in each well.

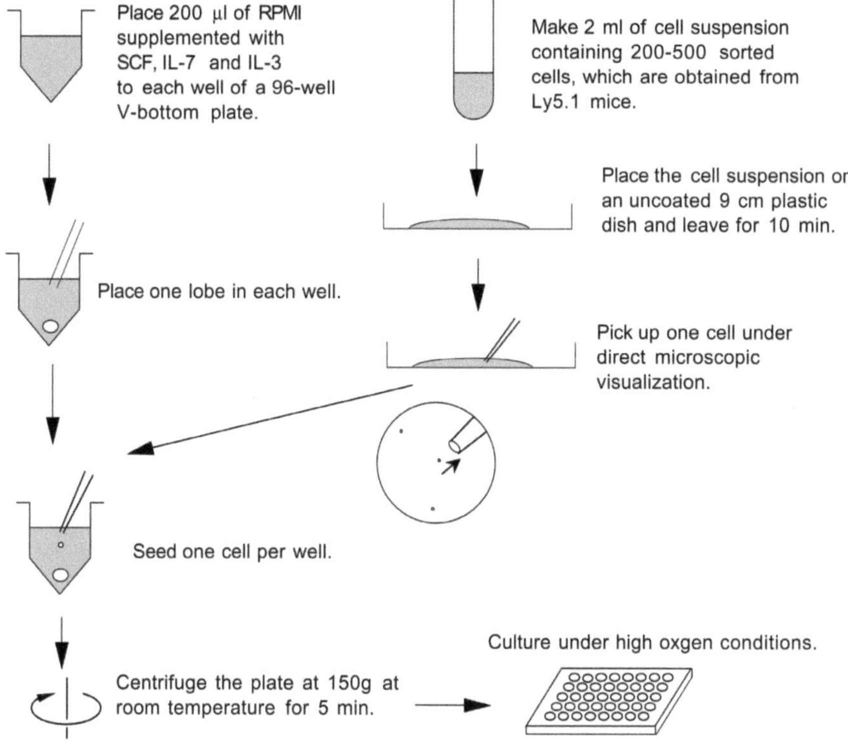

Fig. 3. Seeding of single cells.

3. Wells of the outer lanes of the plate are usually not used for cultures, since the medium in these wells tend to evaporate more rapidly.
4. In order to prevent evaporation of medium in culturing wells, wells of the outer lanes and those not used for culture are filled with medium or PBS.

3 3 2. Preparation of Cells To Be Examined

1. Cells to be examined are stained with appropriate antibodies and collected by flow-cytometrical cell sorting (*see* **Notes 6** and **7**).
2. Prepare 2 mL of cell suspension containing 200 to 400 cells from Ly5.1 mice.
3. Place 2 mL of cell suspension in an uncoated 9-cm plastic dish and leave for 10 min so that all cells sink down to the bottom of the plate.

3.3.3. Seeding of a Single Cell

1. Pick up a single cell under microscopic visualization by using a long fine tip attached to a 20-µL pipettor. Breath-controlled fine glass capillary is also useful for picking up single cells. Be careful not to pick up more than one cell (*see* **Note 8**).
2. Centrifuge the plate at 150*g* at room temperature for 5 min. The plate is then cultured under high oxygen submersion conditions.

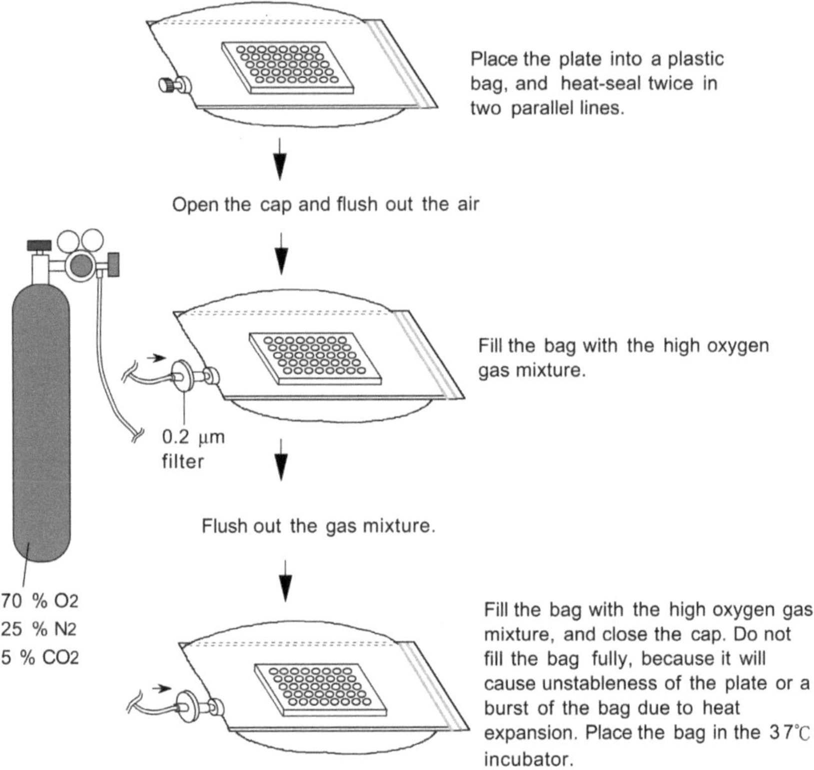

Fig. 4. High oxygen culture.

3.4. *High Oxygen Submersion Culture* (Fig. 4)

1. Prepare a plastic bag that has a cap on one side. The other side is cut open. The bag can be re-used several times. Place the plate into the bag.
2. Heat seal the bag twice in two parallel lines, for extra security.
3. Open the cap and flush out the air.
4. Fill the bag with the high oxygen gas mixture (70% O_2, 25% N_2, 5% CO_2; **ref. *19***) and close the cap. The gas mixture is supplied from a specially ordered gas cylinder.
5. Place the bag in the 37°C incubator. No need to control the CO_2 concentration.
6. The medium is replaced by half every 5 d.
7. The culture period for progenitors of murine fetal tissues is usually 10 d. T-lineage cells live longer, but myeloid cells tend to disappear earlier.

3.5. *Cell Harvest From Each Well* (Fig. 5)

1. Suck up the FT lobes and cells outside the lobe together with 100 μL of medium using 200-μL tip with a large hole. Such a tip can be prepared by cutting back the tip of an ordinary 200-μL tip.
2. Place the lobe, cells and medium into each well of a 96-well U-bottom plate.

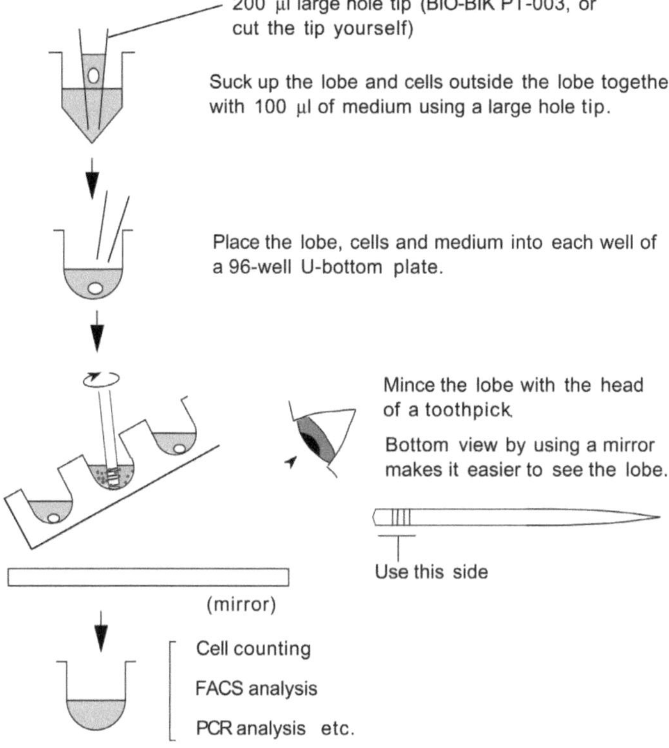

Fig. 5. Cell harvest from culture wells.

3. Mince the lobe with the head of a toothpick. A toothpick with a hemisphere-shaped head is preferable (*see* **Note 9**). Check the appearance of the lobe during mincing by examining it from the bottom, using a mirror.
4. The cell suspension thus made can be used for cell counting, flow cytometric analysis, polymerase chain reaction analysis etc. The cell recovery per well differs depending on progenitor types, ranging from 1000 to 100,000.

3.6. Cell Staining for Flow Cytometric Analysis

1. Place 20 μL of the cell suspension in a 96-well U-bottom plate (*see* **Note 10**).
2. Add 5 μL of monoclonal antibody (MAb) mixture to the side wall of the well.
3. Mix the MAb with the cell suspension by gently tapping the plate, and incubate for 20 min on ice.
4. Add 200 μL of MEM with 1% FCS.
5. Centrifuge the plate at 150*g* at 4°C for 5 min.
6. Discard the supernatant.
7. Add 200 μL of MEM with 1% FCS.
8. Resuspend the cells, and the cell suspension is passed through the nylon mesh into a test tube. The sample is ready for flow cytometric analysis.

3.7. Flow Cytometric Analysis

3.7.1. First Step Screening

As a first step, all wells were screened for the generation of cells from the seeded single Ly5.1 progenitor. For the first screening, cells were stained with two colors with anti-Ly5.1 and anti-Ly5.2. The samples containing Ly5.1$^+$ cells are selected for further analysis.

3.7.2. Staining of Cells for Second-Step Analysis

Samples selected for further analysis are stained with four colors using the combination of anti-Ly5.1, anti-Thy-1, anti-B220, and anti-Mac-1. Staining with three colors using a combination of: 1) anti-Ly5.1, anti-Thy-1, anti-B220, and 2) anti-Ly5.1, anti-Thy-1, and anti-Mac-1 also works.

3.7.3. Judgment of Progenitor Types

Any lineage markers would give some non-specific staining, so the judgment of lineage type of generated cells requires evaluation from several angles. A large gate area is set in forward/side scatter in order to include all viable cells (**Fig. 6A**). Cells showing Ly5.1$^+$Thy-1$^+$B220$^-$ and Ly5.1$^+$Thy-1$^-$B220$^+$phenotypes are tentatively regarded as donor derived T- and B-cells, respectively. Cells in these populations are then checked for forward/side scatter and expression of Mac-1, and those falling within the lymphocyte area of scattergram and negative for Mac-1 expression are judged to be T or B lineage cells. Ly5.1$^+$Mac-1$^+$ cells with myeloid scatter characteristics are considered to be donor derived myeloid lineage cells. Note that these Mac-1$^+$ cells sometimes include B220 low positive or Thy-1 low positive cells. The progenitor type is determined based on the types of cells generated. The progenitor generating T, B and myeloid lineage cells is termed p-Multi. Likewise, other types are termed p-MT, p-MB, p-TB, p-M, p-T, and p-B (*see* **Note 11**). Among these types, p-TB has never been detected in fetal tissues (*see* **Note 12**). Representative flow cytometric profiles of cells derived from each of the six types of progenitors are shown in **Fig. 6B**.

3.7.4. The Distribution of Different Types of Progenitors in Fetal Liver Subpopulations

An example of the distribution of different progenitor types found in fetal liver is shown in **Fig. 7**. As a progenitor source, Sca-1$^+$ and Sca-1$^-$ cells from the Lin$^-$c-kit$^+$ population of 12 dpc murine fetal liver were used (**Fig. 7A**). 124 cells of the Sca-1$^+$ group and 160 cells of the Sca-1$^-$ group were examined (*see* **Fig. 7B**; **ref. *19***; **Note 13**).

4. Notes

1. In hematology, clonal assays have long been used for evaluation of progenitor activity. The CFU-C assay is the most popularly used clonal assay that is effective in determining the developmental potential of individual progenitors towards the erythroid and myeloid lineages ***(1,2)***. In these studies, however, the developmental potential towards the T- or B-cell lineages has not been usually taken into consideration. In contrast, in almost all studies on T- or B-cell development, 10^3 or more cells have been used in the cultures ***(8–12)***. These assays are effective in examining the developmental potential of progenitors towards the single lineage of interest. Problems emerge, however, when trials of modifications are made to determine the developmental potential of a cultured cell towards

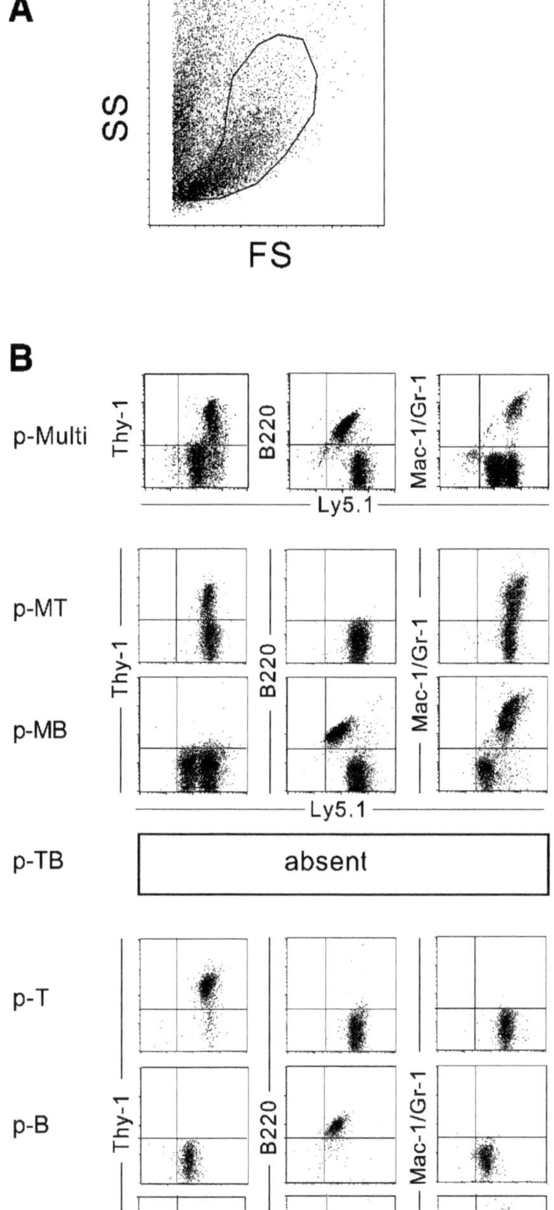

Fig. 6. Flow cytometric profiles of cells derived from six types of progenitors.

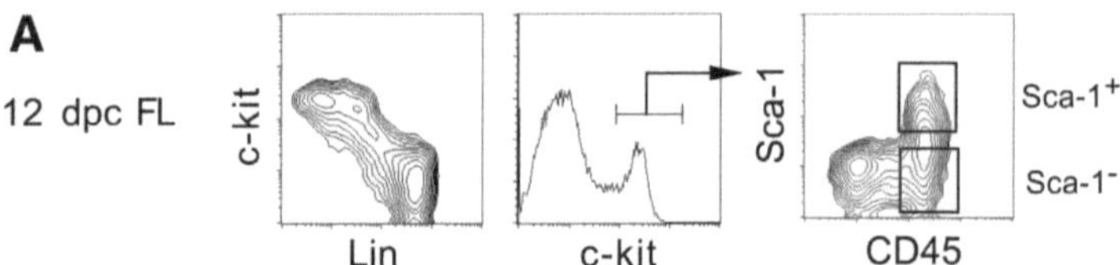

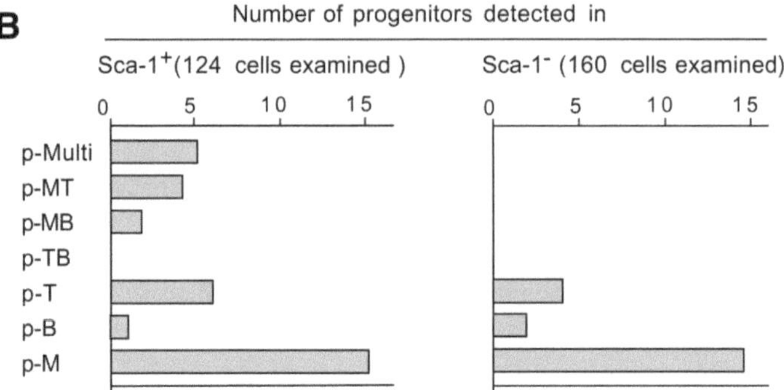

Fig. 7. Distribution of different types of progenitors in fetal liver subpopulations.

more than two lineages. In such experiments, even if the cultured progenitors generated two types of hematopoietic cells, it is impossible to determine whether the cultured cell population included a bipotent progenitor or two types of unipotent progenitors.

2. Trials of single cell assays for examining lymphoid and myeloid potential have been undertaken ***(7,13–18)***. However, the methods applied in these studies could not determine T-cell generating potential at the same time as induction of other lineages. Accordingly, these studies failed to detect T-cell lineage committed progenitors, and provided little information on the branching point towards the T-cell lineage.
3. It is important to select a batch of FCS. We usually select it through several steps. As the 1st screening, hematopoietic progenitor cells (e.g., Lin$^-$c-kit$^+$Sca-1$^+$ FL cells, 100–500 cells per culture) are cultured in the presence of the FCS to be assessed on a monolayer of stromal cells that allows B-cell development, and batches that give high B-cell growth are selected. As the second step, hematopoietic progenitor cells are cultured with a dGuo-treated FT lobe (100 c-kit$^+$Sca-1$^+$ cells per lobe), and a batch that gives the highest T-cell growth is selected. In parallel with the second step selection, we usually perform the MLP assay by adding the FCS of batches to be tested. In this case, cells in the Lin$^-$c-kit$^+$Sca-1 high expressing population, where p-Multi are enriched ***(21)***, are examined at the single cell level, and the batch that gives the highest plating efficiency for p-Multi is selected.
4. B-cell-generating potential tends to be more difficult to detect in the MLP assay than other lineage potentials. If you face this difficulty, we recommend using fetal progenitors of Balb/c mice, because the B-cell growth from progenitors of Balb/c mice is much more efficient than that of other mouse strains. Induction of T-cell differentiation can be carried out using MHC mismatched FT lobes. The disadvantage of using Balb/c mice is that the stem/progenitor cells of this strain do not express Sca-1. In this case, we recommend using Lin$^-$c-kit$^+$FcγRII/III (FcR)$^-$ cells as a progenitor source rather than Lin$^-$c-kit$^+$Sca-1$^+$ cells.

5. Before doing the single cell assay, it is important to determine the culture conditions that evenly support the generation of myeloid, T- and B-cells. In such calibration experiments, as the first step, we recommend culturing 30–100 c-kit$^+$Sca-1$^+$ fetal liver cells per well, but not single cells ***(19)***. If the culture conditions seem to be skewed to a certain lineage, the concentration of one or more cytokines should be changed. In the next step, it is important to check the sensitivity for the detection of progenitor activity of each lineage by your MLP assay in comparison with those detected by other efficient culture systems. For this purpose, c-kit$^+$Sca-1$^+$ cells have to be examined at a single cell level by the MLP assay. The frequency of progenitors expressing B-, myeloid- and T-cell potential should be comparable to those obtained by clonally culturing the c-kit$^+$Sca-1$^+$ cells with monolayered stromal cells (for B-cell potential), in the CFU-C assay (for myeloid cell potential), and with a dGuo-lobe without any added cytokines (for T-cell potential).
6. The MLP assay described here is not yet applicable to studies on progenitors in adult bone marrow. Further studies are necessary to determine the culture conditions required for even induction of bone marrow progenitors towards different lineages.
7. Preparation of cells from liver, blood or thymus of murine fetuses were performed as follows. Embryos (12 dpc) were separated from the placenta by pinching and cutting the umbilical cord using fine forceps. The placenta was not removed from the uterus in order to reduce contamination with maternal blood. The embryo was washed twice to remove any contamination of maternal blood, and then placed in medium to allow bleeding until it became completely pale. The embryo was then removed, and the blood left in the dish was collected. The embryo was washed once and placed in another dish containing medium, where it was dissected to obtain FL and FT. Single cell suspension of FL was prepared by pipetting the FL lobes. FT lobes were minced between glass slides using the frosted portion. All fetal cells were then passed through a 40-μm nylon mesh, washed, and resuspended in medium. Viable cells were counted using Trypan blue exclusion.
8. In our single cell culture, we do not use the clone-sort system of the cell sorter. This is because the hand manipulation system is more reliable to exclude doublet cells or dead cells. We practice this method of picking and placing single cells to each well of a Terasaki Plate. Important points for avoiding picking up two or more cells are that the cells should be suspended at a very low concentration (<200 cells/mL) in a dish, and the cell suspension should sit for a long enough time (more than 10 min) to allow all cells to sink to the bottom of the dish.
9. To efficiently harvest cells from a lobe, we recommend using a small disposable stick for mincing the lobe. It is preferable that the stick has a hemisphere-shaped head (*see* **Fig. 5**). We use toothpicks made in Japan for this purpose.
10. To reduce cell loss, we do not wash the cells prior to staining.
11. In single cell cultures, multipotent or bipotent progenitors do not necessarily generate a comparable number of myeloid, T- and B-cells in a culture well. Numbers or proportions of these cells fluctuate depending upon various unknown or uncontrollable conditions, which include the developmental stage of the progenitors cultured, the combination and concentration of cytokines added, and the area of the dGuo-treated FT lobe where the progenitor is seeded. In some cases, T-cells comprise >95% and myeloid cells comprise <2% of cells recovered from one well. Nevertheless, the progenitor seeded to this well should be judged as a p-MT, provided that the small number of myeloid cells form a clear peak in the flow cytometric analysis.
12. MLP<MTB> assay is effective in classifying progenitors into seven types: p-Multi, p-MT, p-MB, p-TB, p-M, p-T, and p-B. Among them, p-TB has never been detected despite examining 10,000 or more cells. We modified the MLP<MTB> with the addition of erythropoietin allowing the development of erythroid lineage cells, and named this assay in

analogy MLP<METB> assay. With the MLP<METB> assay, progenitors can be classified into 15 types: p-METB, p-MET, p-MEB, p-MTB, p-ETB, p-ME, p-MT, p-MB, p-ET, p-EB, p-TB, p-M, p-E, p-T, and p-B. Among them, p-MET, p-MEB, p-ETB, p-ET, p-EB, and p-TB have never been detected. The failure to detect certain progenitor types may indicate that lineage restriction proceeds through an ordered process but not at random, as has previously been proposed ***(30)***.

13. In any assay system, the progenitor that expressed all the potentials that the assay system is designed to detect can be regarded as a multipotent progenitor. However, it may be unclear whether a given progenitor expressed its full potential under the assay conditions used. Therefore, it is important that such progenitors be isolated as a cell population or detected in cell populations that do not include multipotent progenitors.

References

1. Pluznik, D. H. and Sachs, L. (1965) The cloning of normal "mast" cells in tissue culture. *J. Cell. Physiol.* **66,** 319–324.
2. Bradley, T. R. and Metcalf, D. (1966) The growth of mouse bone marrow cells in vitro. *Aust. J. Exp. Biol. Med. Sci.* **44,** 287–299.
3. Jenkinson, E. J., Franchi, L. L., Kingston, R., and Owen, J. J. (1982) Effect of deoxyguanosine on lymphopoiesis in the developing thymus rudiment in vitro: application in the production of chimeric thymus rudiments. *Eur. J. Immunol.* **12,** 583–587.
4. Watanabe, Y. and Katsura, Y. (1993) Development of T cell receptor alpha beta-bearing T cells in the submersion organ culture of murine fetal thymus at high oxygen concentration. *Eur. J. Immunol.* **23,** 200–205.
5. Anderson, G. and Jenkinson, E. J. (2001) Lymphostromal interactions in thymic development and function. *Nat. Rev. Immunol.* **1,** 31–40.
6. Nishikawa, S., Ogawa, M., Nishikawa, S., Kunisada, T., and Kodama, H. (1988) B lymphopoiesis on stromal cell clone: stromal cell clones acting on different stages of B cell differentiation. *Eur. J. Immunol.* **18,** 1767–1771.
7. Cumano, A., Paige, C. J., Iscove, N. N., and Brady, G. (1992) Bipotential precursors of B cells and macrophages in murine fetal liver. *Nature* **356,** 612–615.
8. Hardy, R. R., Carmack, C. E., Shinton, S. A., Kemp, J. D., and Hayakawa, K. (1991) Resolution and characterization of pro-B and pre-pro-B cell stages in normal mouse bone marrow. *J. Exp. Med.* **173,** 1213–1225.
9. Osmond, D. G., Rolink, A., and Melchers, F. (1998) Murine B lymphopoiesis: towards a unified model. *Immunol. Today* **19,** 65–68.
10. Wu, L., Antica, M., Johnson, G. R., Scollay, R., and Shortman, K. (1991) Developmental potential of the earliest precursor cells from the adult mouse thymus. *J. Exp. Med.* **174,** 1617–1627.
11. Matsuzaki, Y., Gyotoku, J., Ogawa, M., Nishikawa, S., Katsura, Y., Gachelin, G., and Nakauchi, H. (1993) Characterization of c-kit positive intrathymic stem cells that are restricted to lymphoid differentiation. *J. Exp. Med.* **178,** 1283–1292.
12. Moore, T. A. and Zlotnik, A. (1995) T-cell lineage commitment and cytokine responses of thymic progenitors. *Blood* **86,** 1850–1860.
13. Galy, A., Travis, M., Cen, D., and Chen, B. (1995) Human T, B, natural killer, and dendritic cells arise from a common bone marrow progenitor cell subset. *Immunity* **3,** 459–473.
14. Delassus, S. and Cumano, A. (1996) Circulation of hematopoietic progenitors in the mouse embryo. *Immunity* **4,** 97–106.
15. Kondo, M., Weissman, I. L., and Akashi, K. (1997) Identification of clonogenic common lymphoid progenitors in mouse bone marrow. *Cell* **91,** 661–672.

16. Aiba, Y. and Ogawa, M. (1997) Development of natural killer cells, B lymphocytes, macrophages, and mast cells from single hematopoietic progenitors in culture of murine fetal liver cells. *Blood* **90,** 3923–3930.
17. Lacaud, G., Carlsson, L., and Keller, G. (1998) Identification of a fetal hematopoietic precursor with B cell, T cell, and macrophage potential. *Immunity* **9,** 827–838.
18. Hao, Q. L., Zhu, J., Price, M. A., Payne, K. J., Barsky, L. W., and Crooks, G. M. (2001) Identification of a novel, human multilymphoid progenitor in cord blood. *Blood* **97,** 3683–3690.
19. Kawamoto, H., Ohmura, K., and Katsura, Y. (1997) Direct evidence for the commitment of hematopoietic stem cells to T, B and myeloid lineages in murine fetal liver. *Int. Immunol.* **9,** 1011–1019.
20. Kawamoto, H., Ohmura, K., and Katsura, Y. (1998) Presence of progenitors restricted to T, B, or myeloid lineage, but absence of multipotent stem cells, in the murine fetal thymus. *J. Immunol.* **161,** 3799–3802.
21. Kawamoto, H., Ohmura, K., Fujimoto, S., and Katsura, Y. (1999) Emergence of T cell progenitors without B cell or myeloid differentiation potential at the earliest stage of hematopoiesis in the murine fetal liver. *J. Immunol.* **162,** 2725–2731.
22. Ohmura, K., Kawamoto, H., Fujimoto, S., Ozaki, S., Nakao, k., and Katsura, Y. (1999) Emergence of T, B and myeloid lineage-committed as well as multipotent hematopoietic progenitors in the aorta-gonad-mesonephros region of day 10 fetuses of the mouse. *J. Immunol.* **163,** 4788–4795.
23. Kawamoto, H., Ikawa, T., Ohmura, K., Fujimoto, S., and Katsura, Y. (2000) T cell progenitors emerge earlier than B cell progenitors in the murine fetal liver. *Immunity* **12,** 441–450.
24. Katsura, Y. (2002) Redefinition of lymphoid progenitors. *Nat. Rev. Immunol.* **2,** 127–132.
25. Spangrude, G. J. (2002) Divergent models of lymphoid lineage specification: do clonal assays provide all the answers? *Immunol Rev.* **187,** 40–47.
26. Lu, M., Kawamoto, H., Katsube, Y., Ikawa, T., and Katsura, Y. (2002) The common myelolymphoid progenitor: a key intermediate stage in hemopoiesis generating T and B cells. *J. Immunol.* **169,** 3519–3525.
27. Ikawa, T., Kawamoto, H., Fujimoto, S., and Katsura, Y. (1999) Commitment of common T/Natural killer (NK) progenitors to unipotent T and NK progenitors in the murine fetal thymus revealed by a single progenitor assay. *J. Exp. Med.* **190,** 1617–1626.
28. Shen, H.Q., Lu, M., Ikawa, T., Masuda, K., Ohmura, K., Minato, N., Katsura, Y., and Kawamoto, H. (2003) T/NK bipotent progenitors in the thymus retain the potential to generate dendritic cells. *J. Immunol.* **171,** 3401–3406.
29. Kina, T., Ikuta, K., Takayama, E., Wada, K., Majumdar, A. S., Weissman, I. L., and Katsura, Y. (2001) The monoclonal antibody TER-119 recognizes a molecule associated with glycophorin A and specifically marks the late stages of murine erythroid lineage. *Br. J. Haematol.* **109,** 280–287.
30. Ogawa, M., Porter, P. N., and Nakahata, T. (1983) Renewal and commitment to differentiation of hemopoietic stem cells (an interpretive review). *Blood* **61,** 823–829.

23

Hematopoietic and Endothelial Development of Mouse Embryonic Stem Cells in Culture

Kyunghee Choi, Yun Shin Chung, and Weh Jie Zhang

Summary

Embryonic stem (ES) cells differentiate efficiently in vitro and give rise to many different somatic cell types. Hematopoietic progenitors present within differentiated ES cells (embryoid bodies, EBs) can be identified by replating EB cells into semisolid media with hematopoietic growth factors. The developmental kinetics of various hematopoietic lineage precursors within EBs and molecular and cellular studies of these cells have suggested that the sequence of events leading to the onset of hematopoiesis within EBs is similar to that found within the mouse embryo. Thus, the in vitro differentiation model of ES cells provides a unique opportunity to study onset mechanisms involved in hematopoietic development.

Key Words: Embryonic stem cell; in vitro differentiation; embryoid body (EB); hemangioblast; blast colony forming cell (BL-CFC); hematopoietic development.

1. Introduction

Embryonic stem (ES) cells are derived from early stage embryos (blastocysts). When plated onto a feeder layer of fibroblasts, the inner cell mass of blastocysts will give rise to colonies of undifferentiated cells (ES colonies), which can be isolated and further expanded. Once established, ES cells can be maintained as pluripotent stem cells on a feeder layer of fibroblasts. One of the factors responsible for maintaining ES cells as stem cells is leukemia inhibitory factor (LIF; **refs.** *1* and *2*). When introduced back into a blastocyst, ES cells can contribute to all tissues except the extraembryonic endoderm and trophoblast of the developing embryo *(3,4)*. It is this particular trait that makes ES cells a valuable tool for genetic engineering (**Fig. 1**). In addition, ES cells differentiate efficiently in vitro and give rise to many different somatic cell progeny *(5–25)*. Hematopoietic progenitors develop sequentially within EBs. The first to develop is the blast colony-forming cell (BL-CFC). BL-CFCs are transient and develop prior to the primitive erythroid population *(26,27)*. Definitive erythroid and myeloid progenitors develop shortly after primitive erythroid progenitors (**Fig. 2**).

From: *Methods in Molecular Medicine, Vol. 105: Developmental Hematopoiesis: Methods and Protocols.*
Edited by: M. H. Baron © Humana Press Inc., Totowa, NJ

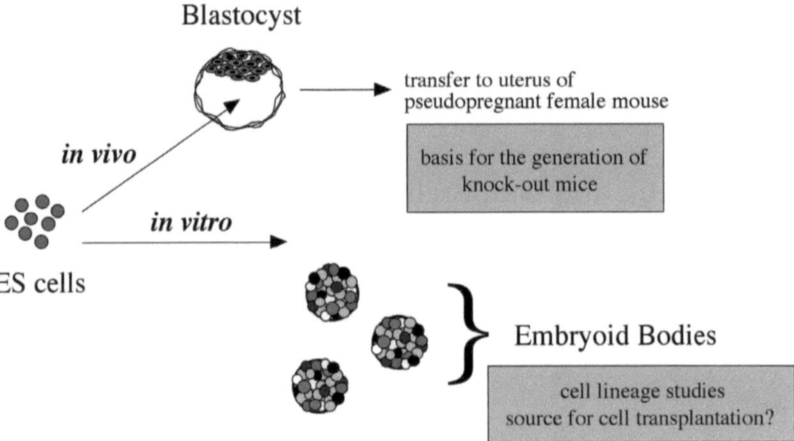

Fig. 1. In vivo and in vitro application of ES cells.

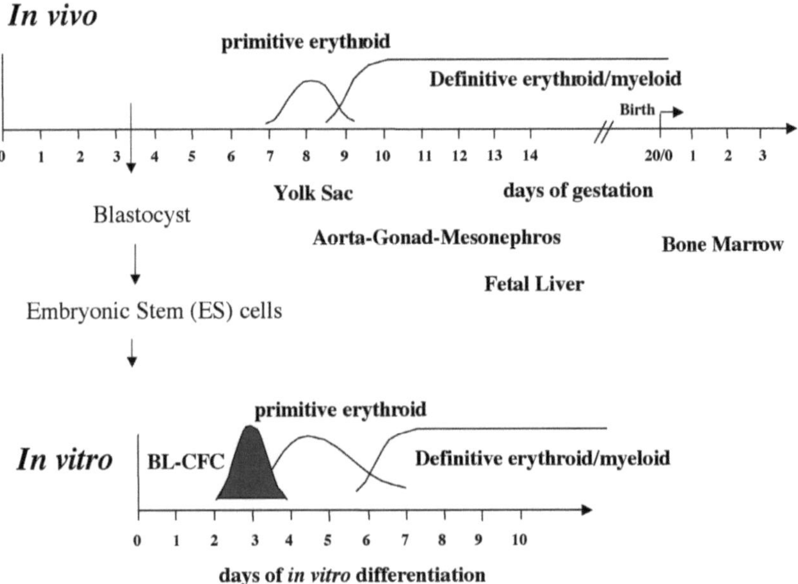

Fig. 2. Hematopoietic development in vivo vs in vitro. Hematopoietic differentiation within EBs recapitulates the in vivo sequence of hematopoietic development. In the developing embryo, primitive erythroid cells develop prior to definitive hematopoietic progenitors. This sequence is preserved in developing EBs. Moreover, BL-CFCs develop in EB before primitive erythoird progenitors. Both BL-CFCs and primitive erythroid progenitors are transient cell types. Scales on the *y*-axis are arbitrary.

BL-CFCs form blast colonies in response to vascular endothelial growth factor (VEGF), a ligand for the receptor tyrosine kinase, Flk-1 ***(28)***. Gene expression analysis indicated that cells within blast colonies (blast cells) expressed a number of genes common to both hematopoietic and endothelial lineages, including *Scl*, *CD34*, and *Flk-1* ***(26)***. In addition, blast cells are clonal and give rise to primitive, definitive hematopoietic, and endothelial cell progenitors when replated in medium containing both hematopoietic and endothelial cell growth factors ***(26,27)***. Collectively, these studies strongly argue that BL-CFCs represent the hemangioblast, a common progenitor of hematopoietic and endothelial cells. In this chapter, we will discuss how to analyze various hematopoietic progenitors developing within EBs. Special emphasis will be given to BL-CFCs.

2. Materials

2.1. ES Culture

1. Tissue culture flasks/dishes should be pretreated with 0.1% gelatin in phosphate-buffered saline (PBS) for at least 20 min at room temperature. Simply add the appropriate amount (i.e., 3 mL per T25 or 7 mL per T75, just to cover the bottom of the flask/dish) of 0.1% gelatin in PBS and keep it at room temperature. Aspirate off gelatin just before adding cells. Flasks/dishes with 0.1% gelatin in PBS can be stored at 4°C as well.
2. 0.1 % Gelatin: dissolve gelatin (Sigma G-1890) at 0.1% in PBS and autoclave.
3. 100X mitomycin C solution: Dissolve mitomycin C (Sigma M-0503) at 1 mg/mL in PBS. Store at 4°C in the dark.
4. Dulbecco's modified Eagle's medium (DMEM): dissolve one package of DMEM (Gibco 12100-046) powder in distilled water. We normally use distilled water from Millipore (Bedford, CA) Milli-Q purification system (QTUM000EX). Add 3.024 g of $NaHCO_3$ (Sigma; cat. no. S5761), 10 mL penicillin/streptomycin (10,000U Gibco/BRL; cat. no. 6005140PG), and 25 mL of 1 *M* HEPES buffer (Gibco/BRL; cat. no. 380-5630 PG). Bring up to 1 L with distilled water, filter through 0.22-micron filter and keep at 4°C.
5. ES-DMEM medium: 15% fetal calf serum (FCS; preselected as described in **step 6**), 1.5% LIF, and 1.5×10^{-4} *M* MTG in DMEM.
6. FCS for ES culture. We normally prescreen FCS for ES culture. Typically, ES cells adapted to grow without feeder cells are used for serum test. ES cells are maintained in test serum for five to six passages and scored for morphology (differentiated or undifferentiated). A good lot of serum should keep the ES cells in an undifferentiated state.
7. Conditioned media from Chinese hamster ovary (CHO) cells transfected with LIF gene (Genetics Institute) is used as a source for LIF. CHO cells are cultured to about 70% confluency. The medium is then changed and the cells are cultured for an additional 3 to 4 d until confluent. Typically, these conditions result in conditioned medium containing LIF at approx 5 μg/mL.
8. 1.5×10^{-4} *M* MTG solution: dilute MTG (Sigma; cat. no. M-6145) 1:10 in DMEM and add 12.4 μL per 100 mL of ES media. Alternatively, β-mercaptoethanol (BME, Sigma; cat. no. M-7522) is used at 1×10^{-4} *M* (prepare a 100X stock solution by adding 72 μL of 14 *M* BME to 100 mL of 1X PBS and add 1 mL per 100 mL of ES media). Make sure that MTG or BME is prepared fresh.
9. Feeder/STO medium: STO cells (*see* **Note 1**) are grown in 10% FCS (the same serum used for ES culture) in DMEM. MTG (add 6.2 μL per 100 mL of media of MTG that is prediluted 1:10 in DMEM) or BME (at 5×10^{-5} *M*, add 0.5 mL of 100X stock per 100 mL media) is also added.

10. Trypsin–ethylene diamine tetraacetic acid: dissolve 2.5 g of trypsin (Sigma; cat. no. T-4799) in 1X PBS. Add 2.16 mL of 0.5 *M* ethylene diamine tetraacetic acid and bring up to 1 L with 1X PBS. Filter sterilize through 0.22-micron filter. Store aliquots at –20°C.
11. 10X PBS: add 160 g of NaCl, 4 g of KCl, 28.8 g of Na_2HPO_4, and 4.8 g of KH_2PO_4 per 2 L of distilled water. Heat dissolve and adjust the pH to 7.4. Make 1X by diluting 1:10 in distilled water and autoclave.
12. ES cell freezing medium: 90% FCS containing 10% DMSO (Sigma; cat. no. D2650). ES cells are frozen at a density of 2–3 × 10^6 cells/mL of freezing medium. Add 1 mL of cells to each freezing vial.

2.2. In Vitro Differentiation of ES Cells

1. IMDM: dissolve one package of IMDM powder (Gibco/BRL; cat. no. 12200-036) in distilled water. Add 3.024 g of $NaHCO_3$ and 10 mL of penicillin/streptomycin. Bring up to 1 L and filter through 0.22-micron filter.
2. ES-IMDM: 15% FCS (the same serum used for ES culture), 1.5% LIF, and 1.5 × 10^{-4} *M* MTG in IMDM.
3. FCS for ES differentiation: we normally prescreen FCS for ES differentiation. Typically, ES cells are differentiated in test serum and analyzed by FACS for Flk-1 staining or by hematopoietic replating. A good lot of serum should give rise to 30 to 50% of Flk-1^+ cells by d 3 to 4 EB stage and should result in good hematopoietic replating.
4. MTG (4.5 × 10^{-4} *M*): dilute 26 μL of MTG into 2 mL of IMDM. Add 3 μL of diluted MTG per 1 mL of differentiation medium.
5. For d 6 EBs that are 6 or more, add Kit-Ligand (KL, final 1%) and IL-3 (final 1%). For EBs that are d 9 or more, feed on d 6 (4–5 mL per 100-mm Petri dish) using the same methylcellulose cocktail as before, but with methylcellulose reduced from 1% to 0.5% (v/v). KL is from media conditioned by CHO cells transfected with a KL expression vector (Genetics Institute, Cambridge, MA). IL-3 is fröu medium conditioned by X63 AG8-653 myeloma cells transfected with a vector expressing IL-3 ***(29)***.
6. Ascorbic acid (Sigma; cat. no. A-4544) solution (*see* **Note 2**): prepare fresh each time you set up a differentiation experiment. Dissolve ascorbic acid at 5 mg/mL in H_2O and filter sterilize (0.22 μm).
7. Differentiation is performed in bacterial Petri dishes (Kond-Valmark Labware, Brampton, Ontario, Canada, 1-800-452-9070; cat. no. 900). Do not use tissue culture dishes because the EBs will adhere to the plastic surface.
8. 2% Methylcellulose is prepared as follows (1-L preparation): 1) weigh a sterile Erlenmeyer flask; 2) add approx 450 mL of sterile water; 3) bring to boil on a hot plate and keep boiling for 3–4 min; 4) add 20 g of methylcellulose, swirl quickly, and return flask to the hot plate; 5) remove from hot plate and swirl again when it starts to boil. Return flask back to the hot plate. Repeat three to four times; 6) weigh and add sterile water (room temperature) up to 500 mL of methylcellulose; 7) cool to room temperature on the bench; 8) in a separate flask, prepare 500 mL of 2X IMDM and filter sterilize; 9) slowly add 2X IMDM to methylcellulose and mix vigorously; 10) put the mixture on ice until the methylcellulose becomes viscous; 11) prepare approx 100-mL aliquots and keep frozen at –20°C. When ready to use, thaw and use a syringe (without needle) to dispense methylcellulose (do not use pipets).

2.3. Hematopoietic Replating

1. 2X Cellulase: dissolve cellulase (Sigma C-1794) in PBS at 2 U/mL. Filter sterilize through 0.45-micron filter. Cellulase is used to digest methylcellulose prior to harvesting EBs.

2. Collagenase: dissolve 1 g of collagenase (Sigma; cat. no. C0310) in 320 mL of 1X PBS. After filter sterilization, add 80 mL of FCS. Prepare aliquots and store at –20°C.
3. D4T-conditioned medium (C.M.): D4T endothelial cells ***(26,27)*** are cultured in 10% FCS in IMDM. Remove medium and change to 4% FCS in IMDM when the culture becomes approx 80% confluent. Culture an additional 72 h and collect the supernatant. Spin down for 5 min at 1000 rpm in a Sorvall RT7 tabletop centrifuge or equivalent, to remove cell debris. Filter sterilize the supernatant using a 0.45-mm filter unit. Prepare 5- to 10-mL aliquots and store at –80°C. Once thawed, D4T C.M. is kept at 4°C for approx 1 wk (*see* **Note 3**).
4. Erythropoietin (Amgen Epogen; cat. no. NDC 55513-126-10).
5. VEGF (R&D Systems; cat. no. 293-VE).
6. KL (kit ligand), R&D Systems; cat. no. 455-MC.
7. IL-1 (R&D Systems; cat. no. 401-ML).
8. IL-3 (R&D Systems; cat. no. 403-ML).
9. IL-6 (R&D Systems; cat. no. 406-ML).
10. IL-11 (R&D Systems; cat. no. 418-ML).
11. G-CSF (R&D Systems; cat. no. 414-CS).
12. GM-CSF (R&D Systems; cat. no. 415-ML).
13. M-CSF (R&D Systems; cat. no. 416-ML).
14. PFHM-II (protein free hybridoma medium), Gibco; cat. no. 12040-077.

3. Methods

3.1. ES Culture

ES cells are routinely maintained on STO feeder cells (*see* **Note 1**). We have used several different ES cell lines (R1, CCE, J1, TC1, and E14). Most of our work is performed using the R1 ES cell line. The various ES cell lines may differ in their growth and differentiation properties. We typically split ES cells every 2 d. STO cells are treated with mitomycin C to inhibit their growth before ES cells are added. Mouse embryo fibroblasts may be used instead of STO cells.

1. Day 1: split STO cells at a density of 50,000 cells/cm^2 (i.e., add 1.25×10^6 cells per T25 flask).
2. Day 2: treat STO cells with mitomycin C for 2 to 3 h, wash, and add fresh new media. Typically, 4 mL of medium containing mitomycin C is added per T25 flask.
3. Day 3: remove media and add ES cells (8×10^5 to 1×10^6 cells per T25 flask) in ES-DMEM medium.

3.2. In Vitro Differentiation of ES Cells

A variety of different methods for in vitro differentiation of ES cells can be used to efficiently generate the progeny of all three primary germ layers: endoderm, ectoderm, and mesoderm. Most often, ES cells are differentiated in a stromal cell-independent manner to give rise to three dimensional, differentiated cell masses called embryoid bodies (EBs, **Figs. 1,5–6**). ES cells can also be differentiated two-dimensionally on stromal cells (typically OP9 cells) or on type IV collagen coated tissue culture plates without intermediate formation of the EB structure ***(7,30)***. The following is a sample protocol for differentiating ES cells via three-dimensional EBs. We found that liquid (suspension) differentiation works well for early EBs (up to d 5–6) and methylcellulose differentiation for late EBs (d 6–14). The methylcellulose (Fluka, 64630) medium contains the same reagents as liquid differentiation medium, with the addition of methylcellulose (*see* **Subheading 2**).

1. Two days prior to setting up the differentiation cultures, split ES cells (4×10^5 ES cells per T25 flask) into an ES-IMDM medium without feeder cells in T-25 flasks. All flasks should be gelatinized.
2. Change medium the next day.
3. Set up differentiation cultures on d 2 as follows:
   a. Aspirate the medium from the flask.
   b. Add 1 mL of trypsin, swirl, and remove quickly.
   c. Add 1 mL of trypsin and wait until cells start to come off the plastic (approx 1–2 min). Do not overtrypsinize cells.
   d. Stop the reaction by adding 1 mL of FCS (same as that used for differentiation) and 4 mL of IMDM and pipet up and down to make a single cell suspension. It is important not to have cell clumps. Transfer to a 14-mL snap cap tube (Falcon; cat. no. 352059).
   e. Centrifuge for 5 to 10 min at 1000 rpm in a Sorvall RT7 tabletop centrifuge or equivalent. Wash the cell pellet in 10 mL of IMDM (without FCS). Spin again at 1000 rpm for 5 to 10 min.
   f. Resuspend the cell pellet in 5 mL of IMDM (with 10% FCS) and count viable ES cells using 2% eosin solution in PBS. Make sure to count ES cells only: the ES cells will appear shiny and smooth, while STO cells are larger and granular. Add 6,000 to 10,000 ES cells per mL of differentiation media to obtain d 2.75-3 EBs. Add 4000 to 5000 cells per mL to obtain d 4–5 EBs. Add 500 to 2000 cells per mL to obtain d 6 to 10 EBs. (**Note:** Use more cells for ES lines that differentiate poorly.)
   g. Primary differentiation is set up based on the cell number required for subsequent (replating) experiments. Total EB cell numbers typically obtained are as follows: d 2.75, approx 0.5–1 × 10^6 EB cells/10 mL of differentiation; d 4, approx 2–3 × 10^6 EB cells/10 mL of differentiation; d 6, approx 3–5 × 10^6 EB cells/10 mL of differentiation.

Differentiation Medium

	Liquid	Methylcellulose
2X methylcellulose	—	1%
FCS (preselected)	15%	15%
Ascorbic acid (5 mg/mL)	50 µg/mL	50 µg/mL
L-glutamine (200 m*M*)	2 m*M*	2 m*M*
MTG	4.5×10^{-4} *M*	4.5×10^{-4} *M*
IMDM	up to 100%	up to 100%

3.3. Hematopoietic Replating

Hematopoietic progenitors present within EBs can be assayed by directly replating EB cells. Day 2.75 to 3 EBs are typically used for the blast colony assay ***(26,27)***, d 4 EBs for primitive erythroid colonies (*see* **Note 4**), and d 6 to 10 EBs for definitive erythroid and myeloid (*see* **Note 4**) progenitor analysis ***(5,6)***. **Figure 3** shows the typical morphology of a blast colony, which normally contains approx 100 to 200 cells.

1. Harvest EBs. 1) EBs in liquid: Transfer media containing EBs into 50-mL tubes. Wash the plate with IMDM. Let it sit at room temperature for approx 10 to 20 min. EBs will settle down to the bottom of the tube. 2) EBs in methylcellulose: Add equal volume of cellulase (2 U/mL, final 1 U/mL) and incubate 20 min at 37°C. Collect EBs in 50-mL tubes. Wash the plate with IMDM and pool with the first EB-containing medium. Let the 50-mL tubes sit at room temperature for about 10 to 20 min. EBs will settle down to the bottom of the tube.
2. Aspirate off the media, add 3 mL of trypsin and incubate for 3 min at 37°C (in a water bath). Vortex quickly and add 1 mL of FCS (same serum as that used for differentiation).

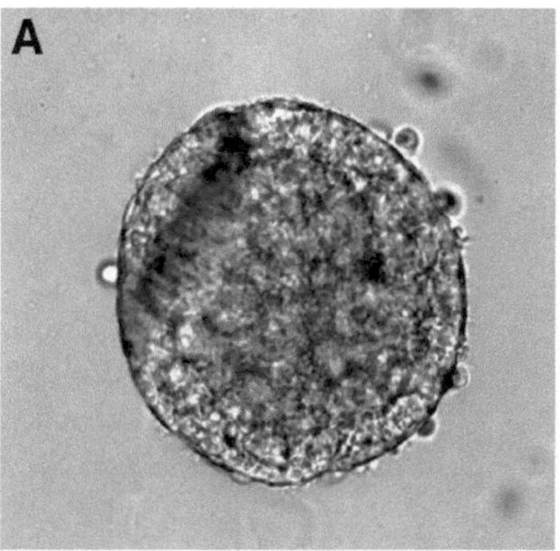

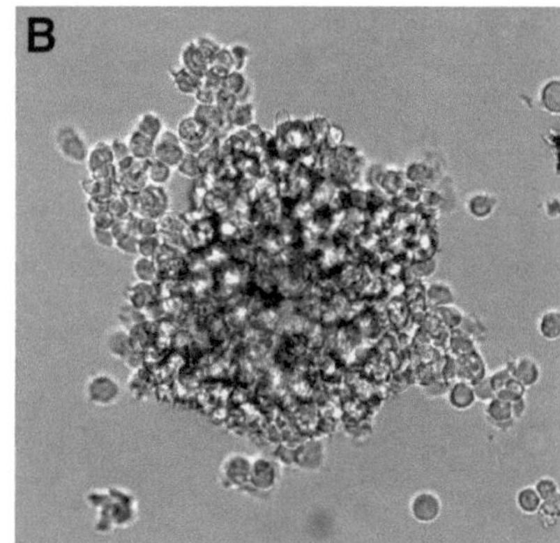

Fig. 3. A typical morphology of EB (**A**) and blast colony (**B**) is shown. Note that individual cells are not visible in EBs, whereas individual cells can be distinguished in blast colonies.

Dissociate through a 20-gage needle by passaging four to five times. Transfer to a 14-mL snap cap tube and spin for 5 to 10 min at 1000 rpm in a Sorvall RT7 tabletop centrifuge or equivalent. Use collagenase for older EBs (>d 9, for example). When collagenase is used, incubate EBs for 1 h at 37°C.

3. Resuspend the cell pellet in 0.3 to 1 mL of IMDM (with 10% FCS). Count the viable cells. At this point, there should be no cell clumps.
4. Add 3–6 × 10^4 EB cells per 1 mL of methylcellulose replating media. Add 1.25 mL of methylcellulose mix to each 35-mm bacterial dish for blast colony assays (*see* **Note 5**). For all other assays, add 1 mL of methylcellulose mixture to each dish. Prepare enough methylcellulose mixture to allow for three replica dishes for each sample plus some extra (to adjust for loss during pipetting). For example, prepare 4.5 mL of methylcellulose replating media for the blast colony assay and 4 mL of methylcellulose replating media for erythroid and myeloid colony assays. (**Note:** use syringes for dispensing methylcellulose. A needle (16 gage) is attached to the syringe when adding methylcellulose-cell mixture to Petri dishes).

Replating

	Blast	Primitive Erythroid	Definitive Erythroid and Myeloid
Methylcellulose	1 %	1 %	1 %
FCS	10 %	—	—
Plasma derived serum (PDS)	—	10 %	10 %
Ascorbic acid	12.5 μg/mL	12.5 μg/mL	12.5 μg/mL
L–glutamine	2 m*M*	2 m*M*	2 m*M*
Transferrin	200 μg/mL	200 μg/mL	200 μg/mL
MTG	4.5×10^{-4} *M*	4.5×10^{-4} *M*	4.5×10^{-4} *M*
D4T C.M.	20%	—	—
VEGF	5 ng/mL	—	—
KL	1%	—	1%
Epo	—	2 U/mL	2 U/mL
PFHM–II	—	5%	5%

(Continued on next page)

Replating *(Continued)*

	Blast	Primitive Erythroid	Definitive Erythroid and Myeloid
IL–1	—	—	5 ng/mL
IL–3	—	—	1%
IL–6	—	—	5 ng/mL
IL–11	—	—	5–25 ng/mL
G–CSF	—	—	2–30 ng/mL
GM–CSF	—	—	3–5 ng/mL or 20 μg/mL
M–CSF	—	—	2–5 ng/mL
IMDM	to 100%	to 100%	to 100%

4. Notes

1. Some workers maintain ES cells in gelatinized flasks without STO feeder cells. We found that ES cells maintained on STO feeder cells give more consistent in vitro differentiation results compared to those maintained in gelatinized flasks.
2. When ES cells differentiate poorly, we check MTG and ascorbic acid. We typically open a new bottle of MTG after 1 to 2 mo. Ascorbic acid needs to be made fresh every time setting up a differentiation.
3. D4T conditioned medium (C.M.) appears to be important to obtain healthy blast colonies. D4T is an endothelial cell line generated from d 4 EBs transformed with polyoma middle T gene ***(26,27)***. We have not checked other endothelial cell conditioned media for their ability to support blast colony formation. Conditioned medium is prepared as follows: D4T endothelial cells are cultured in 10% FCS in IMDM. Medium is changed to 4% FCS in IMDM when the culture becomes approx 80% confluent. Culture an additional 72 h and collect the supernatant. Spin down for 5 min at 1000 rpm in a Sorvall RT7 tabletop centrifuge or equivalent to remove cell debris and filter sterilize the supernatant with 0.45-μm filter unit. Prepare 5- to 10-mL aliquots and store at –80°C. Once thawed, D4T C.M. can be stored at 4°C for about 1 wk.
4. We typically use plasma-derived serum for primitive erythroid and for myeloid colony replating. The red color of erythroid colonies appears to be more vivid in cultures containing plasma-derived serum. Premade methylcellulose mixture (Methocult GF M3434, cat. no. 03434, StemCell Technologies) can successfully be used for replating d 4 and 9 EBs.
5. The blast colony assay is very sensitive. ES cells should look healthy and fresh (shiny and smooth). Mouse ES cells grow rapidly, with an average division time of about 8 h. Therefore, ES cells require frequent splitting. We normally split ES cells every 2 d and do not keep ES cells in culture for a long time after the cells are thawed. Typically, a new vial of cells is thawed after five to six passages. We recommend that ES cells be passed one time right after the thaw before setting up differentiation. In practice, independent differentiation cultures are set up from passages two to five.

References

1. Smith, A. G., Heath, J. K., Donaldson, D. D., Wong, G. G., Moreau, J., Stahl, M., and Rogers, D. (1988) Inhibition of pluripotential embryonic stem cell differentiation by purified polypeptides. *Nature* **336,** 688–690.
2. Williams, R. L., Hilton, D. J., Pease, S., Willson, T. A., Stewart, C. L., Gearing, D. P., et al. (1988) Myeloid leukaemia inhibitory factor maintains the developmental potential of embryonic stem cells. *Nature* **336,** 684–687.

3. Bradley, A., Evans, M., Kaufman, M. H., and Robertson, E. (1984) Formation of germ-line chimaeras from embryo-derived teratocarcinoma cell lines. *Nature* **309,** 255–256.
4. Beddington, R. S. and Robertson, E. J. (1989) An assessment of the developmental potential of embryonic stem cells in the midgestation mouse embryo. *Development* **105,** 733–737.
5. Wiles, M. V. and Keller, G. (1991) Multiple hematopoietic lineages develop from embryonic stem (ES) cells in culture. *Development* **111,** 259–267.
6. Keller, G., Kennedy, M., Papayannopoulou, T., and Wiles, M. V. (1993) Hematopoietic commitment during embryonic stem cell differentiation in culture. *Mol. Cell Biol.* **13,** 473–486.
7. Nakano, T., Kodama, H., and Honjo, T. (1994) Generation of lymphohematopoietic cells from embryonic stem cells in culture. *Science* **265,** 1098.
8. Potocnik, A. J., Nielsen, P. J., and Eichmann, K. (1994) In vitro generation of lymphoid precursors from embryonic stem cells. *EMBO J.* **13,** 5274–5283.
9. Risau, W., Sariola, H., Zerwes, H. G., Sasse, J., Ekblom, P., Kemler, R., et al. (1988) Vasculogenesis and angiogenesis in embryonic-stem-cell-derived embryoid bodies. *Development* **102,** 471–478.
10. Wang, R., Clark, R., and Bautch, V. L. (1992) Embryonic stem cell-derived cystic embryoid bodies form vascular channels: an in vitro model of blood vessel development. *Development* **114,** 303–316.
11. Vittet, D., Prandini, M. H., Berthier, R., Schweitzer, A., Martin-Sisteron, H., Uzan, G., et al. (1996) Embryonic stem cells differentiate in vitro to endothelial cells through successive maturation steps. *Blood* **88,** 3424–3431.
12. Yamashita, J., Itoh, H., Hirashima, M., Ogawa, M., Nishikawa, S., Yurugi, T., et al. (2000) Flk1-positive cells derived from embryonic stem cells serve as vascular progenitors. *Nature* **408,** 92–96.
13. Maltsev, V. A., Rohwedel, J., Hescheler, J., and Wobus, A. M. (1993) Embryonic stem cells differentiate in vitro into cardiomyocytes representing sinusnodal, atrial and ventricular cell types. *Mech. Dev.* **44,** 41–50.
14. Maltsev, V. A., Wobus, A. M., Rohwedel, J., Bader, M., and Hescheler, J. (1994) Cardiomyocytes differentiated in vitro from embryonic stem cells developmentally express cardiac-specific genes and ionic currents. *Circ. Res.* **75,** 233–244.
15. Doetschman, T. C., Eistetter, H., Katz, M., Schmidt, W., and Kemler, R. (1985) The in vitro development of blastocyst-derived embryonic stem cell lines: formation of visceral yolk sac, blood islands and myocardium. *J. Embryol. Exp. Morphol.* **87,** 27–45.
16. Drab, M., Haller, H., Bychkov, R., Erdmann, B., Lindschau, C., Haase, H., Morano, I., Luft, F. C., and Wobus, A. M. (1997) From totipotent embryonic stem cells to spontaneously contracting smooth muscle cells: a retinoic acid and db-cAMP in vitro differentiation model. *FASEB J.* **11,** 905–915.
17. Rohwedel, J., Maltsev, V., Bober, E., Arnold, H. H., Hescheler, J., and Wobus, A. M. (1994) Muscle cell differentiation of embryonic stem cells reflects myogenesis in vivo: developmentally regulated expression of myogenic determination genes and functional expression of ionic currents. *Dev. Biol.* **164,** 87–101.
18. Bain, G., Kitchens, D., Yao, M., Huettner, J. E., and Gottlieb, D. I. (1995) Embryonic stem cells express neuronal properties in vitro. *Dev. Biol.* **168,** 342–357.
19. Strubing, C., Ahnert-Hilger, G., Shan, J., Wiedenmann, B., Hescheler, J., and Wobus, A. M. (1995) Differentiation of pluripotent embryonic stem cells into the neuronal lineage in vitro gives rise to mature inhibitory and excitatory neurons. *Mech. Dev.* **53,** 275–287.
20. Fraichard, A., Chassande, O., Bilbaut, G., Dehay, C., Savatier, P., and Samarut, J. (1995) In vitro differentiation of embryonic stem cells into glial cells and functional neurons. *J. Cell Sci.* **108,** 3181–3188.

21. Liu, S., Qu, Y., Stewart, T. J., Howard, M. J., Chakrabortty, S., Holekamp, T. F., and McDonald, J. W. (2000) Embryonic stem cells differentiate into oligodendrocytes and myelinate in culture and after spinal cord transplantation. *Proc. Natl. Acad. Sci. USA* **97,** 6126–6131.
22. Bagutti, C., Wobus, A. M., Fassler, R., and Watt, F. M. (1996) Differentiation of embryonal stem cells into keratinocytes: comparison of wild-type and beta 1 integrin-deficient cells. *Dev. Biol.* **179,** 184–196.
23. Dani, C., Smith, A. G., Dessolin, S., Leroy, P., Staccini, L., Villageois, P., et al. (1997) Differentiation of embryonic stem cells into adipocytes in vitro. *J. Cell Sci.* **110,** 1279–1285.
24. Buttery, L. D., Bourne, S., Xynos, J. D., Wood, H., Hughes, F. J., Hughes, S. P., et al. (2001) Differentiation of osteoblasts and in vitro bone formation from murine embryonic stem cells. *Tissue Eng.* **7,** 89–99.
25. Kramer, J., Hegert, C., Guan, K., Wobus, A. M., Muller, P. K., and Rohwedel, J. (2000) Embryonic stem cell-derived chondrogenic differentiation in vitro: activation by BMP-2 and BMP-4. *Mech. Dev.* **92,** 193–205.
26. Kennedy, M., Firpo, M., Choi, K., Wall, C., Robertson, S., Kabrun, N., and Keller, G. (1997) A common precursor for primitive erythropoiesis and definitive haematopoiesis. *Nature* **386,** 488–493.
27. Choi, K., Kennedy, M., Kazarov, A., Papadimitriou, J., and Keller, G. (1998) A common precursor for hematopoietic and endothelial cells. *Development* **125,** 725–732.
28. Millauer, B., Wizigmann-Voos, S., Schnurch, H., Martinez, R., Moller, N. P., Risau, W., et al. (1993) High affinity VEGF binding and developmental expression suggest flk-1 as a major regulator of vasculogenesis and angiogenesis. *Cell* **72,** 835–846.
29. Karasuyama, H. and Melchers, F. (1988) Establishment of mouse cell lines which constitutively secrete large quantities of interleukin 2, 3, 4 or 5, using modified cDNA expression vectors. *Eur. J. Immunol.* **18,** 97–104.
30. Nishikawa, S. I., Nishikawa, S., Hirashima, M., Matsuyoshi, N., and Kodama, H. (1998) Progressive lineage analysis by cell sorting and culture identifies FLK1+VE-cadherin+ cells at a diverging point of endothelial and hemopoietic lineages. *Development* **125,** 1747–1757.

24

Analysis of the Vascular Potential of Hematopoietic Stem Cells

Steven M. Guthrie, Sergio Caballero, Robert N. Mames, Maria B. Grant, and Edward W. Scott

Summary

The hematopoietic stem cells residing in the bone marrow have tremendous proliferative and self-renewing capacity, and until recently these cells were thought to produce only progeny of the blood lineages. We have recently demonstrated that these cells are capable of producing endothelial cells of blood vessels. This chapter will outline the methodology for producing chimeric mice through labeled bone marrow transplantation and induction of these donor cells in order to track their plasticity, or their ability to produce nonhematopoietic tissues, specifically blood vessels.

Key Words: Hematopoietic stem cell; hemangioblast; neovascularization; stem cell; retina; hematopoiesis; endothelial cell.

1. Introduction

It has long been known that residing within the bone marrow of adult animals is a pool of cells called hematopoietic stem cells (HSCs), which can divide to produce all the lineages of the blood. HSCs also produce more of themselves, a process called self-renewal. The self-renewal capacity of the HSC has been demonstrated repeatedly in therapeutic settings, such as in patients who receive transplanted stem cells that home to the bone marrow, take up residence, and produce all the blood products for the remainder of the individual's life *(1)*. Until very recently, the role of HSC was limited to the realm of making blood, but new work has greatly broadened the horizons of these cells *(2–10)*. We have demonstrated that adult HSC retain functional hemangioblast activity—producing both blood and blood vessels—and do so clonally *(2)*. Long-term engrafted HSCs are capable of responding to a combination of exogenous growth factor and ischemic injury to regenerate functional blood vessels. This chapter will describe the process of deriving vascular endothelial cells from cells of the hematopoietic lineage. Using a unique model of inducing retinal ischemia, we show that HSC are able to generate new vessels in both the preretinal and intraretinal space of adult mice in parallel with all blood lineages. The HSC, derived from the

From: *Methods in Molecular Medicine, Vol. 105: Developmental Hematopoiesis: Methods and Protocols.*
Edited by: M. H. Baron © Humana Press Inc., Totowa, NJ

adult bone marrow, demonstrates functional hemangioblast activity in that it not only can clonally differentiate into all hematopoietic cell lineages but it also has the ability to play a significant role in neovascularization with substantial contribution to endothelial tissue in various organs. Thus, the differentiation capacity of the HSC can be broadened with specific stimuli. HSC may have the ability to contribute to cells in various other organs and tissues if the appropriate stimuli can be identified. While other studies have demonstrated the ability of HSCs to contribute to other tissues, this is one of the first reports to demonstrate that they do so in a robust and functional manner at a clonal level ***(2)***.

We have also demonstrated that contribution to neovascularization by HSC is not limited to the eye. Various other organs, such as spleen, kidney, muscle, lung, brain, gastrointestinal tract, and liver, have vascular beds, which we believe contain donor-derived endothelial cells. However, further characterization is necessary and ongoing. Neovascularization in these organs and tissues may have tremendous therapeutic potential.

2. Materials

1. Green fluorescent protein (GFP) bone marrow donor mouse (male).
2. BL6 syngeneic "rescue" bone marrow donor mouse (female).
3. BL6 bone marrow recipient mouse (female).
4. Antibodies (list includes antibody and fluorochrome, all from Pharmingen): B220 (CD45R)-PE (cat. no. 553090), CD3-PE (cat. no. 553064), CD4-PE (cat. no. 553730), CD8-PE (cat. no. 01045A), CD11B (Mac-1)-PE (cat. no. 553311), FLK1-PE (cat. no. 555308), Gr1 (Ly6C)-PE (cat. no. 553128), TER119 (Ly-76)-PE (cat. no. 553673), CD117 (c-Kit)-APC (cat. no. 553356), SCA1-biotinylated (cat. no. 553334), streptavadin-PharRed (cat. no. 554067), streptavidin-PE (cat. no. 554061), Factor VIII-PE (Abcam Ab6345), PECAM1-biotinylated (cat no. 553371), and MECA32-biotinylated (cat no. 558773), all stored at 4°C in the dark.
5. O.C.T. embedding medium (Sakura Finetechnical, Tokyo, Japan).
6. Tissue culture treated plates, Dulbecco's modified Eagle's medium (Gibco 11965-084) containing 10% Fetal Bovine Sera (Research Sera RS-50-05), 1X phosphate-buffered saline (PBS).
7. Milteny magnetic-activated cell sorting (MACS) equipment: Sca-1 microbeads (cat. no. 130-057-701) directly conjugated to antibody; stored at 4°C.
8. γ Irradiator.
9. FACSvantage SE/caliber equipment.
10. Ficoll Plaque Plus (Amersham Biosciences, cat. no. 17-1440-02).
11. General anesthetic/inhalant anesthetic.
12. Sulfamethoxazole and trimethoprim oral suspension, 10 mL per 500 mL of water, administered orally.
13. Source of vascular endothelial growth factor (VEGF), such as viral or commercially available recombinant protein, for example, Sigma V-6137 or R&D 494-005.
14. Laser–HGM COMPAC plus model number E-001.
15. Tetramethyl rhodamine isothiocyanate (TRITC)-conjugated dextran (160,000 average. MW, Sigma R-9379), 100 mg dissolved in 100 mL of 4% paraformaldehyde (Sigma P-6148)/phosphate-buffered saline, pH 7.4, prepared fresh each time.
16. Vectashield (Vector Labs H1200) stored at 4°C in the dark; slides and coverslips. A light-proof container that will be stored at 4°C is also needed for the mounted retinas.

17. Confocal microscope.
18. Microtome and slide staining equipment.
19. Sodium fluorescein (10% AK-fluor, Akorn cat. no. NDC-17478-256-10), 50 µL diluted in 50 mL of Avertin, injected subcutaneously.
20. Curved forceps (Roboz, cat. no. RS-5137).
21. Stereo dissecting microscope (Fisher, cat. no. 12-5-62-11).

3. Methods

The following methods described outline: 1) the generation of the GFP/BL6 chimera, 2) the induction of the retinal neovascularization, 3) the enucleation of the eye for mounting, and 4) examination of neovascularization via confocal microscopy and immunohistochemistry staining of serial sections.

3.1. The GFP/BL6 Chimera

The generation of the chimeric GFP/BL6 animal is described in **Subheadings 3.1.1.** through **3.1.5.** This includes 1) the harvesting of bone marrow from the GFP donor animal, 2) the purification and preparation of the marrow for FACS sorting of HSC, 3) the preparation of the BL6 "rescue marrow" (*see* **Subheadings 3.1.4.**) and recipient animals, and 4) the HSC transplant and associated animal husbandry issues.

3.1.1. Harvesting Bone Marrow

1. The GFP transgenic mouse used as the donor strain was obtained from Andras Nagy at Mount Sinai in Toronto, Canada, described in **ref. *11***. The strain carries a GFP transgene driven by a chicken beta-actin promoter and cytomegalovirus (CMV) intermediate early enhancer. All cell types within this animal express GFP (*see* **Note 1**).
2. The BL6 females were obtained from Jackson Laboratories (Bar Harbor, Maine) and should be at least 5-wk-old at the time of bone marrow transplantation (*see* **Note 2**).
3. After fully grown GFP males are euthanized and sacrificed according to proper institutional guidelines, immediately begin surgical removal of the long bones in the legs. Remove all muscle, tendon, and ligature from bone and place the cleaned bone in ice-cold PBS. Each bone end can then be pruned back approx 1 to 2 mm to expose the hollow core of the marrow space. The bone marrow can then be flushed out into a tissue culture treated plate by inserting a 26-gage needle into one end of the bone and flushing 1 to 2 mL of media through the hollow bone core.
4. Repeat until all the bones have been flushed, keeping the cells on ice at all times.
5. Gently triturate the combined volume of cells with a 26-gage needle to break up the cell clumps, and allow to adhere to the plate for 120 min. This step allows for an initial enrichment of HSC away from other adherent progenitor cells such as mesenchymal stem cells. Hematopoietic progenitor stromal cells adhere to the tissue culture treated plastic, whereas HSC will remain suspended in the media.
6. Gently draw up the complete volume of media containing the HSC, wash in >10 mL volume of cold media and pellet. All centrifugation steps are performed at 4°C at 1000*g* unless noted otherwise. Resuspend cells in a proper staining volume as outlined by the protocol of the Milteny MACS system in the following section.

3.1.2. Initial Purification of HSC by MACS

1. Initial purification is done through sorting of the cells by magnetic beads using the Milteny MACS system. Briefly, cells will be stained with an antibody conjugated to a magnetic bead. When these cells are then run over a column in the presence of a magnetic field,

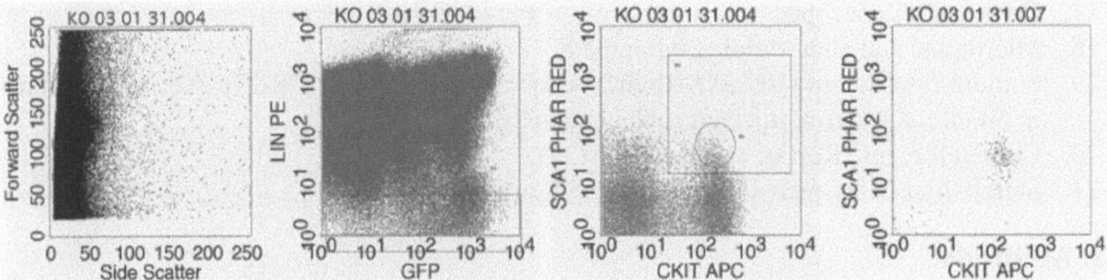

Fig. 1. FACS of stained bone marrow cells. First panel: forward and side scatter of cells and gate R1 drawn. Second panel: cells sorted based on lineage markers and GFP fluorescence. Lineage positive cells are excluded in gate R2. Third Panel: cells sorted based on c-Kit and Sca-1 expression. Cells first sorted in larger gate and then receive another pass through the smaller gate. Fourth panel: reanalysis of doubly sorted cells that will be used for transplantation.

cells which carry the specific surface antigens, and thus have the antibody-bead bound to them, will adhere to the column (termed "positive fraction"). Cells that do not present that surface marker ("negative fraction") will pass directly through the magnetic field and be removed from the positive fraction of cells. The magnetic field can then be removed and the positive fraction collected from the column.

2. To begin MACS enrichment, cell number and viability must be determined from the total marrow flushed from the long bones to ensure that the correct amount of antibody, beads, and staining volume will be used (*see* **Note 3**). To determine the cell number, resuspend the washed cells in Trypan blue and count bright cells using a hemacytometer under a phase-contrast microscope. Wash cells in >10 mL cold PBS and stain with Sca-1 microbeads in appropriate volume. Run the cells over two separate columns, this time discarding the flow-through and keeping the positive fraction. At this time a >90% Sca-1 positive purity typically has been achieved.
3. After enrichment, cells are immediately pelleted and placed back on ice for fluorescent antibody staining for FACS sorting.

3.1.3. Final Purification of HSC by FACS

1. Again all antibody concentrations and incubation times are followed according to the parameters described by the manufacturer guidelines.
2. For our HSC purification we use three different fluorochromes: c-Kit conjugated to APC, biotynylated Sca-1 (with Streptavidin-PharRed secondary antibody), and the lineage markers B220, CD3, CD4, CD8, CD11B, Flk-1, Gr-1, and TER-119, all directly conjugated to PE.
3. The FACSvantage SE is able to isolate single cells based on the surface antigen bound by antibodies and hence the spectrum of absorbance and fluorescence emitted by that cell.
4. Two rounds of purification are necessary to ensure complete removal of all non-HSC cells. *See* **Fig. 1** for of an example of the gates used to isolate single HSC.
5. The flow rate is set at 10,000 events per second with no greater than an 10% abort proportion.
6. The cells are then collected in media immediately after completion of the sort and are isolated and injected into the recipient animals following "rescue" marrow isolation and recipient preparation. *See* **Subheading 3.1.5.**

3.1.4. Harvesting of BL6 Rescue Marrow With HSC Depletion and Irradiation of Recipient Animals

1. The harvesting of non-GFP female BL6 marrow is performed in the same manner as the HSC, except these cells are not given time to adhere to the tissue culture treated plate.
2. Once the marrow has been flushed, washed, and counted, a Sca-1 depletion is done to remove any HSC from the rescue marrow, which would compete with the donor GFP HSC (*see* **Note 4**).
3. Again cells are stained as described in the MACS magnetic bead section, but this time the cells are SCA-1 depleted three times to ensure that the rescue marrow is devoid of HSC.
4. Irradiate recipient BL6 mice with 850-950 RADS of γ radiation to prepare the bone marrow for transplantation.

3.1.5. Purified GFP HSC and Depleted Rescue Marrow Transplantation and Animal Husbandry Concerns

1. Count the rescue marrow and aliquot 1×10^6 cells in a 100 µL of volume into a fresh Eppendorf tube.
2. The highly enriched HSC can be singly isolated in the following manner. A volume of the sorted sample is placed on a glass drop slide and examined under a phase-contrast microscope. The cells must be diluted to a concentration where single cells can be visualized, isolated, and captured one at a time with a micropipet. Under the scope isolate a single, round, bright, viable cell and draw up into a pulled glass micropipet by mouth pipeting with a suction tube. Examine the needle and visualize the cell to ensure that only one cell was drawn. Place the cell into the 100-µL aliquot.
3. Draw the rescue/single HSC mixture into a fresh insulin needle and syringe to ensure no contamination of other samples.
4. Inject an anesthetized, irradiated BL6 animal in the retro-orbital sinus cavity or tail vein. The animals should be monitored until they overcome the effects of the anesthetic and must then be placed on a regime of antibiotics for the next month until multilineage engraftment has been verified (*see* **Note 5**).

3.1.6. Verification of Multilineage Reconstitution

1. The recipient animals are given 1 mo to recover and allow the transplanted HSC sufficient time to begin producing the various hematopoietic cell lineages.
2. Determination of engraftment is resolved by peripheral blood sampling and FACS scanning (*see* **Note 6**). Sample blood from each animal through a tail vein bleed and collect blood in a tube containing PBS and 5 m*M* ethylene diamine tetraacetic acid, which inhibits coagulation.
3. Remove red blood cells through a Ficoll purification as outlined in the instructions. Briefly, layer the blood/PBS volume on top of an equal volume of Ficoll.
4. Centrifuge and remove the "buffy" layer at the interface.
5. Wash the lymphocyte layer containing the nucleated cells and stain with the various lineage marker antibodies conjugated to PE or some other non-GFP fluorochrome.
6. Samples are analyzed by FACS, and animals exhibiting GFP-positive cells of the various lineages are scored positive for engraftment (*see* **Note 7**).
7. The positive animals are then allowed to go an additional three months and multi-lineage engraftment is reconfirmed to demonstrate long-term engraftment by HSC (**Fig. 2**).
8. Exogenous growth factor is then administered as described in **Subheading 3.2.**

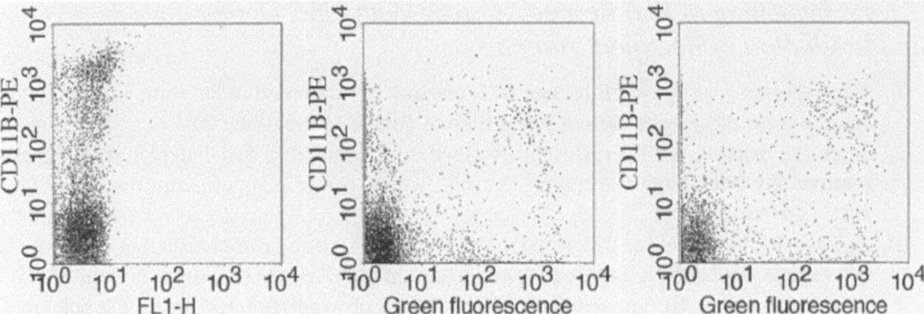

Fig. 2. Confirmation of peripheral GFP blood in recipient animals. First panel is from a nonengrafted animal. The other two panels are typical engraftment levels.

3.2. Induction of Retinal Ischemia

1. The next step involves administration of an endogenous growth factor and vessel damage to promote blood vessel growth in the retina. Fully and robustly engrafted animals are selected and anesthetized.
2. VEGF is administered directly into the vitreous using a 36-gage needle and Hamilton syringe (*see* **Note 8**). Either purified (40 μg/kg) VEGF protein or AAV–VEGF virus (2×10^8 viral particles), where the CMV promotor drives expression of VEGF in an adeno-associated virus (AAV) vector, can be used. VEGF is an endothelial cell-specific mitogen that is transcriptionally regulated by the cytomegalovirus promoter/enhancer when packaged in AAV. AAV mediates the long-term expression in nondividing cells, which allows for stable expression and constant amounts of VEGF to reach the area of ischemia to promote neovascularization (**Fig. 3**; **ref.** ***12***).
3. The study of clinical diseases, such as diabetic retinopathy and retinopathy of prematurity, has led to an understanding of the pathology that occurs in these diseases. In these conditions, the eye "detects" a lack of oxygen, either as a result of the diabetic condition or the removal from the incubator's oxygen-rich environment of a prematurely born baby. As a result, the cells signal new blood vessel growth in the region in an attempt to relieve the perceived ischemia. We take advantage of this neovascularization by creating a local region of ischemia in the eye through cauterizing of large blood vessels with a laser. This induces new blood vessel growth into the region in an attempt to relieve the ischemic pressure.
4. Peak expression of VEGF by AAV has been determined to be at 3 to 6 wk; therefore, the physical disruption of the blood vessels is done during this time (unpublished data). Begin by anesthetizing the mice normally with a general anesthetic, and concurrently administer a 10% sodium fluorescein solution intraperitoneally, which labels blood vessels for facilitating visualization during procoagulation.
5. Dilate the eyes with 1% atropine for 5 min, wash with PBS, and subsequently dilate with 2.5% phenylephrine for 5 min (*see* **Note 9**).
6. Immediately after the two 5-min treatments, the mice undergo laser treatment. An Argon Green laser system (HGM Corporation, Salt Lake City, UT) can be used for retinal vessel photocoagulation with the aid of a 78-diopter lens. The blue-green argon laser (wavelength 488–514 nm) is applied to various venous sites around the optic nerve.
7. Venous occlusions are accomplished with >60 burns of 1-s duration, 50 m*M* spot size, and 50 to 100 mW intensity.

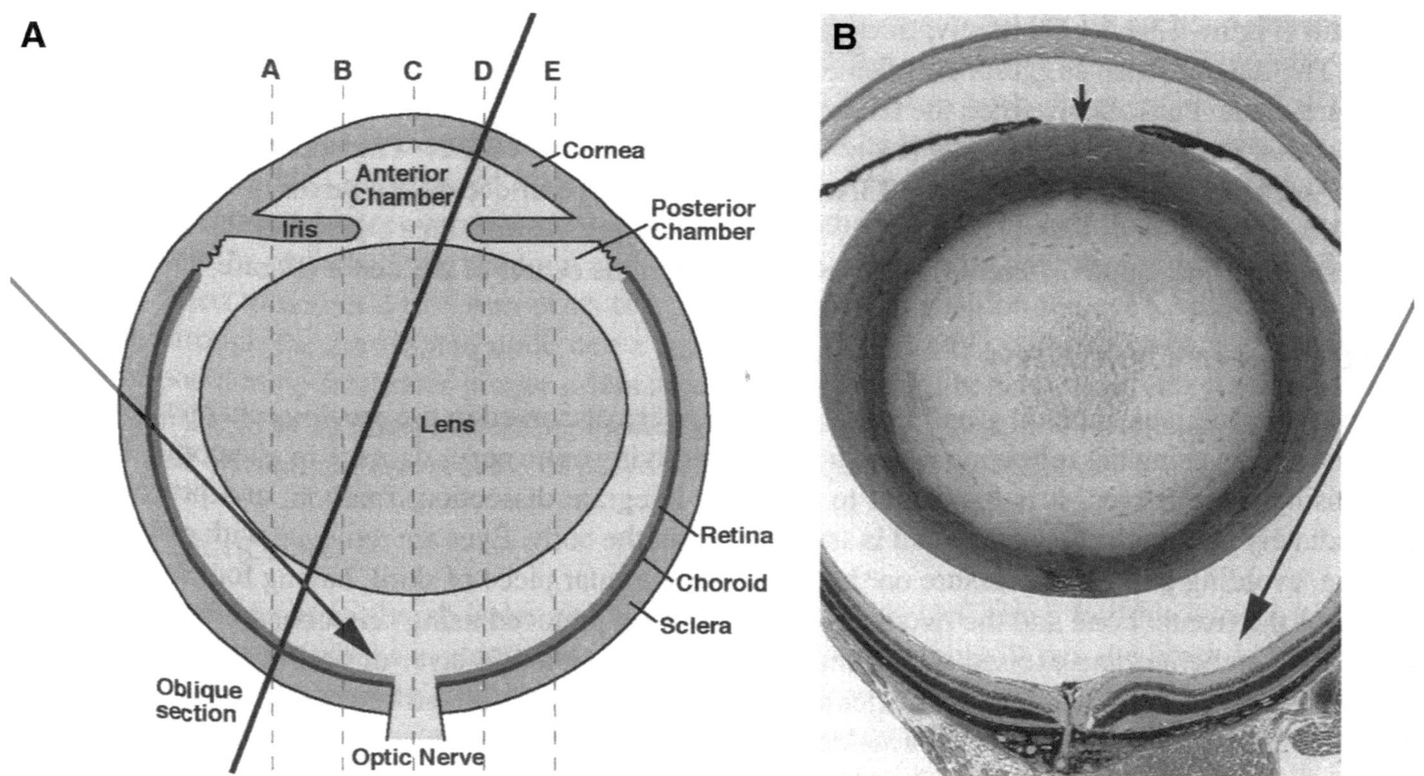

Fig. 3. Illustration and sectional representation of the eye for growth factor administration. Arrows indicate angle and placement of needle for growth factor injection (*see* **Note 8**).

8. Again, allow the animals to recover for 30 d while the transplanted HSC, directed by the ischemia and induced by the VEGF, contribute to the neovascularization to relieve the hypoxia produced by the cauterizing of the existing vessels.

3.3. Eye Removal

1. One month after ischemic injury the eyes are ready to be enucleated and neovascularization imaged by confocal microscopy.
2. Mice are first anesthetized and then perfused while sedated.
3. Peripheral blood and bone marrow should be collected to confirm donor contribution analysis by FACS with lineage specific antibodies conjugated to PE (BD BioSciences, San Jose, CA) similarly to the procedure outlined in **Subheading 3.1.6.** First, the chest cavity is opened and the ribs cut away to expose the heart completely. The left atrium is punctured with a 26-gage needle. Inject >3 mL of 50 mg/mL TRITC-conjugated dextran in 4% paraformaldehyde/PBS slowly into the left ventricle (*see* **Note 10**).
4. Immediately afterwards the eyes are removed by sliding a curved forceps underneath the eyeball and pulling the eye out.
5. Puncture the eye with a 26-gage needle to allow complete perfusion of the eye.
6. Place the eye in fresh phosphate-buffered paraformaldehyde (4%) and shake at room temperature for 30 min.
7. Transfer the eye to 1X PBS and wash by shaking at room temperature for 30 min to overnight.
8. After washing with PBS the eyes are ready for dissection. With the eye positioned on the stage of a stereo dissecting microscope, make an initial incision in the cornea.
9. Enlarge the opening until it is large enough to accommodate the lens of the eye. Gently push the lens forward until it pushes through the hole cut in the cornea. Trim away the remaining cornea until roughly the halfway mark where the sclera and cornea meet. The retina can easily be dissected away from the retinal-pigmented epithelium now.
10. Gently push down on the posterior portion of the retinal-pigmented epithelium and roll the forceps forward. The retina will "pop out" and can readily be mounted (*see* **Note 11**). Place the retina on a glass slide, make five to six cuts around the periphery so that the retina lies flat and place the tissue in Vectashield mounting medium (Vector Laboratories, Burlingame, CA) to inhibit photobleaching. The retinas can immediately be imaged or stored at 4°C in the dark for up to a wk, although immediate imaging is ideal.
11. We used an Olympus IX-70, with inverted stage, attached to the Bio-Rad Confocal 1024 ES system for fluorescence microscopy. A Krypton-Argon laser with emission detector wavelengths of 598 nm and 522 nm differentiated the red and green fluorescence. The lenses used in our system were the (Olympus) 10X/0.4 Uplan Apo, 20X/0.4 LC Plan Apo, 40X/0.85 Uplan Apo, 60X/1.40 oil Plan Apo and 100X/1.35 oil Uplan Apo. The software was OS/2 Laser Sharp. (**Fig. 4**)
12. Immunohistochemistry can be performed on eyes, which are not imaged by confocal microscopy. Enucleate the eyes and place in 4% buffered paraformaldehyde overnight. The next day place the eyes in 30% sucrose until they sink. Place the eyes in O.C.T. embedding medium and flash freeze. Once completely frozen, the eye can be sectioned similarly to other tissues. Once sections are cut, wash in PBS, block, and stain normally. Sections can be imaged immediately by fluorescence or confocal microscopy (**Fig. 5**).

4. Notes

1. GFP expression is driven by the chicken beta actin promoter and is ubiquitously expressed; however, it is present only in actively dividing cells, in the mitotic spindle. It should be

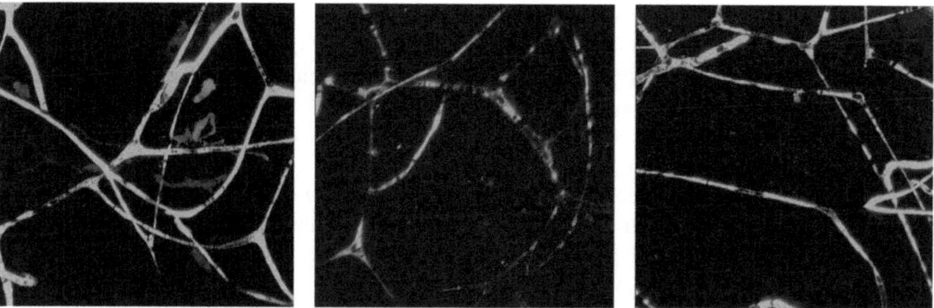

Fig. 4. Areas of neovascularization in the retina. The red channel (TRITC–dextran) and green channel (GFP donor-derived cells) have been merged producing the orange/yellow color indicating areas of colocalization. *See* color insert following p. 80.

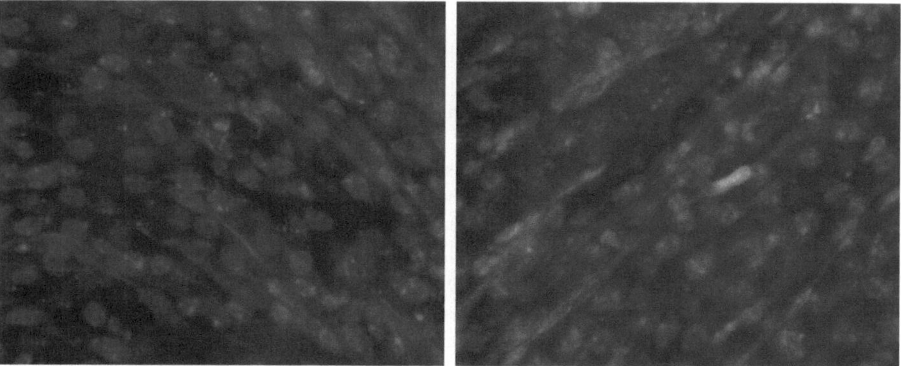

Fig. 5. Immunohistochemistry of kidney tissue sections. The tissues were stained with PECAM1, an endothelial cell specific surface antigen. These cells label red and are lining the blood vessel walls. The green cell is donor-derived, indicating that in rare events, under normal conditions, HSCs contribute to endothelial cells in other tissues. *See* color insert following p. 80.

noted that HSC are generally quiescent. Therefore, GFP expression is not expected to be strong in these cells at the time of HSC harvesting.

2. Recent controversy concerning the events that occur when stem cells contribute to repair has led to the concern and possibility that this may not be an inherent ability of the stem cell but rather a fusion event which occurs between the stem cell and target tissue. Transplantation of male HSC into female recipients directly addresses this issue by allowing for fluorescent *in situ* hybridization of tissue samples to detect X and Y chromosomes and, thus, to determine if a fusion event has occurred.
3. It must be stressed that the correct amount of antibody and volume must be used so that the antibody concentration is optimal for binding to the cells. Unfortunately, a slight miscalculation can cause the complete loss of the desired cell population.
4. HSCs do not adhere to tissue culture treated plastic, but precursors do; therefore, do not allow time for the adherence of the rescue cells.

5. Because the animals received a lethal dose of irradiation their immune systems will experience an interruption and decrease the ability to stave off and combat infection. The antibiotic regime, usually an oral suspension of Bactrim, is sufficient to maintain the animal until the graft immune system has had enough time to recover and begin producing the immune cells of the hematopoietic lineage. Consult veterinary staff for recommended antibiotic regime in use at your institution.
6. The amount of γ irradiation administered is determined by the dose required to kill 90% of the animals without transplantation. Because the radiation dose is not 100% lethal, even without a HSC transplant some animals will recover on their own.
7. Several HSC may have taken up residence in the bone marrow niche, but at any given time only one or two HSC need be cycling to produce the maintenance levels of lineage blood products. As a result some animals may seem to have a greater proportion of GFP cells in the bone marrow than in the peripheral blood.
8. Special care should be taken when injections are done. Any "nicking" or damaging of the lens will result in a cataract making the laser treatment impossible. Also retina and choroid damage from an injection made too deeply will result in bleeding rendering the animal useless for photocoagulation.
9. Unnecessary amounts of atropine should be "blotted" off the eye, and the length of time it is administered should not exceed 5 min. While under the general anesthetic, the mice could experience cardiac difficulties from the systemic absorption of the atropine leading to distress and possible death.
10. Gentle physical massaging of the heart by squeezing with fingers for 60 s after the complete volume of perfusate was injected was found to increase the quality of the vessel perfusion.
11. Technical limitations prevent the use of flat-mounted retinas for both confocal microscopy and for immunocytochemistry. The thickness of the retina (approx 200 μm) prevents adequate diffusion of antibody. If experimental design necessitates, select mice to perfuse with buffer containing Hoechst stain to label nuclei and delineate the vascular lumen. Stain with hematoxylin, and counter-stained with PE-conjugated anti-Factor VIII or Biotin-conjugated anti-PECAM-1 and anti-MECA-32 followed by avidin-PE (BD BioSciences, San Jose, CA). These antibodies bind specifically to endothelial cells, and cells where GFP and PE colocalize are HSC-derived endothelial cells. This methodology, however, prevents the visualization of intact capillary tufts detectable only by confocal microscopy of the whole flat-mounted retina.

Acknowledgments

This work was supported by NIH grants HL70813, HL70738 (E.W.S.), EY12601 (M.B.G.), and a grant from the Juvenile Diabetes Foundation (M.B.G. and E.W.S.). S.M.G. was supported by NIH Training Grant T32AR07603. E.W.S. is a Leukemia and Lymphoma Society Scholar. E.S. is involved with an early stage start-up stem-cell company, RegenMed. This company is virtual, has the possibility to license any patents that might arise from stem-cell studies developed through academic-supported activities, and has the goal of working with other companies to develop stem-cell related products for drug discovery or testing and the development of potential therapeutics.

References

1. Buckner, C. D., Epstein, R. B., Rudolph, R. H., Clift, R. A., Storb, R., and Thomas, E. D. (2001) Allogeneic marrow engraftment following whole body irradiation in a patient with leukemia. *J. Hematother. Stem Cell Res.* **10,** 201–208.

2. Grant, M. B., May, W. S., Caballero, S., Brown, G. A., Guthrie, S. M., Mames, R. N., et al. (2002) Adult hematopoietic stem cells provide functional hemangioblast activity during retinal neovascularization. *Nat. Med.* **8,** 607–612.
3. Petersen, B. E., Bowen, W. C., Patrene, K. D., Mars, W. M., Sullivan, A. K., Murase, N., et al. (1999) Bone marrow as a potential source for hepatic oval cells. *Science* **284,** 1168–1170.
4. Theise, N. D., Nimmakayalu, M., Gardner, R., Illei, P. B., Morgan, G., Teperman, L., et al. (2000) Liver from bone marrow in humans. *Hepatology* **32,** 11–16.
5. Ferrari, G., Cusella-De Angelis, G., Coletta, M., Paolucci, E., Stornaiuolo, A., Cossu, G., et al. (1998) Muscle regeneration by bone marrow-derived myogenic progenitors. *Science* **279,** 1528–1530.
6. Lagasse, E., Connors, H., Al-Dhalimy, M., Reitsma, M., Dohse, M., Osborne, L., et al. (2000) Purified hematopoietic stem cells can differentiate into hepatocytes in vivo. *Nat. Med.* **6,** 1229–1234.
7. Brazelton, T. R., Rossi, F. M., Keshet, G. I., and Blau, H. M. (2000) From marrow to brain: expression of neuronal phenotypes in adult mice. *Science* **290,** 1775–1779.
8. Mezey, E., Chandross, K. J., Harta, G., Maki, R. A. and McKercher, S. R. (2000) Turning blood into brain: cells bearing neuronal antigens generated in vivo from bone marrow. *Science* **290,** 1779–1782.
9. Orlic, D., Kajstura, J., Chimenti, S., Bodine, D. M., Leri, A., and Anversa P. (2001) Bone marrow cells regenerate infarcted myocardium. *Nature* **410,** 701–705.
10. Krause, D. S., Theise, N. D., Collector, M. I., Henegariu, O., Hwang, S., Gardner, R., et al. (2001) Multi-organ, multi-lineage engraftment by a single bone marrow-derived stem cell. *Cell* **105,** 369–377.
11. Hadjantonakis, A.-K. and Nagy, A. (2000) Use of FACS for the isolation of individual cells from transgenic mice harboring a GFP reporter. *Genesis* **27,** 95–98.
12. Fukumura, D., Gohongi, T., Kadambi, A., Izumi, Y., Ang, J., Yun, C. O., et al. (2001) Predominant role of endothelial nitric oxide synthase in vascular endothelial growth factor-induced angiogenesis and vascular permeability. *Proc. Natl. Acad. Sci. USA* **98,** 2604–2609.

25

Dynamic In Vivo Imaging of Mammalian Hematovascular Development Using Whole Embryo Culture

Elizabeth A. V. Jones, Margaret H. Baron, Scott E. Fraser, and Mary E. Dickinson

Summary

The yolk sac is the initial site of hematopoiesis in the mammalian embryo. As the embryo develops, blood vessels form around primitive erythroblasts to connect the yolk sac to the embryo, delivering newly formed blood cells to the embryonic circulation. The limited accessibility of the mammalian embryo has made it difficult to study the dynamic changes in cellular development during the formation of the early hematovascular system. Therefore, we have developed a culture system for studying early hematopiesis, vasculogenesis. and angiogenesis in the mouse embryo. Early embryos (E7.5–E9.5) can be grown on the microscope stage to study the dynamics as vessels form and circulation begins. In addition, this mouse embryo culture system provides an excellent model for understanding the interplay between flow dynamics and cellular development.

Key Words: Post-implantation embryo; embryo culture; microscopy; time-lapse imaging; yolk sac; primitive hematopoiesis; vasculogenesis.

1. Introduction

The mouse hematopoietic system begins to differentiate from the mesodermal germ layer just after E6.5 *(1,2)*. The first site of hematopoiesis, or blood formation, in mammalian embryos is the yolk sac. Clusters of primitive erythroblasts surrounded by endothelial cells emerge from extraembryonic mesoderm as "blood islands." The blood islands initially appear in an extraembryonic ring proximal to the embryo proper and then expand to cover the entire yolk sac surface, forming the capillary plexus *(3)*. As the heart begins to contract, around E8.5, vascular channels become perfused, and the red blood cells lose their attachment and begin to circulate within the vessel *(4)*. During the first few days of blood circulation, the primary plexus is remodeled, into a mature vascular network. Thus, there is a window of development, from E7.0 to E9.5, in which most primitive hematopoiesis and vasculogenesis in the yolk sac is established.

From: *Methods in Molecular Medicine, Vol. 105: Developmental Hematopoiesis: Methods and Protocols.* Edited by: M. H. Baron

Because the early mammalian embryo develops in utero and is inaccessible to experimental manipulation, much of what is known about early blood and endothelial cell differentiation has been gleaned from cells in culture or from observations of embryos made at static time points in development. Although this approach has been successful in identifying key candidate molecules involved in cell fate decisions, this paradigm is not well-suited for studying the dynamic events in hematovascular development. Thus, we have developed a method to study these events in living, intact mouse embryos. Using the embryo culture technique described here, it is possible to image normal development from E7.5 until E9.5 *(5)*, which is ideal for studying early cardiovascular development.

2. Materials

2.1. Media

1. Dulbecco's modified Eagle medium (DMEM)/F-12 Medium (Gibco, Carlsbad, CA, cat. no. 11330032).
2. Heat-inactivated fetal bovine serum (FBS; Gibco, Carlsbad, CA, cat. no. 16140063).
3. Penicillin–streptomycin solution (Irvine Scientific, Santa Ana, CA, cat. no. 9366).
4. HEPES buffer solution 1 *M* (Irvine Scientific, Santa Ana, CA, cat. no. 9319).
5. Syringes (3-mL).
6. Acrodisc Syringe Filters (0.2-μm; VWR, West Chester, PA, cat. no, 28144-040).

2.2. Embryo Dissection

1. CD-1 mouse breeding pairs.
2. CO_2 euthanasia chamber.
3. Pair of watchmaker's forceps, no. 5 (Roboz or Fine Science Tools).
4. Petri dishes (60 × 15 mm).
5. Heated dissecting scope: this can be achieved using a chicken incubator heater (Lyon Electric Company, Chula Vista, CA) to blow hot air over the dissection area.

2.3. Preparation of Rat Serum

1. Male rats, approx 20, at least 8 wk old.
2. Vacutainer tubes (Becton-Dickinson, Franklin Lakes, NJ, cat. no. 366512).
3. Venous Access butterfly needle (Becton-Dickinson, Franklin Lakes, NJ, cat. no. 367283).
4. Absorbent bench protector.
5. Rat guillotine (Braintree Scientific, Braintree, MA, cat. no. RG-100).
6. Ether.
7. 50-mL Falcon tubes (Becton-Dickinson, Franklin Lakes, NJ, cat. no. 352098).
8. Acrodisc syringe filters (0.45 μm; VWR, West Chester, PA, cat. no 28144-007).

2.4. Culture Chamber Components

1. Nunc Lab-tek 2-well, chambered cover glass (Nalge Nunc, Rochester, NY, cat. no. 155380).
2. Soldering iron.
3. Mineral oil, embryo-tested (Sigma, St. Louis, MO, cat. no. M8410).
4. 3/16-in. Silicone Airline Tubing (Hagen, Holm, Germany; cat. no. 11127).
5. Barbed polypropylene fitting, reducing connector, 1/16- to 1/8-in. (Cole-Parmer Instrument,Chicago, IL, cat. no. EW06365-44).
6. Teflon tape.
7. Silicon grease (Dow Corning, Midland, MI).

8. Gas-washing bottle (Fisher Scientific, Springfield, NJ).
9. Pressurized cylinder with regulator with a 5% CO_2, balance air mixture of gas.

2.5. Microscope and Heater Box Components

1. Inverted microscope equipped for time-lapse imaging.
2. Cardboard (approx 4-mm thick).
3. 5/16-in. Thick, foil-foil insulation thermal insulation (Reflectix, Markleville, IN).
4. Velcro adhesive-backed strips (McMaster-Carr, New Brunswick, NJ, cat. no. 9273K33).
5. Egg-incubator heater (Lyon Electric Company, Chula Vista, CA, cat. no. 115-020).

3. Methods

3.1. Preparation of Rat Serum

This procedure is modified from Hogan et al. *(6)*. Note that male rats are used because female rat blood contains hormones that reduces viability of embryos in culture. Ether is the recommended anesthetic because it evaporates completely from the blood once it is collected. Trace amounts of anesthetic can impair embryonic growth.

1. Anesthetize male rats by placing them in a bell jar containing ether. Once the rats are sedated, remove them from the bell jar and place them on their backs on a square sheet of bench protector in a fume hood. Place a 50-mL Falcon tube containing a piece of ether-soaked paper towel over the rat's nose to keep it sedated.
2. Spray the abdomen with 70% ethanol and make a v-shaped incision into the lower abdomen.
3. Move the intestines to expose the dorsal aorta, which can be identified as a small (around 1 mm in diameter) pulsing artery next to the larger, darker vena cava.
4. Puncture this artery using the butterfly needle. Venous Access butterfly needle consists of a butterfly needle connected by tubing to a normal needle. Once blood is seen in the tubing, the other needle should be thrust into a vacutainer tube in order to create a mild suction (*see* **Note 3**). This procedure requires two people since the butterfly needle needs to be held very still to enable good flow.
5. Invert the vacutainer tubes a few times during blood collection to prevent clotting. With practice, 7 to 8 mL of blood per rat can be obtained.
6. After collection, place the blood sample on ice.
7. Sacrifice the rat and place it in a waste bag. It is convenient to collect blood from approx 20 rats per session, yielding around 50 mL of serum.
8. Carcasses must be left in a fume hood overnight to allow the ether to evaporate, particularly if the animal facility incinerates animal waste.
9. After collection, centrifuge the blood at 1300*g* for 20 min at room temperature.
10. Remove and pool the supernatants in 50-mL Falcon tubes.
11. Centrifuged the serum at 1300*g* for 10 min to remove remaining cells.
12. Heat-inactivate the serum at 56°C for 30 min with the lid of the Falcon tube partially unscrewed to allow the ether to evaporate.
13. Slowly filter the serum using a 0.45-μm filter and aliquot into 1-mL samples.
14. Store in a –80°C freezer for up to 1 yr.

3.2. Preparation of Media

Two types of medium are prepared for the static culture technique: a dissecting medium and a culture medium. Media can be prepared the night before, if desired, and stored at 4°C.

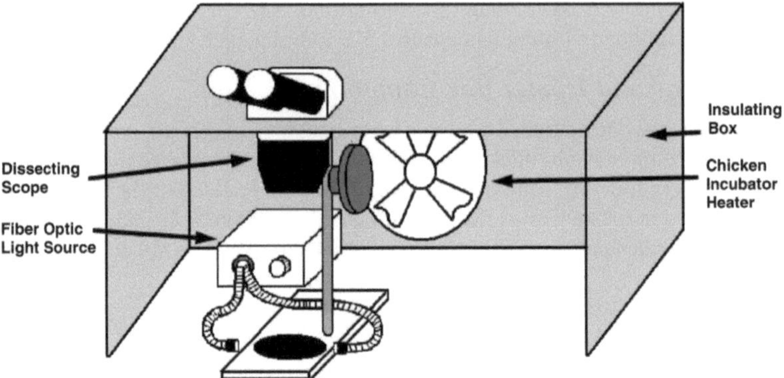

Fig. 1. Heated dissection hood. Dissection microscope can be maintained at 37°C using a chicken incubator heater and an insulated box. The front of the heater box does not need to be enclosed.

3.2.1. Dissection Medium

The dissection medium is composed of 90% DMEM/F-12, 1% HEPES solution, 8% heat-inactivated FBS, and 1% penicillin–streptomycin. Approximately 50 mL of dissection medium is needed per mouse. The FBS and penicillin–streptomycin can be frozen together in aliquots to speed up the medium preparation; however, the HEPES solution should be added fresh. The medium is placed in a water bath at 37°C for at least 1/2 h prior to use.

3.2.2. Culture Medium

The culture medium is 49%DMEM/F-12 (*see* **Note 1**), 49% heat-inactivated rat serum (as described in **Subheading 3.1.**), 1% penicillin–streptomycin solution, and 1% HEPES solution (*see* **Note 2**). Two milliliters of medium are required for a single 21 × 20-mm well of a two-well Lab-tek Chamber slide, with up to three embryos per well. The medium must be sterile-filtered using a 3-mL syringe and a 0.2-μm filter. The tube of medium is then placed in a tissue culture incubator with the lid unscrewed at 37°C for at least 1 h to allow temperature and pH to equilibrate.

3.3. Dissection

1. Set up male and female breeder mice overnight. The presence of a vaginal plug in the morning is considered E0.5.
2. On the E7.5, E8.5 or E9.5, euthanize females with CO_2. Make a v-shaped incision in the lower abdomen and remove the uterine horns. Place these in a Petri dish and cover with warmed dissection medium.
3. Dissect the embryos from the horn in a hood heated to 37°C using a chicken incubator heater (*see* **Fig. 1** and **Note 3**). Techniques for dissection of embryos of various ages have been described elsewhere *(7)*. A small amount of deciduum at the proximal end of the yolk sac should be left in place. Leave the yolk sac intact for E8.5 embryos but remove it for E9.5 embryos (*see* **Note 10**). Change dissecting medium every 15 to 20 min to keep embryos at temperature.

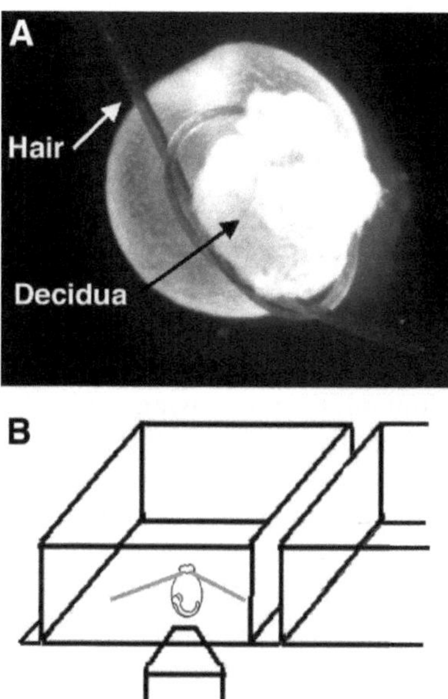

Fig. 2. Immobilization of E8.5 Embryos. E8.5 embryos are immobilized by leaving a small amount of decidua on the ectoplacental cone and tying a piece of human hair around that decidua. The embryos are then positioned on the microscope stage such that the tissue of interest is in view.

4. Using a transfer pipet, move the dissected embryos into Lab-tek chambers, three embryos per well. Add 2 mL of culture medium per well. Place the chamber into the tissue culture incubator for 1 h. Heart rates tend to decrease slightly during dissection since medium is not kept perfectly at 37°C. The time in the tissue culture incubator allows the heart rate to return to normal.

3.4. Immobilization of Embryo

Before imaging the embryos, it is necessary to partially immobilize the E8.5 embryos. At this stage, the yolk sac is more buoyant than the deciduum, causing the embryos to float. They also become very sensitive to small currents in the medium. This is not a concern for earlier stages, in which the yolk sac has not yet expanded. Later-stage embryos (E9.5) are not cultured with the yolk sac and are relatively static.

The embryos are quite sensitive to the method by which they are immobilized. Any attempt to "encase" the embryos, for example, using nitex grating or agar, will exert pressure on the yolk sac, stopping circulation and impeding hematovascular development in the yolk sac. Two methods can be used for immobilization. First, a human hair can be tied in a knot around the deciduum and then used to prop up the embryo in the correct position (**Fig. 2**). Alternatively, an oil micrometer attached to a holding pipet can be used to hold and orient the embryo. The holding pipet requires more effort to set up, but allows a greater amount of control of the embryo.

3.5. The Microscope

The choice of microscope for hematovascular imaging depends on the application and the mode of contrast. Stereo or compound microscopes with transmitted or reflected illumination from a halogen lamp can be used if enough inherent contrast is present in the tissue; however, this is rarely the case. Therefore, most of our imaging work has been performed using a confocal or epifluorescence microscopes in conjunction with a fluorescent label. If fluorescence microscopy is used, care must be taken not to overexpose the embryos because the ultraviolet (UV) or visible range light used for fluorescence excitation can be harmful to the embryos if used for prolonged periods. A confocal microscope with an automated shutter offers precise control over illumination, but microscopes using conventional epifluorescence illumination can be fitted with shutters, triggered by image collection software, to prevent overexposure when images are not being collected (*see* **Note 7**).

For time-lapse imaging, we use an inverted microscope (*see* **Note 8**). The Lab-tek chambers in which the embryos are cultured have cover slip bottoms, a feature that permits the use of either dry, low-magnification objectives, as well as high-magnification, high-numerical aperture, oil- or water-immersion objectives for maximum resolution of single cells. However, the higher the magnification, the more difficult it is to keep the same field of view in focus because of the movement of the embryo. Typically, we use 5X to 20X objectives for imaging, which provide a field of view of 0.2 mm^2 using the LSM 5 PASCAL confocal microscope. Smaller fields of view may require re-alignment of the image to compensate for x-y shifts and/or an autofocus protocol to maintain the plane of imaging along the z-axis.

3.6. Variables in Embryo Culture System

3.6.1. Environmental Control

The most important factor in maintaining normal embryonic development in culture is control of the local environment. For mammalian embryos to develop normally, it is necessary to create a heated and humidified atmosphere, with appropriate gas transfer. Thus, maintaining temperature control, preventing evaporation and regulating gas exchange in the chamber are the most critical aspects of this culture method.

3.6.2. Temperature Control

The hematovascular system is one of the most temperature sensitive systems of the developing embryo. The heart rate is directly influenced by ambient temperature. Therefore, one of the most important factors in maintaining normal development is accurate environmental temperature control.

To keep the temperature constant, we prefer to construct a heater box that surrounds the stage, embryo chamber and microscope optics to ensure stable temperatures and prevent against thermal drift in the optics *(8)*. The heater box is constructed from cardboard to fit snugly around the individual microscope. One side of the box can be fashioned to include a chicken incubator heater or the hot air from a chicken incubator heater can be targeted to the heater box using flexible aluminum duct tubing on the outlet (**Fig. 3**). Holes are cut out in the front so that the eyepieces are external to the heater box.

Once the cardboard box has been fashioned, it is covered with a layer of foiled thermal insulation. Most of the microscope boxes are made with separate sides, so that

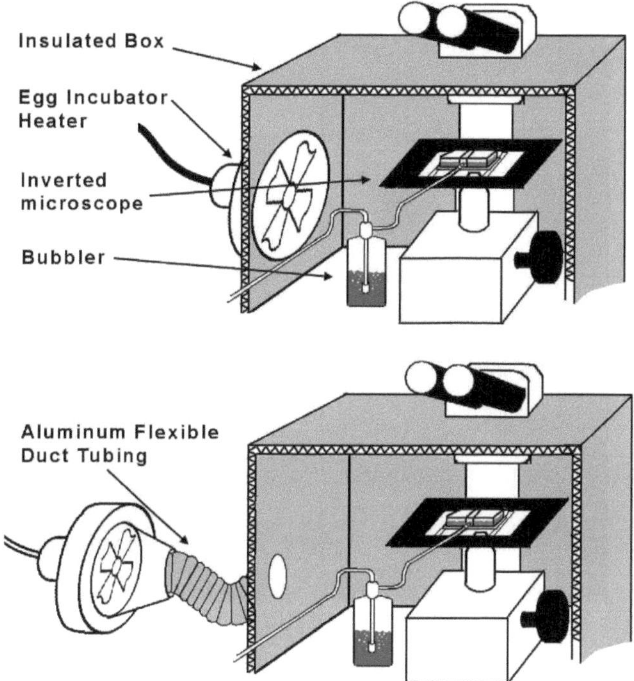

Fig. 3. Microscope configuration. The heater box is constructed around the microscope (shown with front panel cut-away). The box is kept at temperature with a chicken incubator heater. This heater can either be incorporated as one of the heater box walls (top) or placed in a separate location and connected to the box using aluminum ducting (bottom). The inlet of the air needs to be humidified through a gas-washing bottle and connected to the Lab-tek chamber using flexible tubing and a barbed polypropylene fitting.

the box can easily be removed from the microscope. The insulation is attached such that it extends past the cardboard, which allows the edges to be securely sealed. Velcro can be used to connect the various sides of the box, allowing the heater box to be removed from the microscope when not in use.

The chicken incubators have a built-in temperature controller. In most experiments, we required more accurate temperature control than can be obtained with the chicken incubators. This can be achieved using a digital temperature controller (Fischer Scientific, Springfield, NJ; model no. 11-463-47A) to maintain the optimum temperature.

3.6.3. Gas Exchange

Mammalian embryos require both oxygen and carbon dioxide during culture. We have been using a gas mixture consisting of 5% CO_2, 20% oxygen, and 75% nitrogen for stages between E7.5–E9.5. Traditionally, mouse embryos have been cultured in lower levels of oxygen (5%) until they reach E9.5 ***(9)***. In our experiments, cultures were successful at all ages using the higher oxygen concentration.

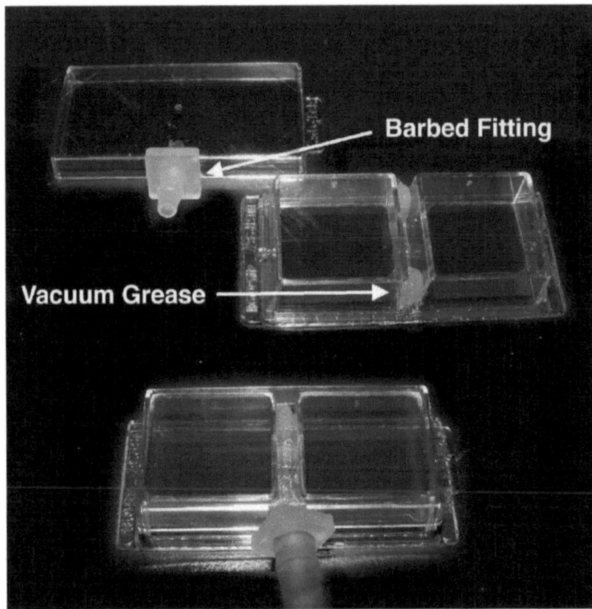

Fig. 4. Modification and aeration of Lab-tek chambers. A small hole is made in the Lab-tek chamber lid and a barbed polypropylene fitting is inserted (top left). The space between the chambers is filled with silicon grease to seal chamber (top right). The lid is placed on top of the chambers and gas is fed to fitting using flexible tubing (bottom).

To deliver the gas to the sealed Lab-tek chamber, it is necessary to introduce an inlet for the gas tubing. A small hole is made in the chamber lid, using a soldering iron to melt the plastic (*see* **Note 5**). The wells of the Lab-tek chambers are separated by a small space, which is a convenient place to introduce the gas inlet. A small barbed polypropylene fitting is inserted into the soldered hole in the chamber lid, allowing the other end to be attached to tubing which supplies the gas. Vacuum grease is used to seal the space where air is introduced between the lid and the bottom of the chamber (**Fig. 4**).

3.6.4. Evaporation Control

Evaporation is the most significant problem with early embryonic culture. Even small amounts of evaporation can cause embryos to develop abnormally. The E8.5 embryos are especially sensitive to this. Therefore, several steps need to be taken to prevent evaporation.

First, the incoming air is humidified by passing it through a bubbler, or gas-washing bottle (**Fig. 3**). The gas flow rate should also be set as low as the regulator allows because insufficient aeration is rarely a problem.

To prevent humidity from escaping the chamber environment, the chambers are also sealed from the outside with Teflon tape. This allows the air/carbon dioxide mix-

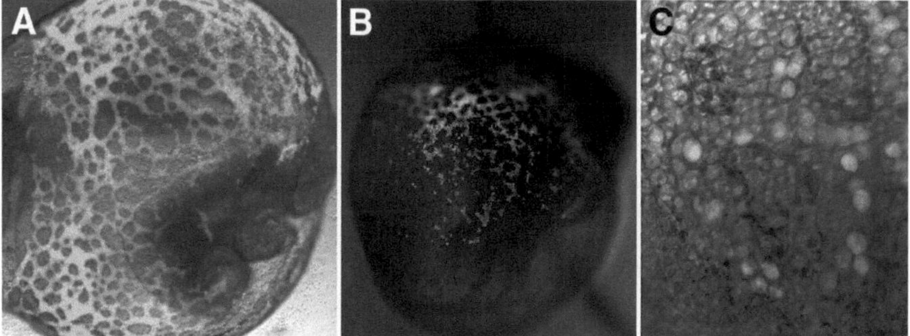

Fig. 5. Expression of GFP in Primitive Erythroblasts. Expression of GFP can be seen throughout the vascular network of an E8.5 embryo (**A**), in the individual erythroblasts of the blood islands in E8.5 embryos (**B**), and in flowing erythroblasts in E9.0 embryos (**C**). Using the ε-globin promoter to drive GFP expression, fluorescence is restricted to primitive red blood cells. In (**A**), the head and developing heart can be seen for the embryo, which is undergoing the process of "turning." *See* color insert following p. 80.

ture to escape, but not the water vapors (*see* **Note 6**). A length of approx 20 to 25 cm of tape is used and wrapped several times around the outside of the chamber.

For E8.5 embryos, the medium should also be covered with a thin layer of "embryo-tested" mineral oil. The mineral oil does not hinder gas exchange significantly, and prevents water from evaporating. Without mineral oil, the yolk sacs of E8.5 embryos tend to shrivel, and yolk sac circulation stops.

3.7. Time-Lapse Imaging

Once the heater box has reached 37°C, which should take around 30 min, the culture chamber is placed on the stage of the microscope, and the inlet gas is attached to the barbed fitting (**Fig. 3**). At this point, time-lapse imaging can begin.

Because most hematovascular development in mouse embryo occurs over several hours, it is sufficient to image once every 5 to 10 min. For confocal imaging, Z-sections or single frames can be taken. For blood flow dynamics, short continuous movies can be taken at each time point.

Because immobilization of the embryo is not complete, the time-lapse needs to be followed to ensure that the embryo does not shift significantly in the x, y, or z planes. If this is occurring, the embryo can be re-positioned or re-focused.

Culture can be sustained for up to 24 h for embryos at E8.5 and for 12 to 18 h for E9.5 embryos (*see* **Notes 9** and **11**).

3.8. Tissue Staining

Although blood in older embryos is auto-fluorescent, no signal is seen at earlier stages, E7.5 to E9.5. A transgenic mouse line in which GFP is expressed in primitive erythroblasts (**Fig. 5**) provides specific labeling of red blood cells ***(10)***. Transgenic mice expressing fluorescent proteins are ideal for dynamic imaging because fluorescent proteins provide a bright, stable, uniform marker that can be directed to specific cells using particular promoter/enhancer combinations (*see* **ref. *11*** for review).

Using stable fluorescent lines is preferred for imaging over other techniques such as the injection of fluorescent dyes, because over-manipulation of the embryos can limit viability. At present, however, only a few fluorescent protein-expressing transgenic lines are available for imaging cardiovascular development at this stage. A Tie2-GFP mouse has been developed that shows expression in all endothelial cells from E8.5 onward *(12)*. Expression of GFP in the Tie1-EGFP mouse is restricted to certain endothelial cells *(13)*. The promoters for several genes involved in hematopoietic development have also been used for the production of fluorescent transgenics, including the GATA-2 promoter *(14)*, and the Flk-1 promoter *(15)*. The ability to visualize the development of both the endothelium and the early hematopoietic cells may help clarify the related lineage of these two cell types and whether they indeed arise from a common precursor, the hemangioblast.

Efforts to find chemical dyes that are specific to endothelial or hematopoietic cells have been unsuccessful. Several lipophilic dyes were tried, including BODIPY Ceramide TR, DiD, DiO, and Hoechst (Molecular Probes, Eugene, OR), but these did not penetrate the tissue significantly. DiD-labeled low-density lipoprotein has some endothelial cell specificity *(16)*, however, our attempts with the dye were unsuccessful. CellTracker Orange CMTMR (Molecular Probes, Eugene, OR) and other self-loading dyes can penetrate the tissue. They are not specific but can be used as a counterstain to provide context for specific stains.

It is possible to label cells using dye injection for cell tracking. This has been achieved for E8.5 embryos (unpublished data), and can be extended to other ages in principle. A fluorescent lipophilic dye, such as DiI or DiO (Molecular Probes, Eugene, OR), is loaded into a pulled glass needle. The dye can be injected into specific cells or specific tissues using a picospritzer, which uses pulsed air, or using iontophoresis, which uses electrical current *(17)*.

3.9. Quantitative Analysis

Embryonic culture can also be used to quantitate various parameters during hematovascular development. 4D-tracking software, such as Volocity (Improvision, Lexington, MA), can perform cell counts or track cell motion in order to measure migration velocity. In our lab, we have been using the ε-globin: GFP mice *(10)*, in combination with the line scanning function of the confocal microscope in order to assess both blood flow rates and hematocrit in the early vasculature.

Blood flow in the early vasculature is much too rapid to be followed using whole field imaging. Blood flow in the dorsal aorta at E8.5 is around 10 mm/s (Jones et al., in press). The blood flow in the yolk sac is much slower, in the range of 1 to 7 mm/s depending on stage and the diameter of the vessel (Jones et al., in press). The yolk sac is the location of extensive remodeling between E8.5 and E9.5, and therefore a very interesting model for angiogenic processes. To image blood flow in the early yolk sac using traditional cell tracking algorithms, imaging rates of at least 400 Hz are required. To overcome the high-speed requirements, line scanning rather than whole field imaging is used. The laser is positioned perpendicular to the blood vessel. In the resultant images, the red blood cells appear as streaks. The time the erythroblast took to pass over the laser line can be calculated from the number of line scans in each "streak" (Jones et al., [5]) and can be used to calculate the velocity of the blood.

The hematocrit, or volume percent red blood cells, affects many important features of hemodynamics, or blood fluid dynamics, and can vary dramatically in diseases such as anemia and polycythemia. The hematocrit also affects the viscosity of the blood, and is therefore central to understanding flow dynamics in the cardiovascular system. The hematocrit of early embryos has not previously been measured directly because of technical difficulties in blood collection. Hematocrit is dependent on vessel size, an effect known as the Fahreus effect ***(18)***. Hematocrit can be calculated from the line scans based on the percentage of pixels within a vessel that are fluorescent. The primitive erythroblasts are labeled with GFP ***(10)*** and the vessel walls can be located with dyes that mark all cells, such as CellTracker Orange CMTMR. The hematocrit is then calculated from the line scans by calculating the number of fluorescent pixels compared with the total number of pixels in the blood vessel. Blood flow in early vessels is parabolic (Jones et al., [***5***]) and radially symmetric; therefore, a line scan through the center of the vessel is a good representation of the red blood cell density within the vessel. Hematocrit was found to rise from around 15% to around 30% between E8.5 and E10.5 (Jones et al., [***5***]).

In summary, by combining the culture of mammalian embryos with quantitative analysis using line scanning, we have been able to investigate aspects of development that were previously inaccessible.

4. Notes

1. If the DMEM/F-12 has a slight pinkish color, it can still be used for dissection but not for culture. DMEM contains a pH indicator called Phenol Red, which is pink when basic and yellow when acidic. The addition of HEPES to already basic medium means that the HEPES is being used to buffer the medium and will not be useful in buffering the changes in pH during culture. As a test, observe whether the DMEM/F-12 changes color upon addition of HEPES solution. If it does, the DMEM/F-12 should be replaced.
2. The second most common cause of failed cultures is the HEPES solution. If cultures begin to fail, try using new HEPES solution.
3. Previous protocols for rat serum production used syringes to gently pull the blood, rather than the Vacutainer system. We have found that this method tends to cause red cell lysis, spoiling the serum.
4. If a heated dissection scope is not available, embryos can be kept warm by more frequent changing of the dissection medium. This approach is, however, not optimal.
5. The soldering iron used to introduce the gas will become covered with plastic and will then be unusable for soldering. If this is unacceptable, any method to introduce a small hole in the plastic lid is suitable, such as a heated syringe needle.
6. It is also possible to use vacuum grease to seal the Lab-tek chambers rather than wrapping the chamber in Teflon tape. This allows embryos to be oriented while on the microscope stage, with no lid on the chamber. When the lid is put on the chamber, vacuum grease in the inner edge of the Lab-tek lid is used to seal chamber. This process is less desirable than sealing with Teflon tape because escaping gas will carry some water vapor with it.
7. Embryos are very sensitive to photo-damage by UV light, especially at higher magnifications. If embryos do not develop normally, static culture on the microscope should first be attempted without imaging or with only white light. In this way, it is possible to ascertain whether the UV light is harming the embryos. If so, reduce the magnification, the number of images acquired, the laser power (for confocal), or ideally, switch to a multiphoton microscope.

8. If imaging is performed from above the culture, it must be kept in mind that even slight pressure on the yolk sac causes circulation to terminate, altering hematopoietic development. It is possible to use dipping lenses if upright imaging is necessary. However, care must be taken to ensure a sealed environment, and constant refocusing will be necessary as the yolk sac expands. The expansion of the yolk sac is less of an issue on inverted microscopes.
9. Embryos that develop in static culture should always be scored for hallmarks of normal development after imaging. This is necessary because not all embryos will develop successfully in static culture *(5)*.
10. Imaging may be hindered by the yolk sac at E8.5 or by the turning motion of the embryo owing to axial rotation. We have had some success culturing embryos without their yolk sac.
11. Embryos as early as E5.5 can also be cultured using this system. Scoring of developmental hallmarks in these embryos is especially critical.

References

1. Baron, M. (2001) Induction of embryonic hematopoietic and endothelial stem/progenitor cells by hedgehog-mediated signals. *Differentiation* **68,** 175–185.
2. Palis, J. and Yoder, M. C. (2001) Yolk-sac hematopoiesis: the first blood cells of mouse and man. *Exp. Hematol.* **29,** 927–936.
3. Yancopoulos, G. D., Klagsbrun, M., and Folkman, J. (1998) Vasculogenesis, angiogenesis, and growth factors: ephrins enter the fray at the border. *Cell* **93,** 661–664.
4. Haar, J. L. and Ackerman, G. A. (1971). A phase and electron microscopic study of vasculogenesis and erythropoiesis in the yolk sac of the mouse. *Anat. Rec.* **170,** 199–223.
5. Jones, E. A., Crotty, D., Kulesa, P. M., Waters, C.W., Baron, M. H., Fraser, S.E., and Dickinson, M. E. (2002) Dynamic in vivo imaging of postimplantation mammalian embryos using whole embryo culture. *Genesis* **34,** 228–235.
6. Hogan, B., et al. (1994) *Manipulating the Mouse Embryo: A Laboratory Manual*, 2nd Ed. Cold Spring Harbor Laboratory Press, Cold Spring Harbor, NY, p. 497.
7. Nagy, A. (2003) *Manipulating the Mouse Embryo : A Laboratory Manual*, 3rd Ed. Cold Spring Harbor Laboratory Press, Cold Spring Harbor, NY, p. 764.
8. Kulesa, P. S. and Fraser, S. E. (1998) Neural crest cell dynamics revealed by time-lapse video microscopy of whole embryo chick explant cultures. *Dev. Biol.* **204,** 327–344.
9. Copp, A. J. and Cockroft, D. L. (1990) *Postimplantation Mammalian Embryos: A Practical Approach*. The Practical approach series. IRL Press, Oxford, p. 357.
10. Dyer, M. A., et al. (2001) Indian hedgehog activates hematopoiesis and vasculogenesis and can respecify prospective neurectodermal cell fate in the mouse embryo. *Development* **128,** 1717–1730.
11. Hadjantonakis, A. K., Dickinson, H. E., Fraser, S. E., and Papaioannov, V. E. (2003) Technicolour Transgenics: Imaging Tools for Functional Genomics in the Mouse. *Nat. Rev. Genet.* **4,** 613–625.
12. Motoike, T., Loughna, S., Perens, E., Roman, B. L., Liao, W., Chau, T. C., et al. (2000) Universal GFP reporter for the study of vascular development. *Genesis* **28,** 75–81.
13. Iljin, K., Petrova, T. V., Veikkola, T. V., Kumar, V., Poutanen, M., and Altitalo, K. (2002) A fluorescent Tie1 reporter allows monitoring of vascular development and endothelial cell isolation from transgenic mouse embryos. *FASEB J.* **16,** 1764–1774.
14. Minegishi, N., Ohta, J., Yamagiwa, H., Suzuki, N., Kawauchi, S., Zhou, Y., et al. (1999) The mouse GATA-2 gene is expressed in the para-aortic splanchnopleura and aorta-gonads and mesonephros region. *Blood* **93,** 4196–4207.

15. Hirai, H., Ogawa, M., Suzuki, N., Yamamoto, M., Breler, G., Mazda, O., et al. (2003) Hemogenic and nonhemogenic endothelium can be distinguished by the activity of fetal liver kinase (Flk)-1 promoter/enhancer during mouse embryogenesis. *Blood* **101,** 886–893.
16. Bkaily, G., Pothier, P., D'Orleans-Juste, P., Simaan, M., Jacques, D., Jaalouk, D., et al. (1997) The use of confocal microscopy in the investigation of cell structure and function in the heart, vascular endothelium and smooth muscle cells. *Mol. Cell. Biochem.* **172,** 171–194.
17. Quinlan, G. A., Trainor, P. A., and Tam, P. P. (1999) Cell grafting and labeling in postimplantation mouse embryos. *Methods Mol. Biol.* **97,** 41–59.
18. Fahraeus, R. and Lindqvist, T. (1931) The viscosity of blood in narrow capillary tubes. *Am. J. Physiol.* **99,** 563–568.

26

Fluorescent Protein–Cell Labeling and Its Application in Time-Lapse Analysis of Hematopoietic Differentiation

Matthias Stadtfeld, Florencio Varas, and Thomas Graf

Summary

Here, we present a computer-controlled time-lapse system for imaging of cultured hematopoietic cells labeled by the expression of different fluorescent proteins. First, we describe experiments to optimize the visualization of three green fluorescent protein variants (cyan-, green-, and yellow-enhanced fluorescent protein) and the red-fluorescent protein (DsRed) by standard wide-field fluorescence microscopy. Then, we describe procedures to best distinguish combinations of cells expressing these proteins using seven commercially available filter sets, based on the relative fluorescence intensities of the individual fluorescent proteins. Finally, we make recommendations about which of these filters to choose when working with specific fluorescent proteins.

Key Words: Green fluorescent proteins (GFP); red fluorescent protein (DsRed); fluorescence microscopy; hematopoietic differentiation; time-lapse experiments.

1. Introduction

The development of fluorescent proteins to label live cells has revolutionized biological experimentation, making it possible to observe processes that otherwise could only be studied indirectly. In the field of hematopoiesis, there are a number of cell culture applications for fluorescent protein labeling, such as observing in real time the onset of differentiation, the dynamics of cell reprogramming, cell interactions, and cell movements. Our laboratory is primarily interested in exploiting fluorescent-labeled proteins as a tool to visualize pathways of hematopoietic differentiation. A "tree" of hematopoietic differentiation, starting with the hematopoietic stem cell and ending with nine major lineages, has been proposed. However, this tree is based largely on indirect experimentation, namely the potential of isolated progenitors to generate uni- or multilineage colonies. What happens in the time between seeding of a single progenitor and the generation of differentiated progeny is a black box that can only be illuminated if individual progenitor cells are followed as they divide and form mature progeny. This has been accomplished by time-lapse microscopy for cultured postimplantation embryos in a study where morphology was combined with

From: *Methods in Molecular Medicine, Vol. 105: Developmental Hematopoiesis: Methods and Protocols.* Edited by: M. H. Baron © Humana Press Inc., Totowa, NJ

fluorescence microscopy *(1)* and in a study of neuronal precursors using morphology *(2)*. Because differentiating hematopoietic cells cannot easily be distinguished by bright field microscopy, similar approaches have so far given only limited insights for blood cells *(3)*.

A way to identify differentiated hematopoietic cells is to use blood cell precursors from genetically modified mice expressing variants of the green fluorescent protein (GFP, from the jellyfish *Aequorea victoria*) in specific lineages. A number of such mouse lines, most of which are transgenics, have been described: RAG-1-enhanced green fluorescent protein (EGFP), labeling B- and T-cells *(4)*; CD2-EGFP, labeling T-cells *(5)*; lysozyme-EGFP (knockin), labeling granulocytes and macrophages *(6)*; CX3CR1 knockin of EGFP, labeling monocytes and natural killer cells *(7)*, epsilon globin EGFP, labeling primitive erythrocytes *(8)*; adult beta globin enhanced cyan fluorescent protein (ECFP), labeling definitive erythroid cells *(9)*; Sca-1-EGFP, labeling early hematopoietic progenitors *(10,11)*; CSF1-R-EGFP, labeling macrophages *(12)*; and GATA-1-EGFP, labeling primitive and definitive erythroid cells *(13)*. Recently, we described a first mouse with two different lineages labeled with distinguishable GFPs, lysozyme-EGFP, and beta globin ECFP *(9)*. To our knowledge, no transgenic mice based on the red-fluorescent protein (DsRed from the sea anemone *Discosoma striata*) have yet been published. In this chapter, we first describe a cell culture system that allows automatic recording of fluorescent protein labeled cells in culture over prolonged periods of time. Then, we discuss a number of parameters that need to be considered to obtain optimal results with fluorescent microscopy: how do cells react when exposed to fluorescent light illumination of different wavelengths for extended periods of time? What is the influence of the medium and the substrate on background and signal sensitivity? What filter sets are best suited to visualize particular GFP variants and combinations of some of these variants?

2. Materials and Methods

2.1. A System That Allows Long-Term Monitoring of Cell Cultures With a Fluorescence Microscope

To monitor the growth of cultured cells, we use a Nikon Eclipse TE200 inverted fluorescence microscope with a 100-W mercury lamp as a light source. The microscope is fitted with a Nikon TE-ICC two door incubator housing. This incubator, which contains the Nikon TE-ICV incubator temperature control unit, maintains the temperature (measured with a gage taped to the stage) at 37°C, with fluctuations of ±0.1°C. Because the housing is large and not air tight, it is difficult to maintain the desired concentration of CO_2 and humidity. We have therefore developed a small chamber that encases the culture vessels and is described in **Fig. 1A,B**. The chamber is fed with a mixture of 5% CO_2 and air through two inlets opposed to each other (a single inlet would lead to the formation of a CO_2 gradient) using Nalgene Premium Tubing (3/16 in. ID; *see* **Note 1**). The gas is moisturized by bubbling through a beaker with water kept at 37°C. Because the chamber is not air tight, the positively pressured gas exits through the spaces between the culture vessel and its support (**Fig. 1C**). We culture the cells on either 96-well plates with a glass bottom (MatTek Corporation) or eight-chamber polystyrene vessel tissue culture treated glass slides (Falcon Plastics, Becton Dickinson), pretreated with gelatin (0.1%) to increase adherence.

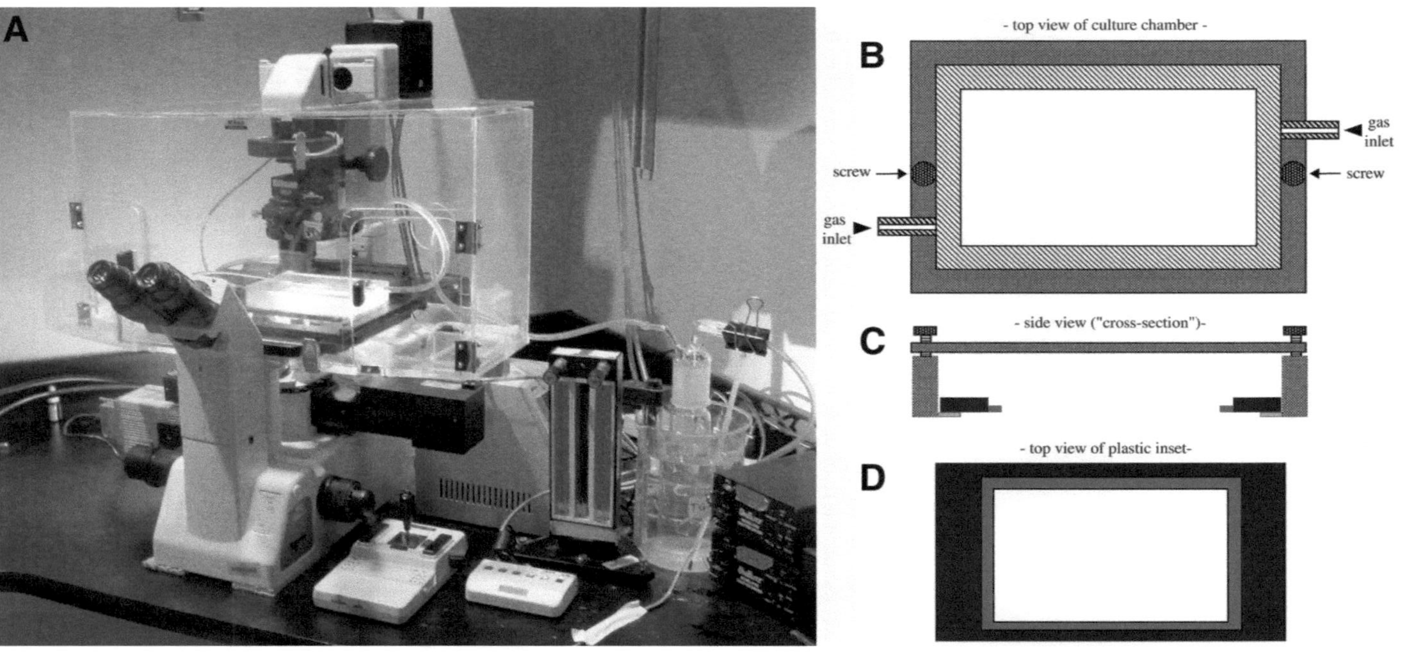

Fig. 1. Microscope set-up and cell culture chamber. (**A**) microscope set-up used to record live images of fluorescent protein expressing cells at different time intervals. The microscope can be seen to be encased by a large Plexiglas chamber and to contain the culture chamber, with two hoses that supply the gas mixture. (**B**) Diagram of the culture chamber (made from Plexiglas) viewed from the top. It measures 16.0 cm wide × 10.8 long × 2.5 cm high and contains two hollow metal insets for the delivery of moistened air/CO_2 mixture (arrowheads), and two screw threads (dark gray circles) to accommodate the lid. The crosshatched area indicates a 1-mm platform carved out from the Plexiglas chamber that can support a 96-well plate or an inset (*see* panel **D**). (**C**) Cross section of the chamber showing the inset (dark grey). The arrows in B indicate the plane of the cross section. (**D**) View of the Plexiglas inset (13.0 cm wide × 8.6 cm long × 0.5 cm high), seen from the top. The crosshatched area indicates a 1-mm platform carved out from the Plexiglas. The platform can support four tissue culture glass slides.

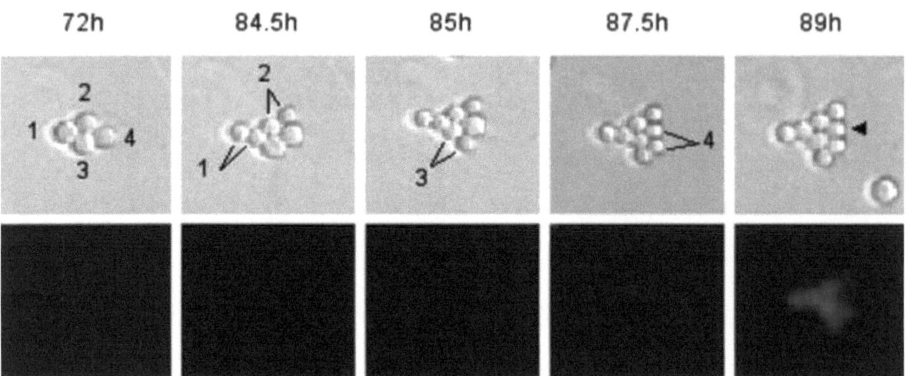

Fig. 2. Differentiation of myeloid progenitors visualized by fluorescence time-lapse microscopy. Nucleated bone marrow cells were isolated from a lysozyme EGFP mouse, in which macrophages and granulocytes are labeled by GFP expression. The cells were cultured in methylcellulose containing stem cell factor, interleukin-3, and interleukin-6. Images were taken 0.5-hour intervals using the Endow GFP filter and both the bright field (upper panel) and fluorescent (lower panel) shutter. Images taken at indicated time points after initiation of the culture are shown. The numbers (1 to 4) label individual cells and their progeny. Maturation of the cells into mature cells of myelo-monocytic lineage is indicated by GFP detection. Note that the first two fluorescence positive cells are visible after 87.5 h, corresponding to the two cells that divided first. At 89 h, all cells are fluorescence positive, except for one (pointed out with an arrowhead in the upper panel). *See* color insert following p. 80.

These slides are placed into the inset described in **Fig. 1A**. We use Iscove's modification of Dulbecco's medium without phenol red (Gibco), with penicillin/streptomycin and 10% fetal calf serum. For culture of hematopoietic progenitor cells appropriate cytokines are added (*see* **Note 2**).

The microscope is connected to a high sensitivity cooled CCD camera (Hamamatsu ORCA 100) and has a motorized stage to allow recording and memorizing of multiple positions and filter holder (Prior). The filter holder can accommodate up to six filter cubes, which will be described subsequently. Filters to be used, stage positions to be imaged, exposure times and exposure intervals are programmed into a PC (2.0 GHz Pentium processor, 1024 KB RAM, 80 GB hard-drive) using Metamorph imaging software (Universal Imaging Corporation, Version 5.6). Image processing is also done using Metamorph software (*see* **Note 3**). The recording is performed automatically, requiring only occasional re-adjustments of the focus (*see* **Note 4**). We use 20X and 40X objectives with high numerical apertures (0.75–0.95) to maximize sensitivity of signal detection. Cells can be cultured in this system for periods exceeding 1 wk (*see* **Note 5**).

As an example illustrating the feasibility of the approach to study differentiation in real time, bone marrow progenitors from a lysozyme EGFP mouse ***(6)*** were cultured under and analyzed by time-lapse. As shown in **Fig. 2**, myelomonocytic differentiation can be demonstrated by GFP expression without the need for staining procedures.

Table 1
Fluorescent Proteins and Filter Sets

A. Fluorescent Proteins

	Excitation maximum	Emission maximum	Rel. brightness	Reference
ECFP (CFP)	434	477	0.32	Clontech, 2003
EGFP (GFP)	489	508	1	Clontech, 2003
EYFP (YFP)	514	527	1.55	Clontech, 2003
DsTedT1 (RFP)	555	584	0.54	Campbell, 2002

B. Filter Sets

	Chroma no.	Purpose	Exciter	Dichroic	Emitter
Cyan GFP	41044	CFP	437/20	455	480/40
Endow GFP	41017	GFP	470/40	490	510/20
Yellow GFP	41028	YFP	500/20	515	535/30
JP2	31040	YFP	510/20	530	560/40
TRITC	41002	Rhodamine	535/50	565	610/75
Texas Red	41004	Texas Red	560/55	595	645/75

A. The table shows a summary of properties of the fluorescent proteins relevant for this article. Names used throughout the text are shown in brackets. Brightness = quantum yield × extinction factor.

B. Names and characteristics of the filter sets used and their Chroma catalogue number. "Purpose" indicates the application for which the filters were originally designed. The numbers in the respective columns indicate the bandwidth of the exciter and emitter filters (*see also* **Note 6**).

2.2. Choosing Appropriate Fluorescent Proteins and Filters

Optimal results with fluorescence microscopy depend on a high signal to noise ratio. This can be achieved either by increasing the specific signal or by decreasing the background noise. To maximize the signal, a strong promoter should be chosen to drive fluorescent protein expression. Using fluorescent proteins with a high relative brightness also enhances signal intensity. **Table 1** lists some of the properties of the four fluorescent proteins described in this article and the filter sets used to analyze them. The three versions of GFP, namely EGFP (here called GFP), ECFP (here, CFP), and enhanced yellow fluorescent protein, (EYFP, here, YFP) are currently the most widely used because of their spectral properties, brightness, and relatively low propensity for bleaching. The blue variant of GFP, BFP, is of limited use as it bleaches very rapidly and therefore was not included in our study. DsRedT1, the particular DsRed protein that we have used for our studies, was originally developed for rapid folding and high signal intensity (Bevis and Glick, 2002). It is here termed red fluorescent protein (RFP). The seven filter sets listed in **Table 1** were purchased from a collection of filters from a single company (Chroma Technologies), although similar filters are available from other sources as well (such as Omega Optical, www.omegafilters.com; Semrock, www.semrock.com). The Cyan GFP, Endow GFP (developed by Dr. Sharyn Endow), and Yellow GFP filters are recommended by Chroma for visualization of CFP, GFP, and YFP, respectively. The TRITC and Texas Red filters were developed for visualization

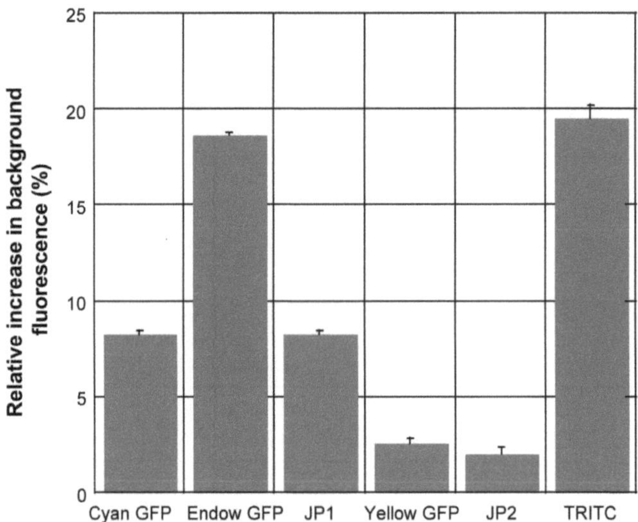

Fig. 3. Phenol red in the culture medium increases the level of background fluorescence. Images of cell culture medium (in Iscove's modification of Dulbecco's medium without phenol red) with and without phenol red (2 mL of medium in 35-mm plastic culture dishes) were acquired with the indicated filters. The relative background fluorescence was calculated as the difference (percentage) between the values obtained with and without phenol red.

of proteins labeled with rhodamine/DiI and Texas Red, but they can also be used for RFP. It has to be noted that the TRITC filter we used here (Chroma 41002) picks up light of slightly shorter wavelengths than other available TRITC filters, leading to a relatively strong signal with YFP expressing cells (*see* **Subheading 2.5.**). Finally, the JP1 and JP2 filter sets were developed by Dr. Jonathon Pines to visualize GFP and YFP in double labeling experiments (*see* **ref. *15***; **Note 6**).

2.3. Phenol Red-Free Medium and Glass Bottom Vessels Improve Image Quality

The second parameter that contributes to image quality is background fluorescence. To test the influence of phenol red in the culture medium on background fluorescence, we acquired a series of images in media with and without this pH indicator. As shown in **Fig. 3**, phenol red dramatically increases the background levels, especially when visualizing GFP and RFP with the Endow GFP and TRITC filters, respectively. As a result, the relative signal intensity is decreased, hampering the detection of weak signals (when visualizing YFP with the Yellow GFP and JP2 filters, this effect is only minor). Therefore, we recommend using phenol red-free medium (we routinely fill a chamber in an eight-chamber slide or a row in a 96-well plate with phenol red-containing medium to visually monitor the pH of the cultures).

In addition, both the intensity and the clarity of fluorescent signals can be significantly improved when working with glass-bottom plates instead of plastic. The signal

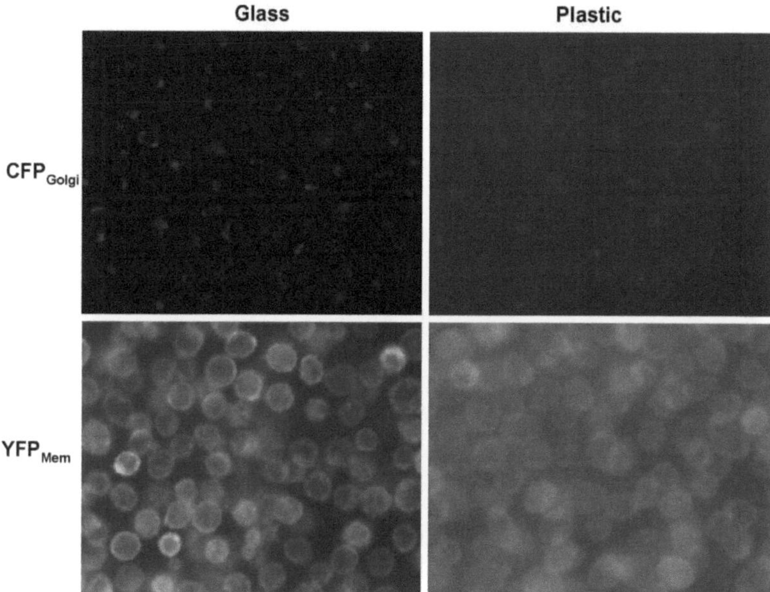

Fig. 4. Plastic culture dishes impair the quality of fluorescence imaging. The 18-81 Pro B cell line expressing membrane-localized YFP and 3T3 cells with Golgi-localized CFP were cultured on plastic dishes and glass-bottom dishes, respectively. Images were taken using the filter sets Cyan GFP (for CFP) and JP2 (for YFP).

to noise ratio increased over 50% for all GFP variants for glass versus plastic, with the most dramatic effect seen with CFP. This is exemplified in **Fig. 4** for CFP and YFP. In conclusion, using medium without phenol red and glass-bottom plates maximizes the sensitivity of signal detection (culture media without phenol red and glass-bottom culture dishes/slides are available from different manufacturers).

2.4. Exposure to Fluorescent Light Can Impair Cell Growth and Viability

Because of the known detrimental effects of ultraviolet light on nucleic acids and proteins, it seemed possible that prolonged exposure of cultures to fluorescent light might impair cell growth and viability. To detect and quantify such potential phototoxic effects, we exposed small colonies of mouse erythroleukemia (MEL) cells for various lengths of time to light passing through four different filters. The impact on cell growth was determined by comparing the cell numbers in the individual colonies after 24 h. As shown in **Fig. 5**, exposures of MEL cells using the Cyan GFP filter for 10, 30, or 60 s led to an essentially complete block of proliferation and extensive cell death. A less dramatic effect was evident using the Endow GFP filter, whereas no phototoxicity was observed with the Yellow GFP and TRITC filters even at the longest exposures (we would expect the JP1, JP2 and Texas Red filters to be comparable with the Endow GFP, Yellow GFP and Texas Red filters, respectively).

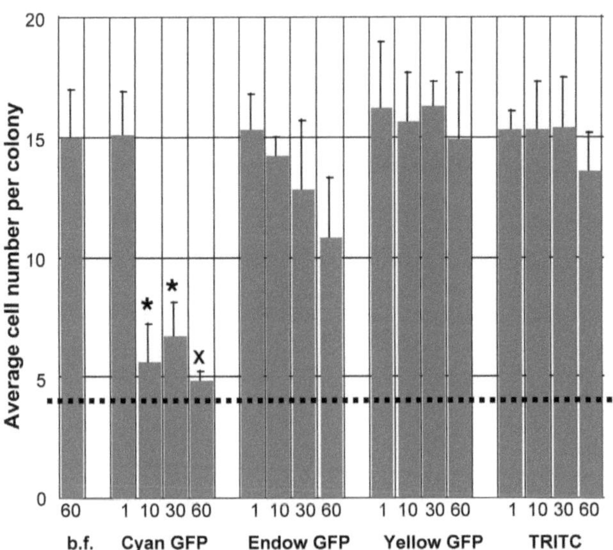

Fig 5. Prolonged short wavelength light exposure is toxic for cultured cells. To determine the impact of illumination on cells in culture, MEL cells were seeded in methylcellulose at clonal density. For each filter and exposure time, five colonies at the four-cell stage were selected and exposed to light. After cultivation for 24 h, the number of cells in each colony was determined and the state of the cells assessed. Colonies exposed to bright field light (b.f.) served as a control. *, Some cells dead; x, all cells dead. Error bars indicate standard deviation. The dotted line marks the four-cell stage, the baseline of this experiment.

Although cells are usually not exposed for more than one or a few seconds during image acquisition, time is needed to focus the image and adjust exposure times. In addition, time-lapse applications require multiple image acquisitions of the same cells, leading to high cumulative exposure times. The problem of phototoxicity associated with prolonged exposure times can be reduced somewhat by using the intensifier function ("gain"), which most imaging software programs offer in their acquisition menu (*see* **Note 7**).

In conclusion, prolonged exposure of cells to short wavelength light can be toxic, especially when using the Cyan GFP filter. Therefore, whenever possible, the use of CFP should be avoided in time-lapse studies or in other applications that require long exposure times.

2.5. Visualizing Individual Fluorescent Proteins With Different Filters

To compare and quantify the relative signal intensities of the different fluorescent proteins, we exposed individual cells expressing CFP, GFP, YFP, or RFP to light of different wavelengths, using the seven filters, for different lengths of time. As can be seen in **Fig. 6**, CFP (top left) can be best visualized by the Cyan GFP filter but also gives a signal with the Endow GFP and the JP1 filter. Thus, the Endow GFP filter

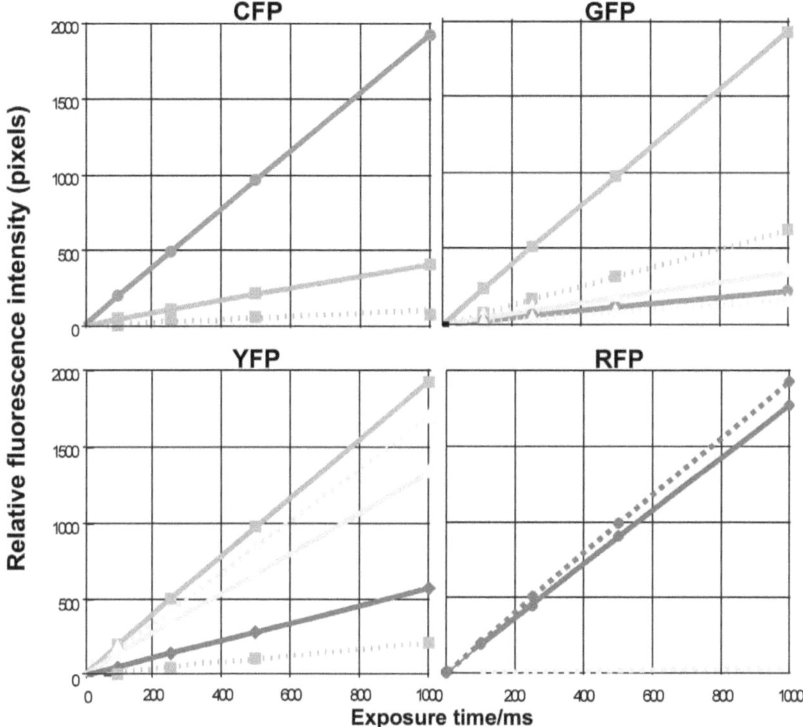

Fig. 6. Fluorescent intensities of three GFP variants and of RFP determined with the different filters. Images were collected from cell lines expressing CFP, GFP, YFP, or RFP. The fluorescence intensity of individual cells was determined by subtracting the background intensity from the signal intensity using the indicated filters and exposure times. Only filters yielding signals above cellular autofluorescence background are shown in the graphs. The fluorescence intensities were normalized to the values obtained with CFP expressing cells. Blue line, CFP; solid green line, Endow GFP; broken green line, JP1; solid yellow line, Yellow GFP; broken yellow line, JP2; solid red line, TRITC; broken red line, Texas Red. *See* color insert following p. 80.

could be of advantage when trying to avoid damage induced by the short wavelengths associated with the Cyan GFP filter (**Fig. 5**). GFP (top right) is approx three times brighter with the Endow GFP filter (solid green line) than with JP1 (broken green line). GFP is also visible in both YFP filters (yellow lines) and in Cyan GFP (blue line). The Endow GFP filter is also well suited to visualize YFP expression (bottom left). In fact, it gave an even stronger signal than both YFP filters. This means that a single filter, Endow GFP, can be used to visualize GFP, YFP, and—with lower efficiency—CFP in single-labeling applications. The figures also show that YFP can be imaged using the TRITC filter (solid red line) albeit with lower efficiency than with Endow GFP or one of the YFP filters. Finally, RFP (bottom right) is best visualized using the Texas Red (broken red line) or TRITC filters.

Table 2
Relative Fluorescence Intensities

Filter Protein	Cyan GFP	Endow GFP	JP1	Yellow GFP	JP2	TRITC	Texas Red
CFP	100	22	6	0	0	0	0
GFP	12	100	33	18	9	0	0
YFP	0	115	13	79	100	34	0
RFP	0	0	0	0	2	92	100

The table summarizes the data shown in **Fig. 6**. The numbers are the relative fluorescence intensities of the individual proteins in the different filters. This value is constant at different exposure times under the experimental conditions used and can therefore serve as a 'fingerprint' for each protein (*see* text for details).

The relative fluorescence intensities of the different fluorescent proteins and filter sets are summarized in **Table 2**. For example, viewing CFP expressing cells with the Endow GFP filter or the JP1 filters gives a signal corresponding to 22% and 6%, respectively, of that observed with the Cyan GFP filter. As long as saturation is avoided, the relative fluorescent intensities are independent of the exposure time although they may vary somewhat with different imaging setups, such as using a Xenon lamp instead of a Mercury lamp.

In conclusion, the recommended filters for individual colors are Cyan GFP for CFP, Endow GFP for both GFP and YFP, and Texas Red for RFP. However, YFP can also be visualized with essentially the same quality with the JP2 and Yellow GFP filters and RFP with the TRITC filter.

2.6. Distinguishing Mixed Populations of Cells Expressing Different Fluorescent Proteins

Partial overlaps in the absorption and emission spectra of some of the fluorescent proteins make an unambiguous identification of a fluorescent signal sometimes difficult (for the spectra, *see* for example http://www.clontech.com/gfp/excitation.shtml and http://www.bdbiosciences.com/spectra/)

In the following, we describe how to distinguish combinations of cells expressing two, three, and four different fluorescent proteins (where each cell type only expresses one protein) by selecting the appropriate filters and in some cases requiring image subtraction procedures (*see* **Note 8**). The recommendations for the filter choice are summarized in **Table 3**. In some cases we mention alternatives because the most appropriate filters may not always be available. Our recommendations are based on the data in **Fig. 6** and **Table 2**, which show the relative intensities of the fluorescent proteins in the different filters.

2.6.1. CFP/YFP, CFP/RFP, GFP/RFP, and YFP/RFP

With the appropriate filters (Cyan GFP plus Yellow GFP or JP2, Cyan GFP plus Texas Red or TRITC, Endow GFP plus Texas Red, or TRITC and Yellow GFP plus Texas Red), these color combinations can be distinguished easily. None of the proteins in the previously mentioned pairs are visible with the filter used to visualize the other.

Table 3
Recommended Filter Sets

Second Protein First Protein	CFP	GFP	YFP	RFP
CFP	Cyan GFP			
GFP	Cyan GFP/Yellow GFP[a]	Endow GFP		
YFP	Cyan GFP/JP2	JP1/JP2[a]	Endow GFP	
RFP	Cyan GFP/Texas Red	Endow GFP/Texas Red	Texas Red/Yellow GFP	Texas Red

The table summarizes the recommendations for filter choice for single and double labeling with fluorescent proteins. Please see the text for additional comments and possible alternatives.

[a] Image processing necessary.

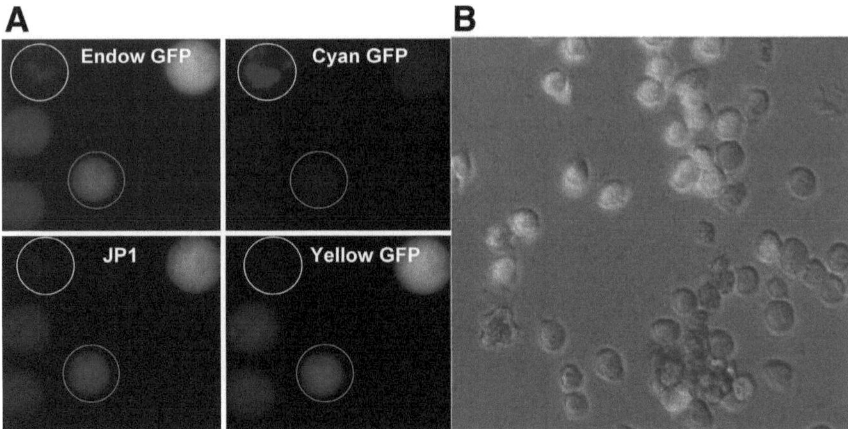

Fig. 7. CFP and GFP can be separated using the Yellow GFP filter. **(A)** A mixed population of cells stably expressing either GFP (18-no. 1 Pro B cells) or Golgi localized CFP (nonadherent 3T3 fibroblasts) were imaged using the Cyan GFP, Endow GFP, JP1, and Yellow GFP filters. The exposure times with Endow GFP, JP1, and Yellow GFP filters were adjusted to achieve a comparable GFP intensity. The white circle indicates a CFP-labeled Golgi apparatus. Note that although the CFP signal (white circles) is detected by both JP1 and Endow GFP filters, it is not observed with the Yellow GFP filter. Also note detection of the signal GFP (red circles) with the Cyan GFP filter. **(B)** Common myeloid progenitors were isolated as previously described ***(16)*** from the bone marrow of a lysozyme M-EGFP/globin-ECFP double-transgenic mouse in which macrophages/granulocytes are labeled by GFP and erythroid cells by CFP expression. The common myeloid progenitors were cultured at clonal density in 0.2% methylcellulose in the presence of SCF, IL3, IL11 and EPO. Six days after start of the culture fluorescent images were taken using the Cyan GFP and Yellow GFP filters. The images were processed as described in **Subheading 2.6.** (CFP/GFP) and overlaid with a brightfield image. Cells expressing lysozyme (macrophages) are green; cells expressing the globin transgene (erythrocytes) are blue. *See* color insert following p. 80.

2.6.2. CFP/GFP

The problem of this combination is that GFP can be detected with the Cyan GFP filter and vice versa CFP is visible in both Endow GFP and JP1 filters. This problem can be partly solved by visualizing GFP with the Yellow GFP filter, which does not detect CFP. Then, the GFP signal detected with the Cyan GFP filter can be removed by subtraction of the Yellow GFP image from the Cyan GFP image. Pictures of CFP and GFP expressing cells imaged with the Cyan GFP, Endow GFP, JP1 and Yellow GFP filters are shown in **Fig. 7A**. Another example, showing a mixed hematopoietic colony consisting of myeloid and erythroid cells (obtained from a lysozyme EGFP × globin ECFP mouse) is shown in **Fig. 7B**.

Alternative 1: use the Cyan GFP plus the Endow GFP filter. Subtract the Cyan GFP image from the Endow GFP image and vice versa ("cross-subtraction," *see* **Note 8**). This approach may be necessary when working with a relatively weak GFP signal that cannot be adequately visualized using the Yellow GFP filter.

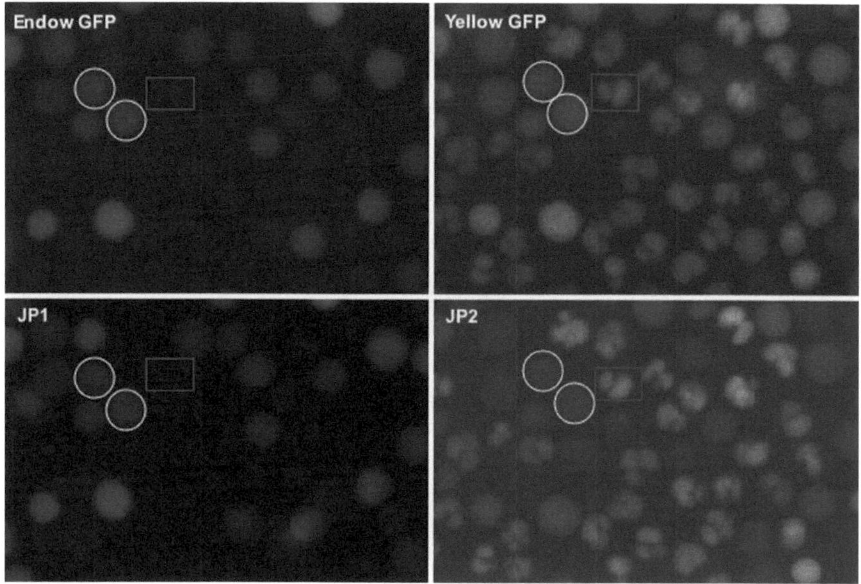

Fig. 8. The JP1/JP2 filter combination facilitates separation of GFP and YFP. A mixed population consisting of 18-81 cells expressing either GFP (strong) or nuclear YFP (weak) was cultured on a glass-bottom 96-well plate. Images were taken with the indicated filter sets. The exposure time was 500 ms for Endow GFP and 1500 ms for JP1 to obtain similar values for the GFP signal (images shown in green). The exposure time with Yellow GFP and JP2 filters was 2500 ms (images shown in yellow). The position of a YFP expressing cell is indicated by a red box and the positions of two GFP expressing cells by white circles. Note that at a similar intensity of GFP expressing cells, the YFP signal is weaker with the JP1 than with the Endow GFP filter. Also note that the separation of YFP from GFP is better with the JP2 filter than with the Yellow GFP filter. *See* color insert following p. 80.

2.6.3. GFP/YFP

Again the problem is that both proteins are visible in the filters routinely used to visualize the other. The best filters for this combination are JP1 for GFP and JP2 or Yellow GFP for YFP, requiring a simple "cross-subtraction." An example of results obtained with this procedure is shown in **Fig. 8**.

Alternative 2: use the JP1 filter for GFP and the TRITC filter, which doesn't detect any GFP signal, for YFP. Only the subtraction of the TRITC image from the JP1 image is necessary. This is a good solution when working with strong GFP and YFP signals.

Alternative 3: use the Endow GFP filter and the TRITC filter. The exposure time with the TRITC filter should be at least 3.5 times longer than with Endow GFP to compensate for the strong YFP signal in Endow GFP (*see* **Table 2**). The images are processed as described for JP1/TRITC.

Alternative 4: use the Endow GFP and Yellow GFP filters. First subtract the Yellow GFP image from the Endow GFP image (image A). Image A is then subtracted from the Yellow GFP image (image B, only YFP signals are visible). Image B in turn is subtracted from image A (image C, only GFP). This more complicated solution maybe helpful if only these two relatively common filters are available.

2.6.4. CFP/YFP/RFP

Use Cyan GFP plus Yellow GFP plus Texas Red filters. No image subtraction is necessary.

2.6.5. CFP/GFP/RFP

Use Cyan GFP plus Yellow GFP plus Texas Red filters. Subtract the Yellow GFP image from the Cyan GFP image to remove GFP detected with the Cyan GFP filter.

2.6.6. CFP/GFP/YFP

Use Cyan GFP plus JP1 plus Yellow GFP filters. Subtract the Yellow GFP image from the Cyan GFP image to remove the GFP signal detected with Cyan GFP (image A, only CFP). Then, subtract the JP1 image from the Yellow GFP image to obtain a pure YFP signal (image B). Finally subtract images A and B one after the other from the JP1 image to remove both CFP and YFP signals detected with the JP1 filter.

2.6.7. GFP/YFP/RFP

Use JP1 plus Yellow GFP plus Texas Red filters. Neither are GFP or YFP detectable with the Texas Red filter nor is RFP visible with the JP1 and Yellow GFP filter. Therefore, this triple combination can be handled as described above for the GFP/YFP pair.

2.6.8. CFP/GFP/YFP/RFP

Use Cyan GFP, JP1, Yellow GFP, and Texas Red filters. RFP is the only of these molecules detectable in the Texas Red filter. Proceed as described for the CFP/GFP/YFP combination.

2.7. Distinguishing Double Expressers From Single Expressers by Spectral "Fingerprinting"

To distinguish cells expressing two or more fluorescent proteins from cells that express only one protein, the same rules apply as for the separation of single expressers (**Subheading 2.6.**). In all cases where no spectral overlap occurs, such as in the CFP/YFP, CFP/RFP, GFP/RFP, or YFP/RFP combinations, double expressers can be unambiguously identified. The same holds true for the CFP/YFP/RFP combination. All other combinations have some overlap and can only be separated by applying a "fingerprinting" technique. The respective fingerprints can be deduced from the relative fluorescent intensities shown in **Fig. 6** and **Table 2**. For the CFP/GFP pair, for example, such a fingerprint corresponds to ratios of 100:22 for CFP and to 12:100 for GFP when using the Cyan GFP and Endow GFP filters. For the GFP/YFP pair and the JP1 plus JP2 filter combination, this ratio is 100:27 for GFP and 13:100 for YFP. A deviation from these ratios indicates the presence of both proteins in the same cell. Fluorescent fingerprinting, which works best when none of the simultaneously expressed proteins is strongly dominant, has been previously described for the detection of tobacco cells expressing multiple fluorescent proteins *(17)*.

2.8. Recommendations for the Purchase of Filters for a Microscope With Four Filter Spaces

On balance, the Cyan GFP, JP1, Yellow GFP, and Texas Red filters represent the best choice in dealing with combinations of the currently most widely used fluorescent proteins.

2.9. Using SubCellular Localization of Fluorescent Proteins to Help Distinguish Labeled Cells

The standard forms of fluorescent proteins are equally distributed throughout the cell. Using localized forms of these proteins can greatly help distinguishing cells expressing different fluorescent proteins. An additional advantage of subcellular localization is the enhancement of the fluorescent signal through its concentration in a smaller area, such as the nucleus. There are now many "addresses" with which fluorescent proteins can be tagged, targeting them to the nucleus, cell membrane, Golgi apparatus, nucleolus, mitochondria. Some of these modified fluorescent proteins are commercially available (Clontech, BD Biosciences. *See* Clontech catalog for references). An example is shown in **Fig. 4**, where cells exhibit CFP localized to the Golgi (**Fig. 4A**) or YFP to the cell membrane (**Fig. 4B**). Another example is shown in **Fig. 8**, where cells with a nuclear localized YFP were mixed with cells expressing nonlocalized GFP. When localizing fluorescent proteins to cellular organelles, their individual pH dependence must be taken into account. For example, YFP is more sensitive to acidic conditions than CFP or RFP *(18)*.

3. Outlook

Imaging fluorescent protein-labeled cells is a rapidly evolving field, with new "colors" and techniques being added continuously. For example, while working on this manuscript, the development of a new series of red and yellow fluorescent proteins from *Anthozoa* coral species was announced (*Clontechniques*, July 2003). Among these new proteins is a yellow-fluorescent protein that is spectrally better separated from GFP than YFP. However, it remains to be seen how well this new protein works in practice. In addition, a YFP variant has been described that, although spectrally similar, folds more rapidly and is 20 to 30 times brighter than the original one *(19)*. It should be noted that more sophisticated imaging techniques for fluorescent protein separation than discussed here have been described, such as fluorescence lifetime imaging microscopy *(20)*, filter free spectral confocal microscopy (Leica, AOBS), and two-photon laser scanning microscopy *(21)*. The latter technique makes it possible to separate GFP from FITC fluorescence, two molecules with almost identical emission spectra. Although these methods are not currently accessible to most researchers, they are likely to become more popular in the future. Finally, readers are directed to a review on fluorescent protein properties and technologies *(22)* and to a paper describing a time-lapse recording system, which describes a number of useful technical details *(1)*.

4. Notes

1. Custom-made gas mixes can be useful for specific applications. For example, erythroid and other hematopoietic progenitors can be expanded best in reduced oxygen tension

(14). Such mixes can be purchased from a number of companies (e.g., Matheson Gas Products, New Jersey) and easily hooked up to the system described.

2. A problem we faced when culturing fast growing hematopoietic progenitors in 1% methylcellulose is the formation of closely packed three-dimensional colonies. This made tracking of individual cells virtually impossible. On the other hand, when using liquid medium, the movement of the stage while acquiring images at multiple positions led to the disturbance of colony formation. Using 0.2% methylcellulose cultures was found to be an acceptable compromise.
3. All image-processing procedures described here can be also performed using ImageJ, a flexible, Java-based software that runs on both Macintosh and PC. ImageJ can be downloaded free of charge at http://rsb.info.nih.gov/ij/. Although camera control for image acquisition is also possible with ImageJ, no time-lapse feature is yet available. However, ImageJ is constantly expanded and the latest updates are also available from the link above.
4. The culture chamber has to be firmly attached to the stage by adhesive tape to prevent undesired dislocations during long term culturing. Likewise, the culture vessel has to be immobilized in the culture chamber. When starting time-lapse movies we routinely check the position and the focus of the images acquired in the first and second rounds. If necessary, we pause the acquisition to adjust position and focus. After these initial adjustments, the system is usually stable.
5. For time-lapse acquisitions longer than 2 to 3 d, we found it necessary to place a sterile gauze sponge soaked in sterile water inside the culture chamber to prevent the cultures from drying. Water in the sponge is replenished every 1 to 2 d with a 3-mL syringe using a thin plastic tube inserted into the chamber through the inlet.
6. A filter set consists of three individual filters: excitation filter, dichroic beamsplitter and emission filter. In Endow GFP, for example, the exciter filter allows only light between 450 and 490 nm to pass through to the beamsplitter, which deflects all wavelengths shorter than 495 nm towards the sample. Only wavelengths longer than 495 nm returning from the excited sample pass the beamsplitter to reach the emitter filter, which in turn only lets pass wavelengths between 500 and 550 nm, the light registered by eye or camera. Although each filter set thus consists of three filters, we refer to them as "filters" throughout the text. More information about filters can be found at www.chroma.com.
7. Using the gain function allows a reduction of the exposure time by a factor that is equivalent to the chosen gain. By this, the overall image resolution is reduced, for example when comparing an image taken with 500 ms exposure at a gain of 4 and an image taken with 2-s exposure a gain of 1 the 500 ms image will be more "noisy." Therefore, we recommend restricting the use of higher gains to the initial focusing of the image, when phototoxicity is not an issue and high image quality is more important than short exposure times.
8. Saturation of the images must be avoided to allow reliable image subtraction. In addition, when "cross-subtraction" (the subtraction of image A from image B and vice versa) is necessary, it is important to acquire both images with the same exposure time. In general, the removal of unspecific background fluorescence by a background subtraction procedure is necessary before doing "cross-subtractions." Overall, the separation of fluorescent proteins by appropriate filter choice (when possible) is preferable to image processing because it is less time consuming and also leads to images of higher quality.

Acknowledgments

We would like to thank members of the Graf lab for supplying cell lines and reagents and for comments. We would also like to thank Todd Evans and Michael Cammer for comments on the manuscript. This work was supported by grant RO1 CA89590-01 from NCI/NIH (T.G.). M.S. was supported by the Boehringer Ingelheim Fonds (BIF).

References

1. Jones, E. A., Crotty, D., Kulesa, P. M., Waters, C. W., Baron, M. H., Fraser, S. E., et al. (2002) Dynamic in vivo imaging of postimplantation mammalian embryos using whole embryo culture. *Genesis* **34,** 228–235.
2. Qian, X., Shen, Q., Goderie, S. K., He, W., Capela, A., Davis, A. A., et al. (2000) Timing of CNS cell generation: a programmed sequence of neuron and glial cell production from isolated murine cortical stem cells. *Neuron* **28,** 69–80.
3. Punzel, M., Liu, D., Zhang, T., Eckstein, V., Miesala, K., and Ho, A. D. (2003) The symmetry of initial divisions of human hematopoietic progenitors is altered only by the cellular microenvironment. *Exp. Hematol.* **31,** 339–347.
4. Yu, W., Misulovin, Z., Suh, H., Hardy, R. R., Jankovic, M., Yannoutsos, N., et al. (1999) Coordinate regulation of RAG1 and RAG2 by cell type-specific DNA elements 5' of RAG2. *Science* **285,** 1080–1084.
5. Singbartl, K., Thatte, J., Smith, M. L., Wethmar, K., Day, K., and Ley, K. (2001) A CD2-green fluorescence protein-transgenic mouse reveals very late antigen-4-dependent CD8+ lymphocyte rolling in inflamed venules. *J. Immunol.* **166,** 7520–7526.
6. Faust, N., Varas, F., Kelly, L. M., Heck, S., and Graf, T. (2000) Insertion of enhanced green fluorescent protein into the lysozyme gene creates mice with green fluorescent granulocytes and macrophages. *Blood* **96,** 719–726.
7. Jung, S., Aliberti, J., Graemmel, P., Sunshine, M. J., Kreutzberg, G. W., Sher, A., and Littman, D. R. (2000) Analysis of fractalkine receptor CX(3)CR1 function by targeted deletion and green fluorescent protein reporter gene insertion. *Mol. Cell Biol.* **20,** 4106–4114.
8. Dyer, M. A., Farrington, S. M., Mohn, D., Munday, J. R., and Baron, M. H. (2001) Indian hedgehog activates hematopoiesis and vasculogenesis and can respecify prospective neurectodermal cell fate in the mouse embryo. *Development* **128,** 1717–1730.
9. Heck, S., Ermakova, O., Iwasaki, H., Akashi, K., Sun, C. W., Ryan, T. M., et al. (2003) Distinguishable live erythroid and myeloid cells in beta-globin ECFP x lysozyme EGFP mice. *Blood* **101,** 903–906.
10. Ma, X., Robin, C., Ottersbach, K., and Dzierzak, E. (2002) The Ly-6A (Sca-1) GFP transgene is expressed in all adult mouse hematopoietic stem cells. *Stem Cells* **20,** 514–521.
11. Hanson, P., Mathews, V., Marrus, S. H., and Graubert, T. A. (2003) Enhanced green fluorescent protein targeted to the Sca-1 (Ly-6A) locus in transgenic mice results in efficient marking of hematopoietic stem cells in vivo. *Exp. Hematol.* **31,** 159–167.
12. Sasmono, R. T., Oceandy, D., Pollard, J. W., Tong, W., Pavli, P., Wainwright, B. J., et al. (2003) A macrophage colony-stimulating factor receptor-green fluorescent protein transgene is expressed throughout the mononuclear phagocyte system of the mouse. *Blood* **101,** 1155–1163.
13. Ohneda, K., Shimizu, R., Nishimura, S., Muraosa, Y., Takahashi, S., Engel, J. D., et al. (2002) A minigene containing four discrete cis elements recapitulates GATA-1 gene expression in vivo. *Genes Cells* **7,** 1243–1254.
14. Koller, M. R., Bender, J. G., Miller, W. M., and Papoutsakis, E. T. (1992) Reduced oxygen tension increases hematopoiesis in long-term culture of human stem and progenitor cells from cord blood and bone marrow. *Exp. Hematol.* **20,** 264–270.
15. Hagting, A., Jackman, M., Simpson, K., and Pines, J. (1999) Translocation of cyclin B1 to the nucleus at prophase requires a phosphorylation-dependent nuclear import signal. *Curr. Biol.* **9,** 680–689.

16. Akashi, K., Traver, D., Miyamoto, T., and Weissman, I. L. (2000) A clonogenic common myeloid progenitor that gives rise to all myeloid lineages. *Nature* **404,** 193–197.
17. Kato, N., Pontier, D., and Lam, E. (2002) Spectral profiling for the simultaneous observation of four distinct fluorescent proteins and detection of protein-protein interaction via fluorescence resonance energy transfer in tobacco leaf nuclei. *Plant Physiol.* **129,** 931–942.
18. Patterson, G., Day, R. N., and Piston, D. (2001) Fluorescent protein spectra. *J. Cell Sci.* **114,** 837–838.
19. Nagai, T., Ibata, K., Park, E. S., Kubota, M., Mikoshiba, K., and Miyawaki, A. (2002) A variant of yellow fluorescent protein with fast and efficient maturation for cell-biological applications. *Nat. Biotechnol.* **20,** 87–90.
20. Pepperkok, R., Squire, A., Geley, S., and Bastiaens, P. I. (1999) Simultaneous detection of multiple green fluorescent proteins in live cells by fluorescence lifetime imaging microscopy. *Curr. Biol.* **9,** 269–272.
21. Lansford, R., Bearman, G., and Fraser, S. E. (2001) Resolution of multiple green fluorescent protein color variants and dyes using two-photon microscopy and imaging spectroscopy. *J. Biomed. Opt.* **6,** 311–318.
22. Lippincott-Schwartz, J., and Patterson, G. H. (2003) Development and use of fluorescent protein markers in living cells. *Science* **300,** 87–91.

27

Analysis of Hematopoietic Development During Human Embryonic Ontogenesis

Manuela Tavian and Bruno Péault

Summary

We describe here diverse methods used to study the onset of hematopoiesis in the human embryo and fetus. In the first part of this chapter, the criteria for estimating developmental stages in human embryos are discussed. This section also presents in detail a refined method for embedding and freezing intact human embryonic tissues that are destined to be analyzed by histology and immunostaining. In the second section, several protocols for the microdissection of human embryos are described in detail, with special attention given to differences encountered between tissues at different ages of gestation. Because of the limited number of cells available at the early stages of human gestation, we have established a miniaturized cell amplification system permitting further development of intact organ rudiments dissected from a human embryo and cultured *in toto*. The last part of the chapter is devoted to the study of myeloid and lymphoid potentials using, respectively, a mouse bone marrow-derived stromal cell line and cultured mouse embryonic thymus rudiments.

Key Words: Human embryo; stem cell; immunohistochemistry; organ culture; T-cell; B-cell; NK cell; aorta; embryonic liver; hematopoiesis.

1. Introduction

Investigations on human developmental hematology were merely limited to incidental observations *(1)* until human embryonic and fetal tissues were made more routinely available to experimentation through voluntary and medical interruptions of pregnancy. Beyond extrapolation of experimental results obtained on animal embryos, direct characterization of human prenatal hematopoietic cells was also stimulated when the transplantation of human fetal liver *(2)* and, to a much larger extent, umbilical cord blood *(3)* came into practice. Even more fundamentally, observations made on human embryos contributed significantly to recent debates pertaining to the very origin of hematopoietic cells in ontogeny, suggesting that stem cells born to the embryo proper, and not derived from the yolk sac, play a central role, if not the only one, in the development of definitive hematopoiesis ***(4,5)***. More than a mere confirmation of conver-

From: *Methods in Molecular Medicine, Vol. 105: Developmental Hematopoiesis: Methods and Protocols.*
Edited by: M. H. Baron © Humana Press Inc., Totowa, NJ

gent observations made in other vertebrates, these studies have documented incipient hematopoiesis in the species where the most extreme temporal restriction of yolk sac blood-forming activity is observed because vitelline hematopoiesis is circumscribed within less than 3 wk of human development. Conversely, embryonic aorta-associated clusters of emerging intraembryonic hematopoietic cells are more conspicuous in human than in animal embryos, which has allowed their more thorough characterization in the former ***(4,6)***. Among other advantages, one must also mention the large array of markers available for human hematolymphoid cells and the usually very high quality of corresponding antibodies because these are commonly used for diagnostic purposes.

Finally, the lack of genuine in vivo assays for human hematopoietic cells has been circumvented by the development of various surrogate xenogeneic systems. Although human early embryonic cells are usually too few in number to be engrafted into immunodeficient mice, the development of small numbers of human stem cells can be efficiently supported by cultured mouse blood-forming stromas, whether they are adherent bone marrow-derived cell lines or thymus embryonic epithelial rudiments maintained in their native three-dimensional arrangement.

2. Materials

2.1. Recovery of Human Tissues

1. Sterile phosphate-buffered saline (PBS) with calcium and magnesium containing antibiotics (penicillin 10 U/mL and streptomycin 10 U/mL).
2. Extra-thin (entomologist-type) pins
3. Wax-bottomed Petri dishes: pour hot paraffin that has been blackened with animal carbon powder (Sigma) into the dishes and allow to solidify.

2.2. Histology and Immunostaining

1. Phosphate buffer: 6.4 g/L $NaH_2PO_4 \cdot H_2O$ and 27 g/L Na_2HPO_4, pH 7.2.
2. Phosphate buffer with 4% paraformaldehyde (w/v; *see* **Note 1**).
3. Phosphate buffer with 15% sucrose (w/v) prepared before use or stored in the refrigerator no longer than 1 wk.
4. Phosphate buffer with 15% sucrose and 7.5% gelatin (w/v). (Store frozen at –20°C for several months and thaw just before use.)
5. Isopentane.
6. Liquid N2.
7. Super frost slides.
8. Antibodies. The first antibody is generally a mouse anti-human antibody; the second one is a biotinylated goat anti-mouse Ig antibody.
9. Horseradish peroxidase-labeled streptavidin (SA-HPR); Alexa 488-labeled streptavidin (SA-Alexa 488); and Alexa 594-labeled streptavidin (SA-Alexa 594; Molecular Probes, Inc., Eugene, OR).
10. Hydrogen peroxide.
11. Diaminobenzidine (DAB; *see* **Note 2**).
12. Harris' hematoxylin for counterstaining.
13. XAM neutral mounting medium (BDH, Poole, UK).
14. Avidin/biotin blocking kit (Vector Laboratories, Burlingame, CA).
15. Mowiol mounting medium (Calbiochem, San Diego, CA; *see* **Note 3**).

2.3. Tissue Dissection

1. Sterile PBS with calcium and magnesium containing antibiotics (penicillin and streptomycin).
2. Sterile small micro-surgical scissors, extra-fine forceps (Dumont no. 5), and custom-made micro-scalpels (*see* **Note 4**).
3. 10-cm Diameter Petri dishes.
4. 50-μm Nylon mesh (Bio Technofix, Bagneux, France).
5. Ficoll-Hypaque (Pharmacia).

2.4. In Vitro Differentiation of Hematopoietic Cells

1. Murine MS-5 stromal cell line *(7,8)*.
2. Trypsin 0.25% (Gibco).
3. α-MEM medium (Gibco).
4. RPMI 1640 medium (Gibco).
5. Human serum, heat-inactivated, AB group (Institut Jacques BOY S.A., Reims, France).
6. Fetal bovine serum (FBS) for use in human myeloid long-term culture medium (Stem Cell Technologies, Vancouver, Canada).
7. Human recombinant cytokines: stem cell factor, Flt3 ligand, thrombopoietin, interleukin (IL)-2, IL-15, IL-7, and IL-3.
8. Nonobese diabetic-severe combined immunodeficient (NOD-SCID) mouse embryonic thymus lobes (d 14).
9. Terasaki cell culture plates.
10. 96-Well and 24-well cell culture plates (Becton-Dickinson).
11. 2-cm Diameter Petri dishes (Greiner Bio-One).
12. Filters (Isopore membrane, 25-mm diameter, 0.8-μm pore size; Millipore).
13. 26-Gage syringe needles.
14. Anti-human antibodies for immunohistochemistry:
    a. CD31 pure JC70A, DAKO; cat. no. M823
    b. CD34 pure Clone QBEN/10, Serotec; cat. no. MCA547
    c. CD45 pure Clone HLe-1, Becton-Dickinson; cat. no. 347460
    d. SMaA pure 1A4, DAKO; cat. no. M851
    e. Gly-A pure JC159, DAKO; cat. no. M819
15. Anti-human antibodies for fluorescence-activated cells sorting (FACS) analysis:
    a. CD4-FITC Clone 13B8.2, Immunotech; cat. no. IM 0448
    b. CD8-PE Clone B9.11, Immunotech; cat. no. IM 0452
    c. CD15-FITC Clone 80H5, Immunotech; cat. no. IM 1423
    d. CD19-PE Clone J4.119, Immunotech; cat. no. IM 1285
    e. CD34-FITC Clone581, Immunotech; cat. no. IM 1870
    f. CD45-PE Clone J33, Immunotech; cat. no. IM 2078
    g. CD56-PE-Cy5 Clone N901, Immunotech; cat. no. IM 2654
    h. CD94-PE Clone HP-3D9, Pharmingen; cat. no. 555889

3. Methods

3.1. Recovery of Human Embryos and Estimation of Gestational Age

Human embryos are obtained immediately after voluntary terminations of pregnancy induced with the RU 486 antiprogestative compound. Portions of fetal liver and long bone marrow are obtained from miscarriages, voluntary terminations by aspiration, and

Table 1
Criteria for Estimating Developmental Stages in Human Embryo. Based on O'Rahilly and Muller, 1987 and Moore, Persaud and Shiota, 1994 *(9,11)*

Carnegie stage	No. of somite pairs	Age (days)	Main external characteristics
8	0	20–21	*Presomite embryo.* The primitive streak extends caudally from the primitive node in the embryonic disc.
9	1–3	20–21	*Flat embryonic disc.* Somites first appear. Head fold evident.
10	4–12	22–23	*Embryo straight or slightly curved.* Neural folds begin to fuse. First and second pairs of branchial arches visible.
11	13–20	24–25	*Embryo curved owing to head and tail folds.* Rostral neuropore closing.
12	21–29	26–27	*Upper limb buds appear.* Three pairs of branchial arches visible. Rostral neuropore closed.
13	30–35	28–30	*Embryo has C-shaped curve.* Lower buds appear. Upper limb buds are flipper-like. Four pairs of branchial arches visible.
14	[a]	31–32	*Upper limbs are paddle-shaped.*
15		33–36	*Hand plates formed.* Lower limbs are paddle-shaped.
16		37–40	*Foot plates formed.* Retinal pigment visible.
17		41–43	*Digital rays clearly visible in hand plates.*
18		44–46	*Digital rays clearly visible in foot plates.*

[a] At this and subsequent stages the number of somites is difficult to determine and so it is not a useful criterion.

medical abortions. Embryos and fetuses are collected in sterile cold PBS containing antibiotics. Embryonic age is estimated based on several anatomic criteria: number of somite pairs at Carnegie stages 9 to 11, limb bud shape and eye pigmentation at stages 12 to 15 and 16 to 17, respectively (*see* **refs. *9,10***; *see* **Table 1**). For fetal tissues, developmental stages are estimated from the duration of the amenorrhea (*see* **Note 5**).

3.2. Histology and Immunostaining

3.2.1. Tissue Fixation

All steps must be conducted at 4°C.

1. Fix tissues overnight in phosphate buffer-4% paraformaldehyde (*see* **Note 6**).
2. Rinse tissues two to three times with phosphate buffer for a total of 24 h.
3. Impregnate tissues twice in phosphate buffer-15% sucrose for at least 24 h (*see* **Note 7**).

3.2.2. Tissue Embedding in Sucrose–Gelatin and Freezing

This protocol is a modified version of the method proposed by Henrique et al. for avian embryos ***(12)***.

1. Immerse tissues in the proper spatial orientation in phosphate buffer-15% sucrose-7% gelatin at 37°C for 1 h, and then let gelatin solidify at 4°C in Petri dishes. A solid block of gelatin-sucrose containing the embryo is formed.
2. Cut out cubes of tissue-containing gelatin and freeze slowly at –60°C in isopentane chilled in liquid N_2. Glue the cubes of tissue-containing gelatin onto a peace of cork (2 × 2 cm) using one to two drops of tissue freezing medium (Jung) to maintain correct orientation of the tissue to be sectioned (the anterior part of the embryo will be at the top of the cube and the posterior at the bottom, near the cork). We use a plastic container with 200 to 300 mL of isopentane immersed in liquid N_2. Check the temperature with a thermometer; when the isopentane reaches –70°C, remove the container from the liquid N_2. Using long forceps, pick up the cork with its attached cube of gelatin. Keep the cube at the surface of the chilled isopentane for about 5 s, and then slowly immerse it into the liquid, in several steps of 5 s each. Once completely immersed, hold the cube in the isopentane for 1 min longer. The cube, now completely white, can be stored for several months at –80°C.
3. Cut 5-μm sections of the embedded tissues on the cryostat at –25 to –28°C. Sections are laid over Super frost slides maintained at room temperature, and can then be stored at –20°C for several months.

3.2.3. Immunostaining by Enzymatic Method

1. Thaw slides at room temperature for about 30 min.
2. Hydrate sections in PBS three times for 5 min each.
3. Inactivate endogenous peroxidases by a passage in PBS containing 0.2% hydrogen peroxide.
4. Rinse slides three times in PBS for 5 min each.
5. Block nonspecific reactions in PBS containing 5% goat serum (PBS-serum) for at least 1 h at room temperature.
6. Incubate overnight at 4°C with the first antibody (generally monoclonal mouse anti-human IgG antibody) diluted to the appropriate concentration in PBS-serum.
7. Wash slides three times in PBS for 5 min each.
8. Incubate for 1 h at room temperature with biotinylated goat anti-mouse IgG antibody diluted in PBS-serum.
9. Wash slides three times in PBS for 5 min.
10. Incubate for 1 h at room temperature with SA-HRP diluted in PBS-serum.
11. Wash slides three times in PBS for 5 min.
12. Use DAB to reveal signal. Dilute DAB to the final concentration of 250 μg/mL in PBS containing 0.03%H_2O_2 (*see* **Note 8**).
13. Wash slides three times in PBS for 5 min.
14. Counterstain sections by covering slide with Harris' hematoxylin until staining is observed. This dye stains the nuclei blue.
15. Wash slides three times in distilled water for 5 min each.
16. Dehydrate the sections successively in 70%, 95%, and 100% ethanol and eventually in toluene for 2 min (each step) and mount the cover slip with XAM.

3.2.4. Immunostaining by Fluorescence

This method is similar to that reported in **Subheading 3.2.3.** In this case, it is not necessary to inactivate endogenous peroxidases (**step 3**), and the streptavidin is directly conjugated to the desired fluorochrome. Slides are then mounted with Mowiol, containing bleaching retardants, before fluorescence microscopy evaluation.

3.2.5. Double Immunofluorescence

Double immunofluorescence is performed using an avidin/biotin blocking step after the first fluorochrome (*see* **Subheading 3.2.4.**).

1. Incubate slides with PBS-serum at room temperature for 1 h.
2. Incubate then with avidin solution for 15 min at room temperature.
3. Wash briefly with PBS and then incubate for 15 min at room temperature with the biotin solution.
4. Proceed following the same protocol as used for simple immunofluorescence (*see* **Subheading 3.2.4.**).

3.3. Tissue Dissection

3.3.1. Embryo Dissection

The dissection procedure on human embryos (3–6 wk of development) changes with the stage of ontogeny. In all cases, the embryo devoid of the amnion is placed dorsally on the bottom of a 10-cm diameter Petri dish filled with cold PBS and the yolk sac is detached (*see* **Fig. 1**). It is possible with experience to leave the embryo free within the dish while carrying out the dissection. However, the latter is easier to perform if the embryo has been fastened to the bottom of the dish. This can be achieved with extra-thin (entomologist-type) pins and a wax-bottomed Petri dish. From 22 to 26 d of development, the para-aortic splanchnopleura, which includes the dorsal aortae, is dissected. At later stages (from 27 to 40 d) the dorsal aorta enclosed in a fine sheath of mesoderm is cut apart with microdissection scissors and fine forceps, from its anterior bifurcation to its caudal end, after the vitelline artery connection (*see* **Note 4**).

3.3.2. Liver Dissection

Embryonic or fetal livers are cut into several small cubes (no more than 2 mm) in a Petri dish containing PBS. These cubes are then disrupted mechanically through grinding between two sterile glass slides. Cell clumps are removed on a 50-μm nylon mesh. Using more advanced stages (after 10 wk of gestation), purification of mononuclear cells is required. In this case cells are centrifuged on a Ficoll–Hypaque gradient. Cells are then washed three times in PBS and can be directly used to perform myeloid and lymphoid potential analyses (*see* **Subheadings 3.4.4.** and **3.4.5.**).

3.4. In Vitro Differentiation of Hematopoietic Stem Cells

The following method described is based on the utilization of MS-5 stroma cells, a murine line that supports, in the presence of added cytokines, the survival, proliferation, and lymphomyeloid differentiation of human hematopoietic stem cells *(7,8)*. Under these conditions, it is possible to develop from embryonic human tissues B lymphocytes ($CD19^+$), NK ($CD56^+$), and myeloid ($CD15^+$) cells and also to maintain T-lymphoid potential as evidenced using fetal thymus organ culture. This is also possible at earlier stages when hematopoietic stem cells cannot be identified by phenotype.

This protocol includes a first step of culture *in toto* (*see* **Subheading 3.4.2.**) where the embryonic explant is cultured intact. It is followed, after mechanical dissociation of tissues, by experiments of lymphomyeloid differentiation (*see* **Subheadings 3.4.4., 3.4.5.,** and **Fig. 2**).

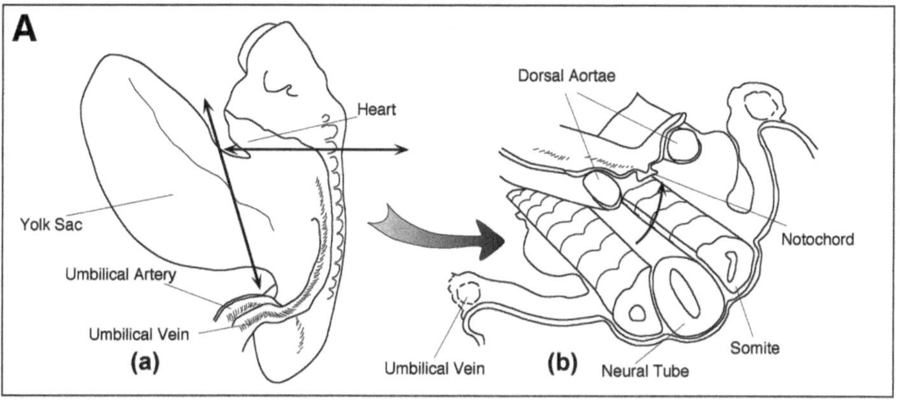

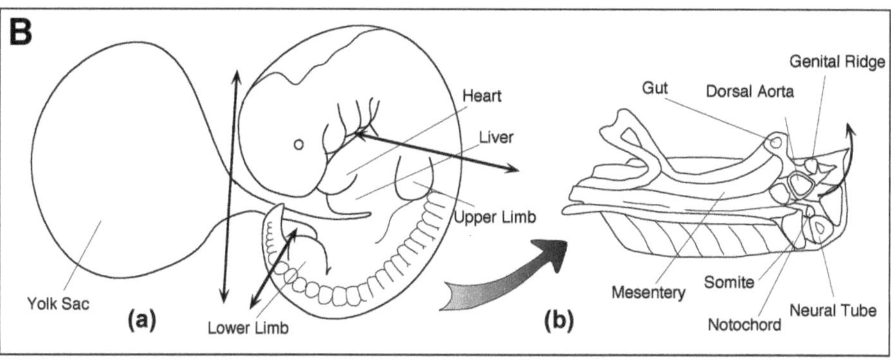

Fig. 1. Embryo dissection. **(A)** 24-d human embryo. After detaching of the yolk sac and upper part including the head and heart (a), the embryo is place dorsally (b). Using extra-fine forceps all the para-aortic region is dissected as shown in (b). **(B)** 32-d human embryo. At this stage also the caudal part is cut out (a), and the truncal region of the embryo is placed dorsally. The mesentery including the dorsal aorta, gut, and genital ridge is then dissected from the embryo (b). From this region, the dorsal aorta is then cut apart.

3.4.1. Stromal Cell Culture

The MS-5 stroma line can be maintained in the incubator for several passages, at 37°C, in a 5% CO_2 atmosphere. However, during prolonged culture, changes in cell morphology occur such as the appearance of lipid vacuoles inside the cytosol. This is accompanied by a gradual loss in the ability of the cell line to support hematopoiesis. In this case it is suggested that a new vial of cells be thawed. MS-5 cells are cultured in α-MEM medium containing 10% FBS and split (1:10) once every 10 d (*see* **Note 9**). The day before co-culture initiation, MS-5 stroma cells are seeded at the concentration of 3000 cells/well and 20,000 cells/well in 96-well and 24-well plates, respectively.

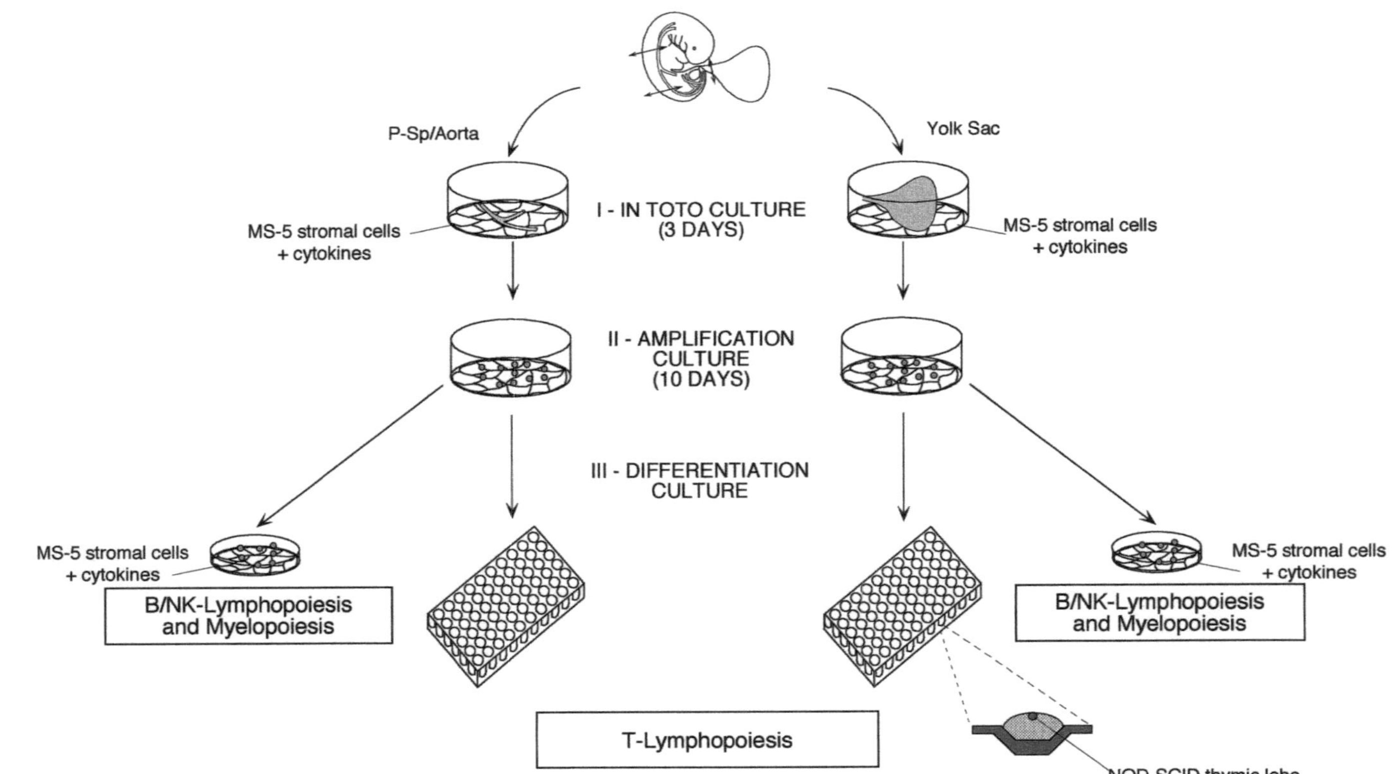

Fig. 2. Human embryo culture. *See* text for details.

3.4.2. *In Toto* Culture

The splanchnopleura, truncal aorta, liver or yolk sac are dissected under sterile conditions under the microscope and seeded undissociated in a 24-well plate containing MS-5 stroma cells. Explants are cultured *in toto* for 2 to 3 d, in RPMI supplemented with human serum, FBS, and human recombinant cytokines: 50 ng/mL stem cell factor, 50 ng/mL Flt3 ligand, 50 ng/mL thrombopoietin, 5 ng/mL IL-2, 10 ng/mL IL-15, 10 ng/mL IL-3, and 20 ng/mL IL-3 (*see* **Note 10**).

3.4.3. Amplification Culture

1. Tissues are then dissociated mechanically by repeated passages through a 26-gage needle, and cells are cultivated for 10 additional days in the same wells (*see* **Fig. 2**).
2. Cells harvested from the well by pipetting are then seeded on fresh MS-5 stromal layers in a 96-well plate. Generally, the contents of one well from a 24-well plate are split into 10 wells in a 96-well plate. At this step, half of the cells can be used to perform T-lymphoid potential analyses (*see* **Subheading 3.4.5.**).

3.4.4. Lymphomyeloid Differentiation Culture

Lymphomyeloid differentiation is performed under the same conditions and in the same medium as described in **Subheading 3.4.2.**

1. Plates are scored visually under the inverted microscope from wk 1 through wk 5 for the presence of hematopoietic cells, and only wells where significant proliferation has occurred are selected.
2. Cells are then collected by pipetting and marked with the hematopoietic cell-specific MoAbs for FACS analysis (*see* **ref. *5*** and **Note 11**). A portion of the cells harvested from a well can be seeded back onto a fresh MS-5 stromal layer.

3.4.5. T-Cell Development in Xenogenic Fetal Thymus Organ Culture

In contrast to myeloid and B-lymphoid differentiation, which takes place in the bone marrow environment and can be sustained on cultured dissociated stromal cells, development of T-cells requires the presence of thymic stromal cells in their intact, native three-dimensional arrangement. The method proposed here to drive T-cell differentiation from human embryonic precursors is based on the use of embryonic thymus lobes from NOD-SCID mice **ref. *13***; *see* **Note 12**).

After in vitro amplification over MS-5 stroma layers (*see* **Subheading 3.4.3.** and **Fig. 2**), cells are collected from the well and incubated with murine embryonic (d 14) thymus lobes (*see* **Note 13**). Colonization of thymic tissue by human cells is facilitated by using the hanging drop procedure:

1. 25 μL of complete medium (RPMI 1640 supplemented with 10% heat-inactivated human serum, 5% fetal calf serum, 5 ng/mL rh-IL2, 20 ng/mL rh-IL7, and 50 ng/mL rh-SCF) containing 50 to 100,000 cells harvested from the amplification culture are dropped in wells of Terasaki plates.
2. One thymus lobe from a 14-d NOD-SCID mouse embryo is carefully added to each well, ensuring that it floats at the top of the drop (*see* **Note 14** and **Fig. 2**).
3. Plates are immediately flipped upside down to allow the formation of hanging drops and incubated undisturbed in a humidified incubator (5% CO_2 in air, 37°C) for 48 h (*see* **Note 15**).

4. After 48 h, Terasaki plates are placed back in the usual orientation and thymuses are transferred with fine forceps onto floating Nucleopore filters in six-well plates containing 2.5 mL of complete medium without cytokines per well. Thymus lobes are cultured under these conditions for a further 18 to 22 d.
5. Thymuses are then recovered and single-cell suspensions are obtained by teasing each individual lobe with two needles under the dissecting microscope.
6. Cells are incubated with anti-human CD4, -CD8, and -CD45 monoclonal antibodies for FACS analysis (*see* **Note 16**).

4. Notes

1. Phosphate-buffered paraformaldehyde is best prepared fresh but may also be stored frozen at –20°C for several months.
2. DAB is a known mutagen; handle with gloves.
3. Mowiol is a mounting medium recommended for use in fluorescence microscopy. To prepare this medium, add 2.4 g of Mowiol 4 to 88 to 6 g of glycerol. Stir to mix. Add 6 mL of water and leave for 2 h at room temperature. Add 12 mL of 0.2 *M* Tris (pH 8.5), and incubate at 53°C until Mowiol has dissolved. Stir occasionally. Clarify by centrifugation at 5000*g* for 15 min. For fluorescence detection, add 2.5% (w/v) 1,4-diazobicyclo-[2.2.2]-octane (DABCO) to reduce fading. Store at –20°C. The solution is stable at this temperature for about a year. Once thawed, it is stable at room temperature for at least 1 mo.
4. Only microsurgery instruments of highest quality and sharpness should be used. Any attempt to use blunt-ended forceps (check under the dissecting microscope) will result in destruction of the embryo. The micro-scalpels are custom-made using normal small sewing needles, which are abraded in oil on a series of abrasive stones (Arkansas stones) with increasingly finer grains in order to obtain a sharp point slanted like a scalpel.
5. Regulations regarding the use in research of human embryonic and fetal tissues vary among countries. Approval must be sought from relevant ethics committees and written consent must be obtained from the patient. All tissues of human origin should be handled at all steps with special care under a laminar flow hood, wearing rubber gloves and a lab coat. Waste should be soaked in diluted bleach before being discarded.
6. If the tissue is very small (2–3 mm), 1 to 2 h of incubation is enough.
7. Because saturation of the tissue with sucrose has a cryo-preservative function, this step is very important and can be also be extended to 48 h.
8. DAB is sensitive to light; cover the tube with dark paper during use.
9. Because MS-5 cells display contact inhibition when confluent, irradiation of the cells is not required prior to performing hematopoietic cell coculture. A layer of confluent MS-5 stromal cells can therefore be maintained in culture for several weeks.
10. The *in toto* culture allows the development of the explant to continue to some extent in vitro. This step is especially important when very early embryos are analyzed. In these tissues blood cells are not yet formed and induction of a hematopoietic cell fate within the mesoderm requires physical contact with the endoderm.
11. It is advisable to perform in parallel, under the same culture conditions, a positive control using a familiar source of hematopoietic stem cells, such as cord blood-sorted $CD34^+$ cells. In some instances, negative results can be caused by poor maintenance in culture of MS-5 stromal cells, rather than to absence of hematopoietic precursors. In this setting, hematopoietic cells proliferate rapidly and are numerous enough to be analyzed after only 7 d of differentiation culture. B-cells usually appear during the third week of co-culture, significantly later than other blood cell types.

12. Since the SCID mutation blocks T-cell development in NOD-SCID mice at an early stage, removal of endogenous thymocytes is not required.
13. As a positive control, mouse thymuses are incubated with 2000 to 5000 cord blood-derived $CD34^+$-sorted cells in each experiment.
14. It should be noted that, although the 16-d thymus is repopulated efficiently by cord blood purified $CD34^+$ progenitors ***(13)***, 14-d mouse thymic lobes are much more efficiently repopulated by T-cell progenitors of human embryonic origin ***(5)***.
15. To avoid dehydration of the wells in the incubator, it is suggested to place the inverted Terasaki plate in a large Petri dish with some small dishes (2 cm in diameter) containing water.
16. Phenotypic analysis of the T-cells produced reveals the presence of both immature $CD4^+CD8^-$ cells and double-positive $CD4^+CD8^+$ T-lymphocytes. However, under these conditions further positive selection resulting in the production of $CD8^+$ single-positive T-cells is compromised by the poor reactivity of murine class I, and to a lesser degree, class II molecules with human cells ***(14)***.

References

1. Bloom, W. and Bartelmez, G. W. (1940) Hematopoiesis in young human embryos. *Am. J. Anat.* **67,** 21–53.
2. Touraine, J. L. (1990) In utero transplantation of stem cells in humans. *Nouv. Rev. Fr. Hematol.* **32,** 441–444.
3. Gluckman, E., Broxmeyer, H. A., Auerbach, A. D., Friedman, H. S., Douglas, G. W., Devergie, A., et al. (1989) Hematopoietic reconstitution in a patient with Fanconi's anemia by means of umbilical-cord blood from an HLA-identical sibling. *N. Engl. J. Med.* **321,** 1174–1178.
4. Tavian, M., Coulombel, L., Luton, D., Clemente, H. S., Dieterlen-Lievre, F., and Peault, B. (1996) Aorta-associated CD34+ hematopoietic cells in the early human embryo. *Blood* **87,** 67–72.
5. Tavian, M., Robin, C., Coulombel, L., and Peault, B. (2001) The human embryo, but not its yolk sac, generates lympho-myeloid stem cells: mapping multipotent hematopoietic cell fate in intraembryonic mesoderm. *Immunity* **15,** 487–495.
6. Labastie, M. C., Cortes, F., Romeo, P. H., Dulac, C., and Peault, B. (1998) Molecular identity of hematopoietic precursor cells emerging in the human embryo. *Blood* **92,** 3624–3635.
7. Berardi, A. C., Meffre, E., Pflumio, F., Katz, A., Vainchenker, W., Schiff, C., et al. (1997) Individual CD34+CD38lowCD19-CD10- progenitor cells from human cord blood generate B lymphocytes and granulocytes. *Blood* **89,** 3554–3564.
8. Robin, C., Pflumio, F., Vainchenker, W., and Coulombel, L. (1999) Identification of lymphomyeloid primitive progenitor cells in fresh human cord blood and in the marrow of nonobese diabetic-severe combined immunodeficient (NOD-SCID) mice transplanted with human CD34(+) cord blood cells. *J. Exp. Med.* **189,** 1601–1610.
9. O'Rahilly, R. and Müller, F. (1987) *Developmental Stages in Human Embryos*, Carnegie Institution of Washington, Washington, DC.
10. Tavian, M., Hallais, M. F., and Peault, B. (1999) Emergence of intraembryonic hematopoietic precursors in the pre-liver human embryo. *Development* **126,** 793–803.
11. Moore, K. L., Persaud, T. V. N., and Shiota, K. (1994) *Color Atlas of Clinical Embryology*, W. B. Saunders Company, Philadelphia, PA.
12. Henrique, D., Adam, J., Myat, A., Chitnis, A., Lewis, J., and Ish-Horowicz, D. (1995) Expression of a Delta homologue in prospective neurons in the chick. *Nature* **375,** 787–790.

13. Robin, C., Bennaçeur-Griscelli, A., Louache, F., Vainchenker, W., and Coulombel, L. (1999) Identification of human T-lymphoid progenitor cells in CD34+ CD38low and CD34+ CD38+ subsets of human cord blood and bone marrow cells using NOD-SCID fetal thymus organ cultures. *Br. J. Haematol.* **104,** 809–819.
14. Blom, B., Res, P., Noteboom, E., Weijer, K., and Spits, H. (1997) Prethymic CD34+ progenitors capable of developing into T cells are not committed to the T cell lineage. *J. Immunol.* **158,** 3571–3577.

28

Hematopoietic Development of Human Embryonic Stem Cells in Culture

Xinghui Tian and Dan S. Kaufman

Summary

The isolation of embryonic stem (ES) cells from human preimplantation blastocytes creates an exciting new starting point to analyze the earliest stages of human blood development. This chapter describes two methods for the promotion of hematopoietic differentiation of human ES cells: stromal cell co-culture and embryoid body formation. Better understanding of basic human hematopoiesis through the study of human ES cells will likely have future therapeutic benefits.

Key Words: Embryonic stem cells; hematopoiesis; embryoid body; stromal cell; differentiation; hematopoietic stem cell.

1. Introduction

Human embryonic stem (ES) cells offer many advantages for studies of basic hematopoiesis. Human ES cells can be maintained for months to years in culture as undifferentiated cells, yet retain the ability to form any cell type within the body *(1,2)*. This potential is presumed from studies with mouse ES cells because definitive studies of human ES cell totipotency cannot be performed. Human ES cells are derived from early blastocysts, and development of these cells into specific lineages likely recapitulates events that occur during normal development. 10^7 or more human ES cells can be easily grown and sampled at any time point during differentiation into specific cellular lineages. These numbers should be sufficient for detailed in vitro and in vivo studies. Perhaps most importantly, twenty years of studies with mouse ES cells clearly demonstrate the value of this developmental system *(3,4)*. Mouse ES cells have been used to define genetic pathways that regulate blood development (and many other lineages), and this knowledge has been shown to translate to human models such as umbilical cord blood or bone marrow-based hematopoietic development. However, only human ES cells allow characterization of the earliest stages of prenatal human hematopoietic development. Specifically, these cells can be used to understand how human hematopoietic stem cells (HSCs) arise from earlier precursors. Although this question has been addressed in murine systems with studies of mouse ES cells and

From: *Methods in Molecular Medicine, Vol. 105: Developmental Hematopoiesis: Methods and Protocols.*
Edited by: M. H. Baron © Humana Press Inc., Totowa, NJ

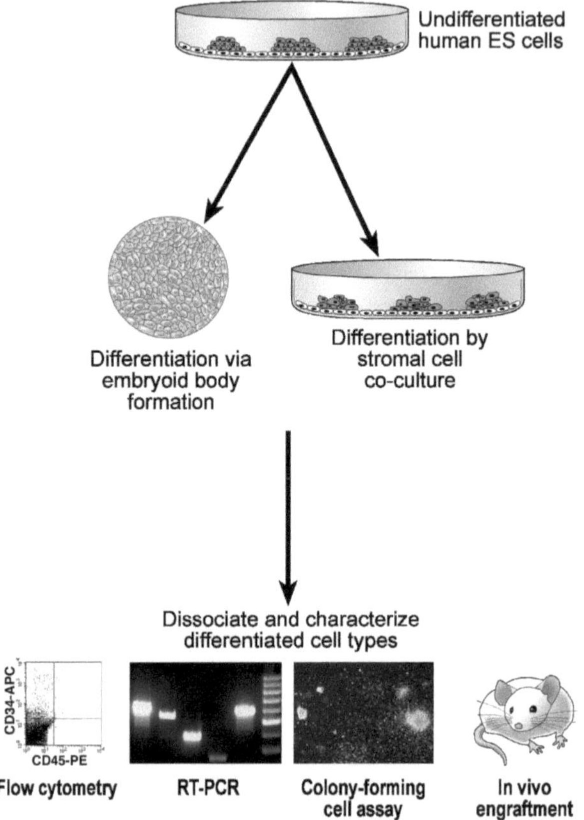

Fig. 1. Schematic of differentiation and analysis of human ES cell-derived hematopoietic cells.

dissection of timed embryos, there are some fundamental differences between mouse and human embryogenesis that suggest that not all developmental pathways may be the same *(5)*. Indeed, mouse and human ES cells have key differences in their phenotype, growth characteristics, and culture requirements that likely translate into unique pathways of development *(1,4,6)*.

This chapter outlines two methods to promote hematopoietic differentiation of human ES cells (**Fig. 1**). Isolation and maintenance of undifferentiated human ES cells will not be discussed in detail. Briefly, human ES cells are routinely maintained in serum-free medium either in direct co-culture with irradiated mouse embryonic fibroblast (MEF) "feeder" cells or in "feeder-free" conditions by culture on Matrigel or laminin-coated plates *(1,7)*. The "feeder-free" growth still requires ES cells to be grown in medium conditioned by MEFs. Therefore, a requirement for feeder cells remains. Some reports have shown other (human) feeder cells can be used to maintain undifferentiated human ES cells, thus potentially avoiding some xenogeneic exposures *(8,9)*.

Original studies of hematopoiesis from human ES cells used co-culture with stromal cells derived from hematopoietic microenvironments to support or promote development of phenotypically and genotypically defined blood cells *(10)*. This co-culture method is technically straightforward and offers the advantage to potentially characterize and modify the stromal cells to define what components they contribute to the hematopoietic process. Indeed, the finding that nonspecific fibroblasts did not support hematopoietic differentiation strongly suggested that interactions between the differentiating ES cells and the stromal cells were important to support blood development. Therefore, in principle, the stromal cells could be engineered to understand better what cell-bound and soluble factors they contribute to hematopoietic development. Because human ES cells were initially thought to be difficult to modify genetically (many methods used for mouse ES cells required modification for use with human ES cells), the ability to analyze inputs from stromal cells offered an important advantage. However, several recent reports have defined methods to stably express exogenous genes in human ES cells *(11–14)*. Differentiation of human ES cells via embryoid body (EB) formation also offers a suitable method to promote hematopoiesis. EB formation is an important method when researchers want to avoid more complex interactions with stromal cells. However, as ES cells differentiate, they rapidly become a diverse mixture of cell types. Typically, only a few percent are blood cells. While understanding all components that contribute development of specific lineages will remain a challenge, human ES cells are now an important resource for the characterization of hematopoietic pathways. Moreover, human ES cells offer the exciting prospect of becoming a suitable source to replace or repair cells, tissues, or organs damaged by disease, trauma, degeneration, or other processes.

In the methods described in this chapter, undifferentiated human embryonic stem (hES) cells were maintained in serum-free medium. To promote hematopoietic differentiation via stromal cell coculture, the human ES cells were typically co-cultured with the mouse bone marrow stromal cell line S17 *(15)*, although other cell lines derived from hematopoietic microenvironments, such as C166 *(16)*, OP9 *(17)*, or primary human bone marrow-derived stromal cells *(18)*, can be used. After a defined number of days in culture, hematopoietic precursor cells derived from human embryonic stem cells are analyzed by fluorescence-activated cell sorting (FACS), colony-forming assays, and reverse transcription polymerase chain reaction. Other assay systems for early hematopoietic progenitors cells, such as the long-term culture initiating cell (LTC-IC) assay *(19)* or injection into non-obese diabetic severe-combined immunodeficient mice, can be used *(20)*.

2. Materials

2.1. Co-Culture of Human ES Cells and S17 Cells

2.1.1. Cell Culture Media

1. hES cell medium: DMEM/F12 (Invitrogen Corporation/Gibco; cat. no. 11330-032) supplemented with 15% knockout SR (Invitrogen Corporation/Gibco; cat. no. 10828-028), 0.1 m*M* β-mercaptoethanol (Sigma; cat. no. M7522), 2 m*M* L-glutamine (Invitrogen Corporation/Gibco; cat. no. 21051-024), 1% MEM nonessential amino acids solution (Invitrogen Corporation/Gibco; cat. no.11140-050), and 4 ng/mL basic fibroblast growth factor (bFGF; Invitrogen; cat. no.13256-029). For culture of undifferentiated hES cells,

L-glutamine is routinely prepared fresh from powder by mixing 0.146 g of L-glutamine and 7 μL of β-mercaptoethanol in 10 mL of phosphate-buffered saline (PBS). L-glutamine-PBS solution (2.5 mL) is added to 250 mL of hES medium, for a final concentration of 2 m*M* L-glutamine and 0.1 m*M* β-mercaptoethanol. bFGF powder (10 μg) is reconstituted in 5 mL of 0.1% Fraction V BSA (prepared in sterile PBS). Aliquot 0.5 mL into sterile tubes and store at –80°C. For the hES medium, add 0.5 mL of the reconstituted bFGF to 250 mL of hES medium.

2. S17 Culture medium: RPMI1640 (Cellgro/Mediatech; cat. no. 10-040-CV) medium containing 10% fetal bovine serum (FBS) certified (Invitrogen Corporation/Gibco; cat. no. 16000-044), 0.055 m*M* β-mercaptoethanol (Invitrogen Corporation/Gibco; cat. no. 21985-023), 1% MEM nonessential amino acids, 1% penicillin–streptomycin (P/S; Invitrogen Corporation/Gibco; cat. no.15140-122), 2 m*M* L-glutamine (Cellgro/Mediatech; cat. no. 25-005-CI).
3. hES/S17 Differentiation medium: Dulbecco's modified Eagle's medium (DMEM) (Invitrogen Corporation/Gibco; cat. no. 11965-092) supplemented with 20% defined FBS (Hyclone; cat. no. SH30070.03), 2 m*M* L-glutamine, 0.1 m*M* β-mercaptoethanol, 1% MEM nonessential amino acids solution, and 1% P/S (same as S17 culture medium).
4. D-10 Medium used for washing: DMEM supplemented with 10% FBS and 1% P/S.
5. Collagenase split medium: DMEM/F12 medium containing 1 mg/mL collagenase type IV (Invitrogen Corporation/Gibco; cat. no.17104-019). Collagenase medium is filter sterilized with a 50-mL, 0.22-μm membrane Steriflip (Millipore; cat. no. SCGP00525).
6. Trypsin–ethylene diamine tetraacetic acid (EDTA) + 2% chick serum: 0.05% trypsin–0.53 m*M* EDTA solution (Cellgro/Mediatech; cat. no. 25-052-CI) with 2% chicken serum (Sigma; cat. no. C5405; *see* **Note 1**).

2.1.2. Cell Culture Supplies

1. Six-well tissue culture plates (NUNC™ Brand Products, Nalgene Nunc; cat. no. 152795).
2. Gelatin (Sigma; cat. no. G-1890): 0.1% (w/v) in water. Autoclave for sterility.
3. Disposable serological pipets (all from VWR Scientific Products): 10 mL (cat. no. 53283-740); 5 mL (cat. no. 53283-738); and 1 mL (cat. no.53283-734; *see* **Note 2**).
4. 70-μm Cell strainer filter (Becton Dickinson/Falcon; ref. 352350).
5. 0.4% Trypan blue stain (Invitrogen Corporation/Gibco; cat. no. 15250).

2.2. EB Formation From Human ES Cells

2.2.1. Cell Culture Media

1. Stemline hematopoietic stem cell expansion medium (Sigma; cat. no. S-0189) supplemented with 4 m*M* L-glutamine and 1% P/S (*see* **Note 3**).
2. Dispase split medium: 0.25 g of dispase powder (Invitrogen Corporation/Gibco; cat. no.17105-041) in 50 mL of DMEM/F-12, then filter sterilized with a 50-mL, 0.22-μm membrane Steriflip (Millipore; cat. no. SCGP00525); dispase final concentration 5 mg/mL.
3. DMEM supplemented with 15% defined FBS (Hyclone; cat. no. SH30070.03), 1% L-glutamine, 1% P/S, 1% MEM nonessential amino acids solution, and 0.1 m*M* 2-mercaptoethanol (Invitrogen Corporation, Gibco; cat. no. 21985-023).

2.2.2. Cell Culture Supplies

1. Poly 2-hydroxyethyl methacrylate (poly-HEME; Sigma; cat. no. P-3932); 1.0 g of poly-HEME powder dissolved in 25 mL of acetone + 25 mL of ethanol in a glass bottle; final concentration 0.02 g/mL.

2. Nontissue culture-treated T25 flasks (Sarstedt; ref. no. 83.1810.502) coated with 2% poly-HEME solution.
3. Blue Max polypropylene 15-mL conical tubes (Becton Dickinson/Falcon; cat. no. 352097).

2.3. Flow Cytometric Analysis (see **Note 4**)

1. FACS wash medium: PBS containing 2% FBS and 0.1% sodium azide (Fisher chemicals; cat. no. S227I).
2. 12 × 75-mm Polystyrene round-bottom tube (Becton Dickinson/Falcon; cat. no. 352054)
3. Propidium iodide (PI; Sigma, P4170) 1 mg/mL dissolved in PBS. Store aliquots at 4°C.

2.4. Hematopoietic Colony-Forming Cell (CFC) Assays

1. MethoCult GF$^+$ H4435 (StemCell Technologies, Vancouver; cat. no. 04435) consisting of 1% methylcellulose, 30% FBS, 1% BSA, 50 ng/mL stem cell factor, 20 ng/mL granulocyte–macrophage colony-stimulating factor, 20 ng/mL interleukin (IL)-3, 20 ng/mL IL-6, 20 ng/mL granulocyte colony-stimulating factor, and 3 U/mL erythropoietin. This medium is optimized for detection of most primitive CFCs. A 100-mL bottle of Methocult can be aliquoted into 2.5-mL samples. Alternatively, Methocult can also be purchased prealiquoted into 3-mL samples.
2. I-2 Medium: Iscove's modified Dulbecco's medium (Invitrogen Corporation, Gibco; cat. no. 12440-053) containing 2% FBS.
3. Nontissue culture-treated 35-mm Petri dish (Greiner Bio-One; cat. no. 627102; *see* **Note 5**).
4. Stripette disposible serological pipet (2 mL; Costar, cat. no. 4021).

2.5. RNA Isolation

1. TRIzol (Invitrogen; cat. no. 15596-026; *see* **Note 6**).
2. Diethyl pyrocarbonate (Sigma; cat. no. D5758).
3. 95% Ethanol.
4. Isopropyl alcohol.

3. Methods

3.1. Culture of Undifferentiated hES Cells

Undifferentiated hES cells were cultured as previously described ***(1,2)***. They were maintained in ES cell medium by co-culture with irradiated MEF cells or in MEF-conditioned medium on matrigel-coated plates (**ref.** *7*; *see* **Note 7**). hES cells are fed daily with fresh medium and are passed onto fresh feeder plates or matrigel-coated plates at approx weekly intervals to maintain undifferentiated growth.

3.2. Preparation of S17 Feeder Layer

Mouse bone marrow S17 cells (3) are maintained in S17 culture medium. To prepare feeder layers, the S17 cells are dissociated with Trypsin–EDTA and irradiated (20 Gy; *see* **Note 7**). Irradiated S17 cells (2.5 mL at 1.0×10^5 cells/mL are plated onto 0.1% gelatin-coated six-well plates (thus, 2.5×10^5 cells per well). Feeder layers should be prepared 1 or more days prior to co-culture with hES cells and remain suitable for use up to 2 wk when kept in a 37°C, 5% CO_2 incubator.

Other stromal cell lines can also be used in a similar manner, although irradiation dose and cell density may vary.

3.3. Co-Culture of hES Cell on S17

For hES cells co-cultures, to improve the viability of human ES cells, small colonies, or clusters of ES cells should be plated onto S17 cell rather than cultured as a single cell suspension. To maintain small colonies rather than single cells, collagenase type IV is used to harvest ES cells.

1. Warm collagenase split medium to 37°C in a water bath.
2. Aspirate medium off of hES cells culture and add 1.5 mL/well collagenase split medium. Place in 37°C incubator for 5 to 10 min, observing at approx 5-min intervals. Cells are ready to be harvested when the edges of the colony are rounded up and curled away from the MEFs or from the matrigel plate.
3. Using 5-mL pipet, scrape and gently pipet to wash the colonies off of the plate, transfer cell suspension to a 15-mL conical tube and add another 3 to 6 mL of hES/S17 differentiation medium. Centrifuge at 400*g* for 5 min. Aspirate medium and wash cells with additional 3 to 6 mL hES/S17 differentiation medium by centrifugation again at 400*g* for 5 min.
4. During this last centrifuge step, prepare the S17 feeder layers by aspirating off the S17 medium and add 2 mL/well of PBS to wash one time.
5. After centrifugation of the hES cells, aspirate medium, resuspend cells in an appropriate volume with hES/S17 differentiation medium. Add 1 mL of cell suspension per well onto S17 plate, then add additional 1.5 to 2 mL of hES/S17 differentiation medium to each well. To evenly distribute cells, gently shake the plate from side to side while placing them in 37°C /5% CO_2 incubator. This will allow hES cells attach evenly within the wells. Do not disturb plates for several hours.
6. During differentiation, culture medium is changed every 2 to 3 d. Typical morphology of cells is shown in **Fig. 2**. For first few days, colonies maintain the appearance of undifferentiated hES cells. They then show obvious evidence of differentiation, forming three dimensional cystic and other loosely adherent structures.

3.4. Dissociation and Harvesting of Differentiated hES Cells

Optimal time required for differentiation into $CD34^+$ cells and CFCs varies somewhat depending on the hES cell line and stromal cells used. In general, a culture period of 14 to 21 d results in the best differentiation. A time course experiment in which cells are sampled every 2 to 3 d is recommended to find the optimal time for formation of specific lineages. For flow cytometry and colony-forming assays, it is necessary to produce a single cell suspension of hES cells that have differentiated on S17 or other stromal cells. Because stromal cells are irradiated prior to coculture with ES cells (*see* **Note 7**), >90% of cells harvested will be derived from hES cells.

To prepare single cell suspension:

1. With differentiated hES cell-derived cells in a six-well plate, aspirate medium and add 1.5 mL of collagenase IV per well for 5 to 10 min until stromal cells layer become more spindle-shaped and break up. Scrape with a 5-mL pipet and transfer hES/S17 cell suspension into 15-mL conical tube. Add another 6 mL of Ca^{2+} and Mg^{2+}-free PBS and break up the colonies by pipetting up and down (vigorously) against the bottom of the tube until there a fine suspension of cells is produced. Centrifuge cell suspension at 400*g* for 5 min.
2. Remove the supernatant and add 1.5 mL of trypsin/EDTA + 2% chick serum solution into the tube. Warm at 37°C in a water bath for 5 to 15 min. Vigorously vortex and observe samples at 3- to 5-min intervals until there are few, if any, clumps of undispersed cells.

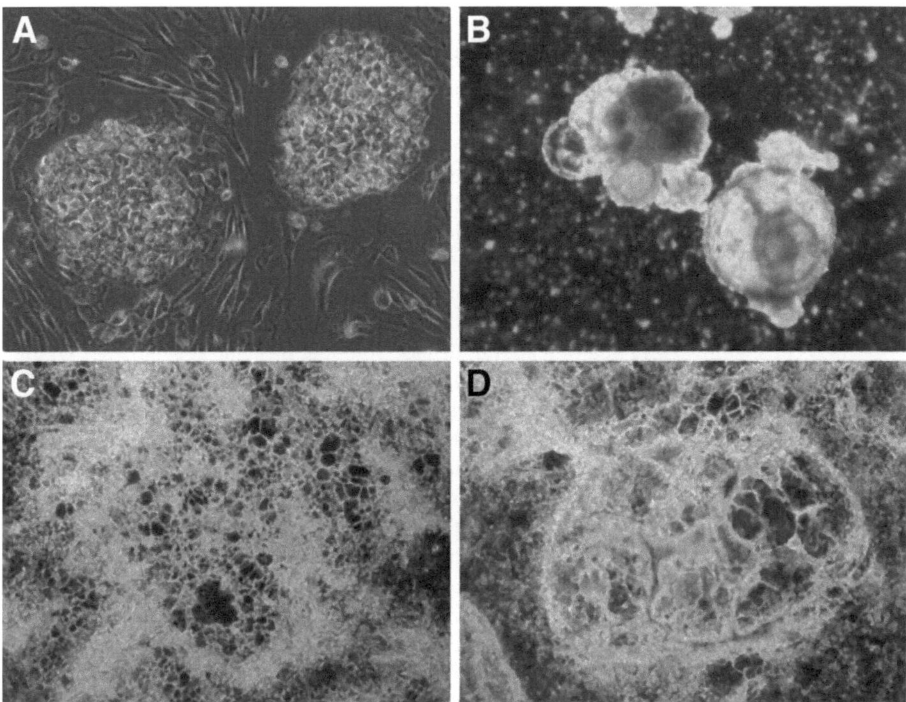

Fig. 2. Hematopoietic differentiation of human ES cells. **(A)** Two colonies of undifferentiated human ES cells grown on MEF feeder layer. These colonies demonstrate uniform morphology with no visible evidence of differentiation. Original magnification 100X. **(B)** Human ES cells induced to form embryoid bodies in suspension for 14 d. Multiple cell types and cystic regions are evident. Original magnification 100X. **(C)** Human ES cells allowed to differentiate on S17 stromal cells for 8 d. The majority of cells in this image are derived from a single colony that has differentiated into multiple cell types, including thin endothelial-type structures and more densely piled-up regions. Original magnification 20X. **(D)** Human ES cells allowed to differentiate on S17 cells for 16 d. These cells are now seen to form spherical, cystic structures, and a variety of other cell types. Original magnification 100X. Some aspects of ES cell differentiation on S17 cells begins to resemble the structure seen in EBs grown in suspension **(B)**.

3. Add 6 mL of DMEM containing 10% FBS (D-10 medium) to neutralize the trypsin–EDTA and pipet up and down to further disperse cells. Centrifuge at 400*g* for 5 min. Resuspend cell pellet with 5 mL of D-10 medium. Filter the cell suspension with 70 μm cell strainer filter to remove any remaining clumps of cells. Count viable cells after staining with 0.4% Trypan blue, using a hemocytometer. From a nearly confluent well, $1–2 \times 10^6$ single hES cells can be obtained.
4. Aliquot cells as needed for FACS, RNA, protein, and hematopoietic CFC assays. Performing multiple assays from the same collection of differentiated ES cells will ensure uniformity of results. Depending on density of cells, two to three wells can be harvested at a single time point to collect enough cells for FACS, CFC, and RNA analysis.

3.5. EB Formation

1. Preparation of hES cells: use human ES cell colonies that contain (by morphological criteria) only undifferentiated cells. EB formation works best when colonies are neither very large nor very small. With experience, one develops a feeling for those colony sizes that work well. If they are too small, the colonies will dissociate within 2 to 4 d. If the colonies are too large, they will not dissociate very easily, and in an attempt to break them apart, they may be damaged. Also, with larger colonies EB formation may not occur efficiently. An ideal time for hES cells to form EBs is typically 6 to 7 d after their last passage date. One six-well plate can generate up to six T25 flasks (one well per flask), although EBs can be pooled into flasks at higher density, as desired.
2. Forming EBs: aspirate the medium from each well, leaving the colonies adherent. Treat hES cells with 1.5 mL/well of 5 mg/mL dispase solution. Incubate at 37°C/5% CO_2 until 50% of the colonies are detached. This usually takes 5 to 10 min with freshly made dispase and can take up to 15 min with an older dispase solution. Gently shake the plate until the remaining colonies detach. If they do not detach, use a 5-mL pipet to wash them off.
3. Add 2 mL of Stemline medium to each well and gently separate the colonies by pipetting up and down. Transfer the cell suspension into a 15-mL conical tube and spin in a centrifuge at 400*g* for 2 min to wash. Aspirate the supernatant, gently flick the tube, and then add 5 mL of fresh Stemline medium. Repeat for three total washes in Stemline medium.
4. Aliquot the cell suspension into untreated T25 flasks, and then add Stemline to a final volume of 7 to 8 mL. Incubate at 37°C/5% CO_2, laying the flask horizontal on the shelf.
5. EB resuspension: the day after EB formation, the cells must be "cleaned-up" to remove remaining stromal and dead cells from the suspension. The EBs should be resuspended in fresh medium and flasks every 3 to 4 d to optimize growth and prevent adhesion. Resuspend the cells in a 15-mL conical tube. If smaller EBs are desired, or the cells have "clumped" together overnight, pipet up and down. Let EBs settle to the bottom. Gently aspirate the supernatant and try to remove the smaller cells that float in the supernatant. Resuspend the cells in 7 to 8 mL of desired medium and add to a T25 flask. Incubate at 37°C/5% CO_2.
6. If the EBs are to be cultured in medium containing FBS, coat the flask with poly-HEME solution to decrease adherence of EBs to plastic. This should be performed approx 45 min before EB resuspension. Using a 1-mL glass pipet, wash 0.5 mL of 2% poly-heme solution over the surface of the untreated T25 flask (Sarstedt) and then aspirate. This poly-HEME can be used to treat another flask. Let the flasks sit in a sterile tissue culture hood with caps completely off for approx 40 min. Wash the poly-heme coated surface with 3 mL of desired medium before adding the EBs. The EBs can then be added and cultured.

3.6. Dissociation of EBs

1. Add EBs to a 15-mL conical tube, let them settle by gravity for approx 1 min, and gently aspirate medium and floating cells that have not yet settled out.
2. Wash with 5 mL of Ca^{2+}- and Mg^{2+}-free PBS, then centrifuge at 400*g* for 3 min.
3. Aspirate supernatant, add 1.5–2 mL of trypsin–EDTA with 2% chick serum, vigorously pipet up and down several times, and vortex to break up EBs.
4. Incubate in 37°C water bath for 5 min, vortex, and pipet vigorously to further dissociate EBs. Return tube to water bath for another 5 min and again remove to vortex and pipet vigorously. Repeat incubation, pipetting, and vortexing at 5-min intervals until EBs seem maximally dissociated (about 10–20 min total). Some clumps may still remain, but longer incubation usually does not improve this digestion.

5. After the EBs have been maximally digested, add 4 mL of D-10 medium and centrifuge at 400*g* for 3 min. Aspirate supernatant and wash twice with additional 5 mL of D-10 medium and centrifuge at 400*g* for 3 min for each wash step.
6. Resuspend cells in desired medium and filter the cell suspension with 70 μm cell strainer filter to remove any remaining clumps of cells. Count viable cells using a hemocytometer, after staining with 0.4% Trypan blue.

3.7. Flow Cytometric Analysis

1. Dissociate the differentiated H1/S17 cells with collagenase and trypsin–EDTA to generate a single cell suspension. Aliquot approx 2×10^5 cells per tube for staining with different antibodies. Wash one or two times with FACS medium before starting staining.
2. Stain with either antigen-specific antibodies and isotype control for at least 15 min on ice. If the first antibodies are unconjugated, the cells should be incubated with conjugated secondary antibodies for another 15 to 30 min after washing with FACS medium between staining steps.
3. Wash one or two times with FACS medium and resuspend the cell pellet in 200 to 500 μL of FACS medium. Perform flow cytometric analysis by standard methods. Importantly, to increase specificity, dead cells should be excluded by PI staining. Staining and fixation of cells is not performed, as this precludes the use of PI staining.

3.8. Hematopoietic CFC Assay

1. hES/S17 cells are cultured for the desired number of days before harvesting. A single cell suspension is prepared. Aliquot 6×10^5 cells into a sterile microfuge tube. Centrifuge at 400*g* for 5 min. Resuspend the cell pellet in 100 μL of I-2 medium. Wash once with I-2 medium.
2. Thaw the MethoCult GF+ medium to room temperature before starting the colony-forming assay. Add cells to 2.5 mL of MethoCult™ GF+ and vortex until they distribute evenly within the medium. Keep the tube of cells in methylcellulose upright at room temperature for approx 15 min to let the bubbles rise and dissipate.
3. Transfer the cells in Methocult GF+ medium into sterile Petri dishes. 2.5 mL of medium should be divided into two 35-mm nontissue culture Petri dishes using a wide blunt 2-mL stripette (1.1 mL cells = 2.5×10^5 cells per dish). Place these two dishes and a third, open dish containing water into a 100-mm culture dish. The third dish helps maintain humidity and thus prevents drying of the methylcellulose-based medium.
4. Incubate at 37°C, 5% CO_2 for 2 wk and score for colony forming units according to standard criteria (22).

3.9. RNA Isolation

1. Spin down aliquots of the single cell suspension as above, remove the medium, and then homogenize in TRIzol by repetitive pipetting (1 mL of Trizol per 5–10 × 10^6 cells). Incubate the samples for 5 min at room temperature (15–30°C). Washing the cells before addition of TRIzol Reagent may increase the possibility of mRNA degradation and should, therefore, be avoided.
2. Add 0.2 mL of chloroform per 1 mL of TRIzol Reagent. Cap the tubes and shake vigorously by hand for 15 s. Incubate at room temperature for 2 to 3 min. Centrifuge at no more than 12,000*g* for 15 min at 2 to 8°C.
3. Transfer the colorless upper aqueous phase to a fresh tube and save the lower red organic phase. Add 0.5 mL of isopropyl alcohol per 1 mL of TRIzol to precipitate the RNA by incubating the samples at room temperature for 10 min. Centrifuge at no more than 12,000*g* at 2 to 8°C.

4. Remove the supernatant. Wash the RNA pellet once with 75% ethanol, adding at least 1 mL of 75% ethanol per 1 mL of TRIzol Reagent used for the initial homogenization. Mix the sample by vortexing and centrifuge at no more than 7500g for 5 min at 2 to 8°C.
5. Dry the RNA pellet (5–10 min) at room temperature; do not dry the RNA by centrifugation under vacuum. Dissolve RNA in RNase-free (diethyl pyrocarbonate treated) water or 0.5% sodium dodecyl sulfate solution by passing the solution a few times through a pipet tip and incubating for 10 min at 55 to 60°C.
6. The purified RNA can be stored at –20°C or –80°C for an extended time prior to reverse-transcription polymerase chain reaction analysis. The protein obtained from the organic phase can be used for the Western blot analysis.

3.10. Protein Isolation

1. Precipitate protein from red organic phase (phenol-ethanol supernatant) with 1.5 ml isopropyl alcohol per 1 mL of TRIzol used in initial homogenization. Incubate for 10 min at room temperature, then centrifuge at 12,000*g* for 10 min at 2 to 8°C.
2. Remove supernatant and wash protein pellet three times with a solution of 0.3 *M* guanidine hydrochloride in 95% ethanol (wash solution). Each wash is performed using 2 mL of wash solution per 1 mL of TRIzol used in original homogenization. Each wash step is incubated at room temperature for 20 min, then centrifuged at 7500*g* for 5 min at 2 to 8°C.
3. After the third wash, resuspend the protein pellet in 2 mL of ethanol, vortex vigorously, and incubate at room temperature for 20 min. Centrifuge at 7500*g* for 5 min at 2–8°C.
4. Vacuum dry protein pellet for 5 to 10 min, then dissolve in 1% sodium dodecyl sulfate. Incubate solution at 50°C if needed to solubilize protein. Centrifuge at 10,000*g* at 2 to 8°C to pellet insoluble material. Transfer cleared supernatant to new tube and use immediately for Western blotting or store at 5 to 10°C.

4. Notes

1. Chick serum is added to trypsin–EDTA solution to improve cell viability, but unlike FBS, chick serum does not contain trypsin inhibitors. Trypsin–EDTA + 2% chick serum should be warmed to 37°C.
2. Disposable glass pipets are used for culture of undifferentiated human ES cells. Some researchers feel these pipets help maintain the ES cells in an undifferentiated state by minimizing exposure to plastics, which may vary between lots, or detergents used to clean reusable glass pipets.
3. Other serum-free media can be used for culture of embryoid bodies. We prefer to culture the dispase-harvested ES cell colonies overnight in serum-free medium to allow optimal formation of EBs with minimal adherence to plastic that occurs with serum containing media, even with poly-HEME-pretreated dishes. Additional cytokines can be added to serum-free media to promote hematopoietic development.
4. We present protocols for assays that are not specific to analysis of human ES cell-derived blood cells. Many variations are possible for flow cytometric analysis, CFC assays, and RNA isolation. We offer these methods as one example.
5. Other nontissue culture treated dishes have been tested. Only Greiner dishes had no adherent cells when this complex mixture of cells was plated in this CFC assay. If cells do adhere and grow, these proliferating cells will likely interfere with results.
6. Other means of RNA and/or protein isolation are also available. For small cell numbers, RNeasy Mini kit (Qiagen; cat. no. 74104) is suitable, especially if protein samples are not desired.

7. Reports using S17 cells to support hematopoietic differentiation of rhesus monkey ES cells did not irradiate or otherwise mitotically inactive the S17 stromal cells *(21)*. These authors felt that growth inhibition of S17 cells when confluent was sufficient to prevent overgrowth when co-cultured with ES cells. We prefer irradiation of stromal cells to prevent growth and proliferation that may complicate interpretation of subsequent assays (such as CFC assay).

Acknowledgments

We thank Julie Morris, Rachel Lewis, and Dong Chen for assistance with embryoid body protocols.

References

1. Thomson, J. A., Itskovitz-Eldor J, Shapiro, S. S., Waknitz, M. A., Swiergiel, J. J., Marshall, V. S., and Jones, J. M. (1998) Embryonic stem cell lines derived from human blastocysts. *Science* **282,** 1145–1147.
2. Odorico, J. A., Kaufman, D. S., and Thomson, J. A. (2001) Multilineage differentiation from human embryonic stem cell lines. *Stem Cells* **19,** 193–204.
3. Keller G, Kennedy M, Papayannopoulou T, and Wiles, M. V. (1993) Hematopoietic commitment during embryonic stem cell differentiation in culture. *Mol. Cell. Biol.* **13,** 473–486.
4. Smith, A. G. (2001) Embryo-derived stem cells: of mice and men. *Annu. Rev. Cell Dev. Biol.* **17,** 435–462.
5. Palis, J. and Yoder, M. C. (2001) Yolk-sac hematopoiesis: the first blood cells of mouse and man. *Exp. Hematol.* **29,** 927–936.
6. Thomson, J. A. and Marshall, V. S. (1998) Primate embryonic stem cells. *Curr. Topics Dev. Biol.* **38,** 133–165.
7. Xu, C., Inokuma, M. S., Denham, J., Golds, K., Kundu, P., Gold, J. D., and Carpenter, M. K. (2001) Feeder-free growth of undifferentiated human embryonic stem cells. *Nat. Biotechnol.* **19,** 971–974.
8. Richards M, Fong, C. Y., Chan, W. K., et al. (2002) Human feeders support prolonged undifferentiated growth of human inner cell masses and embryonic stem cells. *Nat. Biotechnol.* **20,** 933–936.
9. Cheng, L., Hammond, H., Ye, Z., Zahn X., and David, G. (2003) Human adult marrow cells support prolonged expansion of human embryonic stem cells in culture. *Stem Cells* **21,** 131–142.
10. Kaufman, D. S., Lewis, R. L., Hanson, E. T., et al. (2001) Hematopoietic colony-forming cells derived from human embryonic stem cells. *Proc. Natl. Acad. Sci. USA* **98,** 10,716–10,721.
11. Ma Y, Ramezani A, Lewis R, Hawley, R. G, and Thomson, J. A. (2003) High-level sustained transgene expression in human embryonic stem cells using lentiviral vectors. *Stem Cells* **21,** 111–117.
12. Zwaka, T. P. and Thomson, J. A. (2003) Homologous recombination in human embryonic stem cells. *Nat. Biotechnol.* **21,** 319–321.
13. Pfeifer, A., Ikawa, M., Dayn, Y., and Verma, I. M. (2002) Transgenesis by lentiviral vectors: lack of gene silencing in mammalian embryonic stem cells and preimplantation embryos. *Proc. Natl. Acad. Sci. USA* **99,** 2140–2145.
14. Gropp, M., Itsykson, P., Singer, O., Ben-Hur, T., Reinhartz, E., Galun, E., and Reubinoff, B. E. (2003) Stable genetic modification of human embryonic stem cells by lentiviral vectors. *Mol. Ther.* **7,** 281–287.

15. Collins, L. S. and Dorshkind, K. (1987) A stromal cell line from myeloid long-term bone marrow cultures can support myelopoiesis and B lymphopoiesis. *J. Immunol.* **138,** 1082–1087.
16. Wang, S. J., Greer, P., and Auerbach, R. (1996) Isolation and propagation of yolk-sac-derived endothelial cells from a hypervascular transgenic mouse expressing a gain-of-function fps/fes proto-oncogene. In Vitro *Cell. Dev. Biol. Anim.* **32,** 292–299.
17. Nakano, T., Kodama, H., and Honjo, T. (1994) Generation of lymphohematopoietic cells from embryonic stem cells in culture. *Science* **265,** 1098–1101.
18. Simmons, P. J. and Torok-Storb, B. (1991) Identification of stromal cell precursors in human bone marrow by a novel monoclonal antibody, STRO-1. *Blood* **78,** 55–62.
19. Sutherland, H. J., Lansdorp, P. M., Henkelman, D. H., Eaves, A. C., and Eaves, C. J. (1990) Functional characterization of individual human hematopoietic stem cells cultured at limiting dilution on supportive marrow stromal layers. *Proc. Natl. Acad. Sci. USA* **87,** 3584–3588.
20. Dick, J. E., Bhatia, M., Gan, O., Kopp, U., and Wang, J. C. (1997) Assay of human stem cells by repopulation of (NOD)/SCID mice. *Stem Cells* **15(Suppl 1),** 199–203.
21. Eaves, C. and Lambie, K. (1995) Atlas of Human Hematopoietic Colonies. StemCell Technologies, Inc., Vancouver, BC.
22. Li, F., Lu, S, Vida, L. V., Thomson, J. A., and Honig, G. R. (2001) Bone morphogenetic protein 4 induces efficient hematopoietic differentiation of rhesus monkey embryonic stem cells in vitro. *Blood* **98,** 335–342.

IV

Bioinformatics and Functional Genomics

29

A Functional Genomics Approach to Hematopoietic Stem Cell Regulation

Jason A. Hackney and Kateri A. Moore

Summary

Elucidation of the molecular mechanisms that are responsible for regulating the most basic properties of stem cells, self-renewal, and differentiation remains a major challenge in hematopoietic stem cell biology. We have taken a functional genomics approach towards revealing these mechanisms. Previous studies of the fetal liver genetic program led to the development of Stem Cell Database (SCDb, http://stemcell.princeton.edu), a resource for the stem cell community. These studies have been expanded to include the microenvironmental component of hematopoiesis and are the focus herein. In our efforts to study the microenvironmental component we have identified a stromal cell line, AFT024, which serves as a surrogate stem cell niche. The line provides a milieu that facilitates the maintenance of transplantable mouse and human stem cells as well as the generation of large populations of committed progenitors. In a manner mirroring the work done with the SCDb, we provide an online resource, Stromal Cell Database, StroCDB (http://stromalcell.princeton.edu), that is a compendium of information and data derived from biological and molecular studies of this surrogate niche. These include bioinformatic analyses of over 6000 clones derived from a subtracted library enriched for messages expressed in AFT024 as well as data derived from custom expression arrays developed from this library. Herein we describe these efforts and provide a guide for navigating the database and mining the information contained within.

Key Words: Stem cell niche; hematopoietic microenvironment; stromal cell line; AFT024; functional genomics; subtracted library; gene expression; microarrays; bioinformatics; database.

1. Introduction

Despite the completion of whole genome sequencing for mouse, human, and other species, there remains the question of which genes are expressed in specific cell types, that is, what is the molecular profile or genetic program of a particular cell type. Given that hematopoietic stem cells are a particularly interesting cell type, intensive efforts have been undertaken to define the genetic program of these cells. Those studies have

From: *Methods in Molecular Medicine, Vol. 105: Developmental Hematopoiesis: Methods and Protocols.*
Edited by: M. H. Baron © Humana Press Inc., Totowa, NJ

led to the development of Stem Cell Database (SCDb, http://stemcell.princeton.edu) *(1)*. SCDb was first released in 2000 and has continually grown over the years. A newer version of SCDb, to be released in 2004, will contain thousands of gene products containing subtracted complementary deoxyribonucleic acid (cDNA) library sequences from mouse bone marrow and human hematopoietic tissues, including additional libraries from mouse fetal liver. A global analysis of comparative stem cell gene expression using microarrays also has been published recently *(2)*. The reader is invited to peruse these papers and other recent reviews of stem cell gene expression for additional information regarding the genetic program of hematopoietic stem cells *(3,4)*. In the following we have taken a functional genomics approach toward elucidating the molecular mechanisms at play in the hematopoietic microenvironment. Because hematopoietic stem cells (HSCs) undergo their greatest period of self-renewal expansion during their residence in the fetal liver, we created a "snapshot" of the cellular elements mediating this process by developing over 200 cell lines from the d 14 to 14.5 postcoitus fetal liver. The lines were screened for their ability to maintain high levels of stem cell activity in long-term culture. In this screen, long-term supporting lines were very rare *(5)*. AFT024 emerged as the most potent stem cell supporting line and has subsequently been shown to support both mouse and human stem cells in a variety of in vitro and in vivo assays *(6–11)*. We have hypothesized that there is a unique molecular milieu elaborated by AFT024 cells that is not present in nonsupporting lines. To identify the discrete components of this milieu, we have generated a subtracted cDNA library from this cell line. The library was prepared by removing messages in common with a nonsupporting cell line (termed 2018), thereby enriching for transcripts with greater or specific expression by AFT024 cells. We sequenced over 6000 clones from this library and have assembled them into a biological process-oriented database, the Stromal Cell Database (StroCDB) *(12)*. This discourse is intended to serve as a guide that will allow an interested observer to navigate the database effectively and gather as much information as possible. The reader may find it useful to have their Internet browser open to the home page of StroCDB (**Fig. 1**) and peruse the various pages of the database as they are described.

2. Materials

Stromal Cell Database, StroCDB; available at http://stromalcell.princeton.edu

1. Introduction; http://stromalcell.princeton.edu/files/intro.html (*see* **Note 1**)
2. Materials and methods; http://stromalcell.princeton.edu/files/methods.html (*see* **Note 2**)
3. Supplementary data; http://stromalcell.princeton.edu/files/supportive.html (*see* **Note 3**)
4. Figures and tables; http://stromalcell.princeton.edu/files/figures.html (*see* **Note 4**)
5. Informatic classification: http://stromalcell.princeton.edu/files/figures.html
6. Database entry description; http://stromalcell.princeton.edu/files/fields.html
7. Database info query; http://stromalcell.princeton.edu/files/query.html
8. Database Blast query; http://stromalcell.princeton.edu/files/blast.html
9. Predetermined queries; http://stromalcell.princeton.edu

3. Methods

3.1. Development of Stromal Cell Database

The database is built around a sequence set derived from an AFT024 subtracted cDNA library. To make this library, we first made two directionally cloned libraries,

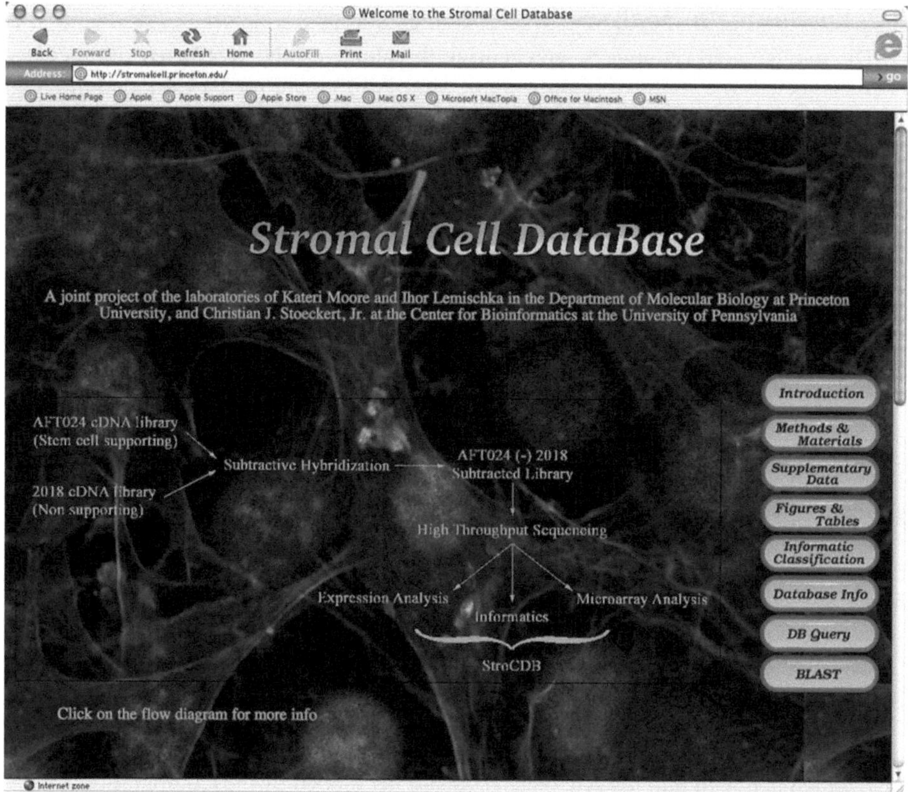

Fig. 1. The home page of StroCDB presents a synopsis of the entire project and links to all other pages contained within the database.

one from the stem cell supporter line AFT024 the other from a nonsupporter line 2018. The subtraction was accomplished by hybridizing single stranded messages generated from a target cDNA library (AFT024 in pSport1) to biotinylated driver RNA transcribed from a cDNA library (2018 in pSport2) with inserts cloned in the opposite (complementary) orientation *(13)*. The complexity of the original library was reduced by two logs, effectively enriching for messages either specific to or overexpressed by AFT024 cells. Messages in common with and unique to the nonsupporting line 2018 were either reduced or removed, effectively eliminating housekeeping and metabolic gene products. Details of the library construction and subtractive hybridization are available at http://stromalcell.princeton.edu/files/methods.html. Directionally cloned cDNAs were sequenced from the 5' end to obtain coding region information from single pass reads. To date, we have sequenced over 6000 clones from the subtracted library. The reader may work his/her way through the flow diagram presented as an interactive map on the Home page of StroCDB (**Fig. 1**). This figure depicts the experimental strategy and the individual elements feeding into StroCDB. Clicking on the elements will open windows that present additional detail about the respective branches.

3.2. Bioinformatic Analyses

The nucleic acid sequences representing the clones in the subtracted library have been subjected to a series of bioinformatic analyses that are roughly divided into two parts. The first comprises automated searches of each clone to determine sequence homology to 1) known mouse proteins, 2) proteins from other species, and 3) expressed sequence tag (ESTs). In addition, a lack of homology to any publicly available sequence will also be revealed. The remaining analyses are undertaken by the individual annotating the clone and are explained subsequently. In short, the hand annotation provides a protein classification, putative function and, most importantly, a summary or notes with insights into the role of the gene product in the biological process. A summary schematic of the bioinformatic processing and hand annotation for each clone in StroCDB is presented (**Fig. 2**).

3.2.1. Automated Searches

On average, each of the sequence entries in StroCDB contains 550 base pairs. The initial analyses comprise batched BLAST (Basic Local Alignment Sequence Tool; ***(14)*** searches of six publicly available databases: 1) GenBank nucleotide (nt), 2) GenBank non-redundant protein (nr) ***(15)***, 3) SWISSPROT ***(16)***, 4) dbEST, 5) mouse, and 6) human DoTS (Database of Transcribed Sequences) ***(17)***. The first three searches reveal homologies to known transcripts and proteins from any species and provide direct links into their corresponding NCBI (National Center for Biotechnology Information) GenBank or SWISSPROT database entries. These data provide a wealth of information about each match and allow the entry to be categorized as to putative cellular role. The remaining searches provide additional information about clones that may not have homology to known proteins. The DoTS alignments are displayed in the BLAST format, which is linked into the AllGenes database developed by the Computational Biology and Informatics Laboratory at the University of Pennsylvania. AllGenes is designed to provide access to an integrated database that describes all the known and predicted mouse and human genes ***(18)***. Homologies to DoTS contigs (assemblies of sequence reads) can extend the length of the clone under study, allowing extension of the coding region and consequently more informative analysis of the structure of the sequence.

The BLAST results are parsed into a separate file for each sequence and stored. A brief synopsis of these results is stored in the database and displayed as depicted (**Fig. 3**). Clicking on the VF (View File) link next to each of the Blast searches displays those results and the links contained within.

3.2.1.1. Database Redundancy

Characterizing the internal redundancy of the database allows us to determine, using Poisson statistics, the approximate complexity of the library from which the transcripts were obtained ***(1)***. This is only an approximation as the libraries were not normalized; there is not an equal chance of choosing any given transcript from the set. Given this caveat, we do believe that this provides at least an estimate of how deeply the library has been sequenced. Thus, StroCDB contains about 35% of the genes represented in the subtracted library. Clicking on the AFT024-2018 Subtracted Library element in the flow diagram on the first page of StroCDB will reveal the calculation and these data. According to this calculation, there are approx 4000 non-redundant entries in StroCDB.

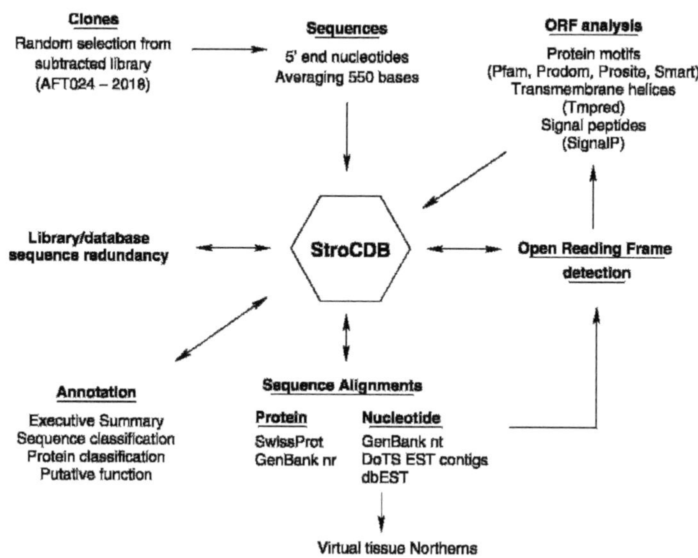

Fig. 2. Schematic of the bioinformatic tools, analyses, and annotation process of individual gene products catalogued in StroCDB.

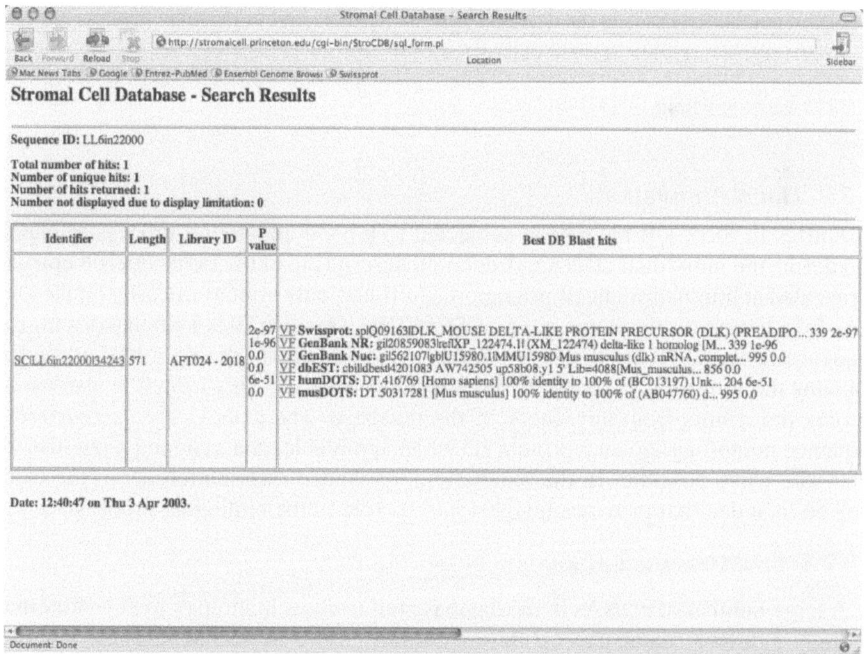

Stromal Cell Database - Search Results

Sequence ID: LL6in22000

Total number of hits: 1
Number of unique hits: 1
Number of hits returned: 1
Number not displayed due to display limitation: 0

<table>
<tr><th>Identifier</th><th>Length</th><th>Library ID</th><th>P value</th><th>Best DB Blast hits</th></tr>
<tr><td>SC|LL6in22000|34243</td><td>571</td><td>AFT024 - 2018</td><td>2e-97
1e-96
0.0
0.0
6e-51
0.0</td><td>VF Swissprot: sp|Q09163|DLK_MOUSE DELTA-LIKE PROTEIN PRECURSOR (DLK) (PREADIPO... 339 2e-97
VF GenBank NR: gi|20859083|ref|XP_122474.1| (XM_122474) delta-like 1 homolog [M... 339 1e-96
VF GenBank Nuc: gi|562107|gb|U15980.1|MMU15980 Mus musculus (dlk) mRNA, complet... 995 0.0
VF dbEST: cbil|dbest|4201083 AW742505 up58b08.y1 5' Lib=4088[Mus_musculus... 856 0.0
VF humDOTS: DT.416769 [Homo sapiens] 100% identity to 100% of (BC013197) Unk... 204 6e-51
VF musDOTS: DT.50317281 [Mus musculus] 100% identity to 100% of (AB047760) d... 995 0.0</td></tr>
</table>

Date: 12:40:47 on Thu 3 Apr 2003.

Fig. 3. Tabular field format of database entries. This half of the table displays the clone identifier, length of sequence tag, *p*-values for and the results of the automated BLAST analyses.

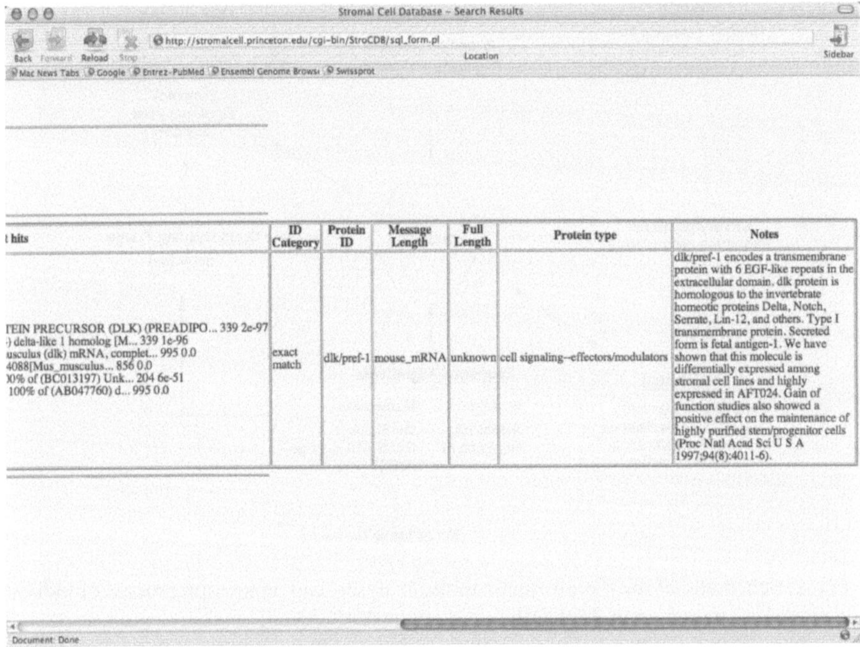

t hits	ID Category	Protein ID	Message Length	Full Length	Protein type	Notes
TEIN PRECURSOR (DLK) (PREADIPO... 339 2e-97 -) delta-like 1 homolog [M... 339 1e-96 usculus (dlk) mRNA, complet... 995 0.0 4088[Mus_musculus... 856 0.0)0% of (BC013197) Unk... 204 6e-51 100% of (AB047760) d... 995 0.0	exact match	dlk/pref-1	mouse_mRNA	unknown	cell signaling--effectors/modulators	dlk/pref-1 encodes a transmembrane protein with 6 EGF-like repeats in the extracellular domain. dlk protein is homologous to the invertebrate homeotic proteins Delta, Notch, Serrate, Lin-12, and others. Type I transmembrane protein. Secreted form is fetal antigen-1. We have shown that this molecule is differentially expressed among stromal cell lines and highly expressed in AFT024. Gain of function studies also showed a positive effect on the maintenance of highly purified stem/progenitor cells (Proc Natl Acad Sci U S A 1997;94(8):4011-6).

Fig. 4. Annotated fields in the database entry table. This half of the table displays the fields that have been hand annotated to classify the information gained from the BLAST searches and bioinformatic analyses. An executive summary of salient points about the gene product is provided in the Notes field.

3.2.2. Hand Annotation

Entries in StroCDB have been subjected to a hand annotation process to classify and define the individual cDNAs. A detailed description of the fields in each entry file is revealed at http://stromalcell.princeton.edu/files/fields.html by clicking on the Database Info button on the home page of StroCDB. The data files associated with each sequence in StroCDB are displayed in this standard format; the right half of the field contains the information added by the annotator (**Fig. 4**). This format is also used to display the results from any query of the database. The cDNAs are categorized by sequence homology, given a protein ID when applicable, and assigned a putative cellular role when possible. In the Notes field, expanded information about the cDNA may be included that provides insights into its role in the biological process.

3.2.2.1. Searching for Information in the Sequence

A large number of cDNAs in the database fail to show homology to any entry in the publicly available databases or show homology only to EST databases. For these entries, the annotator can use a number of Web-based tools to reveal motifs, signal peptides, or transmembrane domains in the ORFs (i.e., open reading frames) for these cDNAs. In these cases, the assembled sequences available from AllGenes are particularly useful, as they effectively extend the sequence read for that particular clone. Identification of certain motifs in a clone can allow their assignment to a family of proteins and a putative cellular role. Examples of these tools are SMART (Simple Modular Architecture Research Tool) ***(19)*** for protein domains and SignalP for signal peptides ***(20)***. Several others are listed under the Biological Sequence Analysis subheading in the Materials and Methods pages of StroCDb.

3.2.3. Informatic Classification Summary

Access to the entire informatic classification of the entries in StroCDB is provided in an easily retrievable format. On the home page of StroCDB the reader may click on the Informatic Classification button to display these data. This retrieves a page containing two pie charts: one showing the sequence homology distribution of the cDNAs and the other their functional categorization. These categories are assigned according to the EGAD cellular roles list (Expressed Genome Anatomy Database from TIGR, The Institute for Genome Research, http://www.tigr.org). Clicking on any section of a pie will retrieve the corresponding cDNAs from the database. In addition, the functional categorization and cellular role subsets are presented in tabular form. Clicking on the entries in the table will retrieve those database files also.

3.3. Querying Stromal Cell Database

For an expression database to be a truly useful tool, it must be provide a format for querying the data. For instance, researchers navigating the database may be interested in finding homologies to individual proteins that they are studying or to whole classes of molecules. We chose to allow queries of the fields displayed in each database entry. These include the sequence identifier, the homology group, the predicted cellular role, the protein name, and the notes fields. Any one or combination of many of these fields can be queried from the main query page at http://stromalcell.princeton.edu/files/query.html. It is also important for an expression database to provide a BLAST interface. This allows an outside investigator to use his/her own sequence strings to retrieve homologies in the StroCDB. Additional information on refining queries is outlined below.

3.3.1. Query by Annotation

We provide a means to perform Boolean queries of the annotation text in the "Notes" and the "Protein Identity" fields. The text search is a regular expression search of these database fields. This means that if you query the "Notes" field with "secret" you will match entries that include the word "secreted" as well as "secretory". Multiple words within a query are considered a Boolean "AND" unless an explicit "OR" or "NOT" is provided between them. Brackets of any type can be used to group more complicated queries, as in: "(secreted OR transmembrane) AND (wnt OR delta)." The query page also allows one to retrieve only unique clones (that is, a group of sisters represented by a single clone), or to retrieve all clones. In general, it is more useful to retrieve unique clones, and to look at sisters of a clone only when indicated, such as if one is seeking to identify putative spliced forms of a gene. In addition, the returned data can be sorted by their homology to any of the six predetermined BLAST searches using the e-value.

3.3.2. Query by Sequence Homology and Functional Category

The database may be queried to retrieve sets of data about sequence homology and functional categories. There is a pull-down menu on the Query page that displays the homology categories, for example, exact match to a mouse protein, homolog of a known protein, novel member of a described protein family, EST from any species. A window displaying all the functional categories and putative cellular roles allows selection of an entire category or a discrete subset within each category. These commands can be concatenated or separated by selecting the category in the window with the appropriate modifier key. As previously indicated, any of these query selections can be combined with the other options available on the Query page. *See* the Informatic Classification Summary section in **Subheading 3.2.3.** for details of an additional graphic display of these data. This graphic is linked and retrieves entire categories or subsets of the annotated clones.

3.3.3. Query by BLAST

This type of query allows the reader to input his/her own cDNA sequence and compare it to the dataset in StroCDB. The query is available by clicking the BLAST button on the Home page to retrieve the http://stromalcell.princeton.edu/files/blast.html page. There are pull down options indicating which types of BLAST analysis can be performed and information explaining each one. In addition, there are parameters that can be chosen to regulate the number and significance of the output data. The sequence homologies are displayed in typical BLAST output format with the StroCDB clone identifiers in a link format. Clicking on the identifier will retrieve the database fields for that entry.

3.3.4. Results From a Query

Having queried the database, the data fields for all the clones that passed the requested criteria are displayed. More information is available for each clone if one clicks on the Identifier. This information includes expression results from array hybridization experiments further explained below. The results from the high-density nylon arrays are presented in the section labeled "Filter Array Expression Profiling Results." A graphical representation of the expression results is displayed, where the intensity of red represents the log2-transformed ratio of signal to background. The section marked "StroChip Expression Profiling Results" displays results from cDNA microarray hybridizations. In this case, the red vs green intensity represents the log2-transformed ratio of AFT024 intensity vs the cell line shown above the figure. Brighter red intensity shows stronger expression in AFT024 than the cell line to which it is compared. Next to both images is a scale bar representing the range of red to green intensities in log2 values.

This information page also lists the sister clones that have been identified for this cDNA. Internal homology is shown as a table of clones and e-values. By clicking "Show All," the data fields for each of these clones are presented. The contiguous sequence or "contig" of these sisters can also be displayed. The contigs were generated using the Cap2 program ***(21)***. We also show a list of the tissue source for each EST homology. This essentially provides a "virtual tissue Northern" of expression data for that particular clone. This information is specific to the individual clone displayed and does not include the sister clone data. Finally, the nucleotide sequence of the clone is shown.

3.4. Development of Expression Arrays From StroCDB

Microarray expression analysis is a widely accepted tool in functional genomics. Arrays have been developed that represent the majority of the publicly available sequence tags and known genes. Nevertheless, there is a high percentage of novel and uncharacterized cDNAs in the StroCDB clone set that are not present on commercially available arrays. In addition, our dataset is highly related to a biological phenotype. It should contain key elements of the molecular networks involved in the microenvironmental regulation of stem cell behavior. We have developed our own custom arrays and, at present, have high-density nylon arrays and cDNA microarrays StroChips available that are representative of the clone set in StroCDB. Details about the construction of the arrays, hybridization, and analyses may be found in the Materials and Methods page of StroCDB under the subheading Array Analyses. Clicking on the Microarray Analysis branch in the flow diagram on the Home page of StroCDB (**Fig. 1**) will reveal the experimental results and the methods of data analyses described in Hackney et al *(12)*. We proposed the hypothesis that a gene expression profile would correlate with a stromal cell line's ability to support stem cells in long-term culture. To test this hypothesis, we profiled five lines from our set of fetal liver stromal cell lines. We have previously shown that, in addition to AFT024, another line (2012) supported highly purified stem cells, albeit half as well, while two others (2018 and BFC012) did not *(6,22)*. An additional line (2058) that had not yet been studied in long-term culture with highly purified cells was chosen as the test line. All five lines were studied for their ability to maintain enriched stem cells in culture, while RNA was isolated from each line and used to interrogate both types of arrays. The cDNA microarrays or StroChips were queried with Cy3 and Cy5 labeled probes; for these experiments, each line was compared to AFT024. The nylon arrays were queried with radiolabeled subtracted cDNA probes; each of the lines was subtracted with BFC012, a nonsupporting line. Both datasets were normalized, transformed, and subjected to k-means clustering *(23)*. The arrays were first analyzed separately and the transcripts in common from the clustering analyses were selected. The test line's gene expression profile predicted that it would have a restricted support capacity. Pearson correlation coefficient analysis showed that the data correlated well with the observed biological phenotypes of the lines, as shown by their ability to maintain long-term cobblestone area forming cells (**Fig. 5**; **ref.** ***24***). These data suggest that restricted or partial supporting lines would be ideal candidates for gain of function experimentation, with "missing" gene products revealed in the array analysis.

We have presented a very brief description of the initial set of experiments that were performed to validate the arrays. There are many additional lines of investigation that can be accomplished with this technology. Future experiments will involve comparison of lines from different developmental time periods (early embryonic vs fetal liver vs adult marrow). In addition, any genetic manipulation of AFT024 that alters its ability to support stem cells could provide source material that would enable us to start defining regulatory networks present on the arrays. There is a myriad of experimental treatments that may be envisaged. Analyses of the possible scenarios mentioned earlier can easily be extended to other types of commercially available oligogonucleotide (e.g., Affymetrix) or long oligo (e.g., Agilent) arrays. The use of these types of arrays would provide a global non-biased gene expression screen that would reveal a great

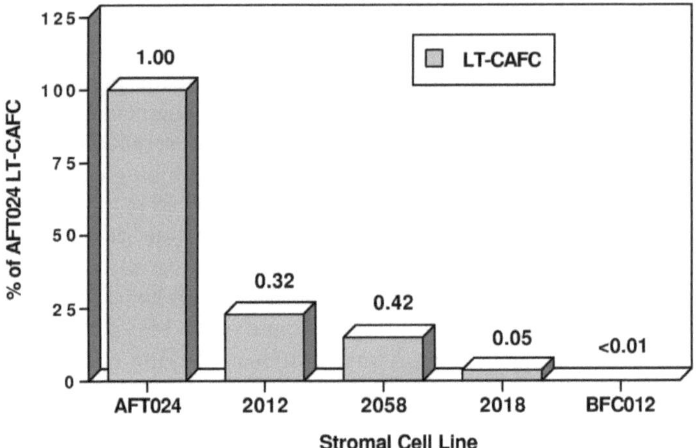

Fig. 5. Maintenance of long-term cobblestone area forming cells (LT-CAFCs) by indicated stromal cell lines compared to AFT024. Pearson correlation coefficients from the cDNA microarray analyses are presented above the bars demonstrating the correlation between the gene expression analyses and the biological support phenotype of the cell lines.

deal of information about gene products that are not contained on the custom arrays. Given the biased and unique set of cDNAs contained on the custom StroChip, this would provide a very complementary approach towards revealing regulatory networks in this system.

Several topics need to be carefully considered prior to using microarrays for these types of studies: 1) the fundamentals of the experimental design: these include the choice of array type, the number of biological and technical replicates necessary to achieve statistically sound data, and the choice of comparison or baseline *(25)*; 2) data normalization and transformation: necessary to minimize "noise" in the data and allow comparison to standards on the array *(26)*; 3) methods of data analysis: it is necessary to determine which algorithms are most applicable to your dataset, examples include but are not limited to, hierarchical clustering, k-means clustering, self-organizing maps, and principal component analysis *(27)*; 4) plans for data storage, retrieval and sharing: experimental protocols and the biological purpose of the study need to be described in adequate detail according to the MIAME (Minimal Information About Microarray Experiments) standards *(28)*; and 5) data validation: differential expression of gene products revealed in the microarray analysis needs to be verified by other methods, for example, Northern blotting or quantitative reverse-transcription polymerase chain reaction. Using the StroChips and stem cell arrays (StemChips) that have been developed from the entries in the Stem Cell Database *(1)* (http://stemcell.princeton.edu), we plan to investigate the molecular crosstalk between stem cells and their supportive microenvironment. Again, many experimental scenarios can be envisaged for these types of experiments, such as a time course study with a variety of conditions and treatments and genetic manipulation of either the stem cell or stromal cell compartments. It is hoped that these functional genomics tools will allow us to unravel the molecular mechanisms of extrinsic stem cell regulatory networks and that these mechanisms will provide insights into all stem cell microenvironments.

4. Notes

The authors intend to use this section to draw the reader's attention to several additional features of the StroCDB, in particular, the pages of the database that have not been discussed yet. These pages provide background information, additional methods, supplemental biological data, and interactive tables.

1. The Introduction button on the home page of StroCDB will retrieve http://stromalcell.princeton.edu/files/intro.html, a page that provides a highly interactive perspective on stem cell biology in vivo and in vitro. Topical subsections of the discussion include the functional properties and origins of HSC, their physical characterization and purification, in vitro cytokine supported systems, stromal cell supported systems, defining the stem cell niche, the plasticity of stem cells, and the molecular definition of a stem cell niche. The various links embedded within the text retrieve PubMed references and additional primary data generated in our laboratory.
2. Additional methods used in these studies but not addressed above are available by clicking on the Methods button of the home page (http://stromalcell.princeton.edu/files/methods.html). This page details methods for the generation of the stromal cell lines, stem cell purification strategies for both fetal liver and adult marrow, stem cell/stromal cell co-cultivation, in vitro hematopoietic progenitor assays, and in vivo transplantation assays for stem cell activity. Again, embedded within the text are links for various references and primary data.
3. Supplementary molecular and biological data are available at http://stromalcell.princeton.edu/files/supportive.html by clicking on the Supplementary Data button on the home page. Links on this page include but are not limited to: 1) experimental design of single cell deposition studies; 2) the developmental potential of single cells deposited on AFT024 cells; 3) reverse-transcriptase polymerase chain reaction expression data of common regulatory cytokines; 4) a retroviral marking strategy; 5) proviral integration data after marking on AFT024 cells; 6) Northern blot expression screen of clones from the library; and 7) cluster analyses from microarray experiments. Also included are studies with highly purified quiescent adult marrow and twice purified fetal liver stem cells.
4. The Figures and Tables button on the home page of StroCDB (http://stromalcell.princeton.edu/files/figures.html) provides access to interactive and expanded figures and tables presented in Hackney et al ***(12)***. These include two web-only tables: one for known secreted, cell surface, matrix and cytoskeletal proteins in StroCDB and the other for molecules regulating both neuronal and hematopoietic systems.
5. A major advantage to a web-based tool like the StroCDB is that it can be continually upgraded and refined. As new data become available, they can be easily integrated into the existing format or the format can be revised to reflect the changing needs of the investigator. We plan to add additional pages to the database that will provide links to a microarray platform under development for array data deposition, analyses and dissemination. We intend to deposit all the primary data related to the existing, published array experiments, including additional information related to the experiments.

References

1. Phillips, R. L., Ernst, R. E., Brunk, B., Ivanova, N., Mahan, M. A., Deanehan, J. K., et al. (2000) The genetic program of hematopoietic stem cells. *Science* **288,** 1635–1640.
2. Ivanova, N. B., Dimos, J. T., Schaniel, C., Hackney, J. A., Moore, K. A., and Lemischka, I. R. (2002) A stem cell molecular signature. *Science* **298,** 601–604.
3. Lemischka, I. (2001) Stem cell dogmas in the genomics era. *Rev. Clin. Exp. Hematol.* **5,** 15–25.
4. Lemischka, I. (1999) Searching for stem cell regulatory molecules. Some general thoughts and possible approaches. *Ann. N Y Acad. Sci.* **872,** 274–287; discussion 287–288.
5. Wineman, J., Moore, K., Lemischka, I., and Muller-Sieburg, C. (1996) Functional heterogeneity of the hematopoietic microenvironment: rare stromal elements maintain long-term repopulating stem cells. *Blood* **87,** 4082–4090.
6. Moore, K. A., Ema, H., and Lemischka, I. R. (1997) In vitro maintenance of highly purified, transplantable hematopoietic stem cells. *Blood* **89,** 4337–4347.
7. Thiemann, F. T., Moore, K. A., Smogorzewska, E. M., Lemischka, I. R., and Crooks, G. M. (1998) The murine stromal cell line AFT024 acts specifically on human CD34+CD38- progenitors to maintain primitive function and immunophenotype in vitro. *Exp. Hematol.* **26,** 612–619.
8. Miller, J. S., McCullar, V., Punzel, M., Lemischka, I. R., and Moore, K. A. (1999) Single adult human CD34(+)/Lin-/CD38(-) progenitors give rise to natural killer cells, B-lineage cells, dendritic cells, and myeloid cells. *Blood* **93,** 96–106.
9. Punzel, M., Wissink, S. D., Miller, J. S., Moore, K. A., Lemischka, I. R., and Verfaillie, C. M. (1999) The myeloid-lymphoid initiating cell (ML-IC) assay assesses the fate of multipotent human progenitors in vitro. *Blood* **93,** 3750–3756.
10. Lewis, I. D., Almeida-Porada, G., Du, J., Lemischka, I. R., Moore, K. A., Zanjani, E. D., et al. (2001) Umbilical cord blood cells capable of engrafting in primary, secondary, and tertiary xenogeneic hosts are preserved after ex vivo culture in a noncontact system. *Blood* **97,** 3441–3449.
11. Nolta, J. A., Thiemann, F. T., Arakawa-Hoyt, J., Dao, M. A., Barsky, L. W., Moore, K. A., et al. (2002) The AFT024 stromal cell line supports long-term ex vivo maintenance of engrafting multipotent human hematopoietic progenitors. *Leukemia* **16,** 352–361.
12. Hackney, J. A., Charbord, P., Brunk, B. P., Stoeckert, C. J., Lemischka, I. R., and Moore, K. A. (2002) A molecular profile of a hematopoietic stem cell niche. *Proc. Natl. Acad. Sci. USA* **99,** 13,061–13,066.
13. Li, W. B., Gruber, C. E., Lin, J. J., Lim, R., D'Alessio, J. M., and Jessee, J. A. (1994) The isolation of differentially expressed genes in fibroblast growth factor stimulated BC3H1 cells by subtractive hybridization. *BioTechniques* **16,** 722–729.
14. Altschul, S. F., Madden, T. L., Schaffer, A. A., Zhang, J., Zhang, Z., Miller, W., et al. (1997) Gapped BLAST and PSI-BLAST: a new generation of protein database search programs. *Nucleic Acids Res.* **25,** 3389–402.
15. Benson, D. A., Karsch-Mizrachi, I., Lipman, D. J., Ostell, J., Rapp, B. A., and Wheeler, D. L. (2002) GenBank. *Nucleic Acids Res.* **30,** 17–20.
16. Boeckmann, B., Bairoch, A., Apweiler, R., Blatter, M. C., Estreicher, A., Gasteiger, E., et al. (2003) The SWISS-PROT protein knowledgebase and its supplement TrEMBL in 2003. *Nucleic Acids Res.* **31,** 365–370.
17. The Computational Biology and Informatics Laboratory. DoTS: a database of transcribed sequences for human and mouse genes. Center for Bioinformatics, University of Pennsylvania. http://www.cbil.upenn.edu/downloads/DoTS/.

18. The Computational Biology and Informatics Laboratory. AllGenes: a web site providing access to an integrated database of known and predicted human and mouse genes. Version 5.0 Ed. Center for Bioinformatics, University of Pennsylvania. http://www.allgenes.org.
19. Ponting, C. P., Schultz, J., Milpetz, F., and Bork, P. (1999) SMART: identification and annotation of domains from signalling and extracellular protein sequences. *Nucleic Acids Res.* **27,** 229–232.
20. Nielsen, H., Engelbrecht, J., Brunak, S., and von Heijne, G. (1997) Identification of prokaryotic and eukaryotic signal peptides and prediction of their cleavage sites. *Protein Eng.* **10,** 1–6.
21. Huang, X. (1996) An improved sequence assembly program. *Genomics* **33,** 21–31.
22. Moore, K. A., Pytowski, B., Witte, L., Hicklin, D., and Lemischka, I. R. (1997) Hematopoietic activity of a stromal cell transmembrane protein containing epidermal growth factor-like repeat motifs. *Proc. Natl. Acad. Sci. USA* **94,** 4011–4016.
23. Tavazoie, S., Hughes, J. D., Campbell, M. J., Cho, R. J., and Church, G. M. (1999) Systematic determination of genetic network architecture. *Nat. Genet.* **22,** 281–285.
24. Ploemacher, R. E., van der Sluijs, J. P., van Beurden, C. A., Baert, M. R., and Chan, P. L. (1991) Use of limiting-dilution type long-term marrow cultures in frequency analysis of marrow-repopulating and spleen colony-forming hematopoietic stem cells in the mouse. *Blood* **78,** 2527–2533.
25. Churchill, G. A. (2002) Fundamentals of experimental design for cDNA microarrays. *Nat. Genet.* **32(Suppl),** 490–495.
26. Quackenbush, J. (2002) Microarray data normalization and transformation. *Nat. Genet.* **32(Suppl),** 496–501.
27. Slonim, D. K. (2002) From patterns to pathways: gene expression data analysis comes of age. *Nat. Genet.* **32(Suppl),** 502–508.
28. Brazma, A., Hingamp, P., Quackenbush, J., Sherlock, G., Spellman, P., Stoeckert, C., et al. (2001) Minimum information about a microarray experiment (MIAME)-toward standards for microarray data. *Nat. Genet.* **29,** 365–371.

Index

A

Agar culture, hematopoietic progenitors
  agar overlay, 295
  agar underlay, 295
  colony identification, 295, 296, 300
  double agar incubation, 295
Avian embryo, grafting studies of hematopoietic cells
  applications, 227
  cell markers
    quail chick combinations, 220, 227
    sex chromosomes, 219, 220
  egg opening, 216, 217, 227
  electroporation for transfection, 224, 225, 227
  embryo manipulation, 218
  heterotopic grafts
    chorioallantoic grafts and chorioallantoic vein injections, 221, 227
    somatopleura, coelum, and dorsal mesentery grafts, 221, 222
  materials, 216, 227
  orthotopic grafts, 222, 223
  overview, 215, 216
  parabiosis, 223, 224
  yolk sac chimeras, 223

B

B-cell multilineage progenitor assay, *see* Multilineage progenitor assay
Bioinformatics, *see* Stromal Cell Database
BL6/green fluorescent protein chimera mouse, *see* Green fluorescent protein
Busulfan, *in utero* myeloablation of mice, 96, 99, 103, 104

C

Cell fate mapping, *see Xenopus* embryo fate mapping
Chimeric mouse
  blastocyst injection and generation, 13
  overview, 8
Collagen culture, megakaryocyte progenitors
  acetylcholinesterase stain, 297
  cytokine mix, 296
  dehydration and fixation of collagen, 296, 297
Confocal microscopy, protein localization in *Drosophila* hemocytes
  antibody reagents, 118
  antibody staining and washing, 118–120
  embryo mounting, 118
  embryo preparation, 113
  Gal4/UAS system to direct gene expression, 117, 118
  imaging and analysis, 119
Congenic mice
  quantitative trait locus identification
    analysis, 57
    generation of mice, 55
  subinterval-specific congenic strain generation and analysis, 58
Cre mouse
  activity analysis in conditionally targeted mice, 14
  gene deletion in adult hematopoietic system, 14, 15
  generation, 12, 13

D

Dextran mini-ruby, *see Xenopus* embryo fate mapping
o-Dianisidine, erythroid cell staining, 173, 176, 193
DIC microscopy, *see* Differential interference contrast microscopy
Differential interference contrast (DIC) microscopy, zebrafish embryos
  contrast enhancement and video magnification, 202, 212
  digitization of video, 204, 213
  embryo preparation and mounting, 200, 201
  image acquisition, 201, 202

macrophage imaging
caudal vein, 209, 213
embryonic tissues, 209, 210
rationale, 204, 205
time-lapse video recording, 210
whole-mount *in situ* hybridization, 210, 211
yolk sac, 205, 207, 208
materials, 200
overview, 199
prospects, 212, 213
video editing, 203, 212
video recording, 202, 203
DNA microarray, Stromal Cell Database for expression array development, 447–449
Drosophila, hemocyte development in embryogenesis
confocal microscopy for protein localization, 117–120
embryos
collection, 112, 119
preparation for hemocyte gene expression analysis, 112, 113
in situ hybridization of messenger RNA, 113–116, 119
materials, 110, 111, 119
overview, 109, 110
strains and maintenance, 111, 112
U-shaped protein immunohistochemistry, 116, 117, 119

E

EB, *see* Embryoid body
Electroporation, avian embryos, 224, 225, 227
Embryoid body (EB)
culture for hematopoietic stem cell development, 34, 37, 40
differentiation culture
human, 434, 435
mouse, 363, 364
Embryonic stem (ES) cell
differentiation culture
human cells
co-culture with feeder cells, 432
dissociation and harvesting of differentiated cells, 432, 433, 437
embryoid body formation and dissociation, 434, 435
feeder cell preparation, 431, 437
flow cytometry, 435
hematopoietic colony-forming cell assay, 435
maintenance, 428, 429
materials, 429–431, 436
protein isolation, 436
RNA isolation, 435, 436
mouse cells
embryoid body differentiation, 363, 364
hematopoietic replating, 364–366
maintenance culture, 363, 366
materials, 361–363, 366
overview, 359, 361
overview, 425, 426
gene expression systems, 24, 25
inducible transgene expression using reverse tetracycline transactivator
embryoid body culture for hematopoietic stem cell development, 34, 37, 40
embryonic stem cell line
characterization, 31–33
generation from Ainv15-targeting cells, 28, 30, 31, 39
HoxB4 induction, 34, 37
materials, 27, 28, 39
overview, 25, 39
therapeutic transplantation of embryonic stem cells, 37, 39
transgene types in hematopoiesis studies, 25–27
manipulation for gene-targeting in mice, 13
research applications and therapeutic prospects, 23, 24
ES cell, *see* Embryonic stem cell
Explant culture, *see* Mouse embryo

F

Fetal thymic organ culture (FTOC)
hematopoietic potential analysis, 283, 284, 286
human/mouse chimeric organ culture
culture conditions, 318
flow cytometry for immunophenotypic analysis, 319, 320
human CD34$^+$ cell isolation and transduction, 318

human T-cell development, 421–423
multilineage progenitor assay, *see* Multilineage progenitor assay
retroviral transduction
CD4/CD8 double-negative thymocyte isolation and transduction, 317, 318
culture conditions, 315, 316
ectopic retroviral supernatant production, 313, 314, 320
expression plasmids, 313
fetal liver collection, 314
fetal thymic lobe collection, 315, 320
materials, 312, 320
retroviral transduction, 315
vesicular stomatitis virus G-pseudotyped supernatant production, 314
T-cell development overview, 311, 312
Flow cytometry
differentiated human embryonic stem cells, 435
erythroid progenitors from humans, 337, 340
fetal thymic organ culture immunophenotypic analysis, 319, 320
hematopietic chimera *Xenopus* embryos
cell harvesting, 163–165
combined surface/DNA staining
Vindlov's reagent, 167
Hoechst 33342, 168
DNA staining, 165
embryo preparation, 161, 162, 168
materials, 160, 161, 168
microsurgery, 162, 163, 168
rationale, 159, 160
surface staining, 165, 168
hematopoietic stem cell enrichment from mouse embryo aorta-gonad-mesonephros region
antibody staining, 260–262, 268
cell cycle analysis
bromodeoxyuridine labeling and staining, 267–269
Hoechst 33258 staining, 266, 267, 269
Ki67 labeling and staining, 268, 269
dead cell discrimination
annexin V, 266
Hoechst 33258, 266, 268
propidium iodide/7-amino-actinomycin D, 265, 266
flow cytometry and cell sorting, 262, 263, 268, 284
materials, 258, 259, 268, 276, 277
overview, 257, 258
single-cell suspension preparation, 260, 268
tissue isolation and dissection, 259, 260, 268
transgene markers and staining, 264, 265, 268
hematopoietic stem cell sorting
development-associated phenotypic changes, 65–67, 72–74
materials, 67
immunostaining, 67, 70, 71, 74
cell sorting, 71, 72
inducible embryonic stem cell line characterization, 31–33
multilineage progenitor assay
first-step screening, 352
progenitor type determination, 352, 355, 356
second-step analysis, 352
staining, 351, 352, 355
peripheral blood analysis in hematopoiesis-transplanted mice
cell sorting, 100, 101, 104
Gpi-1 analysis, 101–103
zebrafish hematopoietic cell purification
adult cells, 191–193, 196
cell sorting, 193, 196
cells expressing fluorescent reporters, 193
embryonic cells, 193, 196
materials, 178
overview, 174
FTOC, *see* Fetal thymic organ culture

G

GFP, *see* Green fluorescent protein
Gpi-1, flow cytometry analysis of peripheral blood in hematopoiesis-transplanted mice, 101–103
Green fluorescent protein (GFP)
BL6 chimera mouse construction for hematopoietic stem cell vascular potential assay
bone marrow harvesting, 371, 376, 377
flow cytometry purification of stem cells, 372
immunomagnetic bead purification of stem cells, 371, 372, 377

multilineage reconstitution verification, 373, 378
rescue marrow harvesting and irradiation of recipient animals, 373, 377
transplantation, 373
hematopoietic cell differentiation studies with imaging of fluorescent protein variants
background fluorescence minimization, 400, 401
distinguishing mixed cell populations expressing different fluorescent protein
cyan/green fluorescent protein, 406, 410
cyan/green/red fluorescent protein, 408
cyan/green/yellow fluorescent protein, 408
cyan/green/yellow/red fluorescent protein, 408
cyan/red fluorescent protein, 404
cyan/yellow fluorescent protein, 404
cyan/yellow/red fluorescent protein, 408
green/red fluorescent protein, 404
green/yellow fluorescent protein, 407, 408
green/yellow/red fluorescent protein, 408
yellow/red fluorescent protein, 404
instrumentation, 396, 398, 409, 410
overview, 395, 396
prospects, 409
relative intensities of variants, 404
spectral fingerprinting for distinguishing double expressers from single expressers, 408
subcellular localization, 409
ultraviolet light effects on cell growth and viability, 401, 402, 410
variants and filter sets, 399, 400, 402–404, 409, 410
inducible embryonic stem cell line characterization, 31–33

H

Hematopoietic progenitors
cell line limitations, 323, 324
clonogenic assays
cytospin preparations from dissociated explants, 253
definitive progenitor assay, 253, 255
Giemsa staining, 253
primitive erythroid progenitor assay, 252, 253
single-cell suspension preparation, 252, 255
culture and analysis from mouse embryo
agar culture
agar overlay, 295
agar underlay, 295
colony identification, 295, 296, 300
double agar incubation, 295
collagen culture of megakaryocyte progenitors
acetylcholinesterase stain, 297
cytokine mix, 296
dehydration and fixation of collagen, 296, 297
dissection and staging of embryos, 294, 300
materials, 290–293, 299
methylcellulose culture
colony identification, 298, 299
plating, 298
reagents, 298
overview, 289, 290
pregnancy timing, 294
single-cell suspension preparation
cell density for culture, 295
collagenase digestion, 294, 295
enzymatic versus mechanical dissociation, 294, 300
trypsin digestion, 294, 300
expansion and differentiation
human cells
erythroid progenitor expansion, 335, 336, 341
flow cytometry, 337, 340
mononuclear cell preparation from umbilical cord blood, 335, 341
terminal erythroid differentiation induction, 337, 339, 340
materials, 326–328, 337, 338
mouse cells
erythroid cell outgrowth, 328, 330, 339, 340
erythroid progenitor development from multipotent cultures, 331
fetal liver isolation, 328, 338

freezing and thawing of cells, 334, 335
multipotent cell outgrowth, 330, 331, 340
p53 knockout erythroblast cloning, 333
p53 knockout erythroid progenitor outgrowth, 332, 333
retroviral gene transfer, 333, 334, 341
terminal erythroid differentiation induction, 331, 332, 339, 340
overview, 324–326
multilineage progenitor assay, *see* Multilineage progenitor assay
Hematopoietic stem cell (HSC)
development-associated phenotypic changes, 65–67, 72–74
embryoid body culture for development, 34, 37, 40
fate mapping, *see Xenopus* embryo fate mapping
flow cytometry, *see* Flow cytometry
genomics databases, *see* Stem Cell Database; Stromal Cell Database
human cell differentiation in vitro
amplification culture, 421
culture *in toto*, 421, 422
lymphomyeloid differentiation culture, 421, 422
materials, 415
stromal cell culture, 419, 422
T-cell development in fetal thymus organ culture, 421–423
in utero transplantation, *see In utero* hematopoietic cell transplantation
mouse embryo enrichment and analysis from aorta-gonad-mesonephros region
antibody staining, 260–262, 268
cell cycle analysis
bromodeoxyuridine labeling and staining, 267–269
Hoechst 33258 staining, 266, 267, 269
Ki67 labeling and staining, 268, 269
dead cell discrimination
annexin V, 266
Hoechst 33258, 266, 268
propidium iodide/7-amino-actinomycin D, 265, 266
dissection
dissections, 277, 279
embryo staging, 277
materials, 274
mating and embryo recovery, 277, 284, 285
explant organ cultures, 276, 281, 285, 286
flow cytometry and cell sorting, 262, 263, 268, 284
hematopoietic potential analysis of organ cultures
culture plate preparation, 281
feeder cell preparation, 281
fetal thymic organ cultures, 283, 284, 286
hematopoietic cultures, 283, 286
materials, 258, 259, 268, 276, 277
overview, 257, 258
single-cell suspension preparation, 260, 268
tissue isolation and dissection, 259, 260, 268
transgene markers and staining, 264, 265, 268
whole-mount *in situ* hybridization
blocking and antibody staining, 280, 281, 285
fixation, storage and processing, 279
materials, 274, 275
riboprobe synthesis and purification, 279
washing and hybridization, 280
neonatal transplantation, *see* Yolk sac cell transplantation, hematopoiesis reconstitution in neonatal mice
quantitative trait loci analysis, *see* Quantitative trait loci
vascular potential assay
eye removal, 376, 378
green fluorescent protein/BL6 chimera mouse construction
bone marrow harvesting, 371, 376, 377
flow cytometry purification of stem cells, 372
immunomagnetic bead purification of stem cells, 371, 372, 377
multilineage reconstitution verification, 373, 378
rescue marrow harvesting and irradiation of recipient animals, 373, 377
transplantation, 373

materials, 370, 371
overview, 369, 370
retinal ischemia induction, 374, 375, 378
yolk sac origins, 95, 96, 273, 274, 289, 290, 391
HoxB4, inducible transgene expression in hematopoietic stem cells, 26, 27, 34, 37
HSC, *see* Hematopoietic stem cell
Human embryo
embryonic stem cells, *see* Embryonic stem cells
hematopietic development investigations, overview, 413, 414
hematopoietic stem cell differentiation in vitro
amplification culture, 421
culture *in toto*, 421, 422
lymphomyeloid differentiation culture, 421, 422
materials, 415
stromal cell culture, 419, 422
T-cell development in fetal thymus organ culture, 421–423
histology and immunostaining
double immunofluorescence, 418
fluorescence immunostaining, 417
materials, 414, 422
peroxidase staining, 417, 422
tissue embedding and freezing, 416, 417
tissue fixation, 416, 422
recovery and gestational age estimation, 414–416
tissue dissection
embryo, 418, 422
liver, 418
materials, 415, 422

I

In situ hybridization, *see also* Whole-mount *in situ* hybridization
messenger RNA in *Drosophila* hemocytes
digoxigenin probe preparation, 114
embryo preparation, 112, 113
embryo staining and analysis, 115, 116, 119
hybridization, 115, 119
precursor marker genes, 113, 114
prehybridization, 114, 115
washing, 115
whole-mount *in situ* hybridization of zebrafish embryos
double hybridization, 181, 182, 195
embryo dechorionation and fixation, 179, 194
hybridization and detection, 180, 181, 194, 195
macrophage studies, 210, 211
materials, 174–176, 194
overview, 179, 194
pigment removal, 179, 180
probe preparation, 182, 183, 195
target genes, 172, 173
Xenopus embryos
probe preparation, 131
sections, 132, 134
whole-mount, 130, 131, 134
In utero hematopoietic cell transplantation (IUHCT)
mouse model
anesthesia, 87
animal husbandry, 84, 85
defective mouse strains, 90, 91
micropipet construction, 83, 84, 91
normal mouse strains, 89, 90
postoperative care, 88
surgical supplies, 86
transplantation, 87, 88, 91, 92
therapeutic applications and rationale, 81–83
IUHCT, *see In utero* hematopoietic cell transplantation

K

Kidney capsule grafting, *see* Thymus organogenesis, mouse assays
Knockdown mouse, overview, 8
Knockin mouse
conditional knockins, 8, 9, 13
generation, 13
inverted conditional, 11
overview, 5, 7
Knockout mouse
conditional knockouts, 8, 12, 14
generation, 11, 12
inverted conditional, 11
overview, 5

L

Larval antigens
tolerance in frog development, 149
Xenopus J strain immune response studies
antiserum preparation, 152, 156
immunohistochemical detection of antibodies, 153, 154, 156, 157
larval skin tissue transplantation into adults, 152, 156
materials, 150, 151
overview, 149, 150
T-cell proliferation assay
adult splenocyte preparation, 155–157
immunohistochemical detection of bromodeoxyuridine-incorporated cells, 156
larval skin tissue preparation for co-culture with adult splenocytes, 154, 155, 157

M

Macrophage, zebrafish embryo imaging
caudal vein, 209, 213
embryonic tissues, 209, 210
rationale, 204, 205
time-lapse video recording, 210
whole-mount *in situ* hybridization, 210, 211
yolk sac, 205, 207, 208
Methylcellulose culture, hematopoietic progenitors
colony identification, 298, 299
plating, 298
reagents, 298
MLP assay, *see* Multilineage progenitor assay
Mouse embryo
explant culture system for analysis of hematopoietic and vascular development
analysis
β-galactosidase activity staining, 249
overview, 248, 249
reverse transcriptase-polymerase chain reaction analysis, 249–251, 255
clonogenic assays for hematopoietic progenitor cells
cytospin preparations from dissociated explants, 253
definitive progenitor assay, 253, 255
Giemsa staining, 253
primitive erythroid progenitor assay, 252, 253
single-cell suspension preparation, 252, 255
cryosectioning, 251
embryo dissection
enzymatic separation of VE and embryo, 244, 245, 254, 255
epiblast transection, 247
harvesting, 242, 243, 254
explant culture
co-culture on cell monolayer, 248
culture with recombinant protein, blocking antibodies, or small molecules, 248, 255
recombinant setup in collagen droplets, 247, 248, 255
materials, 232, 234–242, 253, 254
overview, 231, 232
grafting studies of hematopoietic cells
anesthesia, 225
applications, 227
intrafetal grafting, 225–227
intraplacental injections, 225
markers, 227
materials, 216, 227
overview, 215
uterus exposure, 225, 227
hematopoietic progenitor culture and analysis
agar culture
agar overlay, 295
agar underlay, 295
colony identification, 295, 296, 300
double agar incubation, 295
collagen culture of megakaryocyte progenitors
acetylcholinesterase stain, 297
cytokine mix, 296
dehydration and fixation of collagen, 296, 297

dissection and staging of embryos, 294, 300
materials, 290–293, 299
methylcellulose culture
colony identification, 298, 299
plating, 298
reagents, 298
overview, 289, 290
pregnancy timing, 294
single-cell suspension preparation
cell density for culture, 295
collagenase digestion, 294, 295
enzymatic versus mechanical disociation, 294, 300
trypsin digestion, 294, 300
hematopoietic stem cell enrichment and analysis from aorta-gonad-mesonephros region
antibody staining, 260–262, 268
cell cycle analysis
bromodeoxyuridine labeling and staining, 267–269
Hoechst 33258 staining, 266, 267, 269
Ki67 labeling and staining, 268, 269
dead cell discrimination
annexin V, 266
Hoechst 33258, 266, 268
propidium iodide/7-amino-actinomycin D, 265, 266
dissection
dissections, 277, 279
embryo staging, 277
materials, 274
mating and embryo recovery, 277, 284, 285
explant organ cultures, 276, 281, 285, 286
flow cytometry and cell sorting, 262, 263, 268, 284
hematopoietic potential analysis of organ cultures
culture plate preparation, 281
feeder cell preparation, 281
fetal thymic organ cultures, 283, 284, 286
hematopoietic cultures, 283, 286
materials, 258, 259, 268, 276, 277
overview, 257, 258
single-cell suspension preparation, 260, 268
tissue isolation and dissection, 259, 260, 268
transgene markers and staining, 264, 265, 268
whole-mount *in situ* hybridization
blocking and antibody staining, 280, 281, 285
fixation, storage and processing, 279
materials, 274, 275
riboprobe synthesis and purification, 279
washing and hybridization, 280
thymus organogenesis assays
ectoderm labeling for lineage tracing
embryo isolation, 305, 307, 308
labeling, 305
paraffin embedding and sectioning, 305, 306
recovery and analysis, 305
whole embryo culture, 305, 309
kidney capsule grafting
advantages, 306, 309
anesthesia, 306, 309
graft recovery and analysis, 307, 309
kidney exposure, 307
pharyngeal endoderm isolation, 306, 309
suture and recovery, 307, 309
tissue preparation for transplantation, 306, 309
tissue transplantation, 307, 309
materials, 304
overview, 303, 304
whole embryo culture and in vivo imaging of hematovascular development
culture variables
evaporation control, 388, 389, 391
gas exchange, 387, 388, 391
humidity, 386
temperature, 386, 387

dissection, 384, 385, 391, 392
embryo immobilization, 385
materials, 382, 383
media preparation, 383, 384, 391
microscope, 387, 391, 392
overview, 381, 382
quantitative analysis, 390, 391
rat serum preparation, 383, 391
time-lapse imaging, 389, 392
tissue staining, 389, 390
Multilineage progenitor (MLP) assay
cell harvest from each well, 350, 351, 355
2'-deoxyguanosine treatment of fetal thymus lobes, 346, 347
flow cytometry
first-step screening, 352
progenitor type determination, 352, 355, 356
second-step analysis, 352
staining, 351, 352, 355
high oxygen submersion culture, 350
materials, 346, 354
overview, 345, 346
single-cell seeding, 348, 349, 354, 355
washing of fetal thymus lobes, 347, 348

N

Neovascularization assay, *see* Hematopoietic stem cell
Nomarski microscopy, *see* Differential interference contrast microscopy

O

Oct-3/4, inducible transgene expression in hematopoietic stem cells, 26

P

PCR, *see* Polymerase chain reaction
Polymerase chain reaction (PCR)
reverse transcriptase-polymerase chain reaction analysis of mouse embryo explants
amplification reactions, 250, 251
complementary DNA synthesis, 250, 255
RNA preparation, 249, 250
screening of zebrafish transgene expression, 177, 178, 191, 196

Q

QTL, *see* Quantitative trait loci
Quantitative trait loci (QTL)
candidate genes
confirmation, 59
selection, 58, 59
congenic mice in identification
analysis, 57
generation, 55
definition, 47
fine mapping
strategies, 57, 58
subinterval-specific congenic strain generation and analysis, 58
genetic variation in hematopoietic stem cell compartment of inbred mouse strains, 48, 49
linkage analysis strategies
backcross, intercross, and advanced intercross, 49, 51
chromosome substitution strains, 54
recombinant inbred strains
advantages and limitations, 53, 54
available strains, 51, 52
description, 51
genome-wide significance levels, 52, 53
phenotyping, 52
statistical analysis, 52

R

Retrovirus
erythroid cell transduction, 333, 334, 341
fetal thymic organ culture transduction
CD4/CD8 double-negative thymocyte isolation and transduction, 317, 318
culture conditions, 315, 316
ectopic retroviral supernatant production, 313, 314, 320
expression plasmids, 313
fetal liver collection, 314
fetal thymic lobe collection, 315, 320
flow cytometry for immunophenotypic analysis, 319, 320
human/mouse chimeric organ culture
culture conditions, 318
human $CD34^+$ cell isolation and transduction, 318

materials, 312, 320
retroviral transduction, 315
vesicular stomatitis virus G-pseudo-typed supernatant production, 314
Reverse tetracycline transactivator (rtTA), inducible transgene expression in embryonic stem cells
embryoid body culture for hematopoietic stem cell development, 34, 37, 40
embryonic stem cell line
characterization, 31–33
generation from Ainv15-targeting cells, 28, 30, 31, 39
HoxB4 induction, 34, 37
materials, 27, 28, 39
overview, 25, 39
therapeutic transplantation of embryonic stem cells, 37, 39
transgene types in hematopoiesis studies, 25–27
Reverse transcriptase-polymerase chain reaction, *see* Polymerase chain reaction
rtTA, *see* Reverse tetracycline transactivator

S

SCDb, *see* Stem Cell Database
SCL/tal-1, inducible transgene expression in hematopoietic stem cells, 27
STAT3, inducible transgene expression in hematopoietic stem cells, 26
Stem Cell Database (SCDb), development and contents, 439, 440
StroCDB, *see* Stromal Cell Database
Stromal Cell Database (StroCDB)
AFT024 cell utilization, 439–441
bioinformatic analysis
automated searches, 442
database redundancy, 442
hand annotation, 444, 445
informatic classification summary, 445
contents, 440, 449
development, 440, 441
expression array development, 447–449
querying
annotation, 445
BLAST, 446
results, 446
sequence homology and functional category, 446

T

T-cell
human T-cell development in fetal thymus organ culture, 421–423
multilineage progenitor assay, *see* Multilineage progenitor assay
proliferation assay for frog larval antigen immune response studies
adult splenocyte preparation, 155–157
immunohistochemical detection of bromodeoxyuridine-incorporated cells, 156
larval skin tissue preparation for co-culture with adult splenocytes, 154, 155, 157
thymocyte differentiation, *see* Fetal thymic organ culture
Thymus organogenesis, mouse assays
ectoderm labeling for lineage tracing
embryo isolation, 305, 307, 308
labeling, 305
paraffin embedding and sectioning, 305, 306
recovery and analysis, 305
whole embryo culture, 305, 309
kidney capsule grafting
advantages, 306, 309
anesthesia, 306, 309
graft recovery and analysis, 307, 309
kidney exposure, 307
pharyngeal endoderm isolation, 306, 309
suture and recovery, 307, 309
tissue preparation for transplantation, 306, 309
tissue transplantation, 307, 309
materials, 304
overview, 303, 304
Transgenic mouse
generation
DNA microinjection, 11, 16
transgenic construct, 11
overview, 5

U

U-shaped protein, immunohistochemistry in *Drosophila* hemocytes, 116, 117, 119

W

Whole-mount *in situ* hybridization (WISH)
mouse embryo hematopoietic stem-cell analysis
blocking and antibody staining, 280, 281, 285
fixation, storage and processing, 279
materials, 274, 275
riboprobe synthesis and purification, 279
washing and hybridization, 280
Xenopus embryos, 130, 131, 134
zebrafish embryos
double hybridization, 181, 182, 195
embryo dechorionation and fixation, 179, 194
hybridization and detection, 180, 181, 194, 195
macrophage studies, 210, 211
materials, 174–176, 194
overview, 179, 194
pigment removal, 179, 180
probe preparation, 182, 183, 195
target genes, 172, 173
WISH, *see* Whole-mount *in situ* hybridization

X

Xenopus embryo fate mapping
advantages, 123, 124
β-galactosidase reaction, 129, 134
embedding and sectioning, 131
fixation, 129, 130
fluorescent dextran mini-ruby utilization
assessment, 144, 147
embryo generation, selection, and injection, 141, 143, 144, 146, 147
injection rig, 140, 146
materials, 138–140, 144–146
in situ hybridization
probe preparation, 131
sections, 132, 134
whole-mount, 130, 131, 134
materials, 126, 127
overview, 124, 125, 137, 138
regularly cleaving embryo generation, selection, and culture, 128, 129, 133
reporters, 132, 133
RNA
injection, 129, 134
synthesis for injection, 127, 128
Xenopus laevis
fate mapping, *see Xenopus* embryo fate mapping
flow cytometry of hematopietic chimera embryos
cell harvesting, 163–165
combined surface/DNA staining
Hoechst 33342, 168
Vindlov's reagent, 167
DNA staining, 165
embryo preparation, 161, 162, 168
materials, 160, 161, 168
microsurgery, 162, 163, 168
rationale, 159, 160
surface staining, 165, 168
larval antigen immune response, *see* Larval antigens

Y

Yolk sac cell transplantation, hematopoiesis reconstitution in neonatal mice
busulfan for *in utero* myeloablation, 96, 99, 103, 104
dissection, 98, 99
facial vein injection of neonates, 100, 104
flow cytometry analysis of peripheral blood in transplanted mice
cell sorting, 100, 101, 104
Gpi-1 analysis, 101–103
iradiation of recipient neonates, 99, 100, 103
materials, 97, 98
overview, 95, 96
yolk sac cell digestion and dissociation, 99, 103

Z

Zebrafish
advantages in hematopoiesis studies, 171, 172, 199
differential interference contrast microscopy of embryos
contrast enhancement and video magnification, 202, 212
digitization of video, 204, 213
embryo preparation and mounting, 200, 201
image acquisition, 201, 202

macrophage imaging
caudal vein, 209, 213
embryonic tissues, 209, 210
rationale, 204, 205
time-lapse video recording, 210
whole-mount *in situ* hybridization, 210, 211
yolk sac, 205, 207, 208
materials, 200
overview, 199
prospects, 212, 213
video editing, 203, 212
video recording, 202, 203
erythroid cell staining with *o*-dianisidine, 173, 176, 193
flow cytometry purification of hematopoietic cells
adult cells, 191–193, 196
cells expressing fluorescent reporters, 193
embryonic cells, 193, 196
materials, 178
overview, 174
sorting of cells, 193, 196
hematopoiesis overview, 172
microinjection of embryos
embryo collection, 185, 186
ledge mold, 184, 195
materials, 176, 177
needle preparation, 185, 195
overview, 184
postinjection care, 186
RNA overexpression, 173, 177, 186, 187, 194
technique, 186, 195
microinjection materials, 176, 177
morpholino knockdown of genes, 173, 177, 187–189, 195
transgenic fish preparation
DNA preparation, 177, 190, 195
overview, 173, 189, 190
polymerase chain reaction screening of transgene expression, 177, 178, 191, 196
whole-mount *in situ* hybridization
double hybridization, 181, 182, 195
embryo dechorionation and fixation, 179, 194
hybridization and detection, 180, 181, 194, 195
materials, 174–176, 194
overview, 179, 194
pigment removal, 179, 180
probe preparation, 182, 183, 195
target genes, 172, 173

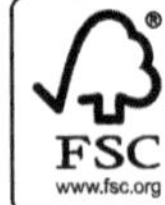

MIX
Papier aus verantwortungsvollen Quellen
Paper from responsible sources
FSC® C105338

If you have any concerns about our products,
you can contact us on
ProductSafety@springernature.com

In case Publisher is established outside the EU,
the EU authorized representative is:
Springer Nature Customer Service Center GmbH
Europaplatz 3, 69115 Heidelberg, Germany

Printed by Libri Plureos GmbH
in Hamburg, Germany